Compliments of Pfizer Inc.

Textbook of
Psychotherapeutic
Treatments

Textbook of Psychotherapeutic Treatments

Edited by

Glen O. Gabbard, M.D.

Brown Foundation Chair of Psychoanalysis and
Professor of Psychiatry
Baylor College of Medicine
Houston, Texas

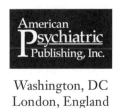

American Psychiatric Publishing, Inc.

Washington, DC
London, England

If you would like to buy between 25 and 99 copies of this or any other APPI title, you are eligible for a 20% discount; please contact APPI Customer Service at appi@psych.org or 800-368-5777. If you wish to buy 100 or more copies of the same title, please e-mail us at bulksales@psych.org for a price quote.

Copyright © 2009 American Psychiatric Publishing, Inc.
ALL RIGHTS RESERVED

Manufactured in the United States of America on acid-free paper
12   11   10   09   08   5   4   3   2   1
First Edition

Typeset in Adobe's Akzidenz Grotesk and Janson Text.

American Psychiatric Publishing, Inc.
1000 Wilson Boulevard
Arlington, VA 22209-3901
www.appi.org

Library of Congress Cataloging-in-Publication Data
Textbook of psychotherapeutic treatments / edited by Glen O. Gabbard. — 1st ed.
    p. ; cm.
  Includes bibliographical references and index.
  ISBN 978-1-58562-304-4 (alk. paper)
  1. Psychotherapy. 2. Psychiatry. I. Gabbard, Glen O. II. American Psychiatric Publishing. III. Title: Psychotherapeutic treatments.
  [DNLM: 1. Mental Disorders—therapy. 2. Psychotherapy—methods. WM 420 T3545 2009]
  RC480.T441 2009
  616.89′14—dc22

                                                                2008018669

British Library Cataloguing in Publication Data
A CIP record is available from the British Library.

Contents

Part 1
Individual Psychodynamic Psychotherapy

Section Editor: Glen O. Gabbard, M.D.

Part 2
Individual Cognitive-Behavioral Therapy

Section Editors: Jesse H. Wright, M.D., Ph.D., and
Judith S. Beck, Ph.D.

Part 3
Individual Interpersonal Psychotherapy

Section Editor: John C. Markowitz, M.D.

Part 4
Individual Supportive Psychotherapy

Section Editor: Arnold Winston, M.D.

Part 5
Group, Family, and Couples Therapy

Section Editor: James Griffith, M.D.

Part 6
Forms of Psychotherapy Integration

Section Editor: Bernard D. Beitman, M.D.

Contributors

Jon G. Allen, Ph.D.
Helen Malsin Palley Chair in Mental Health Research and Professor of Psychiatry, Menninger Department of Psychiatry and Behavioral Sciences, Baylor College of Medicine; Senior Staff Psychologist in The Menninger Clinic, Houston, Texas

Anthony Bateman, M.A., F.R.C.Psych.
Consultant Psychiatrist in Psychotherapy, Halliwick Unit, St. Ann's Hospital, Barnet, Enfield, and Haringey Mental Health Trust; Visiting Professor, University College London, England, and Visiting Consultant, The Menninger Clinic and the Menninger Department of Psychiatry and Behavioral Sciences, Baylor College of Medicine, Houston, Texas

Judith S. Beck, Ph.D.
Director, Beck Institute for Cognitive Therapy and Research; Clinical Associate Professor of Psychology in Psychiatry, University of Pennsylvania, Philadelphia, Pennsylvania

Bernard D. Beitman, M.D.
Professor and Former Chairman, Department of Psychiatry, University of Missouri–Columbia

Richard A. Bermudes, M.D.
Assistant Clinical Professor, Department of Psychiatry and Behavioral Sciences, UC Davis Medical Center, Sacramento, California; Mindful Health Solutions, El Dorado Hills, California

Carlos Blanco, M.D., Ph.D.
Anxiety Disorders Clinic, Columbia University, New York, New York

Peter J. Buckley, M.D.
Professor of Psychiatry, Albert Einstein College of Medicine of Yeshiva University, Bronx, New York; Lecturer in Psychiatry, Columbia University Center for Psychoanalytic Training and Research, New York, New York

David Casey, M.D.
Associate Professor and Vice Chair, Department of Psychiatry and Behavioral Sciences, University of Louisville School of Medicine, Louisville, Kentucky

Andrew Christensen, Ph.D.
Professor of Psychology, University of California, Los Angeles, Los Angeles, California

David A. Clark, Ph.D.
Department of Psychology, University of New Brunswick, Saint John, New Brunswick, Canada

Jean Cottraux, M.D., Ph.D.
Psychiatrist, Lecturer, and Head, Anxiety Disorders Unit, Hôpital Neurologique, Lyon, France

Mantosh Dewan, M.D.
Professor and Chair, Department of Psychiatry, State University of New York Upstate Medical University, Syracuse, New York

Keith S. Dobson, Ph.D.
Professor and Head, Department of Psychology, University of Calgary, Calgary, Alberta, Canada

Amanda M. Epp, B.A.
M.Sc. Student in Clinical Psychology, Department of Psychology, University of Calgary, Calgary, Alberta, Canada

Peter Fonagy, Ph.D., F.B.A.
Freud Memorial Professor of Psychoanalysis and Director, Sub-Department of Clinical Health Psychology, University College London; Chief Executive, Anna Freud Centre, London, England; and Consultant to the Child and Family Program, Menninger Department of Psychiatry, Baylor College of Medicine, Houston, Texas

Edward S. Friedman, M.D.
Associate Professor of Psychiatry and Director, Mood Disorders Treatment and Research Program, Western Psychiatric Institute and Clinic, University of Pittsburgh Medical Center, Pittsburgh, Pennsylvania

Glen O. Gabbard, M.D.
Brown Foundation Chair of Psychoanalysis and Professor of Psychiatry, Baylor College of Medicine, Houston, Texas

Molly F. Gasbarrini
Ph.D. Student, Department of Psychology, Texas A&M University, College Station, Texas

Michael Goldstein, M.D.
Physician-in-Charge, Neuroscience Education, Department of Psychiatry and Behavioral Sciences, Beth Israel Medical Center, New York, New York; Assistant Clinical Professor, Department of Psychiatry and Behavioral Sciences, Albert Einstein College of Medicine, Bronx, New York

James Griffith, M.D.
Residency Training Director and Professor of Psychiatry and Neurology, Department of Psychiatry and Behavioral Sciences, George Washington University School of Medicine, Washington, D.C.

David J. Hellerstein, M.D.
Associate Professor of Clinical Psychiatry, Columbia University College of Physicians and Surgeons, and Research Psychiatrist, New York State Psychiatric Institute, New York, New York

Michael Hollifield, M.D.
Department of Psychiatry and Behavioral Sciences, University of Louisville, Louisville, Kentucky

Susan Johnson, Ed.D.
Professor of Psychology and Psychiatry, University of Ottawa, Ottawa, Ontario, Canada; Director, Ottawa Couple and Family Institute and Center for Emotionally Focused Therapy; Research Professor, Alliant International University, San Diego, California

Jerald Kay, M.D.
Professor and Chair, Department of Psychiatry, Boonschoft School of Medicine, Wright State University, Dayton, Ohio

Melissa C. Kuhajda, Ph.D.
Assistant Professor, Department of Psychiatry and Behavioral Medicine, The University of Alabama School of Medicine, Tuscaloosa, Alabama

Robert Leahy, Ph.D.
American Institute for Cognitive Therapy, New York, New York

Jay L. Lebow, Ph.D.
Clinical Professor of Psychology, The Family Institute at Northwestern and Northwestern University, Evanston, Illinois

Falk Leichsenring, D.Sc.
Department of Psychosomatics and Psychotherapy, University of Giessen, Giessen, Germany

Joshua D. Lipsitz, Ph.D.
Associate Professor of Psychology, Ben Gurion University of the Negev, Beer Sheva, Israel; Associate Professor of Clinical Psychology, Department of Psychiatry, Columbia University College of Physicians and Surgeons, New York, New York

John Manring, M.D.
Associate Professor of Psychiatry, SUNY-Upstate Medical University, Syracuse, New York

John C. Markowitz, M.D.
Research Psychiatrist, New York State Psychiatric Institute, Columbia University, and Clinical Professor of Psychiatry, Weill Medical College, Cornell University, New York, New York

William R. McFarlane, M.D.
Professor, Department of Psychiatry, University of Vermont; Director, Center for Psychiatric Research, Maine Medical Center, Portland, Maine

Meghan McGinn, M.A.
University of California, Los Angeles, Los Angeles, California

John S. Rolland, M.D.
Clinical Professor of Psychiatry and Co-Director, Center for Family Health, University of Chicago, Chicago, Illinois

Richard N. Rosenthal, M.D.
Chairman, Department of Psychiatry, St. Luke's–Roosevelt Hospital Center; Professor of Clinical Psychiatry, Columbia University College of Physicians and Surgeons, New York, New York

Lynn Stormon, Ph.D.
Clinical Psychologist, Private Practice, Syracuse, New York, Candidate in Psychoanalytic Training, International Institute for Psychoanalytic Training, Chevy Chase, Maryland

Holly A. Swartz, M.D.
Assistant Professor, Department of Psychiatry, University of Pittsburgh School of Medicine, Pittsburgh, Pennsylvania

Hillel I. Swiller, M.D., D.L.F.A.P.A., F.A.G.P.A.
Clinical Professor of Psychiatry; and Director, Division of Psychotherapy, Mount Sinai School of Medicine, New York, New York

Mary Target, Ph.D.
Reader in Psychoanalysis, University College London; Professional Director, The Anna Freud Centre, London, United Kingdom

Michael E. Thase, M.D.
Professor of Psychiatry, University of Pennsylvania School of Medicine, Philadelphia Veterans Affairs Medical Center, and University of Pittsburgh Medical Center, Pittsburgh, Pennsylvania

Beverly E. Thorn, Ph.D., A.B.P.P.
Professor of Psychology, Department of Psychology, Editor, *Journal of Clinical Psychology*, The University of Alabama, Tuscaloosa, Alabama

Oriana Vesga-López, M.D.
Anxiety Disorders Clinic, Columbia University, New York, New York

George I. Viamontes, M.D., Ph.D.
Regional Medical Director, Optum Health Behavioral Solutions, Maryland Heights, Missouri

Barbara B. Walker, Ph.D.
Clinical Professor, Department of Psychological and Brain Sciences, Indiana University, Bloomington, Indiana

Froma Walsh, Ph.D.
Mose and Sylvia Firestone Professor Emerita, SSA and Department of Psychiatry, and Co-Director, Center for Family Health, University of Chicago, Chicago, Illinois

Priyanthy Weerasekera, M.D., M.Ed.
Associate Professor and Coordinator, Postgraduate Psychotherapy Program, Department of Psychiatry and Behavioral Neurosciences, McMaster University, Hamilton, Ontario, Canada

Myrna M. Weissman, Ph.D.
Professor, Department of Epidemiology (in Psychiatry), Columbia University Mailman School of Public Health; Chief, Division of Clinical and Genetic Epidemiology, New York State Psychiatric Institute, New York, New York

Joan Wheelis, M.D.
President and Medical Director, Two Brattle Center, Cambridge, Massachusetts

Katherine J. Williams, M.A.
University of California, Los Angeles, Los Angeles, California

Arnold Winston, M.D.
Chairman, Department of Psychiatry and Behavioral Sciences, Beth Israel Medical Center, New York, New York; Professor of Psychiatry, Department of Psychiatry and Behavioral Sciences, Albert Einstein College of Medicine, Bronx, New York

Scott R. Woolley, Ph.D.
Professor and Systemwide Director, Marital and Family Therapy Masters and Doctoral Programs, California School of Professional Psychology, Alliant International University, San Diego, California

Jesse H. Wright, M.D., Ph.D.
Professor and Associate Chairman for Academic Affairs, University of Louisville School of Medicine, Louisville, Kentucky

John Zinner, M.D.
Clinical Professor, Department of Psychiatry and Behavioral Sciences, George Washington University School of Medicine, Washington, D.C.

Disclosure of Interests

The following contributors to this book have indicated a financial interest in or other affiliation with a commercial supporter, a manufacturer of a commercial product, a provider of a commercial service, a nongovernmental organization, and/ or a government agency, as listed below:

Richard A. Bermudes, M.D.—*Speakers' Bureau:* Abbott Laboratories, Bristol-Myers Squibb, Eli Lilly and Company, Pfizer, Inc.

John C. Markowitz, M.D.—*Grant Support:* NARSAD, National Institute of Mental Health.

Richard N. Rosenthal, M.D.—*Grant Support:* Titan Pharmaceuticals, Forest Research Institute; *Advisory Board:* Alkermes, Forest Laboratories; *Speakers' Bureau:* Cephalon.

Holly A. Swartz, M.D.—*Consultant:* Novartis; *CME Speaker:* Bristol-Myers Squibb, AstraZeneca; *Speakers' Bureau:* Bristol-Myers Squibb; *Grant Support:* NARSAD, National Institute of Mental Health.

The following contributors indicated that they had no competing interests during the year preceding manuscript submission:

Anthony Bateman, M.A., F.R.C.Psych.
Bernard D. Beitman, M.D.
Carlos Blanco, M.D., Ph.D.
Peter J. Buckley, M.D.
Andrew Christensen, Ph.D.
Jean Cottraux, M.D, Ph.D.
Mantosh Dewan, M.D.
Keith S. Dobson, Ph.D.
Amanda M. Epp, B.A.
Peter Fonagy, Ph.D., F.B.A.
Glen O. Gabbard, M.D.
David J. Hellerstein, M.D.
Michael Hollifield, M.D.
Susan Johnson, Ed.D.
Melissa C. Kuhajda, Ph.D.
Jay L. Lebow, Ph.D.
Falk Leichsenring, D.Sc.
Joshua D. Lipsitz, Ph.D.
William R. McFarlane, M.D.

Meghan McGinn, M.A.
John S. Rolland, M.D.
Hillel I. Swiller, M.D., D.L.F.A.P.A., F.A.G.P.A.
Mary Target, Ph.D.
Beverly E. Thorn, Ph.D., A.B.P.P.
Oriana Vesga-López, M.D.
Barbara B. Walker, Ph.D.
Priyanthy Weerasekera, M.D., M.Ed.
Joan Wheelis, M.D.
Katherine J. Williams, M.A.
Arnold Winston, M.D.
Scott R. Woolley, Ph.D.
John Zinner, M.D.

Preface

Glen O. Gabbard, M.D.

The relationship between psychotherapy and psychiatry has been strained for some time now. Advances in neuroscience, genetics, and psychopharmacology have skewed psychiatry away from psychotherapy toward a "remedicalization" and an emphasis on medication as the primary tool in the psychiatrist's therapeutic armamentarium. Economic forces have contributed to this trend as well. Managed care companies often look for "quick fixes" and tend to favor pharmacotherapy over "the talking cures."

The result has been unfortunate for the field. In an era in which a sophisticated understanding of the mind–brain interface is possible, psychiatry, at least in some quarters, has become increasingly reductionistic. The hegemony of biological psychiatry has encouraged a Cartesian dualism in which mind and brain are artificially separated from each other. Psychotherapy is seen as the treatment for "psychologically based" disorders, while medication is regarded as the treatment for "brain-based" disorders. This simplistic dualism overlooks the plain facts that psychotherapy must work by changing the brain and that the mind is the activity of the brain.

Nobel Prize winner Eric Kandel (1998) has been at the forefront of an emerging literature that regards psychotherapy as a biological treatment. Working with the marine snail *Aplysia*, Kandel stressed that synaptic connections can be permanently altered and strengthened through the regulation of gene expression when learning takes place. This conceptual understanding can be applied to psychotherapy as well. Learning takes place when psychotherapy is well conducted, and the changes in brain function that result now are being mapped. Goldapple et al. (2004) have even begun to chart the brain regions that are more profoundly affected by psychotherapy as compared with medication. In a study involving cognitive-behavioral therapy

(CBT) and paroxetine for depressed patients, the investigators documented that therapy worked in a "top down" manner, with decreased metabolic activity in the medial, dorsal, and ventral frontal cortices, and increased activity in the anterior cingulate and hippocampus. Paroxetine appeared to work in a "bottom up" way, with decreased activity in the brain stem and subgenual cingulate and increased activity in the prefrontal cortex.

As psychotherapy becomes legitimized as a treatment that affects the brain, rather than mere hand holding or babysitting, a vision of the future emerges in which we can begin to imagine a time when we will be able to predict which patients will do better with psychotherapy, which will respond optimally to medication, and which may require both.

In a landmark study, a group of patients with chronic forms of major depression were treated with nefazodone, a form of CBT, or the combination of both in a randomized controlled trial (Nemeroff et al. 2003). Examined in totality, antidepressants and psychotherapy were roughly equal in their usefulness, but each was significantly less effective than combined treatment. When the data were examined in more detail, however, it became clear that a subgroup of patients did better with psychotherapy alone compared with nefazodone. Specifically, this group had a history of early childhood trauma, including physical or sexual abuse, neglect, or loss of parents at an early age. The combination of psychotherapy and pharmacotherapy was only marginally superior to psychotherapy alone among this group. The investigators concluded that the presence of childhood trauma was a strong indication for psychotherapy as an essential element in the treatment.

Changes have occurred in recent years at the level of psychiatric residency training programs. There has been a growing recognition that psychotherapy is a basic science of psychiatry (Gabbard and Kay 2001). The Residency Review Committee mandated training in several different forms of psychotherapy as part of the core competencies of psychiatry. Even those future psychiatrists who think they would like to treat patients with pharmacotherapy alone will be faced with the task of establishing a therapeutic alliance if they hope to have the patient take the medication as prescribed. Indeed, the quality of the therapeutic alliance has been shown to be a better predictor of outcome than any of the specific treatments or techniques used in the treatment of depression (Krupnick et al. 1996). Hence all residents are now required to be trained up to basic competency in psychotherapy.

While psychotherapy was long criticized as lacking an empirical base, that situation has gradually changed. Some forms of psychotherapy have been more rigorously tested than others in randomized controlled trials, but the rapidly growing base of efficacy studies has been encouraging (Beck 2005; Leichsenring et al. 2004). In addition, research combining medication and psychotherapy has become increasingly common and may be particularly relevant, given that one survey of practitioners found that the majority of patients receive both medication and psychotherapy (Pincus et al. 1999). Whether offered by one treater or two, combined treatment places special demands on the psychotherapist, a topic discussed thoroughly in this volume.

With the expanding literature empirically validating psychotherapy as a treatment, and the plethora of psychotherapies now in the marketplace, a comprehensive textbook of psychotherapeutic treatments in psychiatry has become of central importance, both to practitioners and to trainees in psychiatry and other mental health professions. Hence in one volume we have collected contributions from experts in all of the major psychotherapeutic approaches. The volume begins with a section on psychodynamic psychotherapy, followed by sections on CBT, interpersonal therapy, and supportive psychotherapy.

The section editors have ably assembled a cast of outstanding experts to write each of the chapters. In an effort to provide a consistent format for the student who wishes to study comparative psychotherapy using this textbook, the section editors were asked to organize the sections along similar lines—namely, with chapters on theory, technique, indications and efficacy, and the combination of psychotherapy with medication.

Psychotherapy is not only administered to individuals, of course. Many psychotherapists treat groups, families, and couples. Hence we also include a section that covers these modalities from the standpoint of diverse theories and techniques.

The book ends with a section on forms of psychotherapy integration, given that many psychotherapists are using amalgams of different types of therapy in their own practices. Moreover, specific brands that are integrated and defy easy classification, such as mentalization-based therapy and dialectical behavior therapy, are also included in this section. The integration of neuroscience with psychotherapy is considered to be one of the most exciting areas of research, as it reflects the ongoing effort to build bridges between psychological treatments and our understanding of the brain and neuroscience. Hence a chapter appears on this topic as well. Finally, professional boundaries are an essential component in the practice of all psychotherapy, so we devote a chapter to these risk management issues.

The result is one comprehensive resource that covers all the central psychotherapeutic approaches that are likely to be needed by psychiatrists, psychologists, social workers, and other mental health professionals. The book lends itself to use as a textbook by students as well as a reference book for experienced clinicians to pull off the shelf when needed.

A task of this nature requires a team of experts with special knowledge in diverse areas. I owe a special debt of gratitude to those colleagues who served as section editors: Jesse Wright, Judy Beck, John Markowitz, Arnold Winston, James Griffith, and Bernard Beitman. The assistance of Tina Coltri-Marshall was essential in keeping the project on track—she was the "glue" that kept this sprawling project in a state of cohesiveness throughout the extended period of time that it required. My assistant, Diane Trees-Clay, also was of great support in helping me attend to the multiple tasks inherent in a textbook like this one. Bob Hales and John McDuffie of American Psychiatric Publishing were steady sources of support in the planning and implementation as well. Finally, Greg Kuny worked closely in providing the editorial assistance to see the project fully realized.

I welcome the reader to the pages that follow. I hope you will share our excitement in the growth of the psychotherapy field and the inescapable conclusion that psychotherapeutic treatments are alive and well in psychiatry.

References

Beck AT: The current status of cognitive therapy: a 40-year retrospective. Arch Gen Psychiatry 62:953–959, 2005

Gabbard GO, Kay J: The fate of integrated treatment: whatever happened to the biopsychosocial psychiatrist? Am J Psychiatry 158:1956–1963, 2001

Goldapple K, Segal Z, Garson C, et al: Modulation of cortical-limbic pathways in major depression: treatment-specific effects of cognitive behavior therapy. Arch Gen Psychiatry 61:34–41, 2004

Kandel E: A new intellectual framework for psychiatry. Am J Psychiatry 155:457–469, 1998

Krupnick JL, Sotsky SM, Simmens S, et al: The role of the therapeutic alliance in psychotherapy and pharmacotherapy outcome: findings in the National Institute of Mental Health Treatment of Depression Collaborative Research Program. J Consult Clin Psychol 64:532–539, 1996

Leichsenring F, Rabung S, Leibing E: The efficacy of short-term psychodynamic psychotherapy in specific psychiatric disorders: a meta-analysis. Arch Gen Psychiatry 61:1208–1216, 2004

Nemeroff CB, Heim CM, Thase ME, et al: Differential responses to psychotherapy vs pharmacotherapy in patients with chronic forms of major depression and childhood trauma. Proc Natl Acad Sci 100:14293–14296, 2003

Pincus HA, Zarin DA, Tanielian TL, et al: Psychiatric patients and treatments in 1997: findings from the American Psychiatric Association Practice Research Network. Arch Gen Psychiatry 56:441–449, 1999

PART 1

Individual Psychodynamic Psychotherapy

Section Editor
Glen O. Gabbard, M.D.

Chapter 1

Theoretical Models of Psychodynamic Psychotherapy

Peter Fonagy, Ph.D., F.B.A.
Mary Target, Ph.D.

The psychodynamic approach to psychotherapy is best understood not as a single, readily definable entity, but as an umbrella term for a range of therapeutic strategies underpinned by a variety of theoretical models that are designed to treat psychological disorders. The therapeutic strategies and the underpinning theories share common factors, although there are important differences.

Psychodynamic psychotherapies emphasize the interaction of mental processes in generating problems of subjective experience and behavior. This emphasis contrasts with the focus of descriptive phenomenological psychiatry on accurate categorization of mental disorders. Historically, the psychodynamic approach has been understood to entail a model of the mind that emphasizes wishes and ideas that have been defensively excluded from conscious experience. This is a narrow and somewhat misleading def-

3

inition of psychodynamic approaches. The psychodynamic approach is better understood as a comprehensive account of human subjectivity that aims to understand *all* aspects of an individual's relationship with his or her environment, external and internal.

In our view, *psychodynamic* should refer to the power of the conscious mind to radically alter its position with respect to aspects of its own functions. Freud's categorical statements about the aim of psychoanalysis—"to make the unconscious conscious" (as part of his earlier topographic explanation; S. Freud 1917) and "where id was, there shall ego be" (his updated structural formulation; S. Freud 1933[1932])—were brilliant and succinct aphorisms, drawing attention to the central role of consciousness in mitigating the destructive influence of ideas and feelings that have the capacity to destabilize the personality if they remain outside of the person's awareness. All psychodynamic therapies aim to strengthen patients' ability to understand the motivations for and meanings of their own and others' subjective experiences, behavior, and relationships. The therapist aims to expand patients' conscious awareness of these mechanisms and influences so that they are better able to use their increased emotional awareness to manage continuing pressures.

The following eight assumptions may be considered core to modern psychodynamic therapy. Although some are not unique to the psychodynamic approach, it is unlikely that other therapeutic orientations would embrace all eight of these assumptions wholeheartedly:

1. *Assumption of psychological causation.* At the heart of the psychodynamic approach is the assumption that the problems that people bring to psychotherapy can be usefully discussed in terms of thoughts and feelings. It is assumed that mental disorders can be conceptualized as specific organizations of conscious or unconscious beliefs, thoughts, and feelings.
2. *Assumption of limitations of consciousness and the influence of unconscious mental states.* Psychodynamic clinicians generally assume that to understand conscious experiences, we need to refer to other mental states of which the individual is unaware and, further, that in key instances such a lack of awareness is not coincidental but is motivated by the individual's wish to maximize the experience of safety. This should not be taken to imply a diminution of the emphasis that the theory places on consciousness. Helping patients to become aware of the unconscious expectations underlying their behavior can help them to gain control of previously unmanageable emotions and behavior.
3. *Assumption of internal representations of interpersonal relationships.* Psychodynamic clinicians consider interpersonal relationships, particularly attachment relationships, to be central to the organization of personality.

Mental representations of these intense relationship experiences are assumed to be aggregated across time to form schematic mental structures. These structures are seen as shaping interpersonal expectations and self-representations.

4. *Assumption of ubiquity of psychological conflict.* Psychodynamic approaches assume that wishes, affects, and ideas will sometimes be in conflict. These conflicts are seen as key causes of distress. They are also believed to have the potential to undermine the normal development of key psychological capacities, which may reduce the person's ability to resolve incompatible ideas.

5. *Assumption of psychic defenses.* Historically, the psychodynamic approach has been particularly concerned with defenses: mental operations that distort conscious mental states to reduce their potential to generate anxiety. It is generally accepted that self-serving distortions of mental states relative to an external or internal reality are a ubiquitous feature of human information processing.

6. *Assumption of complex meanings.* Psychodynamic approaches assume that behavior can be understood in terms of mental states that are not explicit in action or within the awareness of the person concerned. In general, the theories specify particular constructions of experience assumed to account for psychological problems (e.g., grandiosity and vulnerable self-esteem associated with narcissistic personality disorder). It is striking that different psychodynamic orientations find different types of meanings "concealed" behind the same symptomatic behaviors. Within a contemporary context, it is the effort to seek further personal meaning, rather than the provision of insight in terms of any particular meaning structure, that would be considered most significant therapeutically.

7. *Assumption of emphasis on the therapeutic relationship.* There is consensus that it is helpful for patients to establish an attachment relationship with a clinician. Different therapeutic schools explain this differently, but converging theorization and research data suggest that engagement with an understanding adult will trigger a basic set of human capacities for relatedness that appear to be therapeutic, apparently almost regardless of content (Alliance of Psychodynamic Organizations 2006). However, controlled trials have repeatedly demonstrated that therapeutic alliance without theoretical content is insufficient (Dew and Bickman 2005); therapeutic impact seems to depend on patient and therapist having a sense of an elaborated rationale in the therapist's mind, which the patient expects to add meaning to his or her experience.

8. *Assumption of the validity of a developmental perspective.* Psychodynamic psychotherapists are invariably oriented to the developmental aspects of

their patients' problems (when and how a problem started, how it relates to an idealized "normal" developmental sequence) and work at least in part to optimize developmental processes. Given this common framework, we shall adopt the developmental perspective in our review of psychodynamic theories.

Most of the above assumptions are central to all psychodynamic theories, although the theories differ in terms of the particular unconscious meanings, developmental periods, patterns of interpersonal relations, qualities of the therapeutic relationship, and even models of mental function that they consider most important to take into account during clinical work with troubled individuals. Historically, the theories developed to fill gaps in the understanding of particular conditions or to justify shifts in therapeutic approaches. The degree to which they gained acceptance was due largely to their usefulness within or to their fitting with the practical approach to therapy adopted by individual psychodynamic clinicians. Although all of these theories aim at providing comprehensive psychological models, the history and development of the psychoanalytic field, and indeed of all science, cautions us against accepting any one of them as definitive statements, since it is the nature of fresh, alternative accounts to highlight the gaps in prior conceptualizations. Were we to consider theories that try to provide comprehensive accounts, we would have to conclude that none can be true. In reality, psychodynamic theory requires multiple theories in much the same way that we need multiple definitions of most complex constructs. Each captures unique aspects of a psychotherapeutic approach to human problems, and by considering each seriously we acquire a more rounded view of both the person and the clinical process.

In this chapter we briefly describe the most popular theoretical models of psychodynamic psychotherapy and establish their unique contributions. In doing so, we hope not only to provide a theoretical framework for the various methods of psychodynamic psychotherapy but also to illustrate the historical contexts and discourses from which they arose and to highlight how these theories differ and borrow from one another.

Freudian Psychoanalysis and Developmental Theory

Sigmund Freud was the first to interpret mental disorder as being linked to childhood experiences (Breuer and Freud 1893–1895) and to the vicissitudes of the developmental process (S. Freud 1900). Freud's discoveries radically altered our perception of the child from one that envisioned him or her in a state of idealized innocence to one that presented the child as a person struggling to achieve control over his or her biological needs and to make them acceptable to society through the microcosm of the family. Freud tried to explain all behavior in terms of the failure of the child's mental apparatus to deal adequately with the pressures inherent in a maturationally predetermined sequence of drive states. Adult psychopathology, dreaming, jokes, and slips of the tongue were all seen as the revisiting of unresolved childhood conflicts over sexuality (S. Freud 1900, 1901, 1905). Freud later gave equal place to aggression as an ultimately unassimilable residue of normal development and, consequently, an explanation of psychological disturbance (S. Freud 1920). Furthermore, Freud's innovative and enduring structural model of the psyche gave a prominent place to the influence of the social environment in analytic theory (S. Freud 1923).

This developmental framework is based on the tripartite structural schema of id, ego, and superego (S. Freud 1923). The hypothesis that conflicts within the human mind are chiefly organized around three themes—1) wish versus moral injunction, 2) wish versus reality, and 3) internal reality versus external reality—has had extraordinary explanatory power. Notably, the ego's capacity to create defenses became the cornerstone of psychoanalytic theorization and clinical work in the United States (Hartmann et al. 1946) and Britain (A. Freud 1936).

Freud's model has many limitations. The sheer variety of later psychoanalytic theories bears witness to the cultural differences that persist in the field, suggesting that to some extent Freud's theories were applicable only to a certain time and place. Although Freud made huge contributions to the field, many others who were at first influenced by him eventually moved away from psychoanalysis—often at the expense of wider recognition, which as a result seemed to be afforded exclusively to Freud. For example, Jung's rejection of libido theory led to a neglect of his undoubted advances in the understanding of narcissism and his development of a theory of the self throughout the life cycle (Jung 1923).

In spite of the diversity of psychoanalytic schools, subsequent psychoanalytic theories have continued the developmental motif. Anna Freud (1965) provided a comprehensive model of psychopathology based on the dimensions of normal and abnormal personality development in which pathology is depicted as or traced to a deviation from normal developmental lines and structural organization. Melanie Klein (1935, 1936) offered a radical alternative to the classical pespectives regarding both severe mental disorders and early child development. Heinz Hartmann and his colleagues focused on the evolution of mental structures necessary for adaptation, and elaborated on the common developmental conflicts between mental structures in early childhood (Hartmann et al. 1946). Margaret Mahler and her colleagues (1975) provided a dynamic map of the first 3 years of life and framed a model for the developmental origins of personality disorders. Otto Kernberg (1975) drew on previous work by Klein, Hartmann (1939), and others to furnish a developmental model of borderline and narcissistic disturbances; Heinz Kohut (1971) constructed a model of narcissistic disturbances based on presumed deficits of early parenting. Although their advocates were initially almost hostile to the developmental model, relational intersubjectivity theories have increasingly emphasized that the earliest experiences create a template for social communication (Mitchell 2000). The emergence and popularity of psychoanalytic schema theories reflects a renaissance of interest in development, particularly infant development (Stern 1985), and is paralleled by the growing following enjoyed by mentalization-based approaches. Mentalization-based approaches originate from an attachment theory perspective (Fonagy et al. 2002), and an overview of these approaches completes our survey of psychodynamic psychotherapy models.

As we can see, then, ever since Sigmund Freud, psychodynamic theoretical accounts have centered on children and childhood experiences: Pathology is believed to be rooted in and made up of recapitulated ontogeny (stages in our origins and development), and disorders of the mind are often understood as maladaptive residues of childhood experience or as developmentally "primitive" modes of mental functioning. The developmental perspective is acknowledged by all genuinely psychoanalytic theories to some degree. Longitudinal, epidemiological birth cohort studies have provided dramatic confirmation that psychoanalysts were on the right track when they emphasized the developmental perspective in their attempts to account for the clinical problems they encountered in their adult patients (e.g., Hofstra et al. 2002; Kim-Cohen et al. 2003). These studies show that in the vast majority of cases, adult psychopathology is antedated by diagnosable childhood disturbance. In a prospective longitudinal cohort, across adult disorders, three-quarters of patients with adult disorders had a diagnosable childhood problem (Kim-Cohen et al. 2003).

Although evidence supports a correlation between problems encountered in early development and disorders acquired in adult life, there are potential problems with using this observed correlation as the basis for a complete acceptance of the theories themselves, and with too readily assuming that later symptoms are the consequence or recurrence of experiences from early childhood. It is arguably an overstatement, based on the evidence at hand, or indeed based on no evidence, to trace particular forms of psychopathology to specific phases (e.g., the link between borderline disorder and Mahler's rapprochement subphase of separation-individuation), and there is likely an overemphasis in psychoanalysis on early experience, which is given an importance within psychoanalysis that is frequently found to be at odds with developmental data (O'Connor 2006). Other fallacies that might be imputed to psychoanalysis include the tendency to *adultomorphize infancy*—that is, to use hypotheses about later states of psychopathology to describe early stages of development. Furthermore, as some argue, because we cannot know what the infant experiences, it is hard to see how empirical evidence in support of psychoanalytic claims can ever be compiled (Green 2000).

In spite of these cogent arguments against the uncritical integration of studies of infant behavior into psychoanalytic theory, to bolster its conclusions, we can still make excellent use of developmental data to deepen our psychoanalytic understanding of psychological disturbance. Empirical evidence provides good support for a developmental model that bears an uncanny resemblance to Freud's model. Westen and Gabbard (2002) have demonstrated that substantial empirical support exists for Freud's core construct: that human consciousness cannot account for its own maladaptive actions. A similar conclusion as to the empirical validity of Freud's central argument has been adopted by the neuroscientist and Freud scholar Mark Solms (Solms and Turnbull 2002). Good evidence exists, for example, for Freud's basic proposition that much of complex mental life is not conscious—that people can think, feel, and experience motivational forces without being aware of them, and can therefore also experience psychological problems that they find puzzling (Mikulincer and Shaver 2007). Freud's claim that unconsciously we are in some ways capable of more complex mental operations than we can consciously perform is supported by literally thousands of research findings, even if the unconscious that such studies point to is composed of processing structures that have little in common with those in Freud's original postulate of a dynamic unconscious.

The Structural Approach

Following Freud's argument that the self has a tripartite structure, comprising id, ego, and superego, the structural approach to psychoanalysis and to psychodynamic psychotherapy concentrates on addressing problems in the ego. Disorder is viewed as originating in faulty ego development (Rangell 1955). The structural approach has come to be referred to as *ego psychology*. Ego psychology proved popular among North American analysts—and there it became a complex, conceptually rigorous, and varied school before, regrettably, waning in its influence in recent years.

In general, the structural model argues that neurosis and psychosis originate at the point when an individual adult's urge to gratify drives reverts to a previously outgrown infantile mode of satisfaction. The symptoms that arise are compromises reflecting the many attempts of the ego to restore equilibrium among the opposing agencies of external reality, superego, and the unacceptable drive representations. As a result of psychological or organic problems, the ego itself may regress, with resultant pathology. In psychosis there is a threat of total dissolution of the ego. If the ego resumes functioning at a level characteristic of early childhood, it will come to be dominated by irrational, magical thoughts and poorly controlled impulses. Mental illness can thus be viewed as a failure of the ego to maintain harmonious interaction between psychic agencies at age-appropriate levels.

Key figures in the history of structural theory include Heinz Hartmann, Erik Erikson, René Spitz, Edith Jacobson, Jacob Arlow, Charles Brenner, and Hans Loewald. Hartmann proposed the key developmental assumption of *change of function*, whereby behavior originating at one point in development may serve an entirely different function later on (Hartmann 1939). Thus persistence of behavior should not be treated as simple repetition. A particular behavior with infantile origin, when observed in an adult, can be independent of the drive originally motivating it, thereby attaining a *secondary autonomy*. Furthermore, Hartmann disagreed with Freud by asserting that the ego evolved out of an undifferentiated matrix from which the id and superego also emerged (as opposed to emerging gradually from the id) (Hartmann et al. 1946); the ego remains linked to the id to some degree because it uses energy from the drives. Hartmann's theory can be seen as psychosocial in that he conceived of development as relying on an "average expectable environment," and thereby Hartmann affirms the importance of the actual parent.

Erikson (1950), meanwhile, was primarily concerned with the interaction of social norms and biological drives in generating self and identity. He also conceived of development as covering the entire life cycle—as seen in his description of eight developmental stages, with later stages assuming the mastery of earlier ones. In his developmental sequence of identity formation, Erikson also described the syndrome of *identity diffusion;* that is, a lack of temporal continuity of self experience in social contexts. With this in mind, Erikson proposed that the organizing construct of self is based not on excitement but on interpersonal dealings and transactions—which he described as a question of developing basic trust over basic mistrust. Westen (1998) considered investigations of Eriksonian concepts of identity (Marcia 1994), intimacy (Orlofsky 1993), and generativity (Bradley 1997) to have been some of the most methodologically sound studies to be inspired by psychoanalytic theories of development.

Spitz (1959) proposed that major shifts in psychological organization, marked by the emergence of new behaviors and new forms of affective expression (organizers), occur when functions are brought into new relation with one another and are linked into a coherent unit. He was also one of the first to ascribe primary importance to the mother–infant interaction as a force in quickening the development of the child's innate abilities. Jacobson (1964) creatively assumed that because early drive states shift continuously between the object and the self, a state of primitive fusion exists between early object representations and self-representation. Finally, Loewald (1973) proposed that *integrative experience* is at the center of development. His fundamental assumption was that all mental activity is relational (both interactional and intersubjective). According to Loewald, internalization (learning) is therefore the basic psychological process that propels development (Loewald 1973). As Friedman (1986) noted, Loewald also shifted emphasis from structures to processes and generated a subtle revision of the classic structural model so that it came to have internalization, understanding, and interpretation at its center.

Modern developmental observations raise questions about the structural approach. For example, structural theorists see psychotic symptoms as regressions to normal but very early functioning, but such assumptions are inconsistent with empirical studies that fail to find a "normal" confusional state between self and object (Gergely 2000). It has been shown that from birth, infants are able to accurately identify their mothers and even to imitate facial gestures (Meltzoff and Moore 1997). Even if putative pathogenic mechanisms such as identity diffusion in some way represented early modes of thought, this in no way implies that the reemergence of these modes of subjectivity in adult mental functioning is indicative of a developmental timetable. For example, infantile modes of cognition may be evoked in relation to later rather than earlier trauma (Fonagy 1996). In a review of psychoanalytic theorization about schizophrenia, Willick (2001) provided a number of examples from the literature illustrating that this criticism applies not only to past psychoanalytic theory but also to some work being done today.

Changes in the notion of the id foreshadowed the demise of structural theory. The original model was criticized in the 1970s and 1980s for its quasi-physiological character, for its homophobic outlook, and for the primacy it gave to sexuality in explanations of psychopathology. As a result, structural theorists had to reinterpret the id as conceived by Freud from being a container of all biologically based, intense physical desires to being a structure related to reality and human figures (e.g., Loewald 1978).

Not all psychoanalysts have accepted the shift of the basic psychoanalytic model from the classic Freudian structural model to object relations theory. In North America a number of psychoanalysts remain fully committed to modifications or updates of the structural approach as proposed, for example, by Brenner (2002). Other influential writers, such as Harold Blum (1983) and Len Shengold (1981), have managed to retain a perspective broadly based on ego psychology while selectively adopting certain object relations ideas. None of these writers, however, have wished to advance a psychoanalytic model that may serve as an alternative to object relations theory. Only relational theorists, self psychologists, and writers in the interpersonalist tradition have aspired to do this.

More recent reviews have tempered the tendency to dismiss the structural approach as reductionist, biologically naive, and overinfluenced by the naïve physiology of nineteenth-century central Europe. For example, experimental work (Birbaumer et al. 2005; Sterzer et al. 2005) confirms Reich and Fenichel's suggestion that the presence of anxiety (autonomic reactivity, amygdala activity) in antisocial youth reduces the risk of adult criminal behavior (Reich 1925; Fenichel 1945). Furthermore, Shevrin has linked the *wanting system*, identified as abnormally sensitized/oversensitive in drug-dependent individuals, to the ego psychology notion of psychic energy and drives (Shevrin 1997)—an argument that has gained support from Panksepp (1998). Finally, the neuropsychological work of Solms (2000) has suggested that the same neural systems activate dreaming and craving. Each and every dream, therefore, starts in the neural structure that most closely fits Freud's concept of instinctual drive states, the ventral tegmental area.

An enduring legacy of the structural approach is found in the work of three psychoanalytic theorists, each of whom drew on the structural approach in elaborating their developmental theories, and each of whom, to a greater or lesser extent, brought psychoanalysis closer to object relations. They are Anna Freud, Margaret Mahler, and Joseph Sandler.

Anna Freud

Sigmund Freud's daughter, Anna Freud, should perhaps be described as a modern structural theorist. Her model is fundamentally developmental, with an emphasis on observational methods; she saw developmental progress as a child coming to terms with developmentally expectable conflicts, where the child has to find a compromise among diverse wishes, needs, perceptions, physical and social realities, and object relations. Although she maintained the classic Freudian position that the individual's drives are the main factor in the construction of the ego and superego, she did carry her father's theories forward by identifying ways that child-rearing contributes to this process (A. Freud 1965).

Anna Freud's theory focused on what she called developmental *lines*, a metaphor that emphasized the continuity and cumulative character of child development. The main lines that she proposed traced a course from dependency to emotional self-reliance and adult relationships, from egocentrism to social partnerships, from sucking to rational eating, and from irresponsibility to responsibility in body management—as well as, in her later work, from attachment only to people, to attachment to other objects, and from irresponsibility to guilt (A. Freud 1974). For Anna Freud, pathology is defined and explained either as the existence of large discrepancies between the lines or notable lags with respect to normal progress along a particular line or lines. Arrest in or regression along a particular developmental line can generate problems.

Anna Freud also identified disturbances of narcissism, object relatedness, and the absence of control over aggressive or self-destructive tendencies alongside a range of deficiencies of development, and later suggested that there is a developmental aspect to the emergence of anxiety problems in childhood. She distinguished between *objective anxiety* (e.g., fear of any aspect of the external world, including parents' real reactions) and fear of the internal world (impulses, wishes, and feelings)—building on her earlier work with infants at the Hampstead war nurseries, where she found that children were less likely to be traumatized by being bombed if during this experience they were with their mothers and if the mothers remained calm (Freud and Burlingham 1944). A carefully conducted study of children's reactions to Scud missile attacks in Israel provides more recent support for this finding (Laor et al. 1996).

Both the development of competence and psychopathology have been traditionally studied throughout the history of psychiatry and psychoanalysis, but they are not commonly integrated. The former has been the concern of developmental psychology, and the latter has been the focus of child and adult psychiatry. Anna Freud's work is notable for bridging the gap between the two.

Margaret Mahler

Margaret Mahler was the first thorough-going developmentalist of the North American tradition. She elaborated a psychoanalytic model of development based on observations of children 6 months to 3 years old. Mahler's developmental model presents object relations and the self as elaborations of instinctual vicissitudes (Mahler et al. 1975). Her focus was on the move from the unity of *I* and *not I* to eventual separation and individuation. *Separation*, in Mahler's model, refers to the child's emergence from a symbiotic fusion with the mother, whereas "individuation consists of those achievements marking the child's assumption of his or her own individual characteristics" (Mahler et al. 1975, p. 4).

Mahler's developmental model involves *normal autism* during the first weeks of life, followed by a symbiotic phase, after which separation-individuation begins with the subphase of differentiation. From 9 to about 15–18 months of age, the second subphase of individuation (*practicing*) occurs, which is followed by a *rapprochement* subphase (the second half of the second year), during which the infant needs to be with the mother. Finally, the fourth subphase of separation-individuation is the consolidation of individuality that begins with the third year of life.

Mahler's work has been extensively used by clinicians working with adults with personality disorders (Kramer and Akhtar 1988; Pine 1985). Narcissistic personality disorders are linked to the inadequate soothing ministrations of the mother during the symbiotic phase and inadequate refueling during separation-individuation. Therefore, the omnipotence characteristic of the child during the practicing subphase is never completely renounced. Cross-cultural research on parent–child relationships, however, suggests that prolonging the symbiotic union between mother and infant does not undermine the individual's capacity to achieve autonomy (Rothbaum et al. 2000). Individuals with borderline personality disorder are often thought to experience residues of the rapprochement subphase conflicts with persistent longings for and dread of fusion with the object, associated with either aggression or withdrawal on the part of the mother. Masterson (1985) suggested that the object, who is desperate to feel needed, rewards the toddler for demanding and clinging behavior. There is limited evidence available to support the suggestion that borderline personality disorder is a transgenerational disorder. A relatively recent study of mothers with borderline personality disorder found that they were more intrusively insensitive toward their 2-month-old infants than were mothers without psychiatric disorder (Crandell et al. 2003).

Mahler described her work as enabling clinicians treating adults to make more accurate reconstructions of the preverbal period, thereby making patients more accessible to psychotherapeutic interventions. However, although Mahler's model has been highly influential, systematic experimental research with infants casts serious doubt on dual notions of normal autism and self-object merger (Gergely 2000). That said, Mahler's developmental framework could well be appropriate for the truly psychological world of the human infant: the infant is aware of itself and the object as separate in the physical (bodily) domain but assumes that psychological states extend beyond physical boundaries (Fonagy et al. 2002). Similarly, Mahler's theories concerning childhood schizophrenia seem unlikely to be explained by the notion of a developmental fixation in the symbiotic phase, but her original contributions to the understanding of borderline personality disorder have been most lasting. Her view of these patients as fixated in a rapprochement—wishing to cling to the other but fearing the loss of their fragile sense of self, wishing to be separate but also fearing to move away from the parental figure—has been crucial to both clinical intervention and theoretical understanding.

Joseph Sandler

Joseph Sandler was a student of Anna Freud's and played an instrumental role in the modernization of psychoanalysis, preparing its integration with the developmental sciences and finding common ground between American ego psychology and British object relations theory. Many of his ideas have been seamlessly integrated into modern core theory. Sandler introduced the frame of reference of the representational world, an approach very similar to the schema theory that has come to dominate social and cognitive behavioral psychology (Sandler and Rosenblatt 1962). He placed feeling states rather than psychic energy at the center of the psychoanalytic theory of motivation. Sandler (1960) introduced the revolutionary concept of *background of safety*, within which the aim of the ego is to maximize safety or security rather than to avoid anxiety. He did not eliminate drives, but explained their influence on behavior through the impact they had on feelings.

Sandler claimed that for patients, the purpose of creating relationships with their therapist (and others) was frequently to actualize unconscious fantasies, and this they carried out by casting themselves and their therapists in specific relationship patterns. By extension of this claim, Sandler offered an entirely new theory of internal object representations. He differentiated the deeply unconscious hypothetical structures—assumed in classic psychoanalysis to develop early in life and to have no chance of directly emerging into consciousness (the past unconscious)—from the present unconscious, which he proposed works as Freud described (irrationally, only partly observing the reality principle but principally concerned with current rather than past experience) (Sandler and Sandler 1984). The second system, the present unconscious, consists of here-and-now adaptations to conflicts and anxieties arising from within the first system, which is a genuine continuation of the past into the present. Sandler linked pleasure in experiencing particular styles of perceptual and cognitive functions with specific forms of pathology. For example, obsessionality, painful though it may be, is also linked to pleasure in childhood. The developmental model of depression that Sandler proposed also makes use of the representational world construct.

In further clinical formulations, Sandler explained the concept of projective identification without making the extravagant assumptions of some Kleinian authors (see the following section, "Object Relations Theory and the Klein-Bion Model"). The "other" can come to enact the patient's fantasy because the patient attempts to modify or control the behavior of the other so that it conforms to the patient's distorted representation of the other. The representation of the other comes to be distorted through the mechanism of projection, in which the other is experienced as owning unwanted aspects of the self-representation. This model is helpful in explaining therapeutic phenomena such as countertransference or phenomena identified by emotional developmental research, such as the transgenerational transmission of patterns of mother–infant interaction (Fraiberg et al. 1975).

Although Sandler's theories were, and are, extensively used, those who use his ideas are often unaware that they are doing so. Thus there is no psychoanalytic school that bears his name. Sandler advanced thinking by clarifying a range of psychoanalytic concepts but was unable to excite his colleagues with the novelty of his contributions.

Object Relations Theory and the Klein-Bion Model

As we shall see, object relations theory has several incarnations, various of which grew to be immensely popular in the 1980s. Broadly speaking, object relations theory moves toward an understanding of psychopathology in terms of mental representations of dyadic self and object relationships, which are rooted in past relationships and which are at first dyadic, are later triadic, and still later encompass multiple relationship representations. The increased interest in relationships is part of an underlying refocusing of psychoanalysis away from the study of intrapsychic conflict toward an experientially based perspective emphasizing the individual's experience of being with others, including being with the therapist during analytic work.

According to object relations theory, the ego is defined in relation to other objects, both internal and external, so it is assumed that the child's mind is initially shaped by early experiences with the caretaker, and that it becomes increasingly complex with development. These early object relations are thought to set patterns that are repeated, and therefore become fixed, in later life. In some versions of object relations theory (e.g., attachment theory), the individual is seen as possessing an *autonomous relationship drive*. Other versions derive relationships from drive theory (Winnicott), and yet others derive drives from object relations (Kernberg). Along the lines of whether drives are derived from relationships or vice versa, Friedman (1988) divided object relations theories into *hard* and *soft* categories, with hard theories exemplified by the work of Melanie Klein, Ronald Fairbairn, and Otto Kernberg, and soft theories by the work of Michael Balint (1968), D.W. Winnicott, and Heinz Kohut.

Central to object relations theories are the ideas of Melanie Klein and Wilfred Bion, who offered highly speculative, often controversial, but remarkably influential accounts of pathology, particularly of self-destructive and persistent behaviors. Klein and Bion both highlighted the negative aspects of emotional development. Klein combined the structural model with an object relations model of development, which in turn lays strong emphasis on constitutional vulnerability rather than caregiver behavior as the prime determinant of developmental pathways. Klein's papers on the depressive position (Klein 1935, 1940), her paper on the paranoid-schizoid position (Klein 1946), and her book *Envy and Gratitude* (Klein 1957) all play a significant part in the Klein-Bion model, which, building on Freud's idea of a self-destructive death drive, postulates two modes of mental functioning: the paranoid-schizoid position and the depressive position.

The paranoid-schizoid position is dominated by tendencies to separate the good and the bad, the idealized and the persecutory; the depressive position entails a more mature, balanced recognition of the bad in the good and one's own role in unrealistically and self-servingly distorting the world into idealized and denigrated components. Klein's metaphor for these two states of mind was the perception of the mother as separately idealized and persecuting in the paranoid-schizoid state and as a whole person who accounts for both good and bad experiences in the depressive state. Recognition in the depressive position that the loved good object and the hated and feared bad object are one and the same gives rise to feelings of guilt and *depressive anxiety*, whereas the paranoid-schizoid position is characterized by *persecutory anxieties.*

An important contribution from the Klein-Bion model is the concept of *projective identification;* that is, the individual externalizes *segments of the ego* and attempts to gain control over these unwanted possessions, often through highly manipulative behavior toward the object (i.e., making the other identify with the projections). Projective identification is best characterized not as a defensive mechanism, but rather as an interpersonal process whereby the self gets rid of feelings by evoking the same feelings in another self (Bion 1962). The roots of this process are found in infancy (Bion 1959). Klein suggested that children innately possess ruthless and sadistic fantasies that are not a reaction to frustration but that pay lip service to the parent's capacity to mitigate the influence of the child's constitutional tendencies. Given its thesis that violent tendencies are innate rather than caused by environmental influences, the Klein-Bion model has been influential in psychological models of the mediation of genetic vulnerability. Recent evidence suggests that physical aggression and destructiveness are indeed particularly marked in the early years and naturally decline in most children over the course of the first decade, with violent children manifesting an absence of this expectable *taming* rather than an emergence of aggression de novo in response to environmental impingement (Shaw et al. 2001; Tremblay 2000; Tremblay et al. 1999).

By and large, the Kleinian model of psychopathology explains mental disorder in terms of the two positions described above. A predominance of the paranoid-schizoid position leads to mental disorder, whereas relative stability of the depressive framework reflects mental health (although Bion [1957] argued that the depressive position is never permanently achieved). In psychotic states, annihilatory/persecutory anxieties are intense and the object with whom the patient attempts to projectively identify is *reintrojected* (i.e., experienced as entering the ego), creating a delusion of the mind or the body being under external control. Neurotic problems are seen as consequences of unresolved, depressive anxiety. For example, depression arises because the experience of loss is a reminder of the damage the person felt he or she caused to the good object. Chronic depression arises when the person cannot escape the fear of injuring the loved object and therefore has to repress all aggressiveness, generating relentless self-persecution. Narcissistic character structure, meanwhile, is considered a defense against envy and dependence. The narcissist's relationships with others are highly destructive; the narcissist makes ruthless use of others and professes not to need them (Rosenfeld 1987).

Klein's ideas have provoked considerable controversy and some ill feeling. Concerns have included her attribution of adult psychological capacities to infants and her dating of pathology to such early stages (Bibring 1947). Because the mental states of infancy are extremely hard to observe, the postulation of crucial pathogenic processes in infancy is extremely unlikely to be proven or disproven. Psychoanalytic infant observation (Bick 1964) permits widely differing interpretations. However, evidence is accumulating that most of the important mental disorders of adulthood are indeed foreshadowed in the biological processes of infancy (e.g., Marenco and Weinberger 2000), and early brain development is increasingly seen as pivotal (Schore 2003).

The British Independent School: Fairbairn and Winnicott

The so-called British Independent School comprises several theorists working individually, all of whom explicitly refrained from establishing schools of followers. Fairbairn and Guntrip were the theory builders, with major contributions from Winnicott, Balint, Klauber, Khan, and Bollas.

The core ideas contained in the theories of this somewhat heterogeneous group of theories might be summarized as follows:

- There is a primary drive for creating object relationships (Fairbairn 1952).
- Insufficient intimacy with the primary object can give rise to a *splitting* in the self, and it is the persistence of incompatible ideas and lack of integration that is at the root of psychological disorders.

- *Holding*, or the capacity to comprehend the infant's mental states, is key to intimacy and integration (Winnicott 1960).
- Holding is communicated by mirroring that neither can nor should be perfect, but is normally good enough, and permits repair (Winnicott 1967).
- The infant "conjures the mother" through the use of a physical object (e.g., a blanket), which is known as a *transitional object* (Winnicott 1953).
- The self emerges through nonintrusive interactions with the mother, which facilitate the baby's illusion that the object/mother is a product of the baby's creative gestures and therefore controlled and controllable.
- If the mother cannot comprehend the infant, a *false (compliant) self* will develop to protect the true self (Winnicott 1960).
- It is lack of (recognition of) love between mother and child, and not a primary destructiveness, that will lead the child to believe that the child's hate has destroyed the object/mother (Fairbairn 1952).

Fairbairn proposed that early trauma is stored in memories that are "frozen" or dissociated from a person's central ego or functional self, an idea of particular relevance to understanding narcissistic and borderline personality disorders. Fairbairn saw the roots of all pathology as being in a schizoid reaction to the trauma of not being known or loved. Winnicott and Fairbairn both associated schizophrenia with total privation—that is, the complete absence of a "good enough mother," which makes the infant view his or her love as bad and destructive and leads the infant to withdraw from emotional contact with the outer world, ultimately creating a highly disturbed sense of external reality. Severe personality disorder could be seen as the result of having had a "good enough mother" who subsequently disappeared. Schizoid personality (Fairbairn 1952) arises out of the baby's feeling that love for the mother is destroying her and therefore has to be inhibited along with all intimacy. Borderline patients were considered by Winnicott to share defenses with psychotic patients; that is, they have no sense of others, and respond with threats of intense anger if their sense of omnipotence is threatened (Winnicott 1960). Empirical studies have shown that borderline patients do indeed have a specific deficit in mental state awareness in the context of attachment relationships (Fonagy et al. 1996).

The Independents' general approach to development—the description of the infant as biologically prepared to attend to environmental events that respond to them—has been very well supported by infant research (Meltzoff and Moore 1998; Watson 2001), and Winnicott's views on the importance of sensitive maternal care are broadly supported by developmental research, although there is general dissatisfaction about the fuzziness of the concept of maternal sensitivity (De Wolff and van Ijzendoorn 1997). Research, such as work on affective interactions between infant and mother, supports the notion of a dual unit of infant and mother, in which the mother and infant mutually create the infant's moods (Jaffe et al. 2001; Tronick 2007). However, the ideas emerging from the British Independent School have only partially stood the test of time. Winnicott, it now seems, was correct to look to environmental influences as a determinant of normal and pathological development, but he might have overstated their importance. For example, research does not support Winnicott's exclusive concern with the infant–mother relationship, because many other factors, particularly genetic influences, shape a child's personality (Bolton et al. 2006). Winnicott's assumption that the relationship between infant and mother provides the basis for all serious mental disorders also flies in the face of accumulating evidence suggesting that genetic factors account for the observed association of environmental deprivation and pathological outcome (Rutter et al. 1999). The greatest problem with Winnicott's framework, however, is its attempt to map adult states of mind onto infant experiences. To some extent this criticism is applicable to the entire British object relations tradition. Human development is far too complex for infantile experiences to have direct links to adult pathology. In fact, longitudinal studies of infancy suggest that personality organization is subject to reorganization throughout development, based on both positive and negative influences (e.g., Emde and Spicer 2000).

Heinz Kohut and Self Psychology

Self psychology emerged from the thinking of Heinz Kohut. Initially concentrating on problems of narcissism, self psychology was soon applied to other mental disorders and involved a specific therapeutic approach foregrounding empathy. Although Kohut's theories changed over time, his key assumptions included the following (Kohut 1977):

- Narcissistic development proceeds along a path of its own, and parents serve as selfobjects (people in the environment who perform particular functions for the self).
- Empathic responses from the mirroring selfobject allow the unfolding of exhibitionism and grandiosity.
- Frustration promotes a gradual modulation of infantile omnipotence through a *transmuting internalization* of this mirroring selfobject, which in turn leads gradually to a consolidation of the nuclear self.
- The idealization of selfobjects, also through internalization, leads to the development of ideals.

Kohut (1984) later believed that a) a cohesive self is a goal to be attained, as opposed to there being a self that changes over time; b) the *enfeebled self* (to whom the selfobject has typically failed to attune emotionally) turns defensively toward pleasure aims (drives); and c) anxiety is primarily the self's experience of a defect or lack of continuity.

It emerges from the foregoing description that self psychology is a theory based on deficiency. A deficiency of facilitating experiences is assumed to lead to a primary psychic deficit, an inadequately developed self. Fear of losing the sense of who one is underlies all pathology. Diagnostic distinctions are made in terms of characteristics of the self: psychosis precludes a cohesive sense of self; patients with personality disorders have an enfeebled self vulnerable to temporary fragmentation, and neurotic pathology is thought to be associated with the robustness of self structure. Narcissistic personality, meanwhile, is a developmental arrest at the stage of the grandiose exhibitionistic self, which fails to be neutralized by the parent's age-specific mirroring responses, and borderline personality disorder results from an inability to psychologically hold on to selfobjects that might otherwise be soothing to the self. Furthermore, drug addiction is thought to fill a missing gap in the psyche (Kohut 1977).

Like Winnicott, Kohut has proven influential, and although some evidence used to support his theories is far-fetched, at other times his work seems prescient. For example, a large body of evidence supports the central role of abnormal self-esteem in the generation of psychological disturbance (Brown et al. 1995). Self psychologists have also felt supported by the identification of so-called mirror neurons in the primate brain (Gallese et al. 2004; Rizzolatti and Craighero 2004). These are cells that appear to be activated when the rhesus monkey identifies a movement analogous to its own in the world. (It should be borne in mind that monkeys do not recognize themselves in the mirror; the suggestion here is that there is a predisposition toward identifying environmental events pertaining to the self.) Although prima facie this is consistent with a developmental emphasis on mirroring, it is somewhat far-fetched to consider it a direct confirmation of self psychological ideas.

Kohut's model has often, and appropriately, been criticized as *parent blaming*—and, again like Winnicott, Kohut is open to criticism for overemphasizing environmental influences, especially in the face of increasing evidence of genetically rooted personality traits. Correlations between characteristics of early parenting and later child behavior can be reinterpreted, given that any manifestation of the behaviors predicted by the parents' nurturing style can as easily be the result of the 50% genetic overlap between parent and child. Thus, while genetic influences contribute to parenting style, they might equally produce those behaviors in a child, or indeed have no small part in determining those qualities of a child's early environment that are predicted to result from that parenting style without the parenting style itself being the cause—an effect called *passive genotype–environment correlation*. In a landmark investigation of genetic and environmental influences on adolescent development, Reiss and colleagues (2000) found that 44 out of 52 statistically significant associations between a family relationship (e.g., parental warmth or sibling relationships) and measures of adjustment (e.g., the presence of depression or antisocial behavior) showed genetic influences that accounted for more than half of the common variance. For almost half of the 52 associations, little correlation between family relations and adolescent functioning remained once genetic influence was taken into consideration. The impact of primarily environmental influences on development is further called into question when we take into account the so-called child-to-parent effect, whereby aspects of the family environment are shaped by the child's genetically rooted characteristics (best shown in adoption studies; see, e.g., Deater-Deckard et al. 1999). Nevertheless, genetically informed studies do repeatedly find that qualities of the family environment moderate genetic influence; this moderating effect is greater in relation to conditions such as antisocial behavior at higher levels of negative parenting (Feinberg et al. 2007). Kohut has been criticized not only for his radical revision of psychoanalytic ideas but also for his failure to recognize the work of others working in similar areas, including Winnicott and Loewald. For these reasons, Kohut's model of self psychology has largely been abandoned.

Structural Object Relations: Otto Kernberg

Advanced primarily by Otto Kernberg, structural object relations theory involves a synthesis of the Klein-Bion model and the models of the modernizers of structural theory (Sandler, Mahler, and Loewald). Through his work, which offers a comprehensive reconsideration of psychological disorders, Kernberg has become the most cited living analyst and one of the most influential analysts in the history of the field.

Following Sandler, Kernberg (1982) considers affects to be the primary element in the motivational system. That is to say, representations of the interactions between self and object, colored by particular affects, constitute the basic building blocks of psychic structure; drives come about from the accumulations of types of self–object–affect triads—not the other way around—although eventually drives do become motivators of behavior and are not replaced by object relations structures. The psychic structures (id, ego, superego) come about through various processes of *internalization*:

a) through introjection, whereby entire interactions between self and others are internalized in their affective context; b) through identifications that recognize the variety of role dimensions that exist in interactions with others; and c) through ego identity, which denotes the overall organization of introjections and identifications (Kernberg 1976). As a child develops, the ego at first separates good images from bad so as to protect one from the other, before these images become integrated into complete object and self representations in the third year of life. Failure to integrate these separated images can lead to pathology, in which splitting (as opposed to repression) remains the principal coping mechanism. As a child develops beyond age 3 years, Kernberg's theory follows the structural model of development. According to Kernberg, all disorders originate in the early stages of the self–object dyadic configurations—that is, before self and object have emerged as integrated units.

The originality of Kernberg's approach to neurotic problems consists in focusing on the current state of the patient's thinking rather than attempting to identify the origin of currently dominant pathogenic conflicts and structural organizations. Kernberg utilizes psychiatric diagnostic categories as predictors of treatment response, arguing that twice-weekly expressive psychotherapy is a better treatment for severe character problems than psychoanalysis. Kernberg's contribution to the understanding of personality disorders is his most distinctive and valuable work. At mild levels of character pathology, not only is the ego poorly organized and unstable, the superego is harsh and sadistic. The patient who feels himself to be the victim of criticism (from the therapist) can suddenly turn into the vicious, unreasonable critic. At severe levels of character pathology, there is marked primitive dissociation or splitting of internalized object relations, with consequent lack of integration of self and object representations. The individual insistently and consistently constructs either idealized or persecutory self and object relations, making relationships with such individuals confused or chaotic (Kernberg 1984). The root cause of personality disorders is the intensity of destructive and aggressive impulses and the relative weakness of ego structures available to handle them. Wisely, Kernberg leaves open the question of whether such excessive aggressiveness is inborn or associated with particularly malevolent early environments. Kernberg's approach to treating borderline personality disorder, *transference-focused psychotherapy*, is well grounded theoretically and fully operationalized, and has been subjected to careful investigation of the process as well as outcomes (Clarkin et al. 1999; Kernberg et al. 1989, 2002). The most recent findings suggest that transference-focused psychotherapy is at least as efficacious as dialectical behavioral therapy and probably more so than supportive psychotherapy (Clarkin et al. 2007; Levy et al. 2006).

Kernberg's genius lies in marrying the structural (or *metapsychological*) to the phenomenological. For example, signs of idealization, devaluation, or denial (phenomena) in a borderline patient also indicate the organization (structure) of intrapsychic relationship representations—and reveal the individual's failure to generate more advanced mental mechanisms. Kernberg also goes beyond traditional ego psychology by rescuing explanations in terms of *ego weakness* from circularity. For Kernberg, ego weakness is coterminous with an active defensive process that leads to the split-ego organizations that cannot withstand close contact with bad object representations.

Because Kernberg's theory leaves a place for innate factors in development, it can accommodate emerging evidence concerning the powerful genetic influences that appear to be present in borderline personality disorder (Livesley et al. 1998; Torgersen 2000; Torgersen et al. 2000). In addition, his hypotheses concerning the ego weakness of patients with borderline personality disorder are receiving support from work within the Personality Disorders Institute and elsewhere (Goldstein et al. 2007; Levy 2005; Rothbart et al. 2000). Clarkin (2001) has shown how borderline patients are high in negative affect and low in effortful control and how they benefit from psychotherapy in the degree to which they improve their capacity to represent mental states in an attachment context. It may be that Kernberg's etiological hypotheses share some of the general weaknesses of psychoanalytic formulations, but his contribution remains a landmark, not only because his work advanced the psychoanalytic developmental framework for personality disorders, but also because it brought about a major shift in the epistemic stance taken by psychoanalysts influenced by him—from a clinical hermeneutic perspective toward an empirical one.

The Interpersonal Relational Approach

Arguably the most radical change in psychoanalytic thinking has been the newfound popularity of the interpersonal relational perspective, which is rooted in part in the work of Harry Stack Sullivan (1953). The relational psychoanalysis of the 1980s and 1990s consolidated several lines of thought that had been initiated in response to a number of justified critiques of traditional analytic theory, including feminism, the hermeneutic-constructivist critique of the analyst's authority, infancy research, and, closely related, the intersubjectivist-phenomenological philosophy of mind, as well as a general political movement to improve and democratize access to analytic ideas and training (Seligman 2003).

Stephen A. Mitchell (1988) introduced the framework for a range of theoretical developments that collectively can be called *relational psychoanalytic theories*. This framework was provided by his *relational matrix*, which consisted of three dimensions—a self pole, an object pole, and an interactional pole—out of whose configurations and reconfigurations multiple new theories can be generated. Taking its lead from Sullivan, and linked to British object relations theory, this approach emphasizes the active role played by both or all parties in relationships; important contributors to the approach include Ogden (1994), McLaughlin (1991), Hoffman (1994), Renik (1993), Benjamin (1998), and Bromberg (1998). Notions of objective truth are supplemented or replaced with subjectivity, the emphasis shifts from intrapsychic to intersubjective experience, and from fantasy (poetics) to pragmatics (descriptions of experience); concepts of truth and distortion are supplemented with perspectivism; and a reliance on strong theories is replaced by attempts to avoid theoretical bias. Each of the major relational theorists has offered a slightly different integration of the relational matrix (e.g., Mitchell's relational-conflict theory [Mitchell 1988], Ogden's intersubjectivity [Ogden 1994], Hoffman's social constructivism theory [Hoffman 1994], and Greenberg's dual-drive theory [Greenberg 2001]), meaning that there is no single, unifying relational psychoanalytic theory. Relational theories are metatheories in which human relations are considered to play a superordinate role in the creation of human character.

Sullivan (1953) felt that psychoanalysis ignored the relationship-seeking aspect of human character, and proposed that mental conflict was produced not in the individual but by conflicting and contradictory signals and values in the environment. For Sullivan, needs are interpersonal in origin, as is anxiety, the development of which leads to psychopathology. Despite the different terminology, Sullivan's concepts have close ties to the psychodynamic domain: *security operations* seem to be the same as defenses, and *parataxic distortions* appear analogous to internal object relationships. In the kind of therapy Sullivan advocated, however, the therapist seeks less to impart understanding than to explore the nature of and the reasons for patterns of behavior in an active and participatory manner. Whereas in self psychology the nuclear self is conceived as intrapsychic, in an interpersonal relational context the individual's mind is a contradiction in terms, since subjectivity is invariably rooted in intersubjectivity.

The relational model starts from the assumption that subjectivity is interpersonal; that is, the intersubjective replaces the intrapsychic (Mitchell 1988). The human mind is thus rendered a contradiction in terms, because subjectivity is invariably rooted in an intersubjective matrix of relational bonds within which personal meanings are embedded (Mitchell 2000)—rather than in biologically based drives. Thus the internal and the external are not discrete, but are anticipated by and subsumed under the interpersonal field; indeed, the primacy of the interpersonal field within a relational model extends even into the realm of biology, as the organism's existence is defined in relation to its environment. However, the relational psychoanalytic model lacks a specific explanation of how relationality and intersubjectivity may develop, unlike most other psychoanalytic theories, which, whatever self-dimension they prioritize (be it the individual or the interpersonal), propose an explanation of its origins and formation.

From a relational perspective, then, sexuality, for example, not only is a powerful biological and physiological force but also emerges from an interpersonal context in which people regulate each other; hence, it is intersubjective or relational. Its power is not derived from pleasure to the organs, but from its meaning in a relational matrix (Mitchell 1988). A result of adopting this approach is that it privileges observable behavior and actuality over fantasy, meaning that reality is not *behind* the appearance (what the individual is imagining), it is *in* the appearance (what the individual is doing).

According to Mitchell (2000), psychiatric disorders can come about in any of four ways:

1. Through nonreflective, presymbolic behavior that leads to the organization of relational fields around reciprocal influences and mutual regulation
2. Through affective permeability, or the shared experience of intense affect across permeable boundaries where direct resonances emerge in interpersonal dyads
3. Through the organization of experience into self-other configurations, as extensively discussed by Kernberg and other object relations theorists
4. Through intersubjectivity, or the mutual recognition of self-reflective agents identified by relationally oriented psychoanalytic feminists such as Chodorow (1989) and Benjamin (1995)

Relational theory embraces the notion that the absence of a sensitive object causes a child to precociously fill a missing parental function, but it is critical of the developmental arrest model. Relational theorists claim that we privilege the earliest periods at the risk of overlooking current relationship needs. Relational theory also finds a middle ground between Kohut and Kernberg in recognizing both that the child needs the narcissistic illusion of grandiosity (Kohut) and that the narcissistic illusion is defensive (Kernberg). Because the approach focuses on the present relationship between patient and therapist, there has been controversy concerning the readiness with which therapists following this approach disclose their own feelings (Ehrenberg 1992).

Relational analysts have adapted infant research to apply the principle of ongoing dyadic regulation to the therapeutic situation (Beebe and Lachmann 1994; Stern et al. 1998). The therapist and the patient supposedly create a dyadic state of consciousness through mutual affect regulation; each patient–therapist dyad is different but will influence future exchanges for both parties—both with each other and with other people. Therapy occurs when already extant states of consciousness are reintegrated and reconfigured for the patient. Current relational thinking often uses psychopathological accounts of trauma to highlight the relational aspects of actual experience (e.g., Davies 1996). Attention is paid not only to "what really happened" but also to the subjective experience of the patient, not in order to separate veridical events from distortions associated with unconscious fantasy, but rather to elaborate the overwhelming nature of the experience itself—especially because it is so difficult to make meaning from traumatic experiences. It is the inherent paradox of attachment trauma (i.e., an apparently unintended trauma perpetrated by a figure on whom one depends) that a stance of "not knowing what one knows" (Bowlby 1988) might be adopted to keep the crucial relationship intact. Relational psychoanalytic and attachment-inspired clinical descriptions provide similar formulations of dissociation linked with traumatic experience.

There is substantial developmental evidence that psychopathology is accompanied by relational problems and that good interpersonal relations have a protective influence (e.g., Laub 1998). Furthermore, the interpersonal approach has presented the strongest evidence so far for the effectiveness of psychodynamic psychotherapy. Relational ideas underpin interpersonal therapy (IPT; Klerman et al. 1984; see also Ablon and Jones 2002; Frank et al. 2000; Shea et al. 1992), which has a strong evidence base in the literature on depression in adults (and a somewhat meager one for its adaptation in treating adolescents; Mufson et al. 2004a, 2004b). IPT might have moved too far from its origins to be considered a genuine psychodynamic approach (even in the broad sense of that term), but there are more clearly psychoanalytic adaptations of the interpersonal psychodynamic tradition that retain the focus on the relationship-seeking aspect of human character. The best controlled studies of relatively brief psychotherapy for patients with mood disorders (Frank et al. 1991; Shapiro et al. 1995; Shea et al. 1992) or eating disorders (Fairburn 1993), as well as for chronic users of health care services (Guthrie et al. 1999), have all shown IPT to be at least as efficacious as other brief therapies.

Psychoanalytic Schema Theories

Some theorists have attempted to combine psychoanalysis with systems theory (e.g., Boesky 1988; Peterfreund 1971; Rosenblatt and Thickstun 1977), whereas others have combined British object relations theory and cognitive science research with systems theory, to create *person schema theory* (Horowitz et al. 1995). Anthony Ryle, for example, has advanced a model of psychotherapy based on the realization that unconscious relationship procedures can be described and that the resulting descriptions can be of considerable value in psychotherapy (Ryle and Kerr 2002). Cognitive analytic therapy identifies and represents a relatively small number of underlying relationship patterns, including issues of care, dependency, control, submission, love, and anger, as *reciprocal role procedures*. Reciprocal role procedures are addressed explicitly by the therapy, including through formal correspondence between therapist and patient. The most widely cited psychoanalytic schema theorist is Daniel Stern.

Although Stern's account of self development (Stern 1985) did not immediately imply a set of clinical applications, it has been widely used in accounts of the development of personality disorders and neurosis. For Stern, there are four phases of the development of the self: 1) the *emerging self* from birth to 2 months; 2) the *core self*, at 2–6 months, characterized by an emergent sense of agency and continuity across time; 3) the *subjective self*, developing between 9 and 18 months, during which the capacity to share intentions has been achieved and awareness arises of emotion in the other; and 4) the *narrative self*, marked by the emergence of language. Prior self stages condition later stages of self development. (Damasio [1999] developed a similar model of development.)

Stern described instances of the subjective integration of all aspects of lived experience as *emergent moments*, which derive from a range of schematic representations (event representations, semantic representations, perceptual schemas, and sensorimotor representations) in conjunction with representations of *feeling shapes* (patterns of arousal across time) and *protonarrative envelopes* that give a protoplot to an event with an agent, an action, instrumentality, and context. Once combined, these elements are conceptualized in combination as the *schema-of-a-way-of-being-with*. Distortions in this basic schema lead to vulnerability to psychopathology. These schemas come closest to providing a neuropsychologically valid way of depicting a psychoanalytic model of the development of interpersonal experience.

Stern's model fits well with developmental data on infancy, but extensions of the model to childhood and adult psychopathology are less solid, and even fanciful. The adult is not an infant, so continuities from infancy at the level of mental representation are quite unlikely, although they are possible at the procedural, implicit level highlighted by Stern and his colleagues. It is in the realm of mental processes that continuity can seemingly be established from early childhood into adulthood.

Mentalization Theory

Mentalization refers to a person's ability (or lack thereof) to conceive of his or her own and others' mental states as explanations of behavior. In the psychodynamic model that we have developed with our colleagues (Fonagy et al. 2002), this capacity is seen as an index of the development of an agentive self. Firmly rooted in attachment theory, the mentalization-focused approach additionally posits an evolutionary rationale for the human attachment system in that proximity to concerned adults affords an opportunity for the development of social intelligence and meaning making. The biologically based capacity for interpretation in psychological terms, which we have labeled the *interpersonal interpretive function*, unfolds within the context of attachment relationships. Unlike the internal working model, the interpersonal interpretive function does not encode representations of experiences; it is not a repository of personal encounters (see also Stern's *schema-of-a-way-of-being-with* in the "Psychoanalytic Schema Theories" section). It is a mechanism for processing and interpreting new interpersonal experiences.

Interpersonal interpretive function develops through several emotional processes and control mechanisms: a) the labeling and understanding of affect; b) arousal regulation; c) effortful control; and d) the development of mentalizing or mind-reading capacities proper (what elsewhere has been operationalized as *reflective function*) (Fonagy and Target 2002). The infant's experience of attachment relationships helps to develop these processes, which, in turn, are useful for many tasks in later life. The absence or disruption of such a relationship can lead to possible lifelong maladaptive patterns (e.g., Hamilton 2000; Waters et al. 2000).

This approach explicitly rejects the classic Cartesian assumption that emotional and other internal mental states are from the start directly experienced introspectively. It is suggested that the mental states that arise in the infant are discovered by him or her through contingent mirroring interactions with the caregiver (Target and Fonagy 1996). Repeated experience with affect-reflective caregiver reactions is seen as essential for the infant to become sensitized to, and to construct, differentiated representations of his or her internal self states—a process termed *social biofeedback* (Gergely and Watson 1996). Such experiences vitally contribute to the emergence of early mentalization capacities, allowing infants to "discover" or "find" their psychological self in the social world.

Two conditions need to be met to enable the infant to discover his or her psychological self: 1) reasonable congruency of mirroring, whereby the caregiver accurately matches the infant's mental state, and 2) "markedness" of the mirroring, whereby the caregiver is able to express an affect while indicating that it is not an expression of the caregiver's own feelings. Consequently, two impingements can occur: 1) in the case of incongruent mirroring, the infant's representation of internal state will not correspond to a constitutional self state (nothing real), and a predisposition to a narcissistic (false-self) structure might be established; and 2) in cases of unmarked mirroring, the caregiver's expression may be seen as externalization of the infant's experience, and a predisposition to experiencing emotion through other people (a borderline personality structure) might be established (Fonagy et al. 2002). The emergence of the capacity for mentalizing follows a well-researched developmental line that identifies *fixation points*.

Application of the mentalization model to psychopathology has focused on clinical problems associated with dysfunctions of the agentive self, which we consider to be the direct or indirect consequences of dysfunctions of the interpersonal interpretive function. These problems are normally described in psychiatric terminology as severe personality disorder or borderline personality organization (Kernberg 1967). Here only the highlights of the mentalization model as applied to psychopathology are presented. The incongruent unmarked mirroring characteristic of an insecure base generates enfeebled affect representations and attentional control systems. The undermining of these major cognitive mechanisms results in disorganization of the attachment system. Disorganized attachment is thought to be coterminous with disorganization of the self; the incongruent unmarked parenting that undermines attachment organization through the mechanisms described above establishes a part within the self structure, called (after Winnicott) the *alien self*, that corresponds to the caregiver (as perceived) rather than to the child but that nevertheless exists within the self. Ideas or feelings are experienced as parts of the self that do not seem to belong to the self. Trauma, when combined with the sequelae of a deeply insecure early environment, which include enfeebled affect representation and poor affect control systems as well as a disorganized self structure, has profound effects on the development of such vulnerable individuals: a) it inhibits playfulness, which is essential for the adequate unfolding of the interpersonal interpretive function (Dunn et al. 2000; Emde et al. 1997); b) it interferes directly with affect regulation and attentional control systems (Arntz et al. 2000); and, most important, c) in vulnerable individuals it can bring about a total failure of mentalization.

The clinical approach recommended for these patients entails presenting a view of the internal world of the patient that is stable and coherent, can be clearly perceived, and may be adopted as the reflective part of the self (Bateman and Fonagy 2004). A randomized controlled trial with 44 patients treated in a partial hospital setting provided tentative evidence for the clinical value of this approach (Bateman and Fonagy 1999, 2001).

Conclusion

In the course of this review we have seen that each psychoanalytic model has produced a perspective on development. In many cases one cannot help concluding that psychoanalytic theoreticians were developmental reductionists, oversimplifying complex developmental processes and omitting a comprehensive exploration of how an early deficit could be expected to affect subsequent development. Even when infantile modes of thought and the adult mind in distress seem to share characteristics, it is unwise to assume that later development would not have altered both the mechanism and function of early structures to a point where similarities are superficial. For this reason, as psychodynamic psychotherapy has evolved, classic psychoanalytic theories have been supplemented by schema theories, systemic approaches, interpersonal approaches, and attachment theory, which have all contributed to the elaboration of more sophisticated developmental models.

Psychoanalysis studies human subjectivity at its most complex and therefore provides an essential counterweight to advances in neuroscience and molecular genetics. In order to reach an adequate understanding of the interaction between genes and environment, we must retain our grasp of the full complexity of how the human mind grapples with the challenges of adaptation. Whether or not specific environmental factors trigger the expression of a gene may depend not only on the nature of those factors but also on the way the infant or child experiences them—an intrapsychic function determined by the conscious or unconscious meanings attributed to these experiences. The quality of this experiential filter may in turn be a function either of genetic or environmental influences or of their interaction (Kandel 1998). In this context, it is essential that we not neglect the unconscious domain of human experience.

Psychoanalysis, with its focus on the representation of subjectivity and on subjectivity's emergence from attachment relationships in early development, has much to contribute to the understanding of how individual differences arise in the quality of basic mental mechanisms' functioning. Cognitive psychology and cognitive-behavioral therapy have increasingly converged with psychoanalytic interest in studying the influence of relationship representation patterns on human conduct. Schema theories, systemic approaches, interpersonal approaches, and attachment theory have converged on this problem since the mid-1980s. A full understanding of the interaction between individual mentalized representations of life experience and the expression of genetic dispositions is the task of psychoanalytic psychopathology in the next decades. As Jacob (1998; cited in Kandel 1999, p. 508) noted: "The century that is ending has been preoccupied with nucleic acids and proteins. The next one will concentrate on memory and desire. Will it be able to answer the questions they pose?"

As it stands, evidence is accumulating in favor of psychodynamic psychotherapies (Fonagy et al. 2005; Leichsenring et al. 2004) as well as most theory-based structured interventions (Roth and Fonagy 2005). Developmental psychopathology will play an increasingly important role, because evidence suggests that adult psychiatric disorders have their roots in abnormalities that are already observable in childhood or adolescence.

Nevertheless, both psychoanalysis and psychodynamic psychotherapy as a whole have possible limitations. For example, it has yet to be proven to what extent cultural context has a bearing not only on possible disorders but also on the treatment thereof. Moreover, there is room for improvement in the measures of outcome used in many trials; because psychodynamic psychotherapy is not symptom oriented, evidence about its efficacy is limited (Gabbard et al. 2002). Perhaps the user (patient) should play a larger part in devising therapies as well.

Once again, neuroscience will undoubtedly play a large role in addressing these issues, in particular if, as seems likely, scanning techniques are developed that allow the simultaneous imaging of two individuals interacting (King-Casas et al. 2005). Molecular biology similarly presents cause for optimism; for example, as molecular genetic findings unfold over the next few years, it is likely that biological vulnerability will become increasingly detectable. Furthermore, large-scale biological investigations will not only help with the prevention of psychiatric disorders (by enabling us to identify persons at risk and offer early treatment), they will also enhance our understanding of biologically indicated psychosocial treatments. As we begin to understand the causal paths that disease processes follow in the vulnerable brain, the need for specific psychosocial treatments to assist individuals with biological vulnerabilities will become acute.

In other words, the future of psychodynamic psychotherapy lies not in rejecting but in embracing developments in biology and neuroscience, which, conversely, might also embrace psychodynamic psychotherapy with more open arms. As it emerges that we cannot treat the brain in the same way that we treat the musculoskeletal system, it is quite possible that psychodynamic psychotherapy will similarly emerge (though in a more evidence-based and empirical form that incorporates imaging techniques, neuroanatomical methods, and human genetics) as the best means of understanding and helping the human mind to help itself.

Key Points

- Clinicians can feel confident that the unconscious is "evidence based"—that referring to complex thoughts and feelings that appear to organize a patient's behavior outside of the person's awareness cannot be rejected out of hand on scientific grounds.

- There is a range of excellent and internally coherent models that specify the kinds of thoughts and feelings outside a person's awareness that specific mental disorders might entail. There seems to be little reason for favoring any one over any of the others from the perspective of clinical work.

- The theoretical models come together in highlighting the significance of mental disorders of early development, current and past relationships with attachment figures, imagination and fantasy (particularly in relation to mental states), and enduring mental structures that derive from these experiences.

- Whereas the late 1980s and early 1990s saw, to some degree, a convergence of models around the so-called Object Relations School of theory, early twenty-first-century dynamic theory has seen a divergence in views. Therapists who focus on facets of the relationships that the patient brings to therapy are more concerned with the experiencing of these relationships than with the understanding that an insightful therapist could offer.

- The interface of psychiatry with neuroscience might create a new role for psychodynamic therapists as experts in the social aspects of brain function, at least at the phenotypic level. These findings need to be reflected on rather than simply incorporated into psychoanalytic theories wholesale either as supporting evidence or as indications of the complexity of the phenomena under scrutiny.

References

Ablon JS, Jones EE: Validity of controlled clinical trials of psychotherapy: findings from the NIMH Treatment of Depression Collaborative Research Program. Am J Psychiatry 159:775–783, 2002

Alliance of Psychodynamic Organizations: Psychodynamic Diagnostic Manual. Silver Spring, MD, Interdisciplinary Council on Developmental and Learning Disorders, 2006

Arntz A, Appels C, Sieswerda S: Hypervigilance in borderline disorder: a test with the emotional Stroop paradigm. J Personal Disord 14:366–373, 2000

Balint M: The Basic Fault. London, Tavistock, 1968

Bateman A, Fonagy P: The effectiveness of partial hospitalization in the treatment of borderline personality disorder—a randomized controlled trial. Am J Psychiatry 156:1563–1569, 1999

Bateman A, Fonagy P: Treatment of borderline personality disorder with psycho-analytically oriented partial hospitalization: an 18-month follow-up. Am J Psychiatry 158:36–42, 2001

Bateman AW, Fonagy P: Psychotherapy for Borderline Personality Disorder: Mentalization Based Treatment. Oxford, UK, Oxford University Press, 2004

Beebe B, Lachmann FM: Representation and internalization in infancy: three principles of salience. Psychoanalytic Psychology 11:127–166, 1994

Benjamin J: Like Subjects, Love Objects. New Haven, CT, Yale University Press, 1995

Benjamin J: The Shadow of the Other: Intersubjectivity and Gender in Psychoanalysis. New York, Routledge, 1998

Bibring E: The so-called English School of Psychoanalysis. Psychoanal Q 16:69–93, 1947

Bick E: Notes on infant observation in psychoanalytic training. Int J Psychoanal 45:558–566, 1964

Bion WR: Differentiation of the psychotic from the non-psychotic personalities. Int J Psychoanal 38:266–275, 1957

Bion WR: Attacks on linking. Int J Psychoanal 40:308–315, 1959

Bion WR: A theory of thinking. Int J Psychoanal 43:306–310, 1962

Birbaumer N, Veit R, Lotze M, et al: Deficient fear conditioning in psychopathy: a functional magnetic resonance imaging study. Arch Gen Psychiatry 62:799–805, 2005

Blum H: The position and value of extratransference interpretation. J Am Psychoanal Assoc 31:587–618, 1983

Boesky D: The concept of psychic structure. J Am Psychoanal Assoc 36(suppl):113–135, 1988

Bolton D, Eley TC, O'Connor TG, et al: Prevalence and genetic and environmental influences on anxiety disorders in 6-year-old twins. Psychol Med 36:335–344, 2006

Bowlby J: A Secure Base: Clinical Applications of Attachment Theory. London, Routledge & Kegan Paul, 1988

Bradley C: Generativity-stagnation: development of a status model. Dev Rev 17:262–290, 1997

Brenner C: Conflict, compromise formation, and structural theory. Psychoanal Q 71:397–417, 2002

Breuer J, Freud S: Studies on hysteria (1893–1895), in The Standard Edition of the Complete Psychological Works of Sigmund Freud, Vol 2. Translated and edited by Strachey J. London, Hogarth Press, 1955, pp 1–319

Bromberg PM: Standing in the Spaces. Hillsdale, NJ, Analytic Press, 1998

Brown GW, Harris TO, Hepworth C: Loss, humiliation and entrapment among women developing depression: a patient and non-patient comparison. Psychol Med 25:7–21, 1995

Chodorow N: Feminism and Psychoanalytic Theory. Cambridge, UK, Polity Press, 1989

Clarkin J: Borderline personality disorder, mind and brain: a psychoanalytic perspective. Paper presented at the plenary presentation of the Seventh International Psychoanalytic Association Research Training Program, London, August 10, 2001

Clarkin JF, Yeomans FE, Kernberg OF: Psychotherapy for Borderline Personality. New York, Wiley, 1999

Clarkin J, Levy KN, Lenzenweger MF, et al: Evaluating three treatments for borderline personality disorder: a multiwave study. Am J Psychiatry 164:922–928, 2007

Crandell LE, Patrick MPH, Hobson RP: 'Still-face' interactions between mothers with borderline personality disorder and their 2-month-old infants. Br J Psychiatry 183:239–247, 2003

Damasio A: The Feeling of What Happens: Body and Emotion in the Making of Consciousness. New York, Harcourt Brace, 1999

Davies JM: Linking the "pre-analytic" with the postclassical: integration, dissociation, and the multiplicity of unconscious processes. Contemp Psychoanal 32:553–576, 1996

Deater-Deckard K, Fulker DW, Plomin R: A genetic study of the family environment in the transition to early adolescence. J Child Psychol Psychiatry 40:769–795, 1999

Dew SE, Bickman L: Client expectancies about therapy. Ment Health Serv Res 7:21–33, 2005

De Wolff MS, van Ijzendoorn MH: Sensitivity and attachment: a meta-analysis on parental antecedents of infant attachment. Child Dev 68:571–591, 1997

Dunn J, Davies LC, O'Connor TG, et al: Parents' and partners' life course and family experiences: links with parent-child relationships in different family settings. J Child Psychol Psychiatry 41:955–968, 2000

Ehrenberg DB: The Intimate Edge: Extending the Reach of Psychoanalytic Interaction. New York, WW Norton, 1992

Emde RN, Spicer P: Experience in the midst of variation: new horizons for development and psychopathology. Dev Psychopathol 12:313–331, 2000

Emde R, Kubicek L, Oppenheim D: Imaginative reality observed during early language development. Int J Psychoanal 78:115–133, 1997

Erikson EH: Childhood and Society. New York, WW Norton, 1950

Fairbairn WRD: An Object-Relations Theory of the Personality. New York, Basic Books, 1952

Fairburn CG: Interpersonal psychotherapy for bulimia nervosa, in New Application of Interpersonal Psychotherapy. Edited by Klerman GL, Weissman MM. New York, Guilford, 1993, pp 353–378

Feinberg ME, Button TM, Neiderhiser JM, et al: Parenting and adolescent antisocial behavior and depression: evidence of genotype × parenting environment interaction. Arch Gen Psychiatry 64:457–465, 2007

Fenichel O: The Psychoanalytic Theory of Neurosis. New York, WW Norton, 1945

Fonagy P: Irrelevance of infant observations. J Am Psychoanal Assoc 44:404–422, 1996

Fonagy P, Target M: Early intervention and the development of self-regulation. Psychoanalytic Inquiry 22:307–335, 2002

Fonagy P, Leigh T, Steele M, et al: The relation of attachment status, psychiatric classification, and response to psychotherapy. J Consult Clin Psychol 64:22–31, 1996

Fonagy P, Gergely G, Jurist E, et al: Affect Regulation, Mentalization and the Development of the Self. New York, Other Press, 2002

Fonagy P, Roth A, Higgitt A: The outcome of psychodynamic psychotherapy for psychological disorders. Clin Neurosci Res 4:367–377, 2005

Fraiberg SH, Adelson E, Shapiro V: Ghosts in the nursery: a psychoanalytic approach to the problem of impaired infant-mother relationships. J Am Acad Child Adolesc Psychiatry 14:387–422, 1975

Frank E, Kupfer DJ, Wagner EF, et al: Efficacy of interpersonal therapy as a maintenance treatment of recurrent depression. Arch Gen Psychiatry 48:1053–1059, 1991

Frank E, Grochocinski VJ, Spanier CA, et al: Interpersonal psychotherapy and antidepressant medication: evaluation of a sequential treatment strategy in women with recurrent major depression. J Clin Psychiatry 61:5157, 2000

Freud A: The ego and the mechanisms of defence (1936), in The Writings of Anna Freud, Vol 2. New York, International Universities Press, 1966

Freud A: Normality and Pathology in Childhood: Assessments of Development. New York, International Universities Press, 1965

Freud A: A psychoanalytic view of developmental psychopathology (1974), in The Writings of Anna Freud, Vol 8. Madison, CT, International Universities Press, 1981, pp 119–136

Freud A, Burlingham D: Infants Without Families. New York, International Universities Press, 1944

Freud S: The interpretation of dreams (1900), in The Standard Edition of the Complete Psychological Works of Sigmund Freud, Vols 4 and 5. Translated and edited by Strachey J. London, Hogarth Press, 1953, pp 1–715

Freud S: The psychopathology of everyday life (1901), in The Standard Edition of the Complete Psychological Works of Sigmund Freud, Vol 6. Translated and edited by Strachey J. London, Hogarth Press, 1960, pp 1–190

Freud S: Jokes and their relation to the unconscious (1905), in The Standard Edition of the Complete Psychological Works of Sigmund Freud, Vol 8. Translated and edited by Strachey J. London, Hogarth Press, 1960, pp 1–236

Freud S: Introductory lectures on psycho-analysis, part III: general theory of the neuroses (1917), in The Standard Edition of the Complete Psychological Works of Sigmund Freud, Vol 16. Translated and edited by Strachey J. London, Hogarth Press, 1963, pp 243–463

Freud S: Beyond the pleasure principle (1920), in The Standard Edition of the Complete Psychological Works of Sigmund Freud, Vol 18. Translated and edited by Strachey J. London, Hogarth Press, 1955, pp 1–64

Freud S: The ego and the id (1923), in The Standard Edition of the Complete Psychological Works of Sigmund Freud, Vol 19. Translated and edited by Strachey J. London, Hogarth Press, 1961, pp 1–59

Freud S: New introductory lectures on psycho-analysis (1933[1932]) (Lectures XXIX–XXXV), in The Standard Edition of the Complete Psychological Works of Sigmund Freud, Vol 22. Translated and edited by Strachey J. London, Hogarth Press, 1964, pp 1–182

Friedman L: An appreciation of Hans Loewald's "On the Therapeutic Action of Psychoanalysis." Panel presentation at the Association for Psychoanalytic Medicine, New York, NY, December 2, 1986

Friedman L: The clinical polarity of object relations concepts. Psychoanal Q 57:667–691, 1988

Gabbard GO, Gunderson JG, Fonagy P: The place of psychoanalytic treatments within psychiatry. Arch Gen Psychiatry 59:505–510, 2002

Gallese V, Keysers C, Rizzolatti G: A unifying view of the basis of social cognition. Trends Cogn Sci 8:396–403, 2004

Gergely G: Reapproaching Mahler: new perspectives on normal autism, normal symbiosis, splitting and libidinal object constancy from cognitive developmental theory. J Am Psychoanal Assoc 48:1197–1228, 2000

Gergely G, Watson J: The social biofeedback model of parental affect-mirroring. Int J Psychoanal 77:1181–1212, 1996

Goldstein M, Brendel G, Tuesche, O, et al: Neural substrates of the interaction of emotional stimulus processing and motor inhibitory control: an emotional linguistic go/no-go fMRI study. Neuroimage 36:1026–1040, 2007

Green A: Science and science fiction in infant research, in Clinical and Observational Psychoanalytic Research: Roots of a Controversy. Edited by Sandler J, Sandler AM, Davies R. London, Karnac Books, 2000, pp 41–73

Greenberg J: The analyst's participation: a new look. J Am Psychoanal Assoc 49:359–381, discussion: 381–426, 2001

Guthrie E, Moorey J, Margison F, et al: Cost-effectiveness of brief psychodynamic-interpersonal therapy in high utilizers of psychiatric services. Arch Gen Psychiatry 56:519–526, 1999

Hamilton CE: Continuity and discontinuity of attachment from infancy through adolescence. Child Dev 71:690–694, 2000

Hartmann H: Ego Psychology and the Problem of Adaptation (1939). New York, International Universities Press, 1958

Hartmann H, Kris E, Loewenstein R: Comments on the formation of psychic structure. Psychoanal Study Child 2:11–38, 1946

Hoffman IZ: Dialectic thinking and therapeutic action in the psychoanalytic process. Psychoanal Q 63:187–218, 1994

Hofstra MB, van der Ende J, Verhulst FC: Child and adolescent problems predict DSM-IV disorders in adulthood: a 14-year follow-up of a Dutch epidemiological sample. J Am Acad Child Adolesc Psychiatry 41:182–189, 2002

Horowitz MJ, Eells T, Singer J, et al: Role-relationship models for case formulation. Arch Gen Psychiatry 52:625–632, 1995

Jacob F: Of Flies, Mice and Men. Cambridge, MA, Harvard University Press, 1998

Jacobson E: The Self and the Object World. New York, International Universities Press, 1964

Jaffe J, Beebe B, Feldstein S, et al: Rhythms of dialogue in infancy: coordinated timing in development. Monogr Soc Res Child Dev 66(2):1–132, 2001

Jung CG: Psychological Types. London, Routledge & Kegan Paul, 1923

Kandel ER: A new intellectual framework for psychiatry. Am J Psychiatry 155:457–469, 1998

Kandel ER: Biology and the future of psychoanalysis: a new intellectual framework for psychiatry revisited. Am J Psychiatry 156:505–524, 1999

Kernberg OF: Borderline personality organization. J Am Psychoanal Assoc 15:641–685, 1967

Kernberg OF: Borderline Conditions and Pathological Narcissism. New York, Jason Aronson, 1975

Kernberg OF: Object Relations Theory and Clinical Psychoanalysis. New York, Jason Aronson, 1976

Kernberg OF: Self, ego, affects and drives. J Am Psychoanal Assoc 30:893–917, 1982

Kernberg OF: Severe Personality Disorders: Psychotherapeutic Strategies. New Haven, CT, Yale University Press, 1984

Kernberg OF, Selzer MA, Koenigsberg HW, et al: Psychodynamic Psychotherapy of Borderline Patients. New York, Basic Books, 1989

Kernberg O, Clarkin JF, Yeomans FE: A Primer of Transference Focused Psychotherapy for the Borderline Patient. New York, Jason Aronson, 2002

Kim-Cohen J, Caspi A, Moffitt TE, et al: Prior juvenile diagnoses in adults with mental disorder: developmental follow-back of a prospective longitudinal cohort. Arch Gen Psychiatry 60:709–717, 2003

King-Casas B, Tomlin D, Anen C, et al: Getting to know you: reputation and trust in a two-person economic exchange. Science 308:78–83, 2005

Klein M: A contribution to the psychogenesis of manic-depressive states (1935), in Love, Guilt and Reparation: The Writings of Melanie Klein, Vol 1. London, Hogarth Press, 1975, pp 236–289

Klein M: The psychotherapy of the psychoses (1936), in Contributions to Psychoanalysis, 1921–1945. New York, McGraw-Hill, 1964, pp 251–253

Klein M: Mourning and its relation to manic-depressive states (1940), in Love, Guilt and Reparation: The Writings of Melanie Klein, Vol 1. London, Hogarth Press, 1975, pp 344–369

Klein M: Notes on some schizoid mechanisms (1946), in Developments in Psychoanalysis. Edited by Klein M, Heimann P, Isaacs S, et al. London, Hogarth Press, 1952, pp 292–320

Klein M: Envy and gratitude (1957), in The Writings of Melanie Klein, Vol 3. London, Hogarth Press, 1975, pp 176–235

Klerman GL, Weissman MM, Rounsaville BJ, et al: Interpersonal Psychotherapy of Depression. New York, Basic Books, 1984

Kohut H: The Analysis of the Self. New York, International Universities Press, 1971

Kohut H: The Restoration of the Self. Madison, CT, International Universities Press, 1977

Kohut H: How Does Analysis Cure? Chicago, IL, University of Chicago Press, 1984

Kramer S, Akhtar S: The developmental context of internalized preoedipal object relations: clinical applications of Mahler's theory of symbiosis and separation-individuation. Psychoanal Q 57:547–576, 1988

Laor N, Wolmer L, Mayes LC, et al: Israeli preschoolers under Scud missile attacks: a developmental perspective on risk-modifying factors. Arch Gen Psychiatry 53:416–423, 1996

Laub JH: The interdependence of school violence with neighborhood and family conditions, in Violence in American Schools: A New Perspective. Edited by Elliot DS, Hamburg B, Williams KR. New York, Cambridge University Press, 1998, pp 127–155

Leichsenring F, Rabung S, Leibing E: The efficacy of short-term psychodynamic psychotherapy in specific psychiatric disorders: a meta-analysis. Arch Gen Psychiatry 61:1208–1216, 2004

Levy KN: The implications of attachment theory and research for understanding borderline personality disorder. Dev Psychopathol 17:959–986, 2005

Levy KN, Meehan KB, Kelly KM, et al: Change in attachment patterns and reflective function in a randomized control trial of transference-focused psychotherapy for borderline personality disorder. J Consult Clin Psychol 74:1027–1040, 2006

Livesley WJ, Jang KL, Vernon PA: Phenotypic and genetic structure of traits delineating personality disorder. Arch Gen Psychiatry 55:941–948, 1998

Loewald HW: On internalization, in Papers on Psychoanalysis. New Haven, CT, Yale University Press, 1973, pp 69–86

Loewald HW: Instinct theory, object relations and psychic structure formation. J Am Psychoanal Assoc 26:453–506, 1978

Mahler MS, Pine F, Bergman A: The Psychological Birth of the Human Infant: Symbiosis and Individuation. New York, Basic Books, 1975

Marcia JE: The empirical study of ego identity, in Identity and Development: An Interdisciplinary Approach. Edited by Bosma HA, Graafsma TLG, Grotevant HD, et al. Thousand Oaks, CA, Sage, 1994, pp 67–80

Marenco S, Weinberger DR: The neurodevelopmental hypothesis of schizophrenia: following a trail of evidence from cradle to grave. Dev Psychopathol 12:501–527, 2000

Masterson JF: The Real Self: A Developmental, Self, and Object Relations Approach. New York, Brunner/Mazel, 1985

McLaughlin J: Clinical and theoretical aspects of enactment. J Am Psychoanal Assoc 39:595–614, 1991

Meltzoff AN, Moore MK: Explaining facial imitation: theoretical model. Early Development and Parenting 6:179–192, 1997

Meltzoff AN, Moore MK: Infant intersubjectivity: broadening the dialogue to include imitation, identity and intention, in Intersubjective Communication and Emotion in Early Ontogeny. Edited by Braten S. Paris, Cambridge University Press, 1998, pp 47–62

Mikulincer M, Shaver PR: Attachment in Adulthood: Structure, Dynamics and Change. New York, Guilford, 2007

Mitchell SA: Relational Concepts in Psychoanalysis: An Integration. Cambridge, MA, Harvard University Press, 1988

Mitchell SA: Relationality: From Attachment to Intersubjectivity. Hillsdale, NJ, Analytic Press, 2000

Mufson L, Dorta KP, Wickramaratne P, et al: A randomized effectiveness trial of interpersonal psychotherapy for depressed adolescents. Arch Gen Psychiatry 61:577–584, 2004a

Mufson L, Gallagher T, Dorta KP, et al: A group adaptation of interpersonal psychotherapy for depressed adolescents. Am J Psychother 58:220–237, 2004b

O'Connor T: The persisting effects of early experiences on social development, in Developmental Psychopathology, 2nd Edition, Vol 3: Risk, Disorder and Adaptation. Edited by Cicchetti D, Cohen DJ. New York, Wiley, 2006, pp 202–234

Ogden T: The analytic third: working with intersubjective clinical facts. Int J Psychoanal 75:3–19, 1994

Orlofsky J: Intimacy status: theory and research, in Ego Identity: A Handbook for Psychosocial Research. Edited by Marcia JE, Waterman AS, Matteson DR, et al. New York, Springer-Verlag, 1993, pp 111–133

Panksepp J: Affective Neuroscience: The Foundations of Human and Animal Emotions. Oxford, UK, Oxford University Press, 1998

Peterfreund E: Information, Systems, and Psychoanalysis: An Evolutionary Biological Approach to Psychoanalytic Theory. New York, International Universities Press, 1971

Pine F: Developmental Theory and Clinical Process. New Haven, CT, Yale University Press, 1985

Rangell L: The borderline case. J Am Psychoanal Assoc 3:285–298, 1955

Reich W: Der triebhafte Charakter. Vienna, Internationaler Psychoanalytische Verlag, 1925

Reiss D, Neiderhiser J, Hetherington EM, et al: The Relationship Code: Deciphering Genetic and Social Influences on Adolescent Development. Cambridge, MA, Harvard University Press, 2000

Renik O: Analytic interaction: conceptualizing technique in the light of the analyst's irreducible subjectivity. Psychoanal Q 62:553–571, 1993

Rizzolatti G, Craighero L: The mirror-neuron system. Annu Rev Neurosci 27:169–192, 2004

Rosenblatt AD, Thickstun JT: Modern Psychoanalytic Concepts in a General Psychology. Part 1: General Concepts and Principles. Part 2: Motivation. Madison, CT, International Universities Press, 1977

Rosenfeld H: Impasse and Interpretation. London, Tavistock, 1987

Roth A, Fonagy P (eds): What Works for Whom? A Critical Review of Psychotherapy Research, 2nd Edition. New York, Guilford, 2005

Rothbart MK, Ahadi SA, Evans DE: Temperament and personality: origins and outcomes. J Pers Soc Psychol 78:122–135, 2000

Rothbaum F, Pott M, Azuma H, et al: The development of close relationships in Japan and the United States: paths of symbiotic harmony and generative tension. Child Dev 71:1121–1142, 2000

Rutter M, Silberg J, O'Connor T, et al: Genetics and child psychiatry, I: advances in quantitative and molecular genetics. J Child Psychol Psychiatry 40:3–18, 1999

Ryle A, Kerr IB: Introducing Cognitive Analytic Therapy: Principles and Practice. Chichester, UK, Wiley, 2002

Sandler J: The background of safety. Int J Psychoanal 41:191–198, 1960

Sandler J, Rosenblatt B: The concept of the representational world. Psychoanal Study Child 17:128–145, 1962

Sandler J, Sandler AM: The past unconscious, the present unconscious, and interpretation of the transference. Psychoanalytic Inquiry 4:367–399, 1984

Schore A: Affect Regulation and the Repair of the Self. New York, WW Norton, 2003

Seligman S: The developmental perspective in relational psychoanalysis. Contemporary Psychoanalysis 39:477–508, 2003

Shapiro DA, Rees A, Barkham M, et al: Effects of treatment duration and severity of depression on the maintenance of gains after cognitive-behavioral and psychodynamic-interpersonal psychotherapy. J Consult Clin Psychol 63:378–387, 1995

Shaw DS, Gilliom M, Ingoldsby EM, et al: Developmental trajectories of early conduct problems from ages 2 to 10. Paper presented in the Symposium on Developmental Trajectories in Antisocial Behavior From Infancy to Adolescence at the Biennial Meeting of the Society for Research in Child Development, Minneapolis, MN, April 19-22, 2001

Shea MT, Elkin I, Imber SD, et al: Course of depressive symptoms over follow-up: findings from the National Institute of Mental Health Treatment of Depression Collaborative Research Program. Arch Gen Psychiatry 49:782–787, 1992

Shengold L: Insight as metaphor. Psychoanal Study Child 36:289–306, 1981

Shevrin H: Psychoanalysis as the patient: high in feeling, low in energy. J Am Psychoanal Assoc 45:841–864, 1997

Solms M: Dreaming and REM sleep are controlled by different brain mechanisms. Behav Brain Sci 23:843–850, 904–1121 (discussion), 2000

Solms M, Turnbull O: The Brain and the Inner World: An Introduction to the Neuroscience of Subjective Experience. New York, Other Press, 2002

Spitz RA: A Genetic Field Theory of Ego Formation: Its Implications for Pathology. New York, International Universities Press, 1959

Stern DN: The Interpersonal World of the Infant: A View From Psychoanalysis and Developmental Psychology. New York, Basic Books, 1985

Stern DN, Sander LW, Nahum JP, et al: Non-interpretive mechanisms in psychoanalytic therapy: the 'something more' than interpretation. Int J Psychoanal 79(part 5):903–921, 1998

Sterzer P, Stadler C, Krebs A, et al: Abnormal neural responses to emotional visual stimuli in adolescents with conduct disorder. Biol Psychiatry 57:7–15, 2005

Sullivan HS: The Interpersonal Theory of Psychiatry. New York, WW Norton, 1953

Target M, Fonagy P: Playing with reality, II: the development of psychic reality from a theoretical perspective. Int J Psychoanal 77:459–479, 1996

Torgersen S: Genetics of patients with borderline personality disorder. Psychiatr Clin North Am 23:1–9, 2000

Torgersen S, Lygren S, Oien PA, et al: A twin study of personality disorders. Compr Psychiatry 41:416–425, 2000

Tremblay RE: The origins of youth violence. ISUMA Canadian Journal of Policy Research 1(2, Autumn):19–24, 2000

Tremblay RE, Japel C, Perusse D: The search for the age of onset of physical aggression: Rousseau and Bandura revisited. Crim Behav Ment Health 9:8–23, 1999

Tronick E: The Neurobehavioral and Social-Emotional Development of Infants and Children. New York, WW Norton, 2007

Waters E, Merrick SK, Treboux D, et al: Attachment security from infancy to early adulthood: a 20 year longitudinal study. Child Dev 71:684–689, 2000

Watson JS: Contingency perception and misperception in infancy: some potential implications for attachment. Bull Menninger Clin 65:296–320, 2001

Westen D: The scientific legacy of Sigmund Freud: toward a psychodynamically informed psychological science. Psychol Bull 124:333–371, 1998

Westen D, Gabbard GO: Developments in cognitive neuroscience, I: conflict, compromise, and connectionism. J Am Psychoanal Assoc 50:53–98, 2002

Willick MS: Psychoanalysis and schizophrenia: a cautionary tale. J Am Psychoanal Assoc 49:27–56, 2001

Winnicott DW: Transitional objects and transitional phenomena. Int J Psychoanal 34:1–9, 1953

Winnicott DW: Ego distortion in terms of true and false self (1960), in The Maturational Processes and the Facilitating Environment. New York, International Universities Press, 1965, pp 140–152

Winnicott DW: Mirror-role of the mother and family in child development, in The Predicament of the Family: A Psycho-Analytical Symposium. Edited by Lomas P. London, Hogarth Press, 1967, pp 26–33

Suggested Readings

Bateman AW, Holmes J: Introduction to Psychoanalysis: Contemporary Theory and Practice. London, Routledge & Kegan Paul, 1995

Budd S, Rusbridger R (eds): Introducing Psychoanalysis: Essential Themes and Topics. London, Routledge & Kegan Paul, 2005

Cooper AM (ed): Contemporary Psychoanalysis in America. Washington, DC, American Psychiatric Publishing, 2006

Fonagy P, Target M: Psychoanalytic Theories: Perspectives From Developmental Psychopathology. London, Whurr, 2003

Gabbard GO: Psychodynamic Psychiatry in Clinical Practice, 4th Edition. Washington, DC, American Psychiatric Publishing, 2005

Gabbard GO, Gunderson JG, Fonagy P: The place of psychoanalytic treatments within psychiatry. Arch Gen Psychiatry 59:505–510, 2002

Holmes J, Bateman A: Integration in Psychotherapy: Models and Methods. Oxford, UK, Oxford University Press, 2002

Person ES, Cooper AM, Gabbard GO (eds): The American Psychiatric Publishing Textbook of Psychoanalysis. Washington, DC, American Psychiatric Publishing, 2005

Chapter 2

Techniques of Psychodynamic Psychotherapy

Glen O. Gabbard, M.D.

Psychodynamic psychotherapy has been characterized by a variety of labels over the years: *psychoanalytic psychotherapy, intensive psychotherapy, insight-oriented psychotherapy, expressive-supportive psychotherapy,* and *exploratory psychotherapy,* to name a few. They are all essentially synonymous. This modality derives from the principles of psychoanalysis. Whereas psychoanalysis is generally conducted at a frequency of three to five times per week, with the patient supine on a couch, psychoanalytic psychotherapy is more typically provided once or twice per week, with the patient sitting up.

Dynamic psychotherapy can be long-term and open-ended or short-term with a set number of sessions. Generally, we define *long-term psychodynamic psychotherapy* as lasting more than 24 sessions or longer than 6 months. *Short-term psychodynamic psychotherapy* entails all therapies of fewer than 24 sessions or less than 6 months. A useful definition of *psychodynamic psychotherapy* is "a therapy that involves careful attention to the therapist-patient interaction, with carefully timed interpretation of transference and resistance embedded in a sophisticated appreciation of the therapist's contribution to the two-person field." (Gunderson and Gabbard 1999, p. 685).

In Chapter 1 ("Theoretical Models of Psychodynamic Psychotherapy"), Fonagy and Target comprehensively lay out the various theoretical models subsumed under psychodynamic therapies. Each model emphasizes different aspects of techniques that follow logically from the theoretical assumptions. Although I will note those emphases in passing as I present the fundamentals of technique in psychodynamic psychotherapy, my primary goal is to provide an introduction to common elements in psychodynamic technique, regardless of one's preferred theoretical model. These include the therapeutic alliance, specific types of interventions, transference, countertransference, resistance, working-through, and termination.

Before discussing these technical principles, however, I first provide an overview of how one assesses the patient's suitability for dynamic therapy, how one formulates the biopsychosocial understanding of the patient, and how one collaborates with the patient on the establishment of treatment goals.

Assessment

In Chapter 4 ("Applications of Psychodynamic Psychotherapy to Specific Disorders: Efficacy and Indications"), Leichsenring reviews the data from outcomes studies of dynamic therapy and formulates indications for this modality. A core feature of psychodynamic thinking is that one must go beyond the DSM-IV diagnosis (American Psychiatric Association 1994) in assessing whether the patient is suitable for exploratory therapy. The patient's personality characteristics, defense mechanisms, motivation, and other capacities must be carefully evaluated before reaching a conclusion about whether dynamic therapy is the optimal treatment. Several factors that go into this assessment are summarized in Table 2–1.

Above all, patients suited to psychodynamic therapy must be curious about themselves. They must be motivated to understand unconscious patterns in their lives that lead to suffering. They must be willing to work with the therapist collaboratively to figure out why they do things that are self-defeating or why they hurt others they don't wish to hurt. These qualities are often referred to as *psychological-mindedness*—in other words, these patients can see the internal origins of their difficulties rather than seeing themselves as simply a leaf buffeted in the wind without a sense of agency.

Defense Mechanisms

In the classic model of ego psychology, defense mechanisms prevent a person from becoming aware of sexual or aggressive wishes or the anxiety that

---

TABLE 2–1. Elements of assessment for psychodynamic psychotherapy

---

DSM-IV diagnoses[a]

Capacity and motivation to actively collaborate with the therapist in pursuit of understanding

Typical defense mechanisms

Mentalizing capacity

Quality of object relations

Ego strengths and weaknesses

Presence of intrapsychic conflicts

Developmental deficits

---

[a]American Psychiatric Association 1994, 2000.

is connected with them. In addition, defenses preserve self-esteem in the face of shame and narcissistic vulnerability and externalize internal threats onto others. Defenses are also embedded in relatedness in that they make relationships more manageable by providing an illusion of control over what happens in an interaction with significant people in the patient's life.

Defense mechanisms are generally divided into those that are primitive or immature and those that are higher level or neurotic. Table 2–2 provides some of the common defenses in these two categories. The lists in Table 2–2 are by no means exhaustive. Moreover, everyone uses primitive defenses, such as denial and splitting, when under stress. There are also mature defenses that are not generally regarded as pathological. These include sublimation, anticipation, humor, suppression, and altruism.

Assessment of the defense mechanisms in Table 2–2 guides the psychodynamic clinician regarding how much support the patient needs versus how much insight the patient can tolerate. Thus, dynamic psychotherapy is practiced with an expressive-supportive continuum in mind (Gabbard 2004, 2005; see Figure 2–1 later in this chapter). The therapist recognizes that there must be a balance of interpretive and supportive comments with most patients, and part of the purpose of a careful assessment is to determine the extent to which the emphasis should be in one direction or the other.

Mentalizing Capacity

As Fonagy and Target stressed in Chapter 1, the capacity for mentalizing grows out of attachment theory and refers to a person's ability to conceive

TABLE 2–2. Primitive and higher-level defense mechanisms

Primitive defenses

Splitting	Compartmentalizing internal representations of self and others so that conflict is avoided and integration is not possible
Projective identification	A defense involving subtle interpersonal pressure so that the target of a projection takes on characteristics of an aspect of the self or the internal object that is being projected
Projection	Externalizing unacceptable inner impulses and their derivatives by attributing them to someone else
Denial	Avoiding awareness of aspects of external realities that are difficult to face by dismissing perceptions that are obvious to everyone in the environment
Schizoid fantasy	Retreating into one's private, internal world to avoid anxiety about interpersonal situations

Higher-level defenses

Displacement	Shifting feelings associated with one idea or object to another that resembles the original in some way
Intellectualization	Using excessive and abstract ideation to avoid difficult feelings
Isolation of affect	Separating an idea from its associated affect states to avoid emotional turmoil
Sexualization	Endowing an object or behavior with sexual significance to turn a negative experience into an exciting and stimulating one
Reaction formation	Transforming an unacceptable wish or impulse into its opposite
Repression	Expelling unacceptable ideas or impulses, thus blocking them from entering consciousness (repression is more closely linked with inner states, whereas denial involves external sensory data)

of his or her own and others' mental states as explanations of behavior. Hence, it too is related to psychological-mindedness. The psychodynamic clinician assesses the ability of a patient to see that his or her behavior grows out of a set of beliefs, feelings, and perspectives that are not necessarily the same as others'. Like empathy, mentalizing requires a capacity to sense what is going on in another's mind and respond accordingly. This capacity to be sensitive to what others are feeling and to know that one's internal states contribute to one's behavior augurs well for a more exploratory or interpretative approach in dynamic psychotherapy.

Object Relations

The cornerstone of dynamic therapy is observing how patterns of relationships in a patient's life recur in the relationship with the therapist. Patients who do not have meaningful outside relationships may be more difficult to treat with a psychodynamic approach. Patients who have more chaotic relationships may also present challenges to the therapist, who seeks to have the patient reflect on the details of difficulties in encounters with intimacy rather than simply react with action. Nevertheless, some data suggest that interpretations of the recurrence of these patterns in patients who have disturbed interpersonal relationships may result in significant improvement (Gabbard 2006; Høglend et al. 2006).

Ego Strengths and Weaknesses

The ego is the executive organ of the psyche and is involved in a host of regulatory functions. Someone with high ego strengths tends to have good control of impulses and the capacity to tolerate intense affects such as anxiety, anger, or grief. Other ego strengths involve the capacity to anticipate consequences of one's actions (judgment) and to sustain activity such as work or school despite setbacks and adversities. Patients with these ego capacities are likely to be able to tolerate the frustration and anxiety brought about by exploration of the darkest corners of the psyche that have long been avoided or defended against. By contrast, those with ego weaknesses, such as impulsivity, impaired judgment, difficulties testing reality, and poor tolerance of affect states, will be less likely to endure the stresses of psychotherapy and may even drop out soon after beginning.

Intrapsychic Conflict and Developmental Deficits

In classic psychoanalytic ego psychology, intrapsychic conflict involves a wish or an impulse opposed by a defense. The id may seek pleasure, whereas the superego prohibits the impulse to enjoy oneself. In object relations theory, conflict may involve the disparate wishes or urges of different representations of the self and other. Whatever theoretical model one uses, internal conflict is a source of a great deal of suffering and often causes one to seek psychodynamic therapy. The conflict is often unconscious and appears as a symptom such as inhibition of love or work relationships.

Developmental deficits may occur through early experiences of abuse, neglect, or parental failure to respond empathically to the child's needs. Self psychology is a deficit model theory that, for example, postulates the absence of mirroring responses from the child's parents or caregiver (see Chapter 1). In the terms of the British object relations theory, the self is intruded on by the mother, resulting in the creation of a false self to protect the true self (Winnicott 1965). Patients who have greater degrees of deficit may require more support to be able to tolerate insight, whereas those whose problems have a greater emphasis on intrapsychic conflict may respond more readily to interpretation and insight. The majority of patients have varying degrees of conflict and deficit that are joined in unique and idiosyncratic ways based on the patient's background, genetic vulnerabilities, and resilience.

Biopsychosocial Formulation

Formulating an understanding of the patient who is beginning psychodynamic psychotherapy provides an initial road map that may be rewritten as the journey progresses. The formulation must involve an understanding of the relative contributions of biology, psychological factors, and sociocultural influences. Psychodynamic therapy cannot occur in a vacuum that emphasizes only the intrapsychic while ignoring such factors as genetic contributions, traumatic brain injury, religious background, and specific cultural beliefs. Most therapists will write a brief formulation or at least have an internal understanding in mind as the therapy begins.

Biopsychosocial formulation generally involves three central components (Gabbard 2004; Kassaw and Gabbard 2002; Sperry et al. 1992): 1) a brief description of the nature of the clinical picture and the stressors that brought the patient to treatment; 2) an attempt to integrate the biological, intrapsychic, and sociocultural factors in terms of their relative contributions to the presenting problems; and 3) a succinct statement about how the contributing factors will inform the treatment and the prognosis. Hence, if one feels that an abusive father is a powerful internal representation, represented as a harsh superego, one might predict that the patient might see a male therapist in that light when the psychotherapy deepens. This perception, conscious or unconscious, may make it difficult for the patient to open up fully.

Goals

Patient and therapist need to work together at the outset to form mutually agreed-on goals that are realistic. A patient may come to a therapist with a goal of getting married and having a baby. A therapist cannot realistically promise that psychotherapy can achieve that goal. The therapist might need to reframe the goal as understanding internal and interpersonal conflicts that might interfere with the patient's achievement of meaningful mutual relationships and the exploration of inhibitions that might be involved in wanting to become a parent. Sometimes goals need to be discussed at some length before therapist and patient can agree on where the therapy is headed. Moreover, therapy often takes unexpected detours and circuitous routes that require the modification and rethinking of therapeutic goals.

Goals may be heavily influenced by the theoretical orientation of a dynamic psychotherapist. Table 2–3 lists a number of goals from the psychoanalytic and psychodynamic literature that reflect the varying theoretical models of psychopathology and therapeutic change.

Resolution of conflict derives from ego psychology and the structural model. By exploring impulses, wishes, and defenses against these impulses and wishes, patients may ultimately master conflicts (but not completely eliminate them). The search for authenticity and the truth about oneself may be central to dynamic therapy, reflecting the work of Winnicott (1962), who spoke of the distinction between the true self and the false self that was adopted to please parental figures during childhood. Self psychology seeks to help the patient function with more appropriate selfobjects that validate the needs of his or her self. Most therapies try to improve relationships. Object relations theory would explicitly argue that those aspects of the self or object representations that are projected onto others must be "re-owned" so that the patient feels a more integrated sense of self and a more satisfying sense of re-

---

TABLE 2–3.   Goals of psychodynamic psychotherapy

Resolution of intrapsychic conflict

A search for truth about oneself

An improved capacity to seek out appropriate selfobjects

Improved relationships as a result of gains in understanding about one's internal object relationships

Generation of meaning in one's life as a result of therapeutic dialogue

Improved mentalizing capacity

Source.   Gabbard 2004.

latedness with others. Meaning is also a goal of many therapies, but some models, such as relational theory (Mitchell 1997), suggest that the therapeutic dialogue is specifically designed to discover unconscious meanings and create new meanings through the conversation of patient and therapist. Finally, enhancement of mentalizing capacity is a central goal for those therapies influenced by attachment theory. One is able to achieve a greater sense of intersubjectivity rather than assuming that one's one way of thinking is endorsed by everyone (Fonagy and Target 2000).

An ever-present peril in all psychotherapies is the imposition of the therapist's goals on the patient. A central tenet of psychodynamic therapy is that therapists must respect the patient's autonomy rather than control how the patient behaves, thinks, and feels. When differences occur, a patient's goals generally trump the therapist's goals, provided the former are reasonable. Too much emphasis on goals may also lead a patient to become oppositional. Many patients need a period without goals to explore themselves in the course of psychotherapy.

The cataloguing of goals in Table 2–3 reflects another feature of psychodynamic psychotherapy technique: it is less geared to removal of symptoms than are other modalities, such as exposure and response prevention, which derive from behavior theory. Although symptoms may be seen as an important target, the broader goal is to achieve fundamental characterological change and change the vulnerabilities inherent in the patient's character or personality. For example, a psychodynamic therapist who treats someone with chronic or recurring depression may emphasize the types of stressors and the reactions to those stressors that constitute a recurrent theme in the patient's susceptibility to depression. Does depression generally follow a breakup in a relationship in which the patient feels diminished by the negative view of a romantic partner? Is there an ongoing perfectionistic expectation of the self that is repeatedly contributing to disappointment? In other words, does the patient always fall short of the expectation of achieving something that is forever out of reach?

This focus on vulnerability has become essential in contemporary discourse about recurrent depression (Ingram and Price 2002). Psychodynamic therapists often refer to "structural change" when they modify inherent vulnerability or conflicts between intrapsychic agencies so that the patient's functioning and subjective experience both globally improve.

The Therapeutic Alliance

The *therapeutic alliance* is the envelope within which dynamic therapy takes place. Good therapists must attend to the therapeutic alliance from early in the treatment to ensure that the therapy is viable. Research repeatedly demonstrates that the role of the therapeutic relationship is more important than any specific technique in producing positive therapeutic outcomes (Butler and Strupp 1986; Horvath 2005; Krupnick et al. 1996; Zuroff and Blatt 2006).

The therapeutic alliance is variously defined, but components commonly linked to a good therapeutic alliance are the following: the patient feels attached to the therapist; the patient feels that the therapist is helpful; and the patient and therapist feel a sense of mutual collaboration in pursuing common therapeutic goals (Hilsenroth and Cromer 2007; Horwitz et al. 1996; Luborsky 1984; Luborsky and Luborsky 2006).

Few dynamic psychotherapy concepts have been more rigorously studied than the therapeutic alliance. An extensive body of research suggests that a strong therapeutic alliance is positively correlated with a good outcome, that the patient's assessments tend to be more predictive of outcome than the assessments by others, and that the early alliance in therapy is a predictor of outcome that is as good as or better than assessments taken later (Horvath 2005; Martin et al. 2000). This research indicates that the therapeutic alliance is formed early in treatment, even as early as the first session, and predicts later outcome. Some research provides guidelines regarding what the clinician can do in the first few sessions to enhance the therapeutic alliance (Hilsenroth and Cromer 2007). First, therapists must listen sensitively and convey trust, warmth, and understanding. Exploring the in-session process and the patient's affect in a nonjudgmental manner also improves the alliance, as does speaking with both emotional and cognitive content. Finally, therapists who identify new clinical issues to foster deeper levels of understanding and insight may enhance the alliance.

The basic strategy of dynamic psychotherapy, once it is launched, is to pay careful attention to ruptures that occur in the alliance. Ruptures are usually defined as some kind of breakdown or strain in the collaborative process between therapist and patient, a deterioration in communication between the two, or a general deterioration in the quality of the relationship (Safran and Muran 1996, 2006). Ruptures may involve the withdrawal of the patient from the therapeutic dialogue or an angry or accusatory statement about the therapy or the therapist. It is essential for therapists to identify these ruptures and fully explore them, lest the patient leave without elaborating on the reasons for the rupture. Therapists who can acknowledge their own contribution to the rupture, rather than blaming it on the patient, tend to be more successful in repairing the damage to the alliance. Ruptures in the alliance often provide a glimpse of underlying concerns about the therapy that have been concealed throughout most of the sessions. Hence, they are a valuable opportunity to address potentially disruptive factors in the therapy.

Therapeutic Interventions

Cinematic stereotypes of psychoanalysis and psychodynamic therapy often portray the therapist as an aloof, silent, and cold figure whose facial expressions never change. The contemporary dynamic therapist is warm, empathic, and spontaneous; the "blank screen" therapist belongs to an earlier era. We now know from studies in nonverbal communication that it is impossible to entirely conceal one's feelings, and probably not helpful even if one could do so. A psychodynamic therapist focuses on the patient, so self-disclosure is kept to a minimum unless saying something about here-and-now feelings or an area of common interest is likely to enhance the therapy. In any case, the therapeutic atmosphere should be one of a spontaneous conversation in which the patient feels understood and helped. Terms such as *neutrality* in describing the therapist's attitude are often misunderstood as cold aloofness. A better understanding of the term would be conveyed by saying that the therapist assumes a nonjudgmental attitude of listening to the patient's concerns.

Although the therapeutic dialogue should have a spontaneous quality to it, it is useful to have in mind a continuum of interventions that are designed to promote therapeutic change. These categories will not encompass all of the therapist's comments, but they serve as useful guideposts to help the therapist tailor the technique to the patient. As noted previously, dynamic psychotherapy usually takes place along an expressive-supportive continuum. Interventions can be conceptualized as residing on that continuum, as shown in Figure 2–1.

Interpretation

The term *expressive* is used synonymously with *exploratory* or *interpretive*. Hence, at the left end of the continuum is *interpretation*, the most expressive or insight-producing comment in the therapeutic armamentarium. The intent is to make patients aware of things that are currently outside of their awareness. Interpretations may bring to consciousness something that was previously unconscious, or they may explain a linkage that was outside of the patient's awareness in a way that produces insight. An example of an interpretation is the following:

> **Therapist:** You seem to hold yourself back from succeeding because you worry that your mother will be envious and retaliate against you.

As this example illustrates, interpretation usually involves explaining something to the patient. An interpretation is more likely to be received with an open mind if presented to the patient in a tentative way, as a possibility rather than as a definitive statement from an oracular source of knowledge.

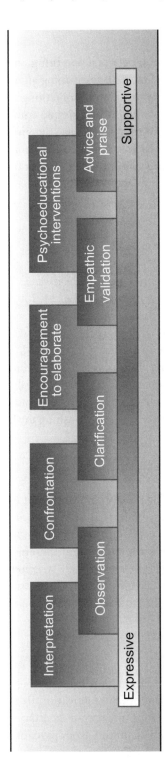

FIGURE 2–1. An expressive-supportive continuum of interventions.

Source. Reprinted from Gabbard GO: *Long-Term Psychodynamic Psychotherapy: A Basic Text.* Washington, DC, American Psychiatric Publishing, 2004, p. 63. Copyright 2004, American Psychiatric Publishing. Used with permission.

Observation

Interpretation, by definition, explains a link between one thing and another. Observation stops short of making a linkage or explaining an underlying motivation. Hence it calls the patient's attention to something that is outside of his or her awareness. An example might be a simple comment such as, "Have you noticed that you almost always yawn as you enter the office and greet me?" Observations frequently focus on nonverbal communications or unconscious enactments that are visible to the therapist but for which the patient has blind spots.

Confrontation

Whereas observations target behavior that is outside of the patient's conscious awareness, confrontation generally points out something that is being avoided but that is within the conscious awareness of the patient. A narcissistic patient came to a psychotherapy session on September 11, 2001, and made no reference to the terrorist attacks on the World Trade Center and the Pentagon that had occurred several hours earlier. As the patient went on and on about how his girlfriend had mistreated him, the therapist said, "I notice that you have not mentioned the terrorist attacks today." The avoidance of that topic led to a productive exploration of how the patient wished to deny the impact of the event on him because it terrified him. Confrontation may also involve the placing of limits for patients who are pushing the limits of the treatment setting.

Clarification

Much of the therapist's activity involves clarifying what the patient is getting at. Patients may be vague or uncertain about what they are feeling or thinking, and therapists often try to summarize or repackage what the patient is saying in a way that clarifies it for both patient and therapist: "It sounds like what you're really saying is that you can't decide whether you really want to stay in this relationship or leave it." Often the therapist's voice has a questioning tone: "Do I understand correctly that you really didn't see your father from the age of 6 to 8?"

Encouragement to Elaborate

In the middle of the continuum is the intervention known as *encouragement to elaborate*. Perhaps the most common form of communication from the therapist, this intervention is designed to elicit further commentary from the patient. The principle of free association stemming from psychoanalysis is applied to dynamic therapy as well. Therapists do whatever they can to stimulate the patient's uncensored, open reporting of whatever comes to mind. Hence, a frequent intervention is, "I'd like to hear more about that." Sometimes the patient is stopped at a moment when the therapist feels more needs to be said: "I'm sure you must have other feelings about it than those you have told me so far. Could you say a little more?" Generally, this kind of intervention is open-ended, but it may also be directed at something specific: "I'd like to hear more about your mother's father. I don't know much about him."

Empathic Validation

While self psychology regards empathy as central to technique, therapists of all persuasions must be alert to patients' need for empathic validation. Often patients have had their internal experiences invalidated or denied by parents as they grew up, leading to a need to present a façade or a false self to the family. Therapists can be particularly helpful when they validate that the patient has a right to certain feelings and that the patient's response is legitimate in light of what has happened to the patient. An empathically validating comment could be, "It is completely understandable to me that you would be angry at your father after he said that to you." Such interventions can also be applied to the here-and-now situation: "You have every reason to be mistrustful of me, given what you've experienced from authority figures in the past."

Psychoeducational Intervention

Near the supportive end of the continuum, psychotherapy becomes more akin to teaching. Dynamic psychotherapy always has an educational aspect because patients learn about themselves in the process of trying to express the nature of their problems. Sometimes patients require specific forms of education about the nature of their illness, the goals of psychotherapy, or the limits of psychotherapy. One patient needed to be told, "I really can't accept your donation to my research because it would be unethical for me to take advantage of our therapeutic relationship by soliciting donations from you." Another dynamic therapist said to a patient with anxiety, "Most of the research on anxiety indicates that there are probably both a genetic component and contributions based on adverse environmental experiences."

Advice and Praise

The most supportive interventions in dynamic psychotherapy are those that directly praise the patient for specific behaviors or comments, or offer advice to the patient on a particular course of action. Patients who are in a state of crisis may need specific advice such as, "You must go to a women's shelter rather than risk your life by staying with your husband." This intervention was needed after a woman who was beaten by her husband had a gun pointed at her. Praise can facilitate the therapeutic alliance and can help the patient feel that he or she is participating in therapy effectively. A typical comment involving praise is, "I think you've come up with a very important insight there that I hadn't thought about before." Praise often involves a therapist's statement of positive regard for the patient: "I'm proud of you for having the courage to speak directly to your mother about this problem instead of concealing it."

Transference

As the definition at the beginning of this chapter reveals, the focus on transference is a hallmark of psychodynamic psychotherapy. A simple definition of *transference* is the displacement of feelings and thoughts associated with a figure in the patient's past onto the therapist. Transference is often unconscious, at least initially, and the patient is bewildered by behavior toward the therapist because it does not make sense, based on who the therapist really is. A patient may say, "I have no idea why I forgot to come today. I'm not aware of any negative feelings about you." Hence the enactment of missing a session or of coming late to a session may reveal unconscious transference. Whereas the original definition assumed that a kind of template in the unconscious was taken from the patient's mind and superimposed on the therapist without much alteration, today the prevailing view is that the therapist's actual behavior is always influencing the patient's experience of the therapist (Hoffman 1998). Hence the transference to the therapist is partly based on real characteristics and partly on figures from the patient's past—a combination of old and new relationships.

Beginning therapists can err on the side of calling too much attention to the transference too soon. As a general principle, one should postpone the interpretation of transference until it becomes a resistance and until it is close to the patient's awareness (Gabbard 2004). In other words, if things are going reasonably well, it makes no sense to interpret transference. If the patient develops, for example, erotized or highly negative feelings, which impede the process of the therapy, interpretation may be essential. Many therapists regard treatment that focuses on transference as more exploratory than therapy geared to extratransference relationships. In supportive therapy, interpretation of the transference may be minimized, although the therapist may silently interpret the transference as a way of increasing his or her understanding of the patient.

The following vignette illustrates the evolution of transference in one therapy session, and its management by the therapist:

Patient: I need to tell you what happened in my conversation with Mom last night. She tries to control everything I do. You've heard of the book *My Mother/My Self*? Well, with her, it's *My Daughter/My Self*. She wants me to be a clone of her, and I can't stand her control.

Therapist *(also female):* What exactly happened last night?

Patient: She said she wanted to take me to dinner, so I went. Then, when I tried to order, I just about lost it. She insisted that I get the special, which was what she was ordering. She told me that she specifically took me to the restaurant so I would try a particular dish. I've told her a hundred times that I'm trying to get red meat out of my diet, and the special was some kind of beef bourguignonne that I simply did not want to eat. So we had an argument right there in front of the people at the next table, who were listening in.

Therapist: I know that you are exasperated right now but, as I've told you before, part of you unconsciously sets up that situation because you get something out of the conflict with your mother. I think you could have written last night's scenario before you went to the restaurant.

Patient: Why would I want to interact with my mother in such an annoying and argumentative way?

Therapist: I don't think we fully understand that yet.

Patient: We don't understand it because it's not true. There's nothing whatsoever appealing about that type of interaction.

Therapist: I think we go through the same type of "dance" here. It's very hard for you to accept what I say because you imagine I'm like your mother, believing that I insist that you think just like I do.

In this vignette, the patient begins to recreate the relationship with her mother in the therapeutic setting. Dynamic therapists assume that patients will reestablish their family situation in therapy, just as they do in intimate relationships outside of therapy. One way that the therapist helps is by *interpreting transference*, a process designed to illustrate to the patient that what happens in the therapeutic relationship is similar to what happens *outside* of therapy. Many patients feel shamed or "caught" when the therapist interprets this type of repetition, so the therapist must be judicious in using transference interpretations.

Transference has many manifestations. Dreams may reveal feelings toward the therapist that otherwise do not enter into the process. Patients may talk about another doctor or professional in highly emotional terms as a way of displacing transference feelings elsewhere. Patients who have concealed erotic feelings toward their therapist may engage in an intense erotic relationship with someone who resembles the therapist.

Transferences also may vary in the course of psychotherapy. In contemporary psychoanalytic and psychodynamic discourse, it is generally recognized that there are multiple transferences—stemming from parents, siblings, and other figures—and not simply one specific transference. Moreover, some patients do not work well within the transference and do not feel intense feelings toward the therapist—a situation known as *resistance to the awareness of transference*—so the therapist will need to work interpretively on outside relationships until the patient feels comfortable enough to bring material into the therapeutic relationship. Other patients go through an entire psychotherapy and benefit greatly without a focus on the transference. Hence one must adapt the types of interventions and the degree of transference work to the specific patient.

Countertransference

The original use of *countertransference*, as described by Freud (1910), was the analyst's transference to the patient. In other words, the patient might remind the therapist of someone from the therapist's past, so that the therapist starts to treat the patient as though he or she *were* that figure. Over time, this view of countertransference was broadened to include the total emotional reaction of the therapist to the patient. Today it is recognized that countertransference is jointly created—it partly involves the therapist's past relationships, but it also involves feelings induced in the therapist by the patient's behavior. The part of the countertransference induced by the patient is generally referred to as *projective identification*. This process involves two steps: 1) a self or object representation within the patient is projectively disavowed by its unconsciously being placed onto someone else, and 2) the projector exerts internal pressure that nudges the other person to experience or unconsciously identify with whatever has been projected. One could say that step 1 is a type of transference, whereas step 2 is a countertransference reaction. In a psychotherapeutic context, a third step occurs: 3) the recipient of the projection, the therapist, contains and tolerates the affective state and the projection of the self or object representation associated with the affect until the patient can take them back and "own" what has been projected. In this manner, projective identification can be regarded as both an interpersonal communication and an intrapsychic defensive operation.

Projective identification often feels obligatory. Therapists may feel that an alien force is taking them over, and feel that they cannot avoid enacting the role that the patient has thrust on them. This state of affairs can be therapeutically useful, however, because the therapist is experiencing something that others in the patient's life experience.

Some therapists may use the countertransference as a step on the road to interpreting something useful to the patient. For example, the therapist might say, "I notice myself feeling a bit frustrated because I keep asking you questions to try to find out what you are thinking or feeling, but you tell me very little. This sounds like what goes on with your husband at home quite frequently." Pointing out the interpersonal process, the therapist can help the patient reflect on how he or she takes an active role in creating a situation that may be unpleasant or difficult in relationships outside of therapy.

The therapist is using self-disclosure of countertransference to promote therapeutic gains in the patient. This type of self-disclosure must be used judiciously, because disclosure of some countertransference feelings may be harmful to the process. For example, it is rarely useful to say, "I hate you," to the patient or "I feel bored by what you are telling me." The patient has no obligation to entertain the therapist, and the revelation of such feelings to the patient may inflict a severe wound that leaves the patient unable to trust the therapist. The revealing of sexual feelings toward the patient is rarely useful. The patient may feel that the therapeutic setting is no longer a safe place if the therapist begins to express sexual desire toward him or her.

Positive countertransference feelings can be present without the therapist knowing it. Positive regard toward the patient may be seen as simply a caring posture that facilitates the therapy. However, countertransference blind spots can grow out of positive feelings. Therapists may be reluctant to confront the patient about aggression or other problems if they do not want to "rock the boat" and cause the patient to have negative feelings toward them. Similarly, a need to rescue the patient may keep the patient from developing his or her own resources for problem solving.

Resistance

The identification and management of *resistance* is also fundamental to the technique of psychodynamic psychotherapy. Dynamic therapists recognize that patients are ambivalent about changing. They unconsciously oppose the therapist's efforts to offer insight and therapeutic change. Defense mechanisms that defend against uncomfortable feelings are activated by the therapy as resistances.

Resistance is not necessarily spoken. It may take the form of a conscious admission of not wishing to go where the therapist wants the patient to go, but it may also appear as a failure to show up on time, a tendency to forget sessions, lapses into silence for no apparent reason, or a preference for discussing matters that appear to be quite irrelevant to the therapeutic goals. However, dynamic therapists know that the way the patient resists is a revelation of something important about the patient—often a highly significant internal object relationship from the patient's past, transported into the present moment with the therapist (Friedman 1991).

In this regard, many resistances are *transference resistances*. The patient may be opposing the therapist's efforts because of unconscious feelings or thoughts about the therapist, based on figures from the patient's past. Patients may feel that the therapist may shame them if they open up, or criticize them for their shortcomings. A good psychodynamic therapist, though, does not directly confront the resistance and try to get the patient to "knock it off." Rather, the therapist attempts to understand why the patient is resisting and encourages the patient to develop a reflectiveness about what is being resisted and why.

When patients say that they cannot think of anything else to talk about or that they cannot reveal certain things about themselves, psychodynamic therapists generally do not directly pursue what is being withheld. Instead, they seek to examine the resistance before the content. Instead of saying, "Tell me what you're withholding," they might say, "Do you have any idea what you're worried about if you were to reveal this to me?" They might also ask, "How do you imagine I'd react if you were to reveal what you're concealing?"

Another form of resistance is acting out rather than talking. Patients often repeat in action what they cannot remember (Freud 1914), and therapists study their nonverbal enactments carefully to understand their meaning.

In self psychology, resistances are regarded in a more positive way, as a way of safeguarding the self. Therapists of this persuasion suggest that it is best to empathize and respect the patient's need for defenses rather than to challenge the patient with his or her defensiveness. Most therapists generally agree with this position, given that confronting resistances head on rarely causes them to fade away.

Most defenses are embedded in character, so characterological resistances are present in many patients. For example, a patient with obsessive-compulsive personality disorder who uses isolation of affect, reaction formation, and intellectualization as characteristic defenses will resist the therapy by intellectualizing and conveying the opposite of what he or she feels. Working on these resistances embedded in the personality is the bread and butter of psychodynamic work. Systematically analyzing these resistances may open a window into the characteristic patterns of relatedness and the underlying anxieties that activate the defenses.

Working Through and Therapeutic Strategies

Working-through in many ways is the heart of psychodynamic psychotherapy. Characteristic patterns of defenses and internal object relations emerge again and again in different contexts, and are repetitively clarified, confronted, observed, and interpreted. By pointing out repetitive patterns that occur in the transference and in outside relationships, as well as their derivation in childhood relationships, the therapist ultimately helps the patient begin to see his or her own responsibility for creating situations in his or her life. Hence one of the outcomes of working-through is an enhanced sense of agency whereby patients start to feel like authors of their own life experiences. Much of working-through involves systematic analysis of the patient's conscious and unconscious fantasies as they emerge in the treatment, as well as recurrent themes in their dreams.

A number of strategies are useful in promoting a productive working-through process. Exploring the Core Conflictual Relationship Theme (CCRT), developed by Luborsky (1984; Luborsky and Luborsky 2006), can be a fruitful course to pursue to help a patient increase self-observation and self-understanding. The CCRT involves a recurrent fantasy of relationships: a statement of the patient's wish, an expected imagined or actual response from the significant other, and a corresponding response from the self. The response from the self involves both behaviors and actions, as well as self states and feelings that may not be expressed. The CCRT emerges as the therapist listens to themes in the patient's narratives about life outside of the therapy. Exploring the specifics of disappointments and expectations often reveals the CCRT. The following example illustrates how these patterns emerge.

> A 28-year-old graduate student had completed all of his coursework but became stuck when it came to completing his dissertation. He told his therapist that he really wanted to get the Ph.D. and couldn't understand why he couldn't make himself sit down and complete the dissertation. He said he had finished about half of it but had lost his motivation and couldn't force himself to concentrate. The therapist asked him what he was afraid of. The patient hesitated and responded, "I'm not exactly sure, but I feel so much pressure from my dissertation advisor and my dad that it's driving me nuts." The therapist asked him to elaborate on the pressure he felt. In both the narrative involving his father and the narrative involving his dissertation advisor, the patient spoke as though they would expect more and more of him if he actually got his Ph.D. He felt his father was never satisfied. He recalled one time when he brought home a report card with all *A*s except one *B*. His father's total focus was why he got a *B* in the one course. The patient described his dissertation advisor as similarly hard driving and demanding. With the help of his therapist, the patient was able to develop the following CCRT: He had a strong wish to succeed to please his father, but he feared that ultimately nothing would please his father (or his dissertation advisor) and that they would only expect more. To avoid placing himself under even greater pressure, he retreated from the task and shut down all his creative efforts. When the therapist pointed this out to the patient, the patient said he instantly felt understood, although he had never put the three aspects of the CCRT together on his own.

Another useful strategy is to follow the patient's affect states and make interventions that facilitate emotional expression. A recent survey of the psychodynamic therapy research literature (Diener and Hilsenroth 2008), showed considerable empirical support for the notion that emotion-focused techniques are positively linked to favorable outcomes. Among these techniques are the following: a) increasing the patient's awareness of his or her emotions; b) facilitating the patient's emotional experience by focusing specifically on affective indicators in the patient, such as crying, or shifts in the patient's mood; and c) making specific references to these indicators. One has to be careful not to intervene too quickly when a patient cries, lest one inadvertently communicate that strong affect is too disturbing to handle. Diener and Hilsenroth recommend sitting with the sadness for a bit before attempting to interpret its meaning for the patient.

Another technique associated with positive outcome is to frame an interpretation as clarification in a manner that increases the patient's affect. An example would be to point out that feelings are not being expressed, or to empathically validate the reason for the feelings.

Yet another strategy is to promote mentalization by helping patients to see situations from an alternative perspective. Goldberg (1999) emphasizes the need to shift from a first-person perspective to a third-person perspective in the course of working through. Therapists need to validate the patient's "I" experience while also bringing to bear their own outside experience from a third-person perspective. The therapist can tactfully bring in his or her own views on what the patient brings up so that the patient gradually begins to appreciate alternative perspectives.

Therapists can enhance mentalization by calling attention to the patient's mental state, even when the patient may not be aware of the nature of that state. If, for example, a patient has a clenched fist, the therapist might observe that the patient appears angry. Then the therapist can illustrate how anger might influence the patient's perception. Moreover, if an impulsive behavior occurs, the therapist may ask the patient what was going on at the time that precipitated the behavior. By calling attention to internal states and specific kinds of actions in order to promote mentalization, the therapist helps the patient track and monitor his or her current state of mind. As Bateman, Fonagy, and Allen note in Chapter 28 ("Theory and Practice of Mentalization-Based Therapy"), therapists must assume a "not knowing" stance with the patient and actively inquire about mental states and alternative perspectives. Helping the patient focus on the therapist's mind is also a useful approach to improve the capacity for mentalization.

Termination

Termination is often mythologized in discussions of ideal cases of psychotherapy or psychoanalysis. The reality is that therapy ends in all different kinds of ways, often with practical considerations such as changes in financial circumstances, relocation of the patient or therapist, or an impasse in the treatment. One of the values of setting goals at the beginning (and later) is that patient and therapist can together gauge the progress of the treatment by assessing how many of the goals have been accomplished and to what extent.

Therapists must avoid the countertransference position of idealizing termination and expecting a perfect outcome. Indeed, a major goal of therapy is to help the patient internalize the process of inquiry that therapy represents so that much of the work can continue on the patient's own. Studies of psychodynamic psychotherapy (Bateman and Fonagy 2001; Svartberg et al. 2004) suggest that there is a "time-release" aspect to dynamic therapy. Patients' improvement continues after termination because the patient–therapist relationship has been internalized so that the work continues.

When patients are dead set on terminating for whatever reasons, it is rarely useful for the therapist to insist that they continue. Psychodynamic psychotherapy is noncoercive. Patients should be there because they want to be there, not because they have to be. It is far better to allow the patient to leave with the idea that "the door is always open." Then the patient can return when he or she feels the need.

Many patients return periodically for a few sessions or for more extended therapy, depending on new challenges in their lives. Still other patients end up as "therapeutic lifers" who see the therapist once every 6 months or so to maintain their gains. Wallerstein (1986) found that in the follow-up of the Menninger Psychotherapy Research Project, some of the patients did well as long as they were never expected to terminate therapy. The ongoing tie to the therapist appeared to have a beneficial effect, rather than simply encouraging dependency. The varieties of termination are multiple and often unexpected (see Table 2–4).

It is important for therapists to remember that we cannot know in advance how a patient will do after termination, and sometimes patients who choose unilateral termination may ultimately benefit as much as those who have mutual termination. Some patients may need to have an ending date established by the therapist, because they feel they can never terminate. Above all, termination must be individualized. Many themes recur in the course of the termination phase of therapy, and psychotherapists themselves often feel a sense of genuine loss, not just in the sense of losing a patient but also in the sense of losing a significant human relationship. For this reason, countertransference must be carefully monitored so that the therapist does not attempt to transform a therapeutic relationship into a personal one (Gabbard 2004).

TABLE 2–4.   Varieties of termination

Mutual agreement of therapist and patient based on achievement of goals

Preplanned termination based on number of sessions

Forced termination because one of the following occurs:

- Therapist graduates or changes clinical assignment

- Patient relocates

- Patient's third-party payer discontinues reimbursement

Unilateral termination in which one of the following occurs:

- Patient feels there is no value in continuing

- Therapist feels there is no value in continuing (and refers patient elsewhere)

Failed attempt at termination, leading to "therapeutic lifer" status

End-setting as a therapeutic strategy

Source.   Adapted from Gabbard GO: *Long-Term Psychodynamic Psychotherapy: A Basic Text.* Washington, DC, American Psychiatric Publishing, 2004, p. 163. Copyright 2004, American Psychiatric Publishing. Used with permission.

Conclusion

Psychodynamic psychotherapy cannot be adequately characterized by its specific techniques. It fundamentally involves a human relationship in which one person tries to understand the other in an empathic, nonjudgmental manner that facilitates increasing levels of disclosure and trust. While most of the therapist's comments can be categorized along the expressive–supportive continuum noted in this chapter, therapists should think about the time with the patient as a form of conversation that has spontaneity and responsiveness. Therapists who simply adhere to the technique as though it were a requirement of the therapy might lose the patient by appearing excessively rigid and scripted. Flexibility is a key feature of a good dynamic therapist, and one must adapt the treatment to the patient rather than the patient to the treatment.

Key Points

- A patient's personality characteristics, defense mechanisms, motivations, and other capacities must be carefully evaluated before a conclusion can be reached about whether dynamic therapy is the optimal treatment.

- A biopsychosocial formulation involving contributions from biology, psychology, and sociocultural influences guides the therapist in the initial stages of the treatment and serves to predict possible developments during therapy.

- Reasonable goals for the therapy must be collaboratively derived from negotiation between patient and therapist.

- Much attention should be paid to the development of the therapeutic alliance, as it is one of the most powerful predictors of outcome in dynamic therapy.

- Interventions used in dynamic psychotherapy reside on an expressive-supportive continuum, and the therapist must shift flexibly along that continuum according to the patient's needs.

- Transference generally is not interpreted until it becomes a resistance.

- Countertransference is a joint creation caused by preexisting issues in the therapist's past and what is induced in the therapist by the patient's behavior.

- Resistance is the manifestation of the patient's defense mechanisms as they are activated in therapy. These manifestations are a major focus of dynamic psychotherapy.

- The working-through process is the heart of dynamic therapy and involves strategies that are tailored to the individual patient.

- Termination occurs in a variety of ways, and the therapist must be flexible in adapting the termination to the patient's situation.

References

American Psychiatric Association: Diagnostic and Statistical Manual of Mental Disorders, 4th Edition. Washington, DC, American Psychiatric Association, 1994

American Psychiatric Association: Diagnostic and Statistical Manual of Mental Disorders, 4th Edition, Text Revision. Washington, DC, American Psychiatric Association, 2000

Bateman A, Fonagy P: Treatment of borderline personality disorder with psycho-analytically oriented partial hospitalization: an 18-month follow-up. Am J Psychiatry 158:36–42, 2001

Butler FF, Strupp HH: Specific and nonspecific factors in psychotherapy: a problematic paradigm for psychotherapy research. Journal of Self Psychotherapy 23:30–39, 1986

Diener MJ, Hilsenroth MJ: Affect-focused techniques in psychodynamic psychotherapy, in Evidence-Based Psychodynamic Psychotherapy. Edited by Levy R, Ablon S. Totowa, NJ, Humana Press, 2008

Fonagy P, Target M: Playing with reality, III: the persistence of dual psychic reality in borderline patients. Int J Psychoanal 81:853–873, 2000

Freud S: The future prospects of psycho-analytic therapy (1910), in The Standard Edition of the Complete Psychological Works of Sigmund Freud, Vol 11. Translated and edited by Strachey J. London, Hogarth Press, 1957, pp 139–152

Freud S: Remembering, repeating and working-through (further recommendations on the technique of psycho-analysis II) (1914), in The Standard Edition of the Complete Psychological Works of Sigmund Freud, Vol 12. Translated and edited by Strachey J. London, Hogarth Press, 1958, pp 145–156

Friedman L: A reading of Freud's papers on technique. Psychoanal Q 60:564–595, 1991

Gabbard GO: Long-Term Psychodynamic Psychotherapy: A Basic Text. Washington, DC, American Psychiatric Publishing, 2004

Gabbard GO: Psychodynamic Psychiatry in Clinical Practice, 4th Edition. Washington, DC, American Psychiatric Publishing, 2005

Gabbard GO: Editorial: when is transference work useful in dynamic psychotherapy? Am J Psychiatry 163:1667–1669, 2006

Goldberg A: Between empathy and judgment. J Am Psychoanal Assoc 47:351–365, 1999

Gunderson JG, Gabbard GO: Making the case for psychoanalytic therapies in the current psychiatric environment. J Am Psychoanal Assoc 47:679–704, 1999

Hilsenroth MJ, Cromer TD: Clinician interventions related to alliance during the initial interview and psychological assessment. Psychotherapy: Theory, Research, Practice, Training 44:205–218, 2007

Hoffman IZ: Ritual and Spontaneity in the Psychoanalytic Process: A Dialectical-Constructivist View. Hillsdale, NJ, Analytic Press, 1998

Høglend P, Amlo S, Marble A, et al: Analysis of the patient-therapist relationship in dynamic psychotherapy: an experimental study of transference interpretations. Am J Psychiatry 163:1739–1746, 2006

Horvath AO: The therapeutic relationship: research and theory: an introduction to the special issue. Psychother Res 15:3–7, 2005

Horwitz L, Gabbard GO, Allen JG, et al: Borderline Personality Disorder: Tailoring the Psychotherapy to the Patient. Washington, DC, American Psychiatric Press, 1996

Ingram RE, Price JM (eds): Vulnerability to Psychopathology: Risk Across the Lifespan. New York, Lippincott Williams & Wilkins, 2002

Kassaw K, Gabbard GO: Creating a psychodynamic formulation from the clinical evaluation. Am J Psychiatry 159:721–726, 2002

Krupnick JL, Sotsky SM, Elkin I, et al: The role of the alliance in psychotherapy and pharmacotherapy outcome: findings in the National Institute of Mental Health Treatment of Depression Collaborative Research Program. J Consult Clin Psychol 64:532–539, 1996

Luborsky L: Principles of Psychoanalytic Psychotherapy: A Manual for Supportive-Expressive Treatment. New York, Basic Books, 1984

Luborsky L, Luborsky E: Research and Psychotherapy: The Vital Link. New York, Jason Aronson, 2006

Martin DJ, Garske JP, Davis KK: Relation of the therapeutic alliance with outcome and other variables: a meta-analytic review. J Consult Clin Psychol 68:438–450, 2000

Mitchell S: Influence and Autonomy in Psychoanalysis. Hillsdale, NJ, Analytic Press, 1997

Safran JD, Muran JC: The resolution of ruptures in the therapeutic alliance. J Consult Clin Psychol 64:447–458, 1996

Safran JD, Muran JC: Has the concept of the therapeutic alliance outlived its usefulness? Psychotherapy: Theory, Research, Practice, Training 43:286–291, 2006

Sperry L, Gudeman JE, Blackwell B, et al: Psychiatric Case Formulations. Washington, DC, American Psychiatric Press, 1992

Svartberg M, Stiles TC, Seltzer MH: Randomized, controlled trial of the effectiveness of short-term dynamic psychotherapy and cognitive therapy for cluster C personality disorders. Am J Psychiatry 161:810–817, 2004

Wallerstein RS: Forty-Two Lives in Treatment: A Study of Psychoanalysis and Psychotherapy. New York, Guilford, 1986

Winnicott DW: The aims of psychoanalytic treatment (1962), in The Maturational Processes and the Facilitating Environment: Studies in the Theory of Emotional Development. London, Hogarth Press, 1976, pp 166–170

Winnicott DW: Ego distortion in terms of true and false self, in The Maturational Processes and the Facilitating Environment: Studies in the Theory of Emotional Development. New York, International Universities Press, 1965, pp 140–152

Zuroff DC, Blatt SJ: The therapeutic relationship in the brief treatment of depression: contributions to clinical improvement and enhanced adaptive capabilities. J Consult Clin Psychol 74:130–140, 2006

Suggested Readings

Basch MF: Doing Psychotherapy. New York, Basic Books, 1980

Gabbard GO: Long-Term Psychodynamic Psychotherapy: A Basic Text. Washington, DC, American Psychiatric Publishing, 2004

Gabbard GO: Psychodynamic Psychiatry in Clinical Practice, 4th Edition. Washington, DC, American Psychiatric Publishing, 2005

McWilliams N: Psychoanalytic Psychotherapy. New York, Guilford, 2004

Chapter 3

Techniques of Brief Psychodynamic Psychotherapy

Mantosh Dewan, M.D.
Priyanthy Weerasekera, M.D., M.Ed.
Lynn Stormon, Ph.D.

All brief therapies, not just brief psychodynamic psychotherapy (BPP), evolved from psychoanalytic roots. Freud reported on psychoanalytic therapies that lasted 1 week (Katherine), 7 weeks (Emmy von N), and 9 weeks (Lucie R) and the cure of Gustav Mahler's impotence in a single, 4-hour session (Breuer and Freud 1893–1895; Jones 1957). Freud's followers defined and formally introduced the key ingredients of brief therapy: increased therapist activity, a limit on the length of treatment and/or number of sessions, narrowed treatment focus, and restricted patient selection criteria (Table 3–1). Today, research validates the efficacy of BPP, and practitioners are extending the reach of this approach by introducing innovative techniques such as block therapy (Davanloo 2004) and by treating new populations. For instance, Milrod et al. (2007) conducted the first randomized

TABLE 3–1. Key techniques of brief psychodynamic psychotherapy: earliest contributions

Technical hallmarks	Contributor(s)	Contribution
Increased therapist activity	Ferenczi (1920)	Advocated "active therapy"
	Alexander and French (1946)	Actively created corrective emotional experiences
Limited time and/or number of sessions	Rank	Set strict 9-month limit; number of sessions not limited
	Malan (1976)	Set firm ending date at first session; number of sessions not limited but averaged 18 sessions
	Mann (1973)	Exact prescription of time: set firm ending date at first session; limited to 12 sessions
Defined, narrow treatment focus	French (1970)	Focal conflict
	Sifneos (1972)	Core neurotic problem
	Balint (Balint et al. 1972), Malan (1976)	Focal psychotherapy
	Luborsky (1984)	Core Conflictual Relationship Theme
Restricted patient selection criteria	Rank	Willing patients
	Sifneos (1972), Malan (1976)	Patient easily forms an alliance; has flexible defenses; is motivated; has circumscribed pathology of recent onset
	Davanloo (1980)	Broadened criteria to include more severe pathology, personality problems

controlled trial of panic-focused psychodynamic psychotherapy in patients with panic disorder and found it to be effective.

In this chapter we address factors that are common to all types of BPP. To be consistent across chapters in this text, we define BPPs as therapies that continue for less than 6 months or involve fewer than 24 sessions. We then describe the three main schools of brief psychodynamic therapies and illustrate how practitioners of each approach would conceptualize and treat the same patient.

Features Common to All Brief Psychodynamic Therapies

The goals of BPP are relief from distressing symptoms, resolution of key conflicts, and, in some cases, changes in character pathology. Research demonstrates that BPP is efficacious in treating a variety of psychiatric disorders (Leichsenring 2005; see also Chapter 4, "Applications of Psychodynamic Psychotherapy to Specific Disorders: Efficacy and Indications") and that specific therapist and patient factors, as well as in-session interventions, predict outcome of BPP (Crits-Christoph and Connolly 1999; Leichsenring 2005).

There are three major schools of brief dynamic psychotherapy: the *drive/structural model*, the *relational model*, and the *integrative/eclectic model* (Messer and Warren 1995). Several features that are common to all BPPs and that differentiate this modality from long-term psychodynamic psychotherapy are listed in Table 3–2. After outlining a generic approach to BPP, we consider variations according to each specific school (Book 1998; Budman 1981; Dewan et al. 2008; Messer and Warren 1995).

Structural Elements

All types of BPP have the following structural elements in common:

- *Engagement*—Rapid formation of a therapeutic alliance and translation of presenting problems into focal goals
- *Discrepancy*—Provision of novel skills, insights, and experiences that challenge patient patterns and facilitate new understandings and actions
- *Consolidation*—Rehearsal of new patterns in varied contexts, accompanied by feedback, to ensure internalization and prevent relapse (Dewan et al. 2008)

Patient Characteristics: Initial Interview and Patient Selection

A full psychiatric and psychodynamic assessment is completed in order to select only those patients who will benefit from this treatment (see Table 3–3).

TABLE 3–2. Differences between brief and long-term psychodynamic psychotherapy

Brief dynamic therapy	Long-term dynamic therapy
Rapid alliance formation	Gradual alliance formation
Narrowed problem focus	Broad range of problems
Increased therapist activity	Moderate therapist activity
Ability to tolerate separation	Variable ability to tolerate separation
Good object relationships	Poor to good object relationships
Less severe pathology	More severe pathology
Here-and-now focus	Past-and-present focus

Several patient characteristics have been identified that are considered essential for BPP. These include motivation for treatment, ability to identify a circumscribed problem, good object relationships (presence of past and current relationships), ability to rapidly form a therapeutic alliance, and capacity to tolerate separation. Patients lacking these characteristics would likely benefit from other approaches or long-term psychodynamic therapy (Book 1998).

Narrowed Problem Focus

After conducting a full assessment, the therapist converts the patient's presenting problem into a psychodynamic formulation, in which major themes center on conflicts that are based on drives, impulses, defenses, relational patterns, wishes, and other universal conflictual situations. Sifneos (1981, p. 49) illustrates an oedipal problem focus from the structural school:

> A graduate student complaining of difficulties with both men and women stated that he had a tendency to cover up his feelings, to wear "a mask," as he put it, so that others would not know what he truly was like. He attributed this tendency to his relationship with his parents. As a result of his strong attachment to his mother, whose favorite he was, and competition with his father, he felt he had to hide his true feelings for both of them. This attitude interfered with his daily life.

Levenson (2004, p. 167) provides an example of a four-part *cyclical maladaptive pattern* (CMP) from the relational school:

1. *Acts of self:* "When I meet strangers, I think they wouldn't want to have anything to do with me."

TABLE 3–3. **Brief dynamic psychotherapy inclusion and exclusion criteria**

	Inclusion	Exclusion
Diagnoses	Depression—mild to moderate[a]	Severe depression, bipolar disorder, psychosis, suicidality
	Anxiety—PTSD, social, panic[a]	OCD
	Somatoform disorders[a]	Severe somatizing disorders
	Eating disorders[a]	Severe eating disorders
	Opiate dependence[a]	
Patient characteristics	Good object relationships (has had at least one relationship)	Poor object relationships
	Highly motivated, "willing" patient	Poor motivation
	Narrow symptom/problem focus	Chronic, severe character pathology; diffuse, ill-defined symptomatology
	Interpersonal difficulties[a]	

Note.   OCD=obsessive-compulsive disorder; PTSD=posttraumatic stress disorder.
[a]Criteria supported by randomized controlled trials (Leichsenring 2005).

2. *Expectations of others' reactions:* "If I go to the dance, no one will ask me to dance."
3. *Acts of others toward self:* "When I went to the dance, guys asked me to dance but only because they felt sorry for me."
4. *Acts of self toward the self (introjection):* "When no one asked me to dance, I told myself that it is because I'm fat, ugly, and unlovable."

Mann (1981, p. 34) gives an example of a problem focus representing the integrated school of BPP:

> **Therapist:** You are a man who has been enormously successful despite many serious difficulties. What hurts you now and has always been a source of hurt to you is the difference you feel between your public image and the private feelings that you have about yourself.

The problem focus is presented to the patient and a therapeutic contract is developed to work through the problem. This is one of the most important variables in the development of the therapeutic alliance (Horvath and Symonds 1991). If the patient does not agree with the problem focus, it is important that the problem be reexamined, reformulated, and presented to the patient for reconsideration (Book 1998). Because therapy is time-limited, the focus is limited to one or two attainable goals. Specific goals could be symptom relief or working through of conflictual relationships (but with limited character change).

Increased Therapist Activity and Techniques

One key therapist variable that differentiates long-term psychodynamic psychotherapy from BPP is *therapist activity level*. Given that BPP typically lasts 4–6 months or less, it is essential that the therapist be active and promote the emergence of material in session. Since the problem focus is presented to the patient in the initial session, subsequent sessions single-mindedly focus on the problem as it is worked through.

Specific techniques utilized depend on the model of therapy followed. The techniques that follow are common to all psychodynamic schools:

Use of Transference

Transference represents unconscious thoughts and feelings the patient has toward his or her primary caretakers "transferred" on to the "blank screen" of the therapist. As therapy progresses, transference deepens. It is the *working through* of the transference that is a key active ingredient of change in both long-term psychodynamic psychotherapy and BPP. Interpretation of transference is one of the means by which working through is accomplished.

> **Patient:** I was here yesterday way before the appointment, but you never came. I waited and waited. No one told me what was happening. I thought I had the wrong date, but I didn't. I thought maybe something had happened to you, but mostly I thought you had something else more important to do.
>
> **Therapist:** Yes, it is unfortunate I was unable to make the appointment. I got held up. I am sorry. I sense you feel quite upset about it, but I think there is something more happening here. There is this feeling of rejection, as though I had something better to do and you aren't important. I think this is a familiar feeling for you. It sounds like this is what you feel all the time, and I think this is what it was like at home with your mother. You never felt she really cared.

Use of Countertransference

Countertransference represents the therapist's thoughts and feelings toward the patient, both conscious and unconscious. It is possible in the example above that the therapist—on further reflection—might become aware that he or she did not want to attend the session because of a feeling of boredom in the previous sessions, or a feeling that the patient was avoiding dealing with important issues. These feelings may indicate important interpersonal themes for the patient, and some therapists consider it important to communicate these feelings back to the patient.

> **Therapist:** I noticed that in our last sessions I was working hard to draw you out. I wonder whether this happens with other people, and I wonder whether this pushes them away and leaves you on your own?

Clarification

A *clarification* is a statement made by the therapist to the patient that is either a restatement or reflection of what the patient has just said. In delivering a clarification, the therapist stays at the descriptive level without going beyond the data.

> **Therapist:** So if I am hearing you correctly, you are saying you felt something strong, something close to anger?

Interpretation

An *interpretation* is a statement made by the therapist to the patient that goes beyond the descriptive level. It provides the patient with a hypothesis about what may be happening, or why he or she may have felt or behaved in a particular way. Psychodynamic therapy focuses on the unconscious meaning of events or situations. When delivering an interpretation to a patient the therapist may encounter some resistance, as these interventions are more difficult for the patient to hear.

> **Therapist:** I wonder whether your anger has something to do with your feeling rejected by your mother, whether in fact the angry feelings are about being hurt, and for you it is easier to tolerate anger than be hurt, because hurt feelings are more painful.

Suggestion/Advice

Through this intervention the therapist tries to bring about certain thoughts, feelings, or behaviors in the patient. This technique is considered controversial, for the therapist is in a position of power over the patient, who is perceived as dependent. An example of appropriate advice (Winston et al. 2004, p. 34) is:

> **Therapist:** People who are interested in what you do usually don't want all the details. They may be interested to know that you enjoyed a movie, but they may not want to hear the whole story. Try stopping and noticing whether the other person asks a question that would tell you he or she wants to know more.

An example of *in*appropriate advice (Winston et al. 2004, p. 35) is:

> **Patient:** My boyfriend humiliated me in public again yesterday. I screamed at him when we got home, and he said I was too sensitive. I can't take it anymore.
> **Therapist:** Tell him that if he does this again, you are leaving him.

These techniques are used in all forms of psychodynamic psychotherapy, although the frequency of use depends on the specific school, as differences exist with respect to what is emphasized in the theory and in the therapeutic encounter with the patient (see Table 3–4).

Termination

Although the end of brief therapy is often defined by time, such as 6 months, or number of sessions, such as 24, therapy ends appropriately only when the identified problem focus has been resolved and when newly acquired psychological skills have been internalized so that they can be readily applied to a variety of other situations.

TABLE 3–4. Brief dynamic models of psychotherapy

Drive/Structural	Relational	Integrative
Focus on drives and conflicts, including oedipal conflicts	Focus on relationships	Focus on both conflicts and relationships and also on loss
Challenging defenses	Focus on interactional patterns	Focus on conflicts, relationships, and self-esteem needs
Confrontational	Nonconfrontational	Nonconfrontational
Anxiety provoking	Non–anxiety provoking	Non–anxiety provoking
Patient experiences seen as conflicts related to impulses connected to the past	Patient experiences accepted at face value	Patient experiences accepted at face value
Addressing intrapsychic conflicts	Addressing deficits and conflicts	Addressing deficits and conflicts
Therapist as objective observer	Therapist as participant	Therapist as participant

Specific Approaches to Brief Psychodynamic Psychotherapy

Although all brief psychodynamic psychotherapeutic approaches have features in common, they differ in their understanding of the nature of psychological problems and in the emphasis they place on the focus of treatment. Three models can be described on the basis of their primary model: the drive/structural model, the relational model, and the integrative model.

Drive/Structural Model

Freud's structural model divides the mind into the id, ego, and superego. A detailed discussion of this model can be found in Chapter 1 ("Theoretical Models of Psychodynamic Psychotherapy"). In brief, the id, housed primarily in the unconscious, contains all the psychic energy and focuses on gratifying instinctual drives. The id's pursuit of pleasure creates tension, and alternative ways to discharge this tension are carried out by the ego (S. Freud 1923). The ego, however, is pragmatic, with no moral sense, thereby requiring the superego to provide a moral code for behavior. Conflict arises as the id's need to gratify all of the senses' desires becomes prohibited by the superego's morality. As described by Anna Freud (1936), the ego uses a variety of defense mechanisms to transform the id's psychic energy into a less threatening form.

Sigmund Freud also described oedipal conflicts that involve the child's attraction to the parent of the opposite sex, which, if not properly resolved, lead to specific interpersonal problems in young adulthood. These unresolved issues become the focus of therapy in later adulthood.

Formal BPP was developed in the 1960s, with Davanloo, Malan, and Sifneos promoting their own brand of BPP according to Freud's drive/structural model (Malan 1979). Patients with adjustment disorders and less severe forms of depression, anxiety, or personality disorders are all considered appropriate candidates for therapy. Malan and Sifneos exclude those patients with more severe pathology whereas Davanloo includes a broader range of patients. Malan added additional exclusion criteria, including a) difficulties in forming an alliance due to severe dependency issues or poor transferences, b) highly rigid defenses, c) poor motivation, and d) complicated ingrained characterological issues. According to Malan, the purpose of therapy is to resolve just one conflict or a few conflicts. The specific conflict typically relates to unacceptable feelings or impulses toward a person in the patient's life; these feelings produce anxiety, which is defended against by a variety of mechanisms.

Malan's approach uses the two traditional psychoanalytic *triangles of insight*—a triangle of conflict and a triangle of persons—which help conceptualize the problem and guide treatment (Figure 3–1). The main goal is to make a connection between the patterns in the triangle of conflict (comprising anxiety, defenses, and impulses or feelings) and a person in the triangle of persons (comprising the therapist, a person in a current relationship with the patient, and a person in a past relationship), until all three persons are linked. Clarifying each pattern in the significant relationships, the therapist moves through both triangles. Malan attends carefully and interprets along the line of the conflict, challenging defenses until the conflict is worked through (Malan 1979).

Sifneos (1992, 2004), in his *short-term anxiety-provoking psychotherapy* (STAPP), emphasizes the importance of presenting the key psychodynamic focus to the patient, which usually involves either oedipal conflicts or separation and grief issues. Using an anxiety-provoking confrontational style, Sifneos addresses the patient's impulses, feelings, defenses, and resistances and clearly deals with transference. Despite the confrontational style of therapy, Sifneos does pay attention to the therapeutic alliance and works to provide a corrective emotional experience for the patient. When the patient is able to demonstrate a clear understanding of his or her difficulties and also a change in behavior, termination is considered (Budman 1981).

Davanloo (1980, 2004), on the other hand, establishes the patient's appropriateness for therapy in an initial 1- to several-hour-long "trial therapy," during which he works on "unlocking the unconscious." He rapidly develops a positive therapeutic alliance by carefully allying with the patient against his or her pathology, which is made ego-dystonic. He consistently

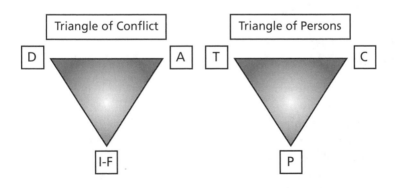

FIGURE 3–1. Traditional psychoanalytic triangles of insight.

Note. A=anxiety; C=person in current relationship; D=defenses; I-F=impulse or feeling; P=person in past relationship; T=therapist.

focuses on the main problem by using a direct, confrontational style, which insistently challenges the patient's defenses and quickly clarifies resistance. Davanloo also uses the psychoanalytic triangles of insight and actively addresses transference but, unlike other theorists, does not rigidly conform to working out one triangle before moving on to the other. He moves from the transference to past and present relationships as he works through the triangle of persons. Davanloo emphasizes providing support and empathy despite his confrontational style, and states that this process facilitates openness, which permits unacknowledged feelings and conflicts to be brought into awareness and worked through. A strong therapeutic alliance is essential if one is to undertake such a confrontational style, and not all patients are able to tolerate this particular approach. Davanloo's inclusion criteria allow patients with more serious character pathology and more severe illness than most other brief psychodynamic therapies allow.

To increase the mobilization of the unconscious, Davanloo (2004) practices *block therapy*, which consists of 5- to 7-hour-long sessions each day in blocks of 3 consecutive days. These blocks are repeated 1–3 months apart.

The drive/structural model of BPP focuses on those key conflicts as originally described by Freud, with Davanloo, Malan, and Sifneos all developing their own brand of brief treatment. Each approach differs with respect to therapeutic style, patient inclusion criteria, and focus of treatment.

We illustrate how the techniques of the traditional drive/structural model would be applied to a patient, Ms. B (see "Case Vignette, Ms. B" and the discussion in "Therapy Approach 1: The Drive/Structural Model"). We also illustrate the treatment of the same patient according to the two other main schools, relational (in "Therapy Approach 2: Relational Time-Limited Dynamic Psychotherapy") and integrative (in "Therapy Approach 3: Mann's Integrative Time-Limited Psychotherapy").

Relational Model

Freud first used the term *object* to represent the aim of an individual's libidinal and aggressive drives. This view was further elaborated by the British Independent School of object relations theory, which gave primacy to the development and pathology of the self within the "relational" matrix between the self and the object. The primary motivating force of human behavior is seen not as pleasure seeking but as "object seeking" or "relationship seeking." From birth, the infant seeks a relationship with the mother, first with parts of her (e.g., voice, touch) and then with the whole, integrated object (Greenberg and Mitchell 1983).

This significant shift in emphasis to the *relationship* between infant and mother was pioneered by Melanie Klein (1959) and later developed by Fairbairn (1949), Winnicott (1965), Mahler (Mahler et al. 1975), and Bowlby (1988). Departing radically from Freud's drive-conflict theory, Fairbairn posited that the motivational force driving human behavior is the fundamental need to relate with the object, a relationship considered necessary for survival. He viewed the primary developmental task of the infant as separating from the object and viewing self and object (or mother) as two distinct whole objects. He developed a sophisticated theory outlining this process and explained how individuals become involved in repeated destructive relationships. He provided a prescription for healthy functioning that permits an individual to participate in a mature relationship where true intimacy—with giving and receiving—is possible (Fairbairn 1949).

Following Fairbairn, Winnicott described the fundamental relational conditions necessary for a child to develop independence, creativity, and a true sense of self that permits creativity and healthy relationships (Winnicott 1965). The emphasis on separation, individuation, and differentiation was further elaborated by Mahler and, later, by Bowlby (1988). Bowlby systematically researched the mother–child relationship and, digressing from the language of the object relations school, focused on the "attachment" between the mother and child. He showed that early attachment patterns (secure, anxious-ambivalent, and anxious-avoidant) produce a template or imprint for future relationships (Daniel 2006).

Object relations theory thereby shifted the focus from intrapsychic conflicts and a drive/structural model to include a deficit model in which specific environmental precursors predict future personality development, psychopathology, and future relationships, including the therapeutic relationship. Although conflict still retains importance in this model, it is conflict between representations of the self and representations of the object within the self. The importance given to the object and the object relationship offers a "relational" and interpersonal dimension, illustrating our inherent human longing to connect and relate with another. Personality is understood in terms of the individual's internal representation of self and other, greater attention is given to current as well as past experiences, and the therapist is viewed as a participant in an interactional process rather than as a passive, objective observer.

The approaches to brief psychodynamic therapy that follow the relational model were developed by Strupp and the Vanderbilt group (Strupp and Hadley 1979; Strupp et al. 1977) and later by Strupp and Binder (1984), Weiss and Sampson (1986), Luborsky and Crits-Christoph (1990), Horowitz (1991), and Levenson (1995). Strupp and colleagues (1977) proposed an interpersonal model that focused on cyclical maladaptive patterns, or CMPs, which are seen as the patient's repetitive maladaptive behaviors that induce negative behaviors from others. This pattern is reenacted in transference and is the focus of treatment, which emphasizes the here and now and the interpersonal dynamics of the session (Messer and Warren 1995).

Strupp and Binder's (1984) time-limited dynamic psychotherapy (TLDP) was further developed by Levenson (1995). As in other brief relational approaches, less emphasis is given to interpretation to promote insight and more to experiential learning in the session. The therapeutic relationship is considered key in resolving dysfunctional interactional patterns, and transference is viewed as the patient's perception of the therapist based on actual previous experiences. Similarly, countertransference is seen as the therapist's natural response to the interpersonal process set up by the patient. According to TLDP, certain past experiences promote maladaptive relationship patterns, which are then reinforced in the present as a result of the patient engaging in similar maladaptive interactions. These patterns become alive in the therapeutic relationship, as the therapist cannot help but become part of the maladaptive interactional dynamics. The therapeutic focus, then, is to help the patient work through these dynamics with the therapist so that what is learned can be transferred to outside relationships. The hope is for the therapist to offer a new relational experience for the patient. When several maladaptive relational patterns exist, it is important to focus on the one that creates the most difficulty (Levenson 1995).

Borrowing concepts from cognitive psychology, Horowitz (1991) described patients' *schemas*, *self-schemas*, and *role relationships*. Psychopathology is conceptualized as developing from the overuse of a maladaptive schema, with the main focus on stress response, loss, and mourning. Supportive as well as explorative techniques are used, with particular attention given to catharsis and the promotion of emotional expression.

The most researched approach is that based on Luborsky's core conflictual relationship theme (CCRT). Luborsky operationalized transference in his CCRT model and demonstrated that interpersonal struggles can be understood in terms of three components: a wish, response from others, and response from self (Luborsky and Crits-Christoph 1990). These components represent the core of the interpersonal struggle in the patient's real world and in the transference relationship, and form the focus of treatment. Luborsky and Mark (1991) have identified key techniques specific to the CCRT method, which are divided into supportive and expressive techniques. Supportive techniques promote the development of a positive therapeutic alliance and include therapist-delivered acceptance, hope and encouragement, respect, and warmth. Expressive techniques focus on listening for the relationship patterns, on subsequent formulation and delivery of the CCRT to the patient as the central focus of treatment, and on the therapist's explanation of the CCRT's connection to the patient's presenting problem.

Book (1998) identified several patient variables as important for treatment, including the following:

- Motivation for treatment
- Capacity to trust
- Ability to explore feelings
- Current experience of emotional suffering
- Ability to examine interpersonal conflicts
- Ability to maintain clear boundaries

In-session techniques emphasize giving greater attention to the present, to current relationships, including the therapeutic relationship, and to the interpersonal process occurring between patient and therapist as a way of understanding the patient's past and current relationship issues. Although interpretation of transference is important, the therapist is seen as providing a "corrective emotional experience" for the patient, which allows the patient to feel safe and explore painful issues. Compared with the drive/structural model, the relational model gives less emphasis to insight and to the interpretation and confrontation of drives and defenses (Messer and Warren 1995).

There is also a very obvious shift in the therapeutic stance of the therapist participating in the process. Patients' accounts of their early developmental years and interpersonal relations are accepted at face value rather than interpreted according to oedipal fantasies (Cashdan 1988).

Hanna Levenson presents a case (see "Case Vignette, Ms. B") and illustrates the techniques used in a relationally oriented brief dynamic psychotherapy, TLDP (in "Therapy Approach 2: Relational Time-Limited Dynamic Psychotherapy").

Integrative Model

Mann (1991), Garfield (1989), Bellak (1992), and Gustafson (1986) all developed eclectic approaches that integrate techniques from a variety of traditions. Mann developed an integrative model of brief dynamic psychotherapy that incorporates concepts from both the structural and the relational models. Using a developmental perspective, he identified separation-individuation as the main theme of brief therapy. His model identifies four universal conflicts that center on the management of loss: 1) independence versus dependence, 2) activity versus passivity, 3) development versus loss of self-esteem, and 4) unresolved versus delayed grief (Mann 1991). After developing a central focus, Mann pays particular attention to the patient's self-esteem needs and to the therapeutic alliance. He helps soothe the patient's anxiety rather than increasing it by confronting the patient about defenses and resistances, akin to the relational rather than the drive/structural model. Individuals with the following are all suitable for this approach:

• Adjustment disorders
• Anxiety reactions
• Maladaptive hysterical, depressive, or obsessional character structures
• Unsatisfactory relationship patterns
• Problems in interpersonal relationships
• Work problems
• Transitions in life

Patients should also have good ego strength, be able to engage in a therapeutic relationship, and be able to tolerate loss (Messer and Warren 1995).

The therapist using Mann's integrative approach is very active, particularly in the early sessions, because therapy lasts only 12 sessions. Fundamental listening and validating skills are used in the early sessions to create a supportive therapeutic environment that facilitates self-disclosure. As therapy progresses, the therapist deals with the patient's disappointment that therapy is limited and unable to provide an answer to all the problems he or she is experiencing. The therapist gently confronts and clarifies, and offers interpretations around the core issues. As termination approaches, increased attention is paid to separation issues, and transference interpretations related to the past and present are offered. Therefore, Mann sees the therapist as providing selfobject functions that reinforce self-esteem and a sense of mastery over the conflictual issue (Mann 1991). Later in this chapter, we illustrate, in a continuation of the following case vignette, how the technique based on Mann's integrative model would be applied to the patient (see "Therapy Approach 3: Mann's Integrative Time-Limited Psychotherapy").

Application of Approaches to a Specific Case

Case Vignette, Ms. B[1]

Ms. B, a 59-year-old, married, white administrative assistant and mother of two grown sons, was sent to therapy by her physician because he suspected that her weight loss, multiple vague symptomatic complaints, and fatigue

---

[1]This case vignette was kindly provided by Hanna Levenson, Ph.D.

were symptoms of depression. While Ms. B compliantly came for her first appointment, she made it very clear that she was "quite happy"; however, she did admit to having "some stress" in her life. Although she was well groomed, her slumped shoulders and monotone voice made her appear lifeless.

Ms. B grew up in a strict, religious household. Her parents focused most of their attention on her "wild" sister because Ms. B "was such an easy child." She married at an early age and supported her husband, Tom, while he finished dentistry school. Their marriage was described as "normal." However, Ms. B and her husband did not spend much time together outside of going to church. Of late, her husband was spending more and more time on the computer.

Ms. B said she was a devoted mother. Although her sons were grown and out of the house, neither of them was yet financially independent, and this caused Ms. B great concern. However, she minimized her worry by saying they "just haven't found themselves yet." Ms. B hesitatingly said she suspected her younger son of having a gambling problem. Further inquiry revealed that over the past 2 years, her parents' health had deteriorated, and Ms. B had become their main source of social, financial, and health care support. Ms. B has worked almost her entire adult life. Recently, she had been experiencing much stress at work, where her duties had markedly increased since the office staff was downsized. Given all of this, she steadfastly maintained that "my life is good and I am blessed."

Therapy Approach 1: The Drive/Structural Model

The therapist (a male) obtains a complete history, paying particular attention to Ms. B's interpersonal relationships. He uses open-ended questions in the first session to find out about her goals for treatment and her expectations of the therapist. It quickly becomes clear that she doesn't feel comfortable taking the initiative but rather expects the therapist to tell her what to do. This early manifestation of transference informs the therapist about patterns of compliance and pleasing behavior in relation to male authority figures.

In the second session, Ms. B reveals that her husband complains about feeling neglected and unappreciated. He spends a lot of time on the Internet, on eBay, and usually doesn't come to bed until after she is asleep. Ms. B rationalizes this by saying that he has a stressful job and deserves to relax after work. The therapist decides to utilize Sifneos's STAPP approach to confront Ms. B's avoidance of the problems in her marriage. He now combines open-ended with forced-choice questions, which arouses Ms. B's anxiety but also reveals Ms. B as "Daddy's little girl" who consults her father on all decisions, which leaves her husband feeling sidelined and unimportant. Ms. B's mother is submissive and passive-aggressive, reacting against her husband's dominance with back pain that leaves her periodically bedridden. Ms. B's father habitually turns to Ms. B for companionship, complaining bitterly about her mother's inadequacies as a wife. When Ms. B talked to her father about her husband's excessive Internet use, her father replied that he never thought that her husband was good enough for her—after all, dentists aren't *real* doctors—but that she shouldn't complain because she has a good life. Ms. B's father had worked long hours in a blue-collar job and always felt envious of her husband's success.

From very early on, Ms. B deployed defenses such as repression, reaction formation, isolation of affect, and rationalization to avoid her negative feelings in order to maintain her parent's positive regard, especially her father's. The therapist's persistent exploration of Ms. B's feelings about her husband's nighttime Internet activity is actively defended against as she continues to maintain that her husband is a good provider and that she is content even as their sex life dwindles to nothing:

> **Therapist:** How do you feel about competing with eBay for your husband's attention?
>
> **Ms. B:** Well (*laughs nervously, somewhat taken aback*), I wouldn't say I am competing! He collects antique toy soldiers, something he enjoys a lot, and he works hard—he should have some fun, too.
>
> **Therapist:** I agree, but it seems that this fun is coming at your expense—you're working extra hard at your job, taking care of your parents and your sons out of your own paycheck, and he's staying up late buying expensive toys while you go to bed alone.
>
> **Ms. B:** It's not that bad…I have a good life, nothing to complain about really…not like some people who have real problems.
>
> **Therapist:** I'd say having no sex life is a "real" problem, wouldn't you?
>
> **Ms. B:** Well…maybe that's normal…after all, we're not young anymore. He's a good, hard-working man…at least he's home and not out like some husbands.
>
> **Therapist:** Sex is a normal part of a healthy marriage throughout the life cycle. Are you really satisfied that while he's home he ignores you?
>
> **Ms. B** (*looking tearful*): We used to be closer that way, I guess, but…I spend most evenings taking care of my mother when she's not feeling well—I feel so horrible when I feel angry and resentful of her. Or I'm out to dinner with my father, who's miserable with her. Then there are the boys, who always need something. I feel wrung out at the end of the day and exhausted. (*She breaks down and cries.*) I feel so lonely…I don't blame him for not wanting to be with me…I look like a wreck and I feel that way, too.

The therapist recognizes the oedipal dynamic and summarizes it for Ms. B:

> **Therapist:** All your life, you have had to distance yourself from your mother in order to protect your special status with your father. Now you distance yourself from your husband—whom your father does not like, just as he does not like your mother—perhaps as a way to maintain closeness with your father.

She is startled when she realizes that she is repeating the relationship that she has with her parents with her sons, in whom she confides and to whom she complains about her husband. Ms. B and the therapist agree that the problems in her marriage stem from her overly close relationship with her father. They agree that the task is to help Ms. B distance herself from her father and limit her involvement with her sons so that she has more time and energy to work on her marriage.

Initially, Ms. B appears compliant with the treatment goal, although she postpones talking to her husband. The therapist sees the positive paternal transference as a resistance, as Ms. B pressures the therapist to reassure her that everything will turn out well, while rationalizing waiting to talk to her husband until he is less stressed at work.

> **Therapist:** I think you want me to be like your father, telling you what to do and how to feel, instead of paying attention to your own thoughts and feelings.
> **Ms. B** (*flustered*): I just want to know that things are going to be OK.
> **Therapist:** I think how things turn out depends on your being able to take a risk in asking for the affection and attention you need from your husband.
> **Ms. B** (*crying helplessly*): But what if he says he's too tired from work to spend time with me at night?

The therapist persistently confronts her resistance while monitoring his countertransference for sadistic impulses or sexual arousal in response to her crying.

Soon, Ms. B begins to interact more with her husband, initiating dinner dates and other activities outside of church attendance, and feels more optimistic about the marriage; the therapist understands this as a reaction formation and a "flight into health" given that she has not initiated a discussion about the Internet activity and their sex life is still nonexistent. The therapist actively confronts Ms. B's avoidance of conflict with her husband and with her father, who continues to make inordinate demands on her time.

> **Therapist:** Have you talked to your husband yet?
> **Ms. B:** Not yet, he's so stressed out…
> **Therapist:** And you're not?
> **Ms. B:** Well, yes, but it's better now that we've been going out to dinner…
> **Therapist:** I think what you've been saying is that you need more—more love and affection, not just dinners out.
> **Ms. B** (*after a long moment of reflection*): That's true…maybe I can come home earlier from work today, just call my parents instead of stopping by, turn off the phone, and make a nice dinner at home…candles and nice music might put us both in a more relaxed mood to talk.

Ms. B's husband reacts warmly. He acknowledges that he has been frustrated by her indifference to him, which makes him feel old and lonely. He tells her that he has enjoyed the extra time they now spend together and is pleasantly surprised that they are talking openly for the first time in their marriage.

As treatment intensifies, Ms. B gets in touch with her anger, first at the therapist and then at her husband, not only for his Internet activity but also for not helping her more with their children and her parents. She then also feels anger at her father for demeaning her husband, for inappropriate demands on her time, and for criticizing her mother. Successfully working through these feelings helps Ms. B create more mature relationships with her parents and husband.

After 5 months of treatment, Ms. B is ready for termination as her attention shifts to her renewed, and increasingly healthy, relationship with her husband. A flexible date for termination is set. The therapist addresses Ms. B's feelings of separation and loss. Ms. B seesaws between feeling ready to go and needing reassurance from her therapist when she experiences conflict with her husband. The therapist encourages her to take on the role he has been playing in questioning her behavior and gives her time to feel ready to terminate treatment. Ms. B resolves her ambivalence and decides that she can handle things on her own. She ends therapy with sadness and gratitude.

Therapy Approach 2: Relational Time-Limited Dynamic Psychotherapy[2]

In keeping with a relational time-limited approach, the first aim is to develop a good working alliance. The therapist tries to acknowledge Ms. B's self-presentation and explore how important it is for her to perform at such a high level with all of her responsibilities. The therapist then begins to discern and to explore the interpersonal context related to Ms. B's story. In order to facilitate deriving a dynamic formulation concerning the relational themes (in content and in process) in her life, a method of organizing clinical information around the CMP (Levenson 1995) is used. With this method, the therapist is particularly interested in what the client has to say about her own thoughts, wishes, feelings, and behaviors toward others (e.g., "I wish I could do a better job at work"); her expectations of others' behaviors (e.g., "My husband would not like it if I interrupted him while he is on the computer"); the behavior of others (e.g., "My sister leaves me to take

---

[2]Discussion of this therapy approach was kindly provided by Hanna Levenson, Ph.D.

care of our parents"); and how she treats and views herself (e.g., "I feel ashamed that sometimes I feel resentful"). These are placed into a narrative that describes the interlocking, interpersonal framework of how one's expectations about how one will be treated by others lead to certain behaviors that then invite others' complementary behaviors, which in turn reinforce a sense of self that leads to further unrewarding actions and expectations, thus becoming a self-fulfilling prophecy—the cyclical pattern of maladaptive behavior.

In addition, as part of the TLDP approach, the therapist needs to be very aware of his or her own internal and external reactions to Ms. B—what the therapist is pulled or pushed to do as he or she interacts with the patient (i.e., interactive countertransference).

Several themes in Ms. B's description of her life and in her style of interacting both in and out of the therapy room emerge, even during the first few sessions, with a recurring interpersonal scenario. Ms. B had always been the good daughter, wife, mother, and worker. Growing up, her place in her family was that of the easy child, for which she got much praise. As she matured, she found that her taking care of everyone else's needs and meeting others' expectations reinforced this role to the extent that she lost touch with what she needed and who she was. Others viewed her as a "can do" type of person and relied on her resourcefulness and consideration. She has seen herself as someone who is ready to make personal sacrifices and this was congruent with her own self-image. But on the cusp of her sixtieth birthday, Ms. B is feeling resentful of how little time she has for herself and how little attention she has received in her life. Whenever her frustrations "leak out" in an abrupt tone of voice or an angry word, she feels guilty and ashamed. As a consequence, she was quite conflicted about exploring other facets of herself and allowing herself to have a broader range of feelings. Thus, she becomes depressed but can only acknowledge it to herself in the form of somatic complaints, for which she has sought medical treatment.

In the initial session, the therapist experiences Ms. B as very willing to be the "good patient." She readily consents to the therapist's request to videotape her and is reluctant to ask for a different appointment time even though the one given to her was not convenient. In terms of interactive countertransference, the therapist is already aware of wanting something more from her (i.e., more congruent affect, more of a sense of entitlement), just as do others in her life. Her smiling affably while talking of how many demands people place on her and how she tries to do them all makes the therapist want to shake her and shout, "Don't be such a doormat!" However, her sad eyes and slumped shoulders also pull for compassion.

The primary experiential goal for the therapy, derived from the CMP, is to make use of experiences within the therapy where she can put her needs first and not be punished or shamed by the therapist. The therapist also tries to encourage Ms. B's risking this new behavior outside of the therapy session and then processing how it goes in the sessions. Consistent with this approach, another goal is to help Ms. B experience and express a wider range of feelings (e.g., anger, joy, pride). In keeping with the relational, recursive model of TLDP, as Ms. B takes a more assertive stance in life, others do not take her as much for granted and come to respect and notice her more. For example, she makes it clear to her husband that she wants to spend more time with him, and he is able to do this, with the result that the marriage is more rewarding for both of them. At work, she is able to set limits on some of her duties and is in the process of asking for a raise when the therapy ends. In session, such changes are also evident. For example, Ms. B becomes irritated with something her therapist says and is able to tell the therapist directly. Ms. B's more active, straightforward behaviors and the resultant changes in how others react to her dramatically affect her sense of self. She comes to see herself as more powerful. She begins to draw again (something she has not done since high school) and is thinking of taking some art classes. Her depression is markedly reduced. Although she is somewhat anxious about "breaking all these old molds," she also leaves therapy after 18 sessions, feeling as if she has a "new lease on life."

The elements of TLDP illustrated in this vignette are the following:

- Need to develop a good alliance quickly
- Delineation of the core cyclical dynamic pattern, which becomes the focus of the work
- Development of experiential goals
- Use of interactive countertransference to inform the formulation as well as to direct the nature of the change
- Opportunity to practice new relational behaviors and attitudes inside and outside the therapy room (i.e., corrective interactive emotional experiences)

Therapy Approach 3: Mann's Integrative Time-Limited Psychotherapy

The therapist using an integrative time-limited approach first conducts several initial interviews to clarify what Ms. B is seeking from therapy and to collect details about her history with which to formulate the central issue, which includes time, affects, and her negative self-image, and which is stated as follows: "You are a competent, capable, hard-working woman whom others have always been able to depend upon. However, you now feel and have always felt unimportant and unworthy." Next, the therapist gauges

Ms. B's reaction to the statement, which, in keeping with her compliant attitude, is to agree with the statement although she says she is surprised and doesn't know why she feels this way because her life is good and she has been blessed. The therapist then asks Ms. B to agree to a 12-session treatment schedule, informs her of the date and duration of each session, including the date of the final session, and asks for her response. Ms. B says that she's worried she won't know what to talk about because she doesn't think she has any real problems compared to other people's suffering.

In the first two sessions, a positive transference develops as the therapist encourages Ms. B to talk about the increased demands on her time at work, in caring for her parents, and in helping her sons, and as the therapist empathizes with her feelings of chronic fatigue and ill health. Ms. B reports that she looks forward to sessions, and by the third or fourth session she starts to feel better and do more for herself, while the therapist maintains a steady focus on the central issue—Ms. B's tendency to sacrifice her own needs to the needs of others, which maintains their dependency and prevents her from experiencing separation and loss through normal developmental phases. During this phase of treatment, the therapist learns a great deal more about the roots of Ms. B's problem in not being allowed to separate and individuate in her original family while growing up. She also begins to talk about her secret fantasy of quitting her job and becoming a travel agent. As the therapist continues to return her attention to the central issue by interrupting Ms. B's fantasies and suggesting they work on the problem at hand, her initial enthusiasm changes to irritation. Now in the middle of the treatment, she experiences the therapist in terms of earlier ambivalence toward her parents, who did not attend to her needs but rather demanded that she be "good" while they focused on her sister, who got the lion's share of their attention while Ms. B was pushed to the sidelines, where she enviously watched her sister's adventures and exploits.

A negatively toned transference develops, and Ms. B begins to resist the treatment. Characteristic defenses such as reaction formation, somatization, and isolation of affect reappear along with denial of the seriousness of her situation, couched in a religious idiom. In the last set of sessions, Ms. B cancels one because of a vague somatic complaint. When the therapist queries her awareness of the impending end of treatment, she denies remembering that a date for termination was scheduled at the outset and becomes uncharacteristically irritable, complaining that there is not enough time left to solve her problems. She begins to talk about being angry with her boss, who has shifted a number of onerous responsibilities to her job description without taking time to teach her new skills or give her direction. The therapist interprets her anger at her boss and at her parents for expecting too much and not helping her more. The therapist observes that this pattern is being repeated at work, where "being good" has resulted in more work for the same pay without adequate support and guidance.

By now it is obvious that Ms. B's problems stem from her inability to say no to the unreasonable demands of others, especially her parents—who have an extensive social network and sufficient financial resources not to have to rely on her exclusively—and her sons—who are well educated and able-bodied. This situation has alienated her husband, who has retreated into online computer games and perusing eBay. The therapist makes interpretations directed to Ms. B's negative self-image, which has developed over years of subordinating her needs to the needs of others while never being recognized or rewarded for her self-sacrifice and hard work.

The termination phase in time-limited psychotherapy typically involves strong affects. In the next-to-last session, Ms. B questions her faith and rails at God as she unconsciously experiences the therapist as abandoning her. In the last session, Ms. B is more sad than angry and has positive feelings about what she has learned in therapy as she separates from the therapist.

During a 6-month follow-up interview, the interviewer discovers that after an initial period of disorganization and emotional upset, Ms. B did make significant changes in her life in terms of being able to set boundaries with her parents and sons, which freed up time to take a long-postponed vacation with her husband. With his support and encouragement, she asked for a raise and got it, which enhanced her self-esteem. Although she still attends church on Sundays, she continues to question her faith and its demands for unquestioning obedience to authority. As she begins to assert herself, Ms. B's somatic complaints, depression, and fatigue subside and she has more energy and enthusiasm for life.

Conclusion

The development of brief dynamic psychotherapy has followed a path similar to that of long-term psychodynamic therapy, with drive/structural models adhering to classic psychoanalysis, relational models adhering to the British object relations theory, and integrative models being connected to contemporary psychodynamic theories. Although these approaches have distinctly different flavors, all of them a) pay attention to the therapeutic relationship, b) have an active therapeutic stance, c) emphasize the development of a clear but narrow focus for treatment, d) have restrictive patient inclusion criteria, and e) limit the length of therapy and/or number of sessions.

Recent reviews of randomized controlled studies (Abbass et al. 2006; Leichsenring et al. 2006) demonstrate the value of brief dynamic psychotherapy across a wide range of mental disorders, with improvements maintained for up to 4 years. New methodologically strong studies are also being presented on the use of BPP in areas previously unreported, such as treating panic disorder (Milrod et al. 2007). This is a positive trend given that not all patients respond to other brief therapies such as cognitive-behavioral therapy, interpersonal psychotherapy, or the experiential therapies. We also need to study whether BPP can be integrated synergistically with these therapies and/or with medications to obtain more robust results. Clearly, BPP has emerged from the shadow of the better-studied cognitive-behavioral and interpersonal therapies. The decision as to which approach to select for a specific patient should be based on the empirical literature rather than personal preference. This literature is emerging at a rapid pace and will no doubt support exciting opportunities for both trainees and patients.

Key Points

- There are various models of brief psychodynamic psychotherapy (BPP).
- Models of BPP differ according to many variables, such as the therapist's involvement as participant versus observer.
- Most therapies consist of fewer than 24 sessions and last less than 6 months.
- Techniques used in long-term dynamic therapy are also used in brief dynamic therapy.
- Attention is given to rapid formation of a therapeutic alliance.
- Drive/structural models adhere to Freud's classic psychoanalytic theory.
- Relational models focus on object relations principles.
- Integrative models attend to both classic and object relations principles.
- Brief therapies can be useful for many patients with a variety of psychiatric problems.
- Randomized controlled trials have demonstrated the efficacy of BPP.

References

Abbass AA, Hancock JT, Henderson J, et al: Short term psychodynamic psychotherapies for common mental disorders. Cochrane Database Syst Rev (4):CD004687, 2006

Alexander F, French TM: Psychoanalytic Therapy: Principles and Application. New York, Ronald Press, 1946

Balint M, Ornstein PH, Blaint E: Focal Psychotherapy, an Example of Applied Psychoanalysis. London, Tavistock, 1972

Bellak L: Handbook of Intensive Brief and Emergency Psychotherapy, 2nd Edition. Larchmont, NY, C.P.S., 1992

Book H: Guidelines for the practice of brief psychodynamic psychotherapy, in Standards and Guidelines for the Psychotherapies. Edited by Cameron P, Ennis J, Deadman J. Toronto, University of Toronto Press, 1998, pp 150–180

Bowlby J: A Secure Base: Parent-Child Attachment and Healthy Human Development. New York, Basic Books, 1988

Breuer J, Freud S: Studies on hysteria (1893–1895), in The Standard Edition of the Complete Psychological Works of Sigmund Freud, Vol 2. Translated and edited by Strachey J. London, Hogarth Press, 1955, pp 1–319

Budman S (ed): Forms of Brief Psychotherapy. New York, Guilford, 1981

Cashdan S: Object Relations Therapy: Using the Relationship. New York, WW Norton, 1988

Crits-Christoph P, Connolly MB: Alliance and technique in short-term dynamic therapy. Clin Psychol Rev 19:687–704, 1999

Daniel SI: Adult attachment patterns and individual psychotherapy: a review. Clin Psychol Rev 26:968–984, 2006

Davanloo H (ed): Short-Term Dynamic Psychotherapy. New York, Jason Aronson, 1980

Davanloo H: Intensive short-term dynamic psychotherapy, in Comprehensive Textbook of Psychiatry, 8th Edition. Edited by Sadock B, Sadock V. Baltimore, MD, Lippincott Williams & Wilkins, 2004, pp 2628–2652

Dewan MJ, Steenbarger BN, Greenberg RP: Brief psychotherapies, in The American Psychiatric Publishing Textbook of Psychiatry, 5th Edition. Edited by Hales RE, Yudofsky SC, Gabbard GO. Washington, DC, American Psychiatric Publishing, 2008, pp 1155–1170

Fairbairn WRD: Steps in the development of an object relations theory of the personality (1949), in Psychoanalytic Studies of the Personality (1959). London, Routledge, 1999, pp 152–161

Ferenczi S: The further development of an active therapy in psycho-analysis (1920), in Further Contributions to the Theory and Technique of Psycho-Analysis. Compiled by Rickman J. Translated by Suttie JI. London, Hogarth Press/Institute of Psycho-Analysis, 1926, pp 198–216

French TM: Psychoanalytic Interpretations: The Selected Papers of Thomas M. French. Chicago, IL, Quadrangle Books , 1970

Freud A: The Ego and the Mechanisms of Defence (1936). New York, International Universities Press, 1966

Freud S: The ego and the id (1923), in On Meta-psychology: The Theory of Psychoanalysis. Pelican Freud Library. London, Penguin Books, 1984, pp 341–406

Garfield SL: The Practice of Brief Psychotherapy. New York, Pergamon, 1989

Greenberg JR, Mitchell SA: Object Relations in Psychoanalytic Theory. Cambridge, MA, Harvard University Press, 1983

Gustafson JP: The Complex Secret of Brief Psychotherapy. New York, WW Norton, 1986

Horowitz M: Short term dynamic therapy of stress response syndromes, in Handbook of Short-Term Dynamic Psychotherapy. Edited by Crits-Christoph P, Barber JP. New York, Basic Books, 1991, pp 166–198

Horvath AO, Symonds BD: Relation between working alliance and outcome in psychotherapy: a meta-analysis. J Couns Psychol 38:139–149, 1991

Jones E: The Life and Work of Sigmund Freud. New York, Basic Books, 1957

Klein M: Our adult world and its roots in infancy (1959), in The Writings of Melanie Klein, Vol 3. London, Hogarth Press, 1975, pp 247–263

Leichsenring F: Are psychodynamic and psychoanalytic therapies effective? A review of empirical data. Int J Psychoanal 86:841–868, 2005

Leichsenring F, Hiller W, Weissberg M, et al: Cognitive behavioral therapy and psychodynamic psychotherapy: techniques, efficacy, and indications. Am J Psychother 60:233–259, 2006

Levenson H: Time-Limited Dynamic Psychotherapy: A Guide to Clinical Practice. New York, Basic Books, 1995

Levenson H: Time-limited dynamic psychotherapy: formulation and intervention, in The Art and Science of Brief Psychotherapies. Edited by Dewan MJ, Steenbarger BN, Greenberg RP. Washington, DC, American Psychiatric Publishing, 2004, pp 157–187

Luborsky L: Principles of Psychoanalytic Psychotherapy: A Manual for Supportive-Expressive Treatment. New York, Basic Books, 1984

Luborsky L, Crits-Christoph P: Understanding Transference: The Core Conflictual Relationship Theme Method. New York, Basic Books, 1990

Luborsky L, Mark D: Short-term supportive-expressive psychoanalytic psychotherapy, in Handbook of Short-Term Dynamic Psychotherapy. Edited by Barber JP, Crits-Christoph P. New York, Basic Books, 1991, pp 110–136

Mahler M, Pine F, Bergman A: The Psychological Birth of the Human Infant: Symbiosis and Individuation. New York, Basic Books, 1975

Malan DH: The Frontier of Brief Psychotherapy: An Example of the Convergence of Research and Clinical Practice. New York, Plenum, 1976

Malan DH: Individual Psychotherapy and the Science of Psychodynamics. Toronto, Butterworths, 1979

Mann J: Time-Limited Psychotherapy. Cambridge, MA, Harvard University Press, 1973

Mann J: The core of time-limited psychotherapy: time and the central issue, in Forms of Brief Therapy. Edited by Budman SH. New York, Guilford, 1981, pp 25–43

Mann J: Time-limited psychotherapy, in Handbook of Short-Term Dynamic Psychotherapy. Edited by Crits-Christoph P, Barber JP. New York, Basic Books, 1991, pp 17–44

Messer SB, Warren CS: Models of Brief Psychodynamic Therapy: A Comparative Approach. New York, Guilford, 1995

Milrod B, Leon AC, Busch F, et al: A randomized controlled clinical trial of psychoanalytic psychotherapy for panic disorder. Am J Psychiatry 164:265–272, 2007

Pine F: Drive, Ego, Object and Self: A Synthesis of Clinical Work. New York, Basic Books, 1990

Sifneos P: Short-Term Psychotherapy and Emotional Crisis. Cambridge, MA, Harvard University Press, 1972

Sifneos P: Short-term anxiety-provoking psychotherapy, in Forms of Brief Therapy. Edited by Budman S. New York, Guilford, 1981, pp 45–81

Sifneos P: Short-Term Anxiety-Provoking Psychotherapy: A Treatment Manual. Cambridge, MA, Harvard University Press, 1992

Sifneos P: Short-Term Dynamic Psychotherapy: Evaluation and Technique, 2nd Edition. New York, Springer, 2004

Strupp H, Binder J: Psychotherapy in a New Key. New York, Basic Books, 1984

Strupp H, Hadley S: Specific versus non-specific factors in psychotherapy: a controlled study of outcome. Arch Gen Psychiatry 36:1125–1136, 1979

Strupp H, Hadley S, Gomes-Schwartz S: Psychotherapy for Better or Worse. New York, Jason Aronson, 1977

Weiss J, Sampson J, Mount Zion Psychotherapy Research Group: The Psychoanalytic Process: Theory, Clinical Observations, and Empirical Research. New York, Guilford, 1986

Winnicott DW: The Maturational Processes and the Facilitating Environment: Studies in the Theory of Emotional Development. New York, International Universities Press, 1965

Winston A, Rosenthal R, Pinsker H: Introduction to Supportive Psychotherapy. Washington, DC, American Psychiatric Publishing, 2004

Suggested Readings

Dewan M, Steenbarger B, Greenberg R (eds): The Art and Science of Brief Psychotherapies: A Practitioner's Guide. Washington, DC, American Psychiatric Publishing, 2004

Messer SB, Warren CS: Models of Brief Psychodynamic Therapy: A Comparative Approach. New York, Guilford, 1995

Chapter 4

Applications of Psychodynamic Psychotherapy to Specific Disorders

Efficacy and Indications

Falk Leichsenring, D.Sc.

Empirical outcome research is needed in psychodynamic and psychoanalytic therapy (Gunderson and Gabbard 1999). In this chapter, I review the available evidence for both short-term and long-term psychodynamic psychotherapy (STPP and LTPP). In the first part, I discuss the procedures of evidence-based medicine and empirically supported treatments with regard

I would like to thank Dr. Gabbard for his helpful comments during review of this chapter.

to their applicability to psychotherapy. I then review the available randomized controlled trials (RCTs) of short-term and moderate-length psychodynamic psychotherapy in specific mental disorders. Because the methodology of RCTs is difficult to apply to LTPP, I close the chapter by reviewing the quasi-experimental effectiveness studies of LTPP.

Evidence-Based Medicine and Empirically Supported Treatments

Several proposals have been made to grade the available evidence of both medical and psychotherapeutic treatments (Canadian Task Force on the Periodic Health Examination 1979; Chambless and Hollon 1998; Clarke and Oxman 2003; Cook et al. 1995; Guyatt et al. 1995; Nathan and Gorman 2002; National Institute for Clinical Excellence 2002). Apart from other differences, all available proposals regard RCTs (efficacy studies) as the "gold standard" for demonstrating the efficacy of a treatment. According to this view, only RCTs can provide the highest level of evidence (i.e., level 1). RCTs are conducted under controlled experimental conditions: they allow the investigator to systematically control for variables that influence the outcome apart from the treatment. The defining feature of an RCT is the random assignment of subjects to the different conditions of treatment (Shadish et al. 2002). Randomization is regarded as indispensable in order to ensure that a priori existing differences among subjects are equally distributed. The goal of randomization is to attribute the observed effects exclusively to the applied therapy. Thus, randomization is used to ensure the internal validity of a study (Shadish et al. 2002).

Gabbard et al. (2002) have discussed different types of RCTs that provide different levels of evidence. The most stringent test of efficacy is achieved by comparing rival treatments while controlling for specific and unspecific therapeutic factors (Chambless and Hollon 1998, p. 8). Furthermore, such comparisons provide explicit information on the relative benefits of competing treatments. Treatments that are found to be superior to rival treatments are more highly valued. Gabbard and colleagues (2002) regard RCTs in which a treatment is compared with a psychological placebo as the second most rigorous type of RCT. However, in my view, comparisons with treatment as usual (TAU), which some consider third in the hierarchy, can provide more stringent tests than placebo-controlled studies because they control for both common factors (e.g., attention) and treatment effects of TAU. A drawback to TAU-controlled studies is that TAU is often poorly defined and differs from one study to another. In one study, for example, TAU may be a routine outpatient psychotherapy in clinical practice; in another study it may be a pure psychopharmacological treatment; and in yet another study it may include counseling or other forms of health care. The fourth most rigorous form of RCT uses control subjects on a waiting list. However, in this type of study it is not clear whether the observed effect in the treatment group is to be attributed to specific or non-specific therapeutic factors (Gabbard et al. 2002). The next level of evidence is provided by prospective open studies, followed by case series and, finally, case reports.

The exclusive position of RCTs in psychotherapy research, however, has recently been challenged (Beutler 1998; Fonagy 1999; Leichsenring 2004; Persons and Silberschatz 1998; Roth and Parry 1997; Rothwell 2005; Seligman 1995; Westen et al. 2004). Following the methodology of pharmacological research in psychotherapy research is questionable. In psychotherapy research, the defining features of RCTs—such as randomization, use of treatment manuals, focus on a specific mental disorder, and frequent exclusion of patients with a poor prognosis—raise the issue of whether RCTs are sufficiently representative of clinical practice (Beutler 1998; Fonagy 1999; Leichsenring 2004; Persons and Silberschatz 1998; Roth and Parry 1997; Rothwell 2005; Seligman 1995; Westen et al. 2004). Furthermore, the methodology of RCTs, with their use of treatment manuals and randomized, controlled conditions, is hardly applicable to long-term psychotherapy lasting several years (Seligman 1995; Wallerstein 1999). Another debatable aspect of the empirically supported treatment approach is the emphasis on disorders and symptoms (Blatt 1995). As Henry (1998, p. 129) noted: "EVTs [empirically validated treatments] place the emphasis on the disorder...and not on the individual...who seeks our services." Furthermore, if a method of psychotherapy has been shown to work under controlled conditions, this does not necessarily imply that it will work equally well under the conditions of clinical practice (Leichsenring 2004). The main reason for this gap is that psychotherapy is not a drug that works equally under different conditions. Difficult-to-quantify factors in the therapist–patient match may influence outcome. Thus, it is questionable whether the methodology for pharmacological research is adequate for research on psychotherapeutic treatments of mental disorders, at least if the effectiveness of a treatment in clinical practice is to be predicted. After all, RCTs serve only a limited function (Roth and Parry 1997, p. 370): "RCTs are...an imperfect tool; almost certainly their results are best seen as one part of a research cycle."

In contrast to RCTs, naturalistic studies (effectiveness studies) are conducted under the conditions of clinical practice. Their results are therefore more representative for clinical practice with regard to patients, therapists, and treatments (external validity) (Shadish et al. 2000). Effectiveness studies cannot control for factors affecting treatment outcome to the same extent that RCTs can (internal validity). However, the internal validity of effectiveness studies can be improved by quasi-experimental designs using methods other than randomization to rule out alternative explanations of the results (Leichsenring 2004; Shadish et al. 2002).

Paradoxically, naturalistic studies are not accepted by, for example, the American Psychological Association as methods for demonstrating that a therapy works (American Psychological Association 1995; Chambless and Hollon 1998; Chambless and Ollendick 2001). The main argument against naturalistic studies refers to threats to the internal validity, that is, to the ability to control factors influencing outcome apart from therapy. However, according to several studies, there is evidence that effectiveness studies do not overestimate effect sizes compared with RCTs (Benson and Hartz 2000; Concato et al. 2000; Shadish et al. 2000).

According to these considerations, efficacy and effectiveness studies address different research questions: RCTs examine the efficacy of a treatment under controlled experimental conditions, whereas effectiveness studies address the effectiveness under clinical practice conditions (Leichsenring 2004). As a consequence, the results of an efficacy study cannot be directly transferred to clinical practice and vice versa (Leichsenring 2004). From this perspective, a distinction is required between empirically supported therapies and RCT methodology (Leichsenring 2004; Westen et al. 2004). The relationship between RCTs and effectiveness studies should not be considered rivalrous; rather, it is complementary.

Evidence for Psychodynamic Psychotherapy in Specific Mental Disorders

One aim of this review is to identify the mental disorders for which RCTs of both STPP and LTPP are available. Here, the criteria proposed by the American Psychological Association Task Force on Promotion and Dissemination of Psychological Procedures (American Psychological Association 1995) to define efficacious treatments, as modified by Chambless and Hollon (1998), were applied. Previous reviews have been written—for example, by Fonagy et al. (2005) and by myself (Leichsenring 2005). Naturalistic (effectiveness) studies of LTPP are reviewed later in this chapter (see "Effectiveness of Long-Term Psychodynamic Psychotherapy in Patients With Complex Mental Disorders: Evidence From Quasi-experimental Naturalistic Studies").

Definition of Psychodynamic Psychotherapy

Psychodynamic psychotherapy operates on an interpretive-supportive continuum. The use of more interpretive or supportive interventions depends on the patient's needs (Gabbard 2004; Gunderson and Gabbard 1999; Waller-stein 1989). Gabbard (2004) has suggested considering therapies of more than 24 sessions or lasting longer than 6 months long-term; in this review, I use this threshold to distinguish between STPP and LTPP. With regard to STPP, different models have been developed, as reviewed by, for example, Messer and Warren (1995). Gabbard's definition of LTPP is the working model of this chapter: LTPP is "a therapy that involves careful attention to the therapist–patient interaction, with thoughtfully timed interpretation of transference and resistance embedded in a sophisticated appreciation of the therapist's contribution to the two-person field" (Gabbard 2004, p. 2).

Thirty-one RCTs providing evidence for psychodynamic psychotherapy have been included in this review (see Table 4–1). Studies examining the combination of psychodynamic therapy and medication are considered in Chapter 5 ("Combining Psychodynamic Psychotherapy With Medication").

Therapy Duration

In the RCTs of psychodynamic psychotherapy, between 7 and 46 sessions of therapy were conducted (Table 4–1). According to the definition of STPP versus LTPP given above, 19 studies (61%) examined STPP (range=7–24 sessions) and 12 studies (39%) examined LTPP (range=24.9–46 sessions, with a treatment duration of up to 3 years). The efficacy studies of LTPP examined time-limited psychodynamic psychotherapy as contrasted to open-ended long-term psychodynamic psychotherapy (for this differentiation, see Luborsky 1984).

Models of Psychodynamic Psychotherapy

In the studies identified, different forms of psychodynamic psychotherapy were applied (Table 4–1). The models developed by Luborsky (1984), M. Horowitz (1976), and Shapiro and Firth (1985) were used most frequently.

Evidence for the Efficacy of Psychodynamic Psychotherapy

The studies included in this review are presented according to the type of mental disorder being treated. However, from a psychodynamic perspective, the results of a therapy for a specific psychiatric disorder (e.g., depression, ag-oraphobia) are influenced by the underlying psychodynamic features (e.g., conflicts, defenses, personality organization), which may vary considerably within one category of psychiatric disorder (Kernberg 1996). These psychodynamic factors may affect treatment outcome and may have a greater impact on outcome than the phenomenological DSM categories (Piper et al. 2001).

TABLE 4–1. Randomized controlled studies of psychodynamic psychotherapy (PP) in specific psychiatric disorders

Disorder	Study	n (PP)	Comparison group	Concept of PP	Treatment duration
Depressive disorders					
Depression	Thompson et al. 1987	24	BT: $n=25$; CBT: $n=27$; waiting list: $n=19$	Horowitz and Kaltreider (1979)	16–20 sessions
Depression	Shapiro et al. 1994	58	CBT: $n=59$	Shapiro and Firth (1985)	8 vs. 16 sessions
Depression	Gallagher-Thompson and Steffen 1994	30	CBT: $n=36$	Mann 1973; Rose and DelMaestro (1990)	16–20 sessions
Depression	Barkham et al. 1996	18	CBT: $n=18$	Shapiro and Firth (1985)	8 vs. 16 sessions
Dysthymic disorder	Maina et al. 2005	10	Supportive therapy: $n=10$; waiting list: $n=10$	Malan 1976	15–30 sessions; mean, 19.6
Anxiety disorders					
Panic disorder	Milrod et al. 2007	26	CBT (applied relaxation): $n=23$	Busch et al. (1999)	24 sessions
Social phobia	Knijnik et al. 2004	15	Credible placebo control group: $n=15$	Knijnik et al. (2004)	12 sessions
Social phobia	Bögels et al. 2003	22	CBT: $n=27$	Malan (1976)	36 sessions

TABLE 4–1. Randomized controlled studies of psychodynamic psychotherapy (PP) in specific psychiatric disorders *(continued)*

Disorder	Study	n (PP)	Comparison group	Concept of PP	Treatment duration
Anxiety disorders *(continued)*					
GAD	Crits-Christoph et al. 2005	15	Supportive therapy: $n=16$	Luborsky (1984); Crits-Christoph et al. (1995)	16 sessions
GAD	Leichsenring et al., unpublished ms., 2008	25	CBT: $n=25$	Luborsky (1984); Crits-Christoph et al. (1995)	30 sessions
PTSD	Brom et al. 1989	29	Desensitization: $n=31$; hypnotherapy: $n=29$	M. Horowitz (1976)	18.8 sessions[a]
Somatoform disorders					
Irritable bowel	Guthrie et al. 1991	50	Supportive listening: $n=46$	Hobson (1985); Shapiro and Firth (1985)	8 sessions
Irritable bowel	Creed et al. 2003	59	Paroxetine: $n=43$; TAU: $n=86$	Hobson (1985); Shapiro and Firth (1985)	8 sessions
Functional dyspepsia	Hamilton et al. 2000	37	Supportive therapy: $n=36$	Shapiro and Firth (1985)	7 sessions
Somatoform pain disorder	Monsen and Monsen 2000	20	TAU/no therapy: $n=20$	Monsen and Monsen (1999)	33 sessions

TABLE 4–1. Randomized controlled studies of psychodynamic psychotherapy (PP) in specific psychiatric disorders *(continued)*

Disorder	Study	n (PP)	Comparison group	Concept of PP	Treatment duration
Eating disorders					
Bulimia nervosa	Fairburn et al. 1986	11	CBT: $n=11$	Bruch (1973); Rosen (1979); Stunkard (1976)	19 sessions
Bulimia nervosa	Garner et al. 1993	25	CBT: $n=25$	Luborsky (1984)	19 sessions
Bulimia nervosa, anorexia nervosa	Bachar et al. 1999	17	Cognitive therapy: $n=17$; nutritional counseling: $n=10$	Barth (1991); Geist (1989); Goodsitt (1985)	46 sessions
Anorexia nervosa	Dare et al. 2001	21	Cognitive-analytic therapy (Ryle 1990): $n=22$; family therapy: $n=22$; TAU: $n=19$	Dare (1995); Malan (1976)	24.9 sessions[a]
Anorexia nervosa	Gowers et al. 1994	20	TAU: $n=20$	Crisp (1980)	12 sessions
Substance-related disorders					
Opiate dependence	Woody et al. 1983, 1990	31	DC: $n=35$; CBT+DC: $n=34$	Luborsky (1984)	12 sessions
Opiate dependence	Woody et al. 1995	57	DC: $n=27$	Luborsky (1984)	26 sessions

TABLE 4–1. Randomized controlled studies of psychodynamic psychotherapy (PP) in specific psychiatric disorders *(continued)*

Disorder	Study	n (PP)	Comparison group	Concept of PP	Treatment duration
Substance-related disorders *(continued)*					
Alcohol dependence	Sandahl et al. 1998	25	CBT: *n*=24	Foulkes (1964)	15 sessions; mean, 8.9
Cocaine dependence	Crits-Christoph et al. 1999, 2001	124	CBT+group DC: *n*=119; group DC: *n*=123; individual DC+ group DC: *n*=121	Mark and Luborsky (1992)	≤36 individual and 24 group DC sessions; 4 months
Personality disorders					
BPD	Munroe-Blum and Marziali 1995	31	Interpersonal group therapy: *n*=25	Kernberg (1975)	17 sessions
BPD	Bateman and Fonagy 1999, 2001	19	TAU: *n*=19	Bateman and Fonagy (1999)	18 months
BPD	Clarkin et al. 2007	30	Dialectical behavioral therapy: *n*=30; supportive therapy: *n*=30	Clarkin et al. (1999b)	12 months

TABLE 4–1.   Randomized controlled studies of psychodynamic psychotherapy (PP) in specific psychiatric disorders *(continued)*

Disorder	Study	n (PP)	Comparison group	Concept of PP	Treatment duration
Personality disorders *(continued)*					
BPD	Giesen-Bloo et al. 2006	42	CBT: $n=44$	Clarkin et al. (1999b)	3 years with sessions twice a week
Cluster C personality disorders	Svartberg et al. 2004	25	CBT: $n=25$	Malan (1976); McCullough Vaillant (1997)	40 sessions
Cluster C personality disorders	Muran et al. 2005	22	Brief relational therapy: $n=33$; CBT: $n=29$	Pollack et al. (1992)	30 sessions
Avoidant personality disorder	Emmelkamp et al. 2006	23	CBT: $n=21$; waiting list: $n=18$	Luborsky (1984); Luborsky and Mark (1991); Malan (1976); Pinsker et al. (1991)	20 sessions

Note.   BPD=borderline personality disorder; BT=behavior therapy; CBT=cognitive–behavioral therapy; DC=drug counseling; GAD=generalized anxiety disorder; PTSD=posttraumatic stress disorder; TAU=treatment as usual.
[a]Mean.

Major Depression

Cognitive-behavioral therapists increase patients' activity and help them work through depressive cognitions. Psychodynamic therapists focus on the conflicts or ego functions associated with the depressive symptoms. As of this writing, four RCTs are available that provide evidence for the efficacy of STPP compared with cognitive-behavioral therapy (CBT) in depression (Barkham et al. 1996; Gallagher-Thompson and Steffen 1994; Shapiro et al. 1994; Thompson et al. 1987). Different models of STPP were applied (Table 4–1). In a meta-analysis of these studies, STPP and CBT proved to be equally efficacious with regard to reducing depressive symptoms and general psychiatric symptoms and improving social functioning (Leichsenring 2001). A more detailed discussion of these results has been presented elsewhere (Leichsenring 2006). In the meta-analysis, STPP achieved large pre-post effect sizes for depressive symptoms, general psychiatric symptoms, and social functioning (Leichsenring 2001). Furthermore, the results proved to be stable in follow-up studies (Gallagher-Thompson et al. 1990; Shapiro et al. 1995). The results are also consistent with the findings of the meta-analysis by Wampold et al. (2002), in which there were no significant differences between CBT and "other therapies" in the treatment of depression. In a small RCT, Maina et al. (2005) examined the efficacy of STPP and brief supportive therapy in the treatment of minor depressive disorders (dysthymic disorder, depressive disorder not otherwise specified, or adjustment disorder with depressed mood). Both treatments were superior to a waiting-list condition at the end of treatment. At 6-month follow-up, STPP was superior to brief supportive therapy.

Pathological Grief

In two RCTs by McCallum and Piper (1990) and Piper et al. (2001), the use of short-term psychodynamic group therapy to treat prolonged or complicated grief was studied. In the first study, short-term psychodynamic group therapy was significantly superior to a waiting-list condition (McCallum and Piper 1990). In the second study, a significant interaction was found between the quality of patients' object relations and the success of different types of therapy in improving different types of symptoms. With regard to grief symptoms, patients with high-quality object relations improved more with interpretive therapy, whereas patients with low-quality object relations improved more with supportive therapy. For general symptoms, clinical significance favored interpretive therapy over supportive therapy (Piper et al. 2001). In both studies (McCallum and Piper 1990; Piper et al. 2001) a considerable proportion of patients received psychopharmacological treatments (45% and 55%, respectively). The treatment conditions compared, however, did not differ with regard to the use of medication. Thus, internal validity was not impaired. The results of these studies apply to the combined treatment of short-term psychodynamic group therapy and medication.

Anxiety Disorders

Results from five RCTs of psychodynamic psychotherapy for anxiety disorders are currently available (Table 4–1). With regard to *panic disorder* (with or without agoraphobia), Milrod et al. (2007) showed in a recent RCT that STPP was more successful than applied relaxation. For *social phobia*, two RCTs of psychodynamic therapy exist: In one study (Knijnik et al. 2004), short-term psychodynamic group treatment for generalized social phobia was superior to the use of a credible placebo control. In the other RCT, LTPP proved to be as efficacious as CBT in the treatment of generalized social phobia (Bögels et al. 2003). In a randomized, controlled feasibility study of *generalized anxiety disorder*, STPP and a supportive therapy were equally efficacious with regard to continuous measures of anxiety, but STPP was significantly superior in terms of symptomatic remission rates (Crits-Christoph et al. 2005). However, the sample sizes of that study were relatively small ($n=15$ vs. $n=16$), and the study was not sufficiently powered to detect more of the possible differences between treatments.

In another RCT, STPP was compared with CBT in the treatment of generalized anxiety disorder (F. Leichsenring, C. Winkelbach, E. Leibing: "Short-Term Psychodynamic Psychotherapy and Cognitive-Behavioral Therapy in Generalized Anxiety Disorder: A Randomized Controlled Study," unpublished manuscript, 2008). Thus far, STPP and CBT have been equally efficacious with regard to the primary outcome measure; however, in some secondary outcome measures, CBT seemed to be superior. The results of the 1-year follow-up are not yet available, so it is not known whether the differences persist in the long run. Furthermore, a large-scale multicenter RCT comparing STPP and CBT in the treatment of social phobia is currently being carried out (Leichsenring et al., in press).

The fifth RCT of psychodynamic psychotherapy for anxiety disorders is a study of *posttraumatic stress disorder* (PTSD). Brom et al. (1989) compared the effects of STPP, behavior therapy (desensitization), and hypnotherapy in patients with PTSD. All of the treatments proved to be equally efficacious and were superior to no treatment as shown in a waiting-list control group. Results of STPP not only were maintained but continued to improve at the 3-month follow-up. However, further studies of psychodynamic psychotherapy in PTSD are required.

Somatoform Disorders

As of this writing, four RCTs of STPP in somatoform disorders are available (Table 4–1). In the RCT by Guthrie et al. (1991), patients with *irritable bowel syndrome* who had not responded to standard medical treatment over the previous 6 months were treated with STPP in addition to standard medical treatment. This approach was compared with standard medical treatment alone. STPP was found to be efficacious in two-thirds of the patients. In another RCT, STPP was significantly more efficacious than routine care and as efficacious as medication (paroxetine) in the treatment of severe irritable bowel syndrome (Creed et al. 2003). During the follow-up period, however, STPP—but not paroxetine—was associated with a significant reduction in health care costs compared with routine care. In an RCT by Hamilton et al. (2000), STPP was compared with supportive therapy in the treatment of patients with chronic, intractable *functional dyspepsia* who had failed to respond to conventional pharmacological treatments. At the end of treatment, STPP was significantly superior to supportive therapy, and the effects were stable during the 12-month follow-up. Monsen and Monsen (2000) compared psychodynamic psychotherapy of 33 sessions versus no treatment or TAU in the treatment of patients with chronic pain. Psychodynamic psychotherapy had significantly superior results as shown on measures of pain, psychiatric symptoms, interpersonal problems, and affect consciousness. The results remained stable or even improved during the 12-month follow-up. Thus, psychodynamic psychotherapy can be recommended for the treatment of somatoform disorders.

Eating Disorders

Bulimia nervosa. Three RCTs of STPP in the treatment of bulimia nervosa are available (Table 4–1). Significant and stable improvements in bulimia nervosa after STPP were demonstrated by Fairburn et al. (1986, 1995) and Garner et al. (1993). In the primary disorder–specific measures (bulimic episodes, self-induced vomiting), STPP was as efficacious as CBT (Fairburn et al. 1986, 1995; Garner et al. 1993). Apart from this, CBT was superior to STPP in some specific measures of psychopathology (Fairburn et al. 1986). However, in a follow-up of the Fairburn et al. 1986 study, in which a longer follow-up period (5.8±2.0 years) of was used, both forms of therapy proved to be equally efficacious and were partly superior to a behavioral form of therapy (Fairburn et al. 1995). Accordingly, longer-term studies are necessary for a valid evaluation of the efficacy of STPP in bulimia nervosa. In another RCT, STPP was significantly superior to both TAU (nutritional counseling) and cognitive therapy (Bachar et al. 1999).

This was true for patients with bulimia nervosa and a mixed sample of patients with bulimia nervosa or anorexia nervosa.

Anorexia nervosa.   Very few evidence-based treatments for the psychotherapeutic treatment of anorexia nervosa, either psychodynamic psychotherapy or CBT, are available (Fairburn 2005). In an RCT by Gowers et al. (1994), STPP combined with four sessions of nutritional advice yielded significant improvements in patients with anorexia nervosa (Table 4–1). Changes in weight and body mass index were significantly better than in a control group (patients receiving TAU). Dare et al. (2001) compared psychodynamic psychotherapy lasting a mean of 24.9 sessions with cognitive-analytic therapy, family therapy, and routine treatment in patients with anorexia nervosa (Table 4–1). Psychodynamic psychotherapy yielded significant symptomatic improvements, and STPP and family therapy were significantly superior to the routine treatment with regard to weight gain. However, the improvements were modest—several patients were undernourished at the follow-up. Thus, the treatment of anorexia nervosa remains a challenge, and more effective treatment models are required.

Substance-Related Disorders

Woody et al. (1983, 1990) studied the effects of STPP and of CBT given in addition to drug counseling versus drug counseling alone in the treatment of opiate dependence (Table 4–1). STPP plus drug counseling yielded significant improvements on measures of drug-related symptoms and general psychiatric symptoms. At the 7-month follow-up, the STPP and CBT treatments were equally efficacious, and both treatments were superior to drug counseling alone. In another RCT, psychodynamic psychotherapy (26 sessions) used in addition to drug counseling was also superior to drug counseling alone in the treatment of opiate dependence (Woody et al. 1995). At 6-month follow-up, most of the gains made by the patients who had received psychodynamic therapy remained.

In an RCT conducted by Crits-Christoph et al. (1999, 2001), psychodynamic psychotherapy of up to 36 individual sessions was combined with 24 sessions of group drug counseling in the treatment of cocaine dependence. The combined treatment yielded significant improvements and was as efficacious as CBT combined with group drug counseling. However, neither CBT plus group drug counseling nor psychodynamic psychotherapy plus group drug counseling was more efficacious than group drug counseling alone. Furthermore, individual drug counseling was significantly superior to both forms of therapy with regard to measures of drug abuse. With regard to psychological and social outcome variables, all treatments were equally efficacious (Crits-Christoph et al. 1999, 2001).

In an RCT, Sandahl et al. (1998) compared STPP and CBT in regard to their efficacy in the treatment of alcohol abuse. STPP yielded significant improvements on measures of alcohol abuse, which remained stable at a 15-month follow-up. STPP was significantly superior to CBT in terms of the number of abstinent days and the improvement of general psychiatric symptoms.

Personality Disorders

Borderline personality disorder. In an RCT conducted by Munroe-Blum and Marziali (1995), STPP yielded significant improvements on measures of borderline-related symptoms, general psychiatric symptoms, and depression, and was as efficacious as interpersonal group therapy (Table 4–1). Bateman and Fonagy (1999, 2001) studied psychoanalytically oriented partial hospitalization treatment for patients with borderline personality disorder. The major difference between the treatment group and the control group was the provision of individual and group psychotherapy in the former. The treatment lasted a maximum of 18 months, with LTPP defined by the criteria used in this review. LTPP was significantly superior to standard psychiatric care, both at the end of therapy and at the 18-month follow-up.

Giesen-Bloo et al. (2006) compared LTPP based on Kernberg's model (transference-focused psychotherapy, TFP; Clarkin et al. 1999b) with schema-focused therapy (SFT), a form of CBT. Treatment duration was 3 years, with two sessions a week. The authors reported statistically and clinically significant improvements with both treatments. However, SFT was found to be superior to TFP in several outcome measures. Furthermore, a significantly higher dropout risk was reported with TFP. This study, however, has serious methodological flaws. The authors used scales for adherence and competence for both treatments for which they adopted an identical cutoff score of 60 to indicate competent application. According to the data published by the authors (Giesen-Bloo et al. 2006), the median competence level for applying SFT methods was 85.7. For TFP, a value of 65.6 was reported. While the competence level for SFT clearly exceeded the cutoff, the competence level for TFP just surpassed it. Furthermore, the competence level for SFT was clearly higher than that for TFP. Accordingly, both treatments were not equally applied in terms of therapist competence. The results of this study are therefore questionable. The difference in competence was not taken into account by the authors, neither in the analysis of resulting data nor in the discussion of the results. Thus, this study raises serious concerns about an investigator allegiance effect (Luborsky et al. 1999).

Another RCT (Clarkin et al. 2007; Levy et al. 2006) compared psychodynamic psychotherapy (TFP), dialectical behavioral therapy (DBT), and psychodynamic supportive psychotherapy (SPT). All three modalities led to general improvement. However, TFP was shown to produce improvements not demonstrated by either DBT or SPT. Those participants who received TFP were more likely to move from an insecure attachment classification to a secure one. They also showed significantly greater changes in mentalizing capacity and narrative coherence compared with the other two groups. TFP was associated with significant improvement in 10 of the 12 variables across the six symptomatic domains compared with 6 for SPT and 5 for DBT. Only TFP led to significant changes in impulsivity, irritability, verbal assault, and direct assault. TFP and DBT reduced suicidality to the same extent.

A meta-analysis addressing the effects of psychodynamic psychotherapy and CBT in personality disorders found that psychodynamic psychotherapy yielded large effect sizes not only for comorbid symptoms but also for core personality pathology (Leichsenring and Leibing 2003). This was true for personality disorders in general and for borderline personality disorder in particular.

Cluster C personality disorders.   There is also evidence for the efficacy of psychodynamic psychotherapy in the treatment of patients with Cluster C personality disorders. In an RCT conducted by Svartberg et al. (2004), psychodynamic psychotherapy of 40 sessions in length was compared with CBT (Table 4–1). Both psychodynamic psychotherapy and CBT yielded significant improvements in patients with DSM-IV Cluster C personality disorders (i.e., avoidant, compulsive, and dependent personality disorders) (American Psychiatric Association 1994). Improvement was assessed in terms of reductions in symptoms, interpersonal problems, and core personality pathology. The results were stable at 24-month follow-up. No significant differences in efficacy were found between psychodynamic psychotherapy and CBT.

Muran et al. (2005) compared the efficacy of psychodynamic therapy, brief relational therapy, and CBT in the treatment of Cluster C personality disorders and personality disorder not otherwise specified. Treatments lasted for 30 sessions. With regard to mean changes in outcome measures, no significant differences were found among the treatments, either at termination or at follow-up. Furthermore, there were no significant differences among the treatments with regard to the patients' achieving clinically significant changes in symptoms, interpersonal problems, features of personality disorders, or therapist ratings of target complaints. At termination, CBT and brief relational therapy were superior to psychodynamic psychotherapy in one outcome measure, patient ratings of target complaints. However, this difference did not persist at 6-month follow-up. With regard to the percentage of patients showing change, no significant differences were found, either at termination or at follow-up, except in one comparison: at termination, CBT showed superiority to STPP on the Inventory of Interpersonal Problems (L.M. Horowitz et al. 2000). Again, this difference did not persist at follow-up. Thus, only a few significant differences were found among the treatments, and the differences did not remain at follow-up.

Avoidant personality disorder is among the cluster C personality disorders mentioned above. In a recent RCT, Emmelkamp et al. (2006) compared CBT with STPP or no treatment (a waiting-list condition) for avoidant personality disorder. The authors reported that CBT was more efficacious than no treatment and more effective than STPP. However, the study has several methodological shortcomings (Leichsenring and Leibing 2006), and the study's design, statistical analyses, and reporting of the results raise serious concerns about an investigator allegiance effect (Luborsky et al. 1999).

Effectiveness of Long-Term Psychodynamic Psychotherapy in Patients With Complex Mental Disorders: Evidence From Quasi-experimental Naturalistic Studies

As discussed earlier, the methodology of RCT does not lend itself well to long-term psychotherapy lasting several years. For these long-term treatments, effectiveness studies (naturalistic studies) are the appropriate method of research (de Maat et al. 2006; Leichsenring 2004; Seligman 1995; Wallerstein 1999; Westen et al. 2004). The National Institute of Mental Health (NIMH) has specifically called for more effectiveness research (Krupnick et al. 1996).

Pre-Post Effect Sizes

With regard to LTPP lasting several years, several effectiveness studies that used reliable and valid outcome measures (Brockmann et al. 2001; Dührssen and Jorswieck 1965; Grande et al. 2006; Leichsenring et al. 2005; Luborsky et al. 2001; Rudolf et al. 1994; Sandell et al. 1999, 2000) have provided evidence that LTPP yields large pre-post or pre-follow-up effect sizes according to the definition given by Cohen (Cohen 1988; Kazis et al. 1989). Some of these studies included control or comparison groups, whereas others reported only pre-post or pre-follow-up effect sizes (Leichsenring et al. 2005; Luborsky et al. 2001). These effect sizes refer to symptoms, interpersonal problems, social adjustment, the number of inpatient days, and other outcome criteria. According to the hierarchy proposed by Gabbard et al. (2002), these studies provide level 5 evidence. Another hierarchy of evidence proposed specifically for naturalistic studies would have these studies correspond to level 2 or level 3 evidence (Leichsenring 2004). Controlled studies are reviewed below.

Recently, a proposal has been made for an alternative approach to the question of control groups in psychotherapy outcome research (Leichsenring and Rabung 2006). The mean changes that occurred in control groups of RCTs of psychodynamic therapy were assessed in a meta-analysis. Both waiting-list and TAU control groups were included. According to the results, the mean changes occurring in waiting-list and TAU control groups corresponded to a small effect size of $d = 0.12$. The effect sizes of some open studies of psychodynamic therapy significantly exceeded the changes found in control groups (Leichsenring and Rabung 2006). This was also true for the studies of LTPP by Rudolf et al. (1994), Luborsky et al. (2001), and Leichsenring et al. (2005). Certainly further research is required to assess the changes occurring in specific mental disorders as assessed by specific diagnostic instruments.

Quasi-experimental Studies: Superiority to Control Groups

As mentioned earlier, the internal validity of effectiveness studies can be improved by quasi-experimental designs (Leichsenring 2004; Shadish et al. 2002). By definition, quasi-experimental studies do not use random assignment; they use other principles to show that alternative explanations of the observed effect are implausible (see Shadish et al. 2002 for details). For effectiveness studies, levels of evidence must be defined by criteria different from those mentioned earlier (see section "Evidence-Based Medicine and Empirically Supported Treatments") (Chambless and Hollon 1998; Clarke and Oxman 2003; Cook et al. 1995; Guyatt et al. 1995; Nathan and Gorman 2002; National Institute for Clinical Excellence 2002), which regard RCTs as the gold standard (Leichsenring 2004). A proposal has been made to define levels of evidence of effectiveness studies (Leichsenring 2004).

The criteria of the American Psychological Association Task Force on Promotion and Dissemination of Psychological Procedures (American Psychological Association 1995; Chambless and Hollon 1998) require that a treatment be proven a) to be superior to a control condition (placebo or no treatment) or b) to be as effective as an already established treatment. In several controlled quasi-experimental effectiveness studies, LTPP met one or both of these criteria. The studies included control groups for which comparability with the LTPP group was ensured by measures of matching or stratifying or by statistical control of initial differences. In all of these studies, LTPP was significantly superior to the respective control condition. The results can be summarized as follows:

- LTPP yielded effect sizes that significantly exceeded those for the untreated and low-dose comparison groups (Dührssen and Jorswieck 1965; Sandell et al. 1999, 2000, 2001).
- LTPP was significantly more effective than shorter forms of psychodynamic psychotherapy (Grande et al. 2006; Rudolf et al. 1994, 2004; Sandell et al. 1999, 2000, 2001).
- According to the studies by Rudolf et al. (2004) and Grande et al. (2006), LTPP was significantly more effective than shorter forms of psychodynamic psychotherapy with respect to the very dimension of outcome for which a superiority of LTPP is to be expected, that is, with respect to structural changes of personality (Grande et al. 2006).
- The results refer to the treatment of multimorbid patients who are not characterized by only one specific mental disorder.

Randomized controlled studies and quasi-experimental studies of LTPP are currently ongoing (Huber et al. 2001; Knekt et al. 2004; Leichsenring et al. 2005).

In a recent study, data from several naturalistic studies were aggregated in order to allow for disorder-specific evaluations (Jakobsen et al. 2007). The data of four effectiveness studies on LTPP carried out in Germany were used (Jakobsen et al. 2007). In a controlled quasi-experimental design, patients treated with LTPP were compared with a matched group of patients treated with shorter-term psychodynamic therapy. This study is a step toward the multisite process and outcome study proposed by Gabbard et al. (2002). With LTPP, Jakobsen et al. (2007) reported large pre-post effect sizes for depressive disorders, anxiety disorders, and personality disorders. LTPP was as effective as shorter-term psychodynamic therapy with regard to symptomatic improvements in these three disorders. As mentioned earlier, however, LTPP was significantly superior to shorter-term psychodynamic therapy with regard to structural changes of personality (Grande et al. 2006).

Process–Outcome Relationship: Mechanisms of Change

The studies discussed above focused on outcome rather than on process variables in psychodynamic psychotherapy. Studies of psychotherapeutic processes have provided data regarding mechanisms of change in psychodynamic therapy. The results can be summarized as follows:

1. Evidence indicates that the outcome of psychodynamic therapy is related to psychotherapeutic techniques and the therapist's skillfulness (Crits-Christoph et al. 1999; Messer 2001): accuracy of interpretation

(Crits-Christoph et al. 1988), adherence of therapist's interventions to the "plan" (Messer et al. 1992), and competent delivery of expressive (but not of supportive) techniques predicted the outcome of STPP and of moderate-length psychodynamic psychotherapy (Barber et al. 1996). These findings suggest that specific techniques of psychodynamic psychotherapy, as contrasted with nonspecific factors of psychotherapy, account for a significant proportion of variance in outcome (Crits-Christoph and Connolly 1999). Less evidence suggests that frequency of psychodynamic techniques is related to outcome (Crits-Christoph and Connolly 1999).

2. There is evidence for an interaction of technique, outcome, and patient variables: frequency of transference interpretations seems to be associated with both a poor outcome and alliance in STPP of patients who are rated low on quality of object relations, with higher frequency associated with poorer outcome and alliance (Connolly et al. 1999; Høglend and Piper 1995; Ogrodniczuk and Piper 1999; Ogrodniczuk et al. 1999; Piper et al. 2001). Although patients with a high quality of object relations may benefit from low to moderate levels of transference interpretations in STPP, results suggest that even they do not benefit from high levels of transference interpretations (Connolly et al. 1999; Piper et al. 1991a, 1991b). By contrast, in a study of LTPP, patients with poor object relations improved more from therapy with transference interpretations than from therapy with no transference interpretations (Høglend et al. 2006). Different techniques seem to be helpful for patients with low quality of object relations in STPP as compared with LTPP.

3. With regard to the therapeutic alliance, some evidence indicates that alliance is a modest predictor of treatment outcome (Barber et al. 2000; Beutler et al. 2004; Crits-Christoph and Connolly 1999; Horvath 2005; Stiles et al. 1998). Accuracy of interpretations was found to correlate significantly with therapeutic alliance in moderate-length treatments (Crits-Christoph et al. 1993). Thus, one way in which accuracy of interpretation may exert its effect is by fostering the therapeutic alliance (Crits-Christoph et al. 1993).

4. With regard to patient process variables, changes in the focus of psychodynamic psychotherapy were shown to correlate with changes in symptoms (Crits-Christoph and Luborsky 1990). Results from a study by Piper et al. (2003) suggest that expression of affect is a mediating variable of outcome in short-term interpretive group therapy of patients with pathological grief.

5. With regard to patient characteristics, the following variables were found to predict a good outcome of STPP: high motivation, realistic expectations, circumscribed focus, high quality of object relations, and ab-

sence of personality disorder (Høglend 1993; Messer 2001; Piper et al. 2001). Contrary to findings from STPP, in LTPP the presence of personality disorder, high initial severity of mental disorder, chronicity, and less optimistic expectations seem to have no predictive power (Lorentzen and Høglend 2005).

Future research should attempt to identify the forms of psychodynamic psychotherapy and the types of mental disorders for which the associations about the mechanisms of change hold true. Barber et al. (2001), for example, did not find a correlation between the therapeutic alliance and the drug-related outcome of psychodynamic psychotherapy. Furthermore, the caveat of Ablon and Jones (2002, p. 780)—"Brand names of therapy can be misleading"—may also apply to psychodynamic psychotherapy. The question as to whether the "different" models of psychodynamic psychotherapy differ empirically is open to further research. Answering this question requires empirical studies of actual therapy sessions that relate process variables to outcome. With this kind of research, empirically supported change processes can be identified (Ablon and Jones 2002). In a review of empirical studies, Blagys and Hilsenroth (2000) identified seven features that were observed significantly more frequently in psychodynamic, psychodynamic-interpersonal, or interpersonal psychotherapy than in CBT—namely, a focus on patients' affects, on resistance, on patterns of behavior, on past experiences, on patients' interpersonal experiences, on the therapeutic relationship, and on patients' wishes, dreams, or fantasies.

Indications for Short- and Long-Term Psychodynamic Psychotherapy

According to the results of the studies presented in this chapter, there is evidence from RCTs that STPP and LTPP are efficacious treatments for the following mental disorders:

- Depressive disorders
- Anxiety disorders
- Somatoform disorders
- Eating disorders
- Substance-related disorders
- Borderline personality disorder
- Cluster C personality disorders

With regard to STPP, the following patient features have a positive impact on treatment outcome (Høglend 1993; Messer 2001; Piper et al. 2001):

- High motivation
- Realistic expectations
- Circumscribed focus
- High quality of object relations
- Absence of personality disorder

However, these variables seem to have no impact on the outcome of LTPP (Lorentzen and Høglend 2005). According to these results, LTPP seems to be more appropriate for more severely disturbed patients (Lorentzen and Høglend 2005). The same relationship seems to apply to the use of transference interpretations: while patients with low quality of object relations do not benefit from a high frequency of transference interpretations in STPP, transference interpretations seem to be useful for these patients in LTPP (Høglend et al. 2006; Piper et al. 1991a, 1991b, 2001).

According to a study reported by Kopta et al. (1994), in which symptom checklists were administered to 854 psychotherapy outpatients at the start of the study and during treatment, about 50% of patients with acute distress were rated as clinically significantly improved after 2 sessions of psychotherapy, 70% after 21 sessions, and 75% after 29 sessions. For patients with chronic distress, the investigators found that 50% of the patients showed clinically significantly improvement after about 11 sessions, and 70% after about 50 sessions. More than 52 sessions were necessary for 75% of these patients to be rated as clinically significantly improved. For patients with characterological distress (i.e., personality disorders), the data of Kopta et al. (1994) suggest that more than 52 sessions are required for about half of the patients to be clinically significantly improved. However, these data do not allow for exact predictions of how many sessions are required for the response rates to surpass the 50% rate.

Perry et al. (1999) estimated the length of treatment necessary for patients with personality disorder to no longer meet the full criteria for a personality disorder (i.e., recovery). Using the available data, they estimated that half of patients with personality disorder would recover by 1.3 years, or 92 sessions, and three-quarters of them would recover by 2.2 years, or about 216 sessions. According to these data, the majority of patients with acute distress benefit significantly from STPP, whereas patients with chronic distress and personality disorders require long-term psychotherapy; such patients do not benefit sufficiently from short-term treatments. In particular, patients with more severe forms of personality disorders seem to need treatment lasting 2 years or longer.

These data are consistent with clinical experience in, for example, the treatment of narcissistic or borderline personality disorder (Gabbard 2005). With regard to depressive disorders, an NIMH study of depression showed that only 24% of patients in the total sample of 239 patients were free of symptoms both 8 weeks after the end of therapy and during the 18-month follow-up period (no major depressive disorder [MDD] according to Research Diagnostic Criteria) (Shea et al. 1992). In this study, no significant differences among CBT, interpersonal therapy, and pharmacotherapy were found (Shea et al. 1992). According to these results, 16–20 sessions of interpersonal therapy or CBT and pharmacotherapy of a comparable duration are insufficient for most patients to achieve lasting remission. Further studies are necessary to assess for which patients short-term treatments are sufficient and for which patients long-term treatments are required.

Personality disorders have been found to have a negative prognostic impact on depressive disorders (Gunderson et al. 2004; Shea et al. 1990). For example, the rate of MDD remissions seems to be significantly reduced by co-occurring borderline personality disorder (Gunderson et al. 2004). Improvements in borderline personality disorder are often followed by improvements in MDD. For this reason, Gunderson and colleagues recommended that clinicians avoid focusing on the treatment of MDD and hoping that improvements in MDD will be followed by improvements in borderline personality disorder; they should primarily treat the personality disorder (Gunderson et al. 2004).

Conclusion

Under the requirements of the criteria proposed by the American Psychological Association Task Force on Promotion and Dissemination of Psychological Procedures and modified by Chambless and Hollon (American Psychological Association 1995; Chambless and Hollon 1998), 31 RCTs are currently available that provide evidence for the efficacy of psychodynamic psychotherapy in specific mental disorders. In these studies, psychodynamic psychotherapy was either a) more efficacious than placebo therapy, supportive therapy, or treatment as usual, or b) as efficacious as CBT. These results are consistent with the most recent meta-analysis of psychodynamic psychotherapy, which reported psychodynamic psychotherapy to be superior to TAU or no treatment (in waiting-list control groups) and equally efficacious compared with other psychotherapies (Leichsenring et al. 2004). Using the data of this meta-analysis, it can be shown that no differences in efficacy exist if psychodynamic psychotherapy is compared to CBT alone. No significant differences were found between psychodynamic psychotherapy and CBT with regard to target problems, general psychiatric symptoms, and social functions, either at the end of treatment or at follow-up (post: Wilks $\lambda = 0.88$, F $= 0.68$, $P = 0.58$; follow-up: Wilks $\lambda = 0.93$, F $= 0.18$, $P = 0.91$). This meta-analysis reported large effect sizes for psychodynamic psychotherapy in target problems, general psychiatric problems, and social functioning. These effects were stable at follow-up and tended to increase (Leichsenring et al. 2004).

On the other hand, it is important to remember that there are mental disorders for which no RCTs of psychodynamic psychotherapy have been performed, such as dissociative disorders and some specific forms of personality disorders (e.g., narcissistic). In the absence of data from RCTs, there is clinical experience suggesting that long-term dynamic therapy or analysis may be helpful for histrionic/hysterical personality disorder and narcissistic personality disorder (Gabbard 2004, 2005; Kernberg 1975; Kohut 1971). Clinical wisdom suggests that dynamic therapy is contraindicated in most cases of antisocial personality disorder, but some data suggest that the presence of depression may increase the likelihood that patients with antisocial personality disorder will respond positively to dynamic therapy (Woody et al. 1985). For patients with PTSD, although one RCT indicated efficacy for STPP, further studies of psychodynamic psychotherapy are needed. For the treatment of children and adolescents, only a few randomized controlled studies currently exist that provide evidence for the efficacy of specific psychodynamic treatments in specific mental disorders (Fonagy and Target 2005). Further studies are urgently required.

Several effectiveness studies reviewed in this chapter have demonstrated that LTPP can yield large pre-post effect sizes and be superior to little or no treatment and to shorter forms of therapy. In these studies, patients with multiple morbidities were treated. Further studies should examine both the efficacy and the effectiveness of LTPP in specific, though comorbid, mental disorders. Toward this end, an RCT examining the efficacy of LTPP in treating depressive disorders is currently being carried out (Huber et al. 2001).

The results of this review indicate that further research of psychodynamic psychotherapy in specific mental disorders is necessary and should include studies of both the outcome and the active ingredients of psychodynamic psychotherapy in each disorder. Measures more specific to psychodynamic psychotherapy should be applied. In many of the studies reviewed in this chapter, psychodynamic psychotherapy and CBT were equally efficacious. Thus, future studies should address the common and specific factors of psychodynamic psychotherapy, CBT, and other forms of psychotherapy (e.g., interpersonal therapy). They should also examine whether some gains are achieved only by psychodynamic psychotherapy; that is, they should address the question of whether there is "added value" from a treatment with ambitious goals. Furthermore, effectiveness studies should be performed to ascertain how effective various methods of therapy that have proven to work under experimental conditions of RCTs are in actual clinical practice.

Key Points

- In evidence-based medicine, randomized controlled trials (RCTs) are regarded as the "gold standard" for demonstrating that a treatment is efficacious.

- The exclusive position of RCTs is increasingly discussed critically.

- RCTs are useful to show that a treatment works under controlled experimental conditions.

- Naturalistic (effectiveness) studies can provide evidence that a treatment works under the conditions of clinical practice.

- RCTs have provided evidence that psychodynamic psychotherapy is efficacious in specific mental disorders.

- The methodology of an RCT is difficult to apply to long-term psychodynamic psychotherapy (LTPP) lasting several years. For these long-term treatments, naturalistic studies are more appropriate.

- Quasi-experimental designs can be used to improve the internal validity of naturalistic (effectiveness) studies.

- Quasi-experimental studies have provided evidence that LTPP lasting several years is effective.

- Process-outcome research has corroborated central assumptions regarding mechanisms of change in psychodynamic therapy.

- Further research of both processes and outcomes of psychodynamic psychotherapy is needed.

References

Ablon J, Jones E: Validity of controlled clinical trials of psychotherapy: findings from the NIMH Treatment of Depression Collaborative Research Program. Am J Psychiatry 159:775–783, 2002

American Psychiatric Association: Diagnostic and Statistical Manual of Mental Disorders, 4th Edition. Washington, DC, American Psychiatric Association, 1994

American Psychological Association, Task Force on Promotion and Dissemination of Psychological Procedures: Training in and dissemination of empirically validated psychological treatments: report and recommendations. Clin Psychol (New York) 48:3–23, 1995

Bachar E, Latzer Y, Kreitler S, et al: Empirical comparison of two psychological therapies: self psychology and cognitive orientation in the treatment of anorexia and bulimia. J Psychother Pract Res 8:115–128, 1999

Barber JP, Crits-Christoph P, Luborsky L: Effects of therapist adherence and competence on patient outcome in brief dynamic therapy. J Consult Clin Psychol 64:619–622, 1996

Barber JP, Connolly MB, Crits-Christoph P, et al: Alliance predicts patients' outcome beyond in-treatment change in symptoms. J Consult Clin Psychol 68:1027–1032, 2000

Barber JP, Luborsky L, Gallop R, et al: Therapeutic alliance as a predictor of outcome and retention in the National Institute on Drug Abuse Collaborative Cocaine Treatment Study. J Consult Clin Psychol 69:119–124, 2001

Barkham M, Rees A, Shapiro DA, et al: Outcomes of time-limited psychotherapy in applied settings: replication of the Second Sheffield Psychotherapy Project. J Consult Clin Psychol 64:1079–1085, 1996

Barth D: When the patient abuses food, in Using Self Psychology in Psychotherapy. Edited by Jackson H. Northvale, NJ, Jason Aronson, 1991, pp 223–242

Bateman A, Fonagy P: The effectiveness of partial hospitalization in the treatment of borderline personality disorder: a randomized controlled trial. Am J Psychiatry 156:1563–1569, 1999

Bateman A, Fonagy P: Treatment of borderline personality disorder with psychoanalytically oriented partial hospitalization: an 18-month follow-up. Am J Psychiatry 158:36–42, 2001

Benson K, Hartz AJ: A comparison of observational studies and randomized, controlled trials. N Engl J Med 342:1878–1886, 2000

Beutler L: Identifying empirically supported treatments: what if we didn't? J Consult Clin Psychol 66:113–120, 1998

Beutler L, Malik M, Alomohamed S, et al: Therapist variables, in Bergin and Garfield's Handbook of Psychotherapy and Behavior Change. Edited by Lambert M. New York, Wiley, 2004, pp 227–306

Blagys MD, Hilsenroth MJ: Distinctive features of short-term psychodynamic-interpersonal psychotherapy: a review of the comparative psychotherapy process literature. Clinical Psychology: Science and Practice 7:167–188, 2000

Blatt S: Why the gap between psychotherapy research and clinical practice: a response to Barry Wolfe. Journal of Psychotherapy Integration 5:73–76, 1995

Bögels S, Wijts P, Sallaerts S: Analytic psychotherapy versus cognitive-behavioral therapy for social phobia. Paper presented at the European Congress for Cognitive and Behavioural Therapies, Prague, Czech Republic, September 2003

Brockmann J, Schlüter T, Eckert J: The Frankfurt-Hamburg study of psychotherapy—results of the study of psychoanalytically oriented and behavioral long-term therapy [in German], in Langzeit-Psychotherapie. Perspektiven für Therapeuten und Wissenschaftler. Edited by Leuzinger-Bohleber M, Stuhr U, Beutel M. Stuttgart, Germany, Kohlhammer, 2001, pp 271–276

Brom D, Kleber RJ, Defares PB: Brief psychotherapy for posttraumatic stress disorders. J Consult Clin Psychol 57:607–612, 1989

Bruch H: Eating Disorders: Obesity, Anorexia Nervosa, and the Person Within. New York, Basic Books, 1973

Busch FN, Milrod BL, Singer MB: Theory and technique in psychodynamic treatment of panic disorder. Journal of Psychotherapy Practice and Research 8:234–242, 1999

Canadian Task Force on the Periodic Health Examination: The Periodic Health Examination. Can Med Assoc J 121:1193–1254, 1979

Chambless DL, Hollon SD: Defining empirically supported treatments. J Consult Clin Psychol 66:7–18, 1998

Chambless DL, Ollendick TH: Empirically supported psychological interventions: controversies and evidence. Annu Rev Psychol 52:685–716, 2001

Clarke M, Oxman AD (eds): Cochrane reviewers' handbook 4.1.6 (updated January 2003), in The Cochrane Library. Oxford, UK, Update Software, 2003

Clarkin JF, Kernberg OF, Yeomans F: Transference-Focused Psychotherapy for Borderline Personality Disorder Patients. New York, Guilford, 1999a

Clarkin JF, Yeomans F, Kernberg OF: Psychotherapy of Borderline Personality. New York, Wiley, 1999b

Clarkin JF, Levy KN, Lenzenweger MF, et al: Evaluating three treatments for borderline personality disorder: a multiwave study. Am J Psychiatry 164:922–928, 2007

Cohen J: Statistical Power Analysis for the Behavioral Sciences. Hillsdale, NJ, Erlbaum, 1988

Concato J, Shah N, Horwitz RI: Randomized, controlled trials, observational studies, and the hierarchy of research designs. N Engl J Med 342:1887–1892, 2000

Connolly MB, Crits-Christoph P, Shappell S, et al: Relation of transference interpretation to outcome in the early sessions of brief supportive-expressive psychotherapy. Psychother Res 9:485–495, 1999

Cook D, Guyatt GH, Laupacis A, et al: Clinical recommendations using levels of evidence for antithrombotic agents. Chest 108 (suppl 4):227S–230S, 1995

Creed F, Fernandes L, Guthrie E, et al; North of England IBS Research Group: The cost-effectiveness of psychotherapy and paroxetine for severe irritable bowel syndrome. Gastroenterology 124:303–317, 2003

Crisp AH: Anorexia Nervosa: Let Me Be. London, Academic Press, 1980

Crits-Christoph P, Connolly MB: Alliance and technique in short-term dynamic therapy. Clin Psychol Rev 6:687–704, 1999

Crits-Christoph P, Luborsky L: Changes in CCRT pervasiveness during psychotherapy, in Understanding Transference: The CCRT Method. Edited by Luborsky L, Crits-Christoph P. New York, Basic Books, 1990, pp 133–146

Crits-Christoph P, Cooper A, Luborsky L: The accuracy of therapists' interpretations and the outcome of dynamic psychotherapy. J Consult Clin Psychol 56:490–495, 1988

Crits-Christoph P, Barber JP, Kurcias J: The accuracy of therapists' interpretations and the development of the therapeutic alliance. Psychother Res 3:25–35, 1993

Crits-Christoph P, Crits-Christoph, K, Wolf-Palacio D, et al: Brief supportive-expressive psychodynamic therapy for generalized anxiety disorder, in Dynamic Therapies for Psychiatric Disorders: Axis I. Edited by Barber JP, Crits-Christoph P. New York, Basic Books, 1995, pp 43–83

Crits-Christoph P, Siqueland L, Blaine J, et al: Psychosocial treatments for cocaine dependence: National Institute on Drug Abuse Collaborative Cocaine Treatment Study. Arch Gen Psychiatry 56:493–502, 1999

Crits-Christoph P, Siqueland L, McCalmont E, et al: Impact of psychosocial treatments on associated problems of cocaine-dependent patients. J Consult Clin Psychol 69:825–830, 2001

Crits-Christoph P, Gallop R, Connolly Gibbons MB, et al: Interpersonal problems and the outcome of interpersonally oriented psychodynamic treatment of GAD. Psychotherapy: Theory, Research, Practice, Training 42:211–224, 2005

Dare C: Psychoanalytic psychotherapy [of eating disorders], in Treatments of Psychiatric Disorders, 2nd Edition, Vol 2. Edited by Gabbard GO. Washington, DC, American Psychiatric Press, 1995, pp 2129–2151

Dare C, Eisler I, Russell G, et al: Psychological therapies for adults with anorexia nervosa: randomised controlled trial of out-patient treatments. Br J Psychiatry 178:216–221, 2001

de Maat S, Dekker J, Schoevers R, et al: The effectiveness of long-term psychotherapy: methodological research issues. Psychother Res 17:59–65, 2006

Dührssen A, Jorswieck E: An empirical-statistical study of the effectiveness of psychoanalytic treatment [in German]. Nervenarzt 36:166–169, 1965

Emmelkamp P, Benner A, Kuipers A, et al: Comparison of brief dynamic and cognitive-behavioral therapies in avoidant personality disorder. Br J Psychiatry 189:60–64, 2006

Fairburn CG: Evidence-based treatment of anorexia nervosa. Int J Eat Disord 37(suppl):26–30, 2005

Fairburn C, Kirk J, O'Connor M, et al: A comparison of two psychological treatments for bulimia nervosa. Behav Res Ther 24:629–643, 1986

Fairburn C, Norman PA, Welch SL, et al: A prospective study of outcome in bulimia nervosa and the long-term effects of three psychological treatments. Arch Gen Psychiatry 52:304–312, 1995

Fonagy P: Process and outcome in mental health care delivery: a model approach to treatment evaluation. Bull Menninger Clin 63:288–304, 1999

Fonagy P, Target M: The psychological treatment of child and adolescent psychiatric disorders, in What Works for Whom? A Critical Review of Psychotherapy Research, 2nd Edition. Edited by Roth A, Fonagy P. New York, Guilford, 2005, pp 385–424

Fonagy P, Roth A, Higgitt A: Psychodynamic psychotherapies: evidence-based practice and clinical wisdom. Bull Menninger Clin 69:1–58, 2005

Foulkes SH: Therapeutic Group Analysis. London, Allen & Unwin, 1964

Gabbard GO: Long-Term Psychodynamic Psychotherapy: A Basic Text. Washington, DC, American Psychiatric Publishing, 2004

Gabbard GO: Psychodynamic Psychiatry in Clinical Practice, 4th Edition. Washington, DC, American Psychiatric Publishing, 2005

Gabbard GO, Gunderson JG, Fonagy P: The place of psychoanalytic treatments within psychiatry. Arch Gen Psychiatry 59:505–510, 2002

Gallagher-Thompson D, Steffen AM: Comparative effects of cognitive-behavioral and brief psychodynamic psychotherapies for depressed family caregivers. J Consult Clin Psychol 62:543–549, 1994

Gallagher-Thompson D, Hanley-Peterson P, Thompson LW: Maintenance of gains versus relapse following brief psychotherapy for depression. J Consult Clin Psychol 58:371–374, 1990

Garner D, Rockert W, Davis R, et al: Comparison of cognitive-behavioral and supportive-expressive therapy for bulimia nervosa. Am J Psychiatry 150:37–46, 1993

Geist RA: Self psychological reflections on the origins of eating disorders. J Am Acad Psychoanal 17:5–28, 1989

Giesen-Bloo J, van Dyck R, Spinhoven P, et al: Outpatient psychotherapy for borderline personality disorder: randomized trial of schema-focused therapy vs transference-focused psychotherapy. Arch Gen Psychiatry 63:649–658, 2006

Goodsitt A: Self psychology and the treatment of anorexia nervosa, in Handbook of Psychotherapy for Anorexia Nervosa and Bulimia. Edited by Garner DM, Garfinkel DE. New York, Guilford, 1985, pp 55–82

Gowers D, Norton K, Halek C, et al: Outcome of outpatient psychotherapy in a random allocation treatment study of anorexia nervosa. Int J Eat Disord 15:165–177, 1994

Grande T, Dilg R, Jakobsen TH, et al: Differential effects of two forms of psychoanalytic therapy: results of the Heidelberg-Berlin study. Psychother Res 16:470–485, 2006

Gunderson JG, Gabbard GO: Making the case for psychoanalytic therapies in the current psychiatric environment. J Am Psychoanal Assoc 47:679–704, 1999

Gunderson JG, Morey LC, Stout RL, et al: Major depressive disorder and borderline personality disorder revisited: longitudinal interactions. J Clin Psychiatry 65:1049–1056, 2004

Guthrie E, Creed F, Dawson D, et al: A controlled trial of psychological treatment for the irritable bowel syndrome. Gastroenterology 100:450–457, 1991

Guyatt G, Sacket DL, Sinclair JC, et al: User's guides to the medical literature, IX: a method for grading health care recommendations. JAMA 274:1800–1804, 1995

Hamilton J, Guthrie E, Creed F, et al: A randomized controlled trial of psychotherapy in patients with chronic functional dyspepsia. Gastroenterology 119:661–669, 2000

Henry WP: Science, politics, and the politics of science: the use and misuse of empirically validated treatment research. Psychother Res 8:126–140, 1998

Hobson RF: Forms of Feeling: The Heart of Psychotherapy. London, Tavistock, 1985

Høglend P: Suitability for brief dynamic psychotherapy: psychodynamic variables as predictors of outcome. Acta Psychiatr Scand 88:104–110, 1993

Høglend P, Piper WE: Focal adherence in brief dynamic psychotherapy: a comparison of findings from two independent studies. Psychother Res 32:618–628, 1995

Høglend P, Amlo S, Marble A, et al: Analysis of the patient-therapist relationship in dynamic psychotherapy: an experimental study of transference interpretations. Am J Psychiatry 163:1739–1746, 2006

Horowitz LM, Alden LE, Wiggins JS, et al: IIP, Inventory of Interpersonal Problems Manual. San Antonio, TX, Psychological Corporation, 2000

Horowitz M: Stress Response Syndromes. New York, Jason Aronson, 1976

Horowitz M, Kaltreider N: Brief therapy of the stress response syndrome. Psychiatr Clin North Am 2:365–377, 1979

Horvath AO: The therapeutic relationship, research and theory: an introduction to the special issue. Psychother Res 15:3–7, 2005

Huber D, Klug G, von Rad M: The Munich process-outcome study: a comparison between psychoanalyses and psychotherapy [in German], in Langzeit-Psychotherapie. Perspektiven für Therapeuten und Wissenschaftler. Edited by Leuzinger-Bohleber M, Stuhr U, Beutel M. Stuttgart, Germany, Kohlhammer, 2001, pp 260–270

Jakobsen T, Rudolf G, Staats H, et al: Results of psychoanalytic long-term psychotherapy: improvements in symptoms and interpersonal relations [in German]. Z Psychosom Med Psychother 53:87–110, 2007

Kazis LE, Anderson JJ, Meenan RF: Effect sizes for interpreting changes in health status. Med Care 27 (suppl 3):S178–S189, 1989

Kernberg OF: Borderline Conditions and Pathological Narcissism. New York, Jason Aronson, 1975

Kernberg OF: A psychoanalytic model for the classification of personality disorders, in Implications of Psychopharmacology to Psychiatry: Biological, Nosological, and Therapeutical Concepts. Edited by Ackenheil M, Bondy B, Engel R, et al. Berlin, Springer, 1996

Knekt P, Lindfors O, Renlund C: A randomized trial of the effect of four forms of psychotherapy on depressive and anxiety disorders, in Studies in Social Security and Health, Vol 77. Edited by Knekt P, Lindfors O. Helsinki, Edita Prima, 2004, pp 1–112

Knijnik DZ, Kapczinski F, Chachamovich E, et al: Psychodynamic group treatment for generalized social phobia [in Portuguese]. Rev Bras Psiquiatr 26:77–81, 2004

Kohut H: The Analysis of the Self. New York, International Universities Press, 1971

Kopta SM, Howard KI, Lowry JL, et al: Patterns of symptomatic recovery in psychotherapy. J Consult Clin Psychol 62:1009–1016, 1994

Krupnick JL, Sotsky SM, Simmens S, et al: The role of the therapeutic alliance in psychotherapy and pharmacotherapy outcome: findings in the National Institute of Mental Health Treatment of Depression Collaborative Research Program. J Consult Clin Psychol 64:532–539, 1996

Leichsenring F: Comparative effects of short-term psychodynamic psychotherapy and cognitive-behavioral therapy in depression: a meta-analytic approach. Clin Psychol Rev 21:401–419, 2001

Leichsenring F: Randomized controlled vs. naturalistic studies: a new research agenda. Bull Menninger Clin 68:115–129, 2004

Leichsenring F: Are psychodynamic and psychoanalytic therapies effective? A review of empirical data. Int J Psychoanal 86:841–868, 2005

Leichsenring F: A review of meta-analyses of outcome studies of psychodynamic therapy, in Psychodynamic Diagnostic Manual (PDM). Edited by Alliance of Psychodynamic Organizations. Silver Spring, MD, Interdisciplinary Council on Developmental and Learning Disorders, 2006, pp 819–837

Leichsenring F, Leibing E: The effectiveness of psychodynamic psychotherapy and cognitive-behavioral therapy in personality disorders: a meta-analysis. Am J Psychiatry 160:1223–1232, 2003

Leichsenring F, Leibing E: Fair play, please! (letter) Br J Psychiatry 190:80, 2006

Leichsenring F, Rabung S: Control groups in psychotherapy outcome research: a complementary approach. Psychother Res 16:604–616, 2006

Leichsenring F, Rabung S, Leibing E: The efficacy of short-term psychodynamic psychotherapy in specific psychiatric disorders: a meta-analysis. Arch Gen Psychiatry 61:1208–1216, 2004

Leichsenring F, Biskup J, Kreische R, et al: The Göttingen study of psychoanalytic therapy: first results. Int J Psychoanal 86:433–455, 2005

Leichsenring F, Hoyer J, Beutel M, et al: The Social Phobia Psychotherapy Research Network (SOPHO-NET)—The first multi-center randomized controlled trial for psychotherapy of social phobia: rationale, methods and patient characteristics. Psychother Psychosom (in press)

Levy KN, Meehan KB, Kelly KM, et al: Change in attachment patterns and reflective function in a randomized control trial of transference-focused psychotherapy for borderline personality disorder. J Consult Clin Psychol 74:1027–1040, 2006

Lorentzen S, Høglend P: Predictors of change after long-term analytic group psychotherapy. J Consult Clin Psychol 61:1541–1553, 2005

Luborsky L: Principles of Psychoanalytic Psychotherapy: A Manual for Supportive-Expressive Treatment. New York, Basic Books, 1984

Luborsky L, Mark D: Short-term supportive-expressive psychoanalytic psychotherapy, in Handbook of Short-Term Dynamic Psychotherapy. Edited by Crits-Christoph P, Barber J. New York, Basic Books, 1991, pp 110–136

Luborsky L, Diguer L, Seligman DA, et al: The researcher's own therapy allegiances: a "wild card" in comparisons of treatment efficacy. Clinical Psychology: Science and Practice 6:95–106, 1999

Luborsky L, Stuart J, Friedman S, et al: The Penn Psychoanalytic Treatment Collection: a set of complete and recorded psychoanalyses as a research resource. J Am Psychoanal Assoc 49:217–234, 2001

Maina G, Forner F, Bogetto F: Randomized controlled trial comparing brief dynamic and supportive therapy with waiting list condition in minor depressive disorders. Psychother Psychosom 74:3–50, 2005

Malan DH: Toward the Validation of Dynamic Psychotherapy. New York, Plenum, 1976

Mann J: Time-Limited Psychotherapy. Cambridge, MA, Harvard University Press, 1973

Mark D, Luborsky L: A Manual for the Use of Supportive-Expressive Psychotherapy in the Treatment of Cocaine Abuse. Philadelphia, University of Pennsylvania, Department of Psychiatry, 1992

McCallum MP, Piper WE: A controlled study of effectiveness and patient suitability for short-term group psychotherapy. Int J Group Psychother 40:431–452, 1990

McCullough Vaillant L: Changing Character: Short-Term Anxiety-Regulating Psychotherapy for Restructuring Defenses, Affects, and Attachment. New York, Basic Books, 1997

Messer SB: What makes brief psychodynamic therapy time efficient. Clinical Psychology: Science and Practice 8:5–22, 2001

Messer SB, Warren CS: Models of Brief Psychodynamic Therapy: A Comparative Approach. New York, Guilford, 1995

Messer SB, Tishby O, Spillman A: Taking context seriously in psychotherapy research: relating therapist interventions to patient progress in brief psychodynamic therapy. J Consult Clin Psychol 60:678–688, 1992

Milrod B, Leon AC, Busch F, et al: A randomized controlled clinical trial of psychoanalytic psychotherapy for panic disorder. Am J Psychiatry 164:265–272, 2007

Monsen K, Monsen TJ: Affects and affect consiousness—a psychotherapy model of integrating Silvan Tomkins' affect and script theory within the framework of self psychology. Progress in Self Psychology 15:287–306, 1999

Monsen K, Monsen JT: Chronic pain and psychodynamic body therapy. Psychotherapy 37:257–269, 2000

Munroe-Blum H, Marziali E: A controlled trial of short-term group treatment for borderline personality disorder. J Personal Disord 9:190–198, 1995

Muran JC, Safran JD, Samstag L, et al: Evaluating an alliance-focused treatment for personality disorders. Psychotherapy: Theory, Research, Practice, Training 42:532–545, 2005

Nathan PE, Gorman JM (eds): A Guide to Treatments That Work, 2nd Edition. New York, Oxford University Press, 2002

National Institute for Clinical Excellence: Schizophrenia: core interventions in the treatment and management of schizophrenia in primary and secondary care. Clinical Guideline 1. London, National Institute for Clinical Excellence, 2002

Ogrodniczuk JS, Piper WE: Use of transference interpretations in dynamically oriented individual psychotherapy for patients with personality disorders. J Personal Disord 13:297–311, 1999

Ogrodniczuk JS, Piper WE, Joyce AS, et al: Transference interpretations in short-term dynamic psychotherapy. J Nerv Ment Dis 187:571–578, 1999

Perry J, Banon E, Floriana I: Effectiveness of psychotherapy for personality disorders. Am J Psychiatry 156:1312–1321, 1999

Persons J, Silberschatz G: Are results of randomized trials useful to psychotherapists? J Consult Clin Psychol 66:126–135, 1998

Pinsker H, Rosenthal R, McCullough L: Dynamic supportive psychotherapy, in Handbook of Short-Term Dynamic Psychotherapy. Edited by Crits-Christoph P, Barber J. New York, Basic Books, 1991, pp 220–247

Piper WE, Azim HF, Joyce AS, et al: Quality of object relations versus interpersonal functioning as predictors of therapeutic alliance and psychotherapy outcome. J Nerv Ment Dis 179:432–438, 1991a

Piper WE, Azim HF, Joyce AS, et al: Transference interpretations, therapeutic alliance, and outcome in short-term individual psychotherapy. Arch Gen Psychiatry 48:946–953, 1991b

Piper WE, McCallum M, Joyce AS, et al: Patient personality and time-limited group psychotherapy for complicated grief. Int J Group Psychother 51:525–552, 2001

Piper WE, Ogrodniczuk JS, McCallum M, et al: Expression of affect as a mediator of the relationship between quality of object relations and group therapy outcome for patients with complicated grief. J Consult Clin Psychol 71:664–671, 2003

Pollack J, Flegenheimer W, Kaufman J, et al: Brief Adaptive Psychotherapy for Personality Disorders: A Treatment Manual. San Diego, CA, Social & Behavioral Documents, 1992

Rose JM, DelMaestro SG: Separation-individuation conflict as a model for understanding distressed caregivers: psychodynamic and cognitive case studies. Gerontologist 30:693–697, 1990

Rosen B: A method of structured brief psychotherapy. Br J Med Psychol 52:157–162, 1979

Roth A, Parry G: The implications of psychotherapy research for clinical practice and service development: lessons and limitations. Journal of Mental Health 6:367–380, 1997

Rothwell P: External validity of randomised controlled trials: "to whom do the results of this trial apply?" Lancet 365:82–92, 2005

Rudolf G, Manz R, Öri C: Outcome of psychoanalytic therapy [in German]. Z Psychosom Med Psychother 40:25–40, 1994

Rudolf G, Dilg R, Grande T, et al: Effectiveness and efficiency of long-term psychoanalytic therapy: the practice study of long-term psychoanalytic therapy [in German], in Psychoanalyse des Glaubens. Edited by Gerlach A, Springer A, Schlösser A. Giessen, Germany, Psychosozial Verlag, 2004

Ryle A: Cognitive-Analytic Therapy: Active Participation in Change. London, Wiley, 1990

Sandahl C, Herlitz K, Ahlin G, et al: Time-limited group psychotherapy for moderately alcohol dependent patients: a randomized controlled clinical trial. Psychother Res 8:361–378, 1998

Sandell R, Blomberg J, Lazar A: Repeated long-term follow-up of long-term psychotherapy and psychoanalysis: first findings of the Stockholm Outcome of Psychotherapy (STOP) Project [in German]. Z Psychosom Med Psychother 45:43–56, 1999

Sandell R, Blomberg J, Lazar A, et al: Varieties of long-term outcome among patients in psychoanalysis and long-term psychotherapy: a review of findings in the Stockholm Outcome of Psychoanalysis and Psychotherapy Project (STOPP). Int J Psychoanal 81:921–942, 2000

Sandell R, Blomberg J, Lazar A, et al: Different long-term results of psychological analysis and long-term psychotherapies: from the research of the Stockholm psychoanalysis and psychotherapy project [in German]. Psyche (Stuttg) 55:273–310, 2001

Seligman ME: The effectiveness of psychotherapy: the Consumer Reports study. Am Psychol 50:965–974, 1995

Shadish WR, Matt G, Navarro A, et al: The effects of psychological therapies under clinically representative conditions: a meta-analysis. J Consult Clin Psychol 126:512–529, 2000

Shadish WR, Cook TD, Campbell DT: Experimental and Quasi-experimental Designs for Generalized Causal Inference. Boston, MA, Houghton Mifflin, 2002

Shapiro DA, Firth JA: Exploratory Therapy Manual for the Sheffield Psychotherapy Project (SAPU Memo 733). Sheffield, UK, University of Sheffield, 1985

Shapiro DA, Barkham M, Rees A, et al: Effects of treatment duration and severity of depression on the effectiveness of cognitive-behavioral and psychodynamic-interpersonal psychotherapy. J Consult Clin Psychol 62:522–534, 1994

Shapiro DA, Rees A, Barkham M, et al: Effects of treatment duration and severity of depression on the maintenance of gains after cognitive-behavioral and psychodynamic-interpersonal psychotherapy. J Consult Clin Psychol 63:378–387, 1995

Shea MT, Pilkonis PA, Beckham E, et al: Personality disorders and treatment outcome in the NIMH Treatment of Depression Collaborative Research Program. Am J Psychiatry 147:711–718, 1990

Shea MT, Elkin I, Imber SD, et al: Course of depressive symptoms over followup: findings from the National Institute of Mental Health Treatment of Depression Collaborative Research Program. Arch Gen Psychiatry 49:782–787, 1992

Stiles WB, Agnew-Davis R, Hardy GE, et al: Relations of the alliance with psychotherapy outcome: findings in the Second Sheffield Psychotherapy Project. J Consult Clin Psychol 66:791–802, 1998

Stunkard AJ: The Pain of Obesity. Palo Alto, CA, Bull Publishing, 1976

Svartberg M, Stiles TC, Seltzer MH: Randomized, controlled trial of the effectiveness of short-term dynamic psychotherapy and cognitive therapy for cluster C personality disorders. Am J Psychiatry 161:810–817, 2004

Thompson L, Gallagher D, Breckenridge JS: Comparative effectiveness of psychotherapies for depressed elders. J Consult Clin Psychol 55:385–390, 1987

Wallerstein R: The psychotherapy research project of the Menninger Foundation: an overview. J Consult Clin Psychol 57:195–205, 1989

Wallerstein R: Comment on Gunderson and Gabbard. J Am Psychoanal Assoc 47:728–734, 1999

Wampold B, Minami T, Baskin TW, et al: A meta-(re)analysis of the effects of cognitive therapy versus 'other therapies' for depression. J Affect Disord 68:159–165, 2002

Westen D, Novotny CM, Thompson-Brenner H: The empirical status of empirically supported psychotherapies: assumptions, findings, and reporting in controlled clinical trials. Psychol Bull 130:631–663, 2004

Woody GE, Luborsky L, McLellan AT, et al: Psychotherapy for opiate addicts: does it help? Arch Gen Psychiatry 40:639–645, 1983

Woody GE, McLellan AT, Luborsky L, et al: Sociopathy and psychotherapy outcome. Arch Gen Psychiatry 42:1081–1086, 1985

Woody G, Luborsky L, McLellan AT, et al: Corrections and revised analyses for psychotherapy in methadone maintenance patients. Arch Gen Psychiatry 47:788–789, 1990

Woody GE, McLellan AT, Luborsky L, et al: Psychotherapy in community methadone programs: a validation study. Am J Psychiatry 152:1302–1308, 1995

Suggested Readings

Ablon J, Jones E: Validity of controlled clinical trials of psychotherapy: findings from the NIMH Treatment of Depression Collaborative Research Program. Am J Psychiatry 159:775–783, 2002

Benson K, Hartz AJ: A comparison of observational studies and randomized, controlled trials. N Engl J Med 342:1878–1886, 2000

Concato J, Shah N, Horwitz RI: Randomized, controlled trials, observational studies, and the hierarchy of research designs. N Engl J Med 342:1887–1892, 2000

Crits-Christoph P, Luborsky L: Changes in CCRT pervasiveness during psychotherapy, in Understanding Transference: The CCRT Method. Edited by Luborsky L, Crits-Christoph P. New York, Basic Books, 1990, pp 133–146

Gabbard GO: Psychodynamic Psychiatry in Clinical Practice, 4th Edition. Washington, DC, American Psychiatric Publishing, 2005

Gabbard GO: Long-Term Psychodynamic Psychotherapy: A Basic Text. Washington, DC, American Psychiatric Publishing, 2004

Gabbard GO, Gunderson JG, Fonagy P: The place of psychoanalytic treatments within psychiatry. Arch Gen Psychiatry 59:505–510, 2002

Grande T, Dilg R, Jakobsen TH, et al: Differential effects of two forms of psychoanalytic therapy: results of the Heidelberg-Berlin study. Psychother Res 16:470–485, 2006

Gunderson JG, Gabbard GO: Making the case for psychoanalytic therapies in the current psychiatric environment. J Am Psychoanal Assoc 47:679–704, 1999

Leichsenring F, Rabung S, Leibing E: The efficacy of short-term psychodynamic psychotherapy in specific psychiatric disorders: a meta-analysis. Arch Gen Psychiatry 61:1208–1216, 2004

Luborsky L: Principles of Psychoanalytic Psychotherapy: A Manual for Supportive-Expressive Treatment. New York, Basic Books, 1984

Messer SB, Warren CS: Models of Brief Psychodynamic Therapy: A Comparative Approach. New York, Guilford, 1995

Psychodynamic Diagnostic Manual (PDM). Edited by Alliance of Psychodynamic Organizations. Silver Spring, MD, Interdisciplinary Council on Developmental and Learning Disorders, 2006

Roth A, Fonagy P (eds): What Works for Whom? A Critical Review of Psychotherapy Research, 2nd Edition. New York, Guilford, 2005

Shadish WR, Matt G, Navarro A, et al: The effects of psychological therapies under clinically representative conditions: a meta-analysis. J Consult Clin Psychol 126:512–529, 2000

Shadish WR, Cook TD, Campbell DT: Experimental and Quasi-experimental Designs for Generalized Causal Inference. Boston, MA, Houghton Mifflin, 2002

Wampold B, Minami T, Baskin TW, et al: A meta-(re)analysis of the effects of cognitive therapy versus 'other therapies' for depression. J Affect Disord 68:159–
165, 2002

Westen D, Novotny CM, Thompson-Brenner H: The empirical status of empirically supported psychotherapies: assumptions, findings, and reporting in controlled clinical trials. Psychol Bull 130:631–663, 2004

Chapter 5

Combining Psychodynamic Psychotherapy With Medication

Jerald Kay, M.D.

The age of psychopharmacology was not met with enthusiasm by all. In the last half of the twentieth century, many psychoanalytically oriented clinicians maintained that medications somehow submerged important conflicts and feelings, making psychotherapy and psychoanalysis less effective. Another concern was that using medication would impart to patients a sense of being exceptionally ill, making them less suitable subjects for psychotherapy or psychoanalysis because they would then have inadequate ego strength. Some therapists even argued that assisting the patient through medication eventuates in symptom substitution wherein new symptoms appear as the initial symptoms subside. The possibility of premature treatment termination because of immediate symptom relief was also discussed. Analysts acknowledged that although medication could be effective, ultimately such treatment would never address core conflictual and characterological issues. Others expressed concern that the analysands would view the introduction of pharmacotherapy as a reflection that they were unresponsive patients, especially if medication were introduced well into the analytic treatment.

As early as 1974, researchers verified that combination therapy was not detrimental to the patient (Klerman et al. 1974). Now such arguments about the negative consequences of utilizing medication and psychodynamic psychotherapies have all but disappeared. A very small group of psychiatrist psychoanalysts, however, continues to express caution on this matter. These clinicians, even when medications appear to be indicated, often have another psychiatrist provide and monitor the use of medication because they do not wish that medication receive a central position in treatment. (Others, of course, refer because they may feel less qualified in the prescription of medicine.) This practice can increase treatment complexity, especially because younger psychiatrists are often providing the pharmacotherapy, some of whom may be former analytic patients of, or may have been residents under the supervision of, the referring analyst.

The stigma about medication endures in this country and throughout the world (see Kay 2005 for a more in-depth discussion on the international situation). A recent study examined the attitudes of psychiatric trainees who were seeking psychiatric treatment in New York City (Fogel et al. 2006). Anonymous questionnaires were sent to nearly 300 residents. With a return rate of nearly 50%, the completed questionnaires indicated that 57% of respondents were in treatment, yet only 18% stated that their therapists had prescribed medication. Residents stated that, in their opinion, psychiatry department members strongly advocated psychotherapy or psychoanalysis but not treatment with medication. Moreover, residents were more apt to share the information with faculty and peers that they were receiving the former, but not the latter (Fogel et al. 2006). If these findings are reflective of training programs across the United States, training directors and faculty have much work to do to decrease this important source of stigma for future practitioners.

This chapter addresses the recent findings about the neurobiology of psychotherapy that have elucidated how psychotherapy changes both brain function and structure. The literature describing the effectiveness and efficacy of using psychotherapy with pharmacotherapy is reviewed, as are the challeneges to the provision of integrated, combined, and split treatment. The importance of the clinician's appreciation of the meaning of medication to the patient and its centrality in treatment compliance are also discussed and illustrated through clinical vignettes.

The Fallacy of Biology Versus Psychology

Although the combined use of psychotherapy and medication in the treatment of patients with mental disorders is ubiquitous, many clinicians persist in a rigid conceptualization of the brain and the mind, believing that disorders of the brain should be treated by medication and psychological problems should be treated with psychotherapy (Gabbard and Kay 2001). Maintaining such a dichotomy has, unfortunately, done a great disservice to our patients. In the last 15 years, some striking studies have illustrated that psychotherapy, when compared with psychopharmacological therapy, can change both brain structure and brain function with equal efficacy and often in an identical fashion. Studies also now point to the benefits of using medication and psychotherapy simultaneously.

This appreciation of the neurobiology of psychotherapy has been furthered by studies demonstrating that in head-to-head comparisons, the psychotherapies produce effects similar to those of medication treatment. Studies have examined the treatment of obsessive-compulsive disorder, major depression, social phobia (social anxiety disorder), and borderline personality disorder. Table 5–1 summarizes these studies. Note, however, that only preliminary data exist with respect to treatment by psychoanalytic psychotherapy. (Milrod et al. [2007] are examining posttreatment neurobiological changes in their large randomized controlled studies of a manual-based psychoanalytic psychotherapy to treat panic disorder utilizing no medication.)

Only one of these studies demonstrated a differential response to medication versus psychotherapy. In a positron emission tomography study, Goldapple et al. (2004) compared the findings at baseline and posttreatment in patients with unipolar depression treated with either 16–20 sessions of cognitive-behavioral therapy (CBT) or paroxetine. Psychotherapy appeared to increase metabolic activity in different locations than the medication did, namely, the dorsal cingulate and hippocampus, and appeared to decrease activity in the frontal cortex. Treatment with paroxetine appeared to increase metabolic activity in the prefrontal cortex, and decreased activity was noted in the subgenual cingulate and hippocampus. The authors advocate that psychotherapy seems to work anatomically from the "top down" and medication from the "bottom up."

These initial imaging studies portend a time when it may be possible to use imaging for the differential treatment of disorders, and they begin to illustrate the helpfulness of psychotherapy. They also emphasize the futility of taking an either-or position regarding the use of psychotherapy and medication. Indeed the possibility exists, at least in the case of depression, that medication and psychotherapy have an additive effect; moreover, some neurovegetative symptoms may respond differentially to medication, and psychotherapy may be more helpful in treating despair and hopelessness (Mayberg 2006).

TABLE 5–1. Neurobiological studies of psychotherapy

Investigators	Imaging technique	Treatment	Disorder	N	Findings
Baxter et al. 1992	PET	Fluoxetine vs. ERP therapy	OCD	18	Decreased activity in head of the right caudate nucleus in responders to psychotherapy (6/9) and pharmacotherapy (7/9)
Joffe et al. 1996	—	CBT	Major depression	30	Increased T_4 levels in all 17 responders Decreased T_4 levels in nonresponders
Schwartz et al. 1996	PET	ERP therapy	OCD	18[a]	Decreased caudate activity (R>L) in responders
Thase et al. 1998	EEG	CBT	Major depression	78	Restored normal sleep architecture
Viinamaki et al. 1998	SPECT	Psychodynamic psychotherapy vs. no treatment	BPD + depression	2[b]	Increased 5-HT metabolism in PFC and thalamus
Brody et al. 2001	PET	IPT vs. paroxetine	Major depression	24	Normalized metabolism in PFC, AC, and temporal lobe with both treatments
Martin et al. 2001	SPECT	IPT vs. venlafaxine	Major depression	28	Increased (R) CBF to basal ganglia with both treatments Increased (R) CBF in limbic system with IPT only

TABLE 5–1.   Neurobiological studies of psychotherapy *(continued)*

Investigators	Imaging technique	Treatment	Disorder	N	Findings
Furmark et al. 2002	PET	Citalopram vs. CBT	Social phobia	18	Decreased (R) CBF in public speaking task bilaterally in AMG, hippo, periamygdaloid, rhinal, and parahippocampal cortices with both treatments Degree of attenuation was associated with clinical improvement
Goldapple et al. 2004	PET	CBT vs. paroxetine	Major depression	31	CBT: increased activity in hippo and DC, decreased in frontal cortex Paroxetine: increased activity in PFC, decreased in hippo and SC
Saarinen et al. 2005	SPECT	Dynamic psychotherapy	Major depression	1	Normalized midbrain level of SERT binding

Note.   AC=anterior cingulate; AMG=amygdala; BPD=borderline personality disorder; CBF=cerebral blood flow; CBT=cognitive-behavioral therapy; DC=dorsal cingulate; EEG=electroencephalography; ERP=exposure and response prevention; hippo=hippocampus; 5-HT=5-hydroxytryptamine (serotonin); IPT=interpersonal psychotherapy; L=change on left side; OCD=obsessive-compulsive disorder; PET=positron emission tomography; PFC=prefrontal cortex; R=change on right side; SB=subgenual cingulate; SERT=serotonin transporter; SPECT=single-photon emission computed tomography; T_4=thyroxine.
[a]Nine new, 9 from previous study.
[b]Ten control subjects.
Source.   Reprinted from Kay J, Kay RL: "Individual Psychoanalytic Psychotherapy," in *Psychiatry*, 3rd Edition. Edited by Tasman A, Kay J, Lieberman JA, et al. Chichester, UK, Wiley, 2008, p. 1871.

Benefits of Combining Medication and Psychotherapy

Pharmacotherapy can diminish uncomfortable symptoms of anxiety and depression, permitting the patient greater access to, expression of, and understanding of his or her feelings, wishes, and behavior while undergoing psychotherapeutic treatment. There are other potential benefits of combining medication and psychotherapy:

- Medication may increase the patient's sense of safety in the doctor–patient relationship, thereby allowing less constricted expression of troubling feelings.
- Through the reduction of acute symptoms, medication may enhance the patient's self-esteem by decreasing passivity and the sense of helplessness.
- Medication may provide the patient with additional psychological resources that make psychotherapy more effective, such as improved concentration and recall.
- Medication has the potential to strengthen the doctor–patient relationship and, for some, may decrease the stigma associated with mental health treatment.
- Medication may increase not only the likelihood of a response to psychotherapy but also the speed and magnitude of the response.
- Feelings about medication-related side effects provide valuable insight into aspects of the patient's personality and emotional experiences, which are often outside of the patient's awareness, and can assist in clarifying both transference and countertransference issues.
- A patient's feelings toward medication can often provide clues to patterns of self-defeating behavior as well as to conflicts about achievement and success.
- When treatment must be interrupted, medication may serve as an important link to the treatment relationship.

The following vignette (modified from Kay 2001, p. 7) demonstrates the helpfulness of medication in initiating a trauma-focused dynamic psychotherapy on a consultation-liaison basis:

> Mr. N was a 32-year-old factory employee who had undergone liver transplantation. Eight months postoperatively he began to reject his new organ and became severely depressed; his depression was manifested by symptoms of uncontrollable crying, sleeplessness, weight loss, anhedonia, suicidal ideation, and pervasive despair. He was difficult to engage, spoke very softly, and avoided nearly all eye contact. The transplant team requested consultation

because Mr. N adamantly refused another necessary operation. Given his significant depression, the psychiatrist suggested, and the patient agreed to, a trial of antidepressant medication with the hope that the alleviation of some of his depressive symptoms would permit a more in-depth exploration of the patient's refusal. Ten days after medication was begun, the patient's depression began to lift, but he remained steadfast in his refusal to consider another surgical procedure, and the transplant surgeons became increasingly irritated with the patient.

The psychiatrist ascertained that the patient was less fearful of dying than he was of the surgical procedure itself. During the brief psychotherapy, the basis for this fear became clear: Mr. N recalled a highly traumatic incident as a teenager in which he nearly drowned while swimming in a hazardous rock quarry. When the psychiatrist asked what the most frightening aspect of the event was, the patient described intense panic after swallowing large amounts of water and being unable to breathe. When questioned about the possible relationship between this event and his position on retransplantation, the patient shared that the most terrifying aspect of the first transplant operation had been his perceived inability to breathe postoperatively because of the numerous tubes in his mouth and nose. Psychoanalytically oriented focal psychotherapy allowed the patient to appreciate his resistance and he subsequently agreed to a second operation, provided that the surgical team was aware of and sensitive to the nature of his fear.

When psychotherapy is added to ongoing pharmacotherapy, significant benefits can accrue as well:

- Because some patients respond only to psychotherapy or medication alone, a favorable outcome is more likely when both are employed (Pampallona et al. 2004).
- Medication compliance is strengthened when psychotherapy is added (Basco and Rush 1996; de Jonghe et al. 2001; Vergouwen et al. 2003).
- Psychotherapy promotes improved coping and adaptation.
- Psychotherapy decreases the likelihood that symptoms will recur, even in the most severe disorders (Fava et al. 1998; Kay 2001).
- Psychotherapy decreases relapse rates when pharmacotherapy is discontinued, because patients often continue to maintain the gains achieved during psychotherapy (Bateman and Fonagy 2001; Teasdale et al. 2001; Wiborg and Dahl 1996).
- Joint psychotherapy and pharmacotherapy improves long-term social functioning (Klerman et al. 1974).
- Psychotherapy and medication together produce faster responses (Bowers 1990) and greater patient satisfaction (de Jonghe et al. 2001; Seligman 1995).
- Psychotherapy and medication may be associated with lower direct and indirect health care costs (Andreoli et al. 2000; Burnand et al. 2002).

- Psychotherapy with medication may reduce treatment dropout rates (de Jonghe et al. 2001).
- Sequential or stepped treatment can provide an option in treatment planning wherein, for example, medication is employed in the acute phase of major depression and psychotherapy is utilized in the continuation phase to prevent relapse and improve quality of life by addressing residual symptoms (Fava 1999; Pava et al. 1994).

Potential Disadvantages of Combination Therapy

In general, employing medication and psychotherapy jointly has few disadvantages. Although the data are very limited, some researchers have expressed concerned about the use of medication in the treatment of panic disorder. Marks et al. (1993) noted that combination therapy with some anxiolytics (benzodiazepines) may negatively influence the outcome. They reported that patients who received combination therapy demonstrated higher relapse rates than patients who were provided psychotherapy as a monotherapy. Similarly, Barlow et al. (2000) noted that long-term outcome was better when panic disorder was treated with CBT alone than with CBT plus imipramine. In a more recent study (Westra et al. 2002), in which panic and agoraphobia patients were treated with group CBT with or without benzodiazepines, those receiving benzodiazepines and group treatment had poorer outcomes than those treated only with the group psychotherapy.

Some clinicians have argued that the treatment of anxiety disorders, such as posttraumatic stress disorder (PTSD), requires an optimal level of discomfort to facilitate motivation and the working through of traumatic events, and have cautioned against using medication that sedates the patient and interferes with this process. In their view, patients with trauma are assisted in recovery through repeated experience, within psychotherapy, of intensely painful feelings of danger, catastrophe, and/or fragmentation. Therapists of most persuasions place great importance not only on the re-experiencing of the trauma to detoxify memories but also on the creation of new memories that produce change in emotions and behavior. Scraps of memories of overwhelming experiences uncovered over time can lead to the formation of a new narrative that can be discussed and understood. New explicit memory is then formed from the parallel retrieval of implicit and explicit memories. It should also be noted that the use of beta-blockers immediately after a traumatic experience may prevent PTSD, but this remains to be proven and the role of psychotherapy in such an approach has yet to be determined.

Economics of Integrated Treatment

At the present time in the United States, the simultaneous treatment of patients with medication and psychotherapy by a psychiatrist is referred to as *integrated treatment* (Kay 2001). If a psychiatrist, or any other physician, is responsible for managing only the medication and the patient is seen by another professional for psychotherapy, the terms *combined, split,* and *collaborative treatment* are used to describe the treatment situation. Split treatment is common in large part due to the economic pressures from managed health care companies, which advocate split treatment as a more cost-effective approach. However, there are few data to support that such a model is more effective. Some preliminary studies suggest it may be more cost-effective when a psychiatrist is responsible for both the psychotherapeutic and pharmacologic treatment of the patient (Dewan 1999; Goldman et al. 1998). Nevertheless, both integrated and split treatments are common, each with their own challenges, and the psychiatrist is obligated to function in both situations for the betterment of patient care.

Unfortunately, not all psychiatrists are following the treatment guidelines published by the American Psychiatric Association (APA), which uniformly advocate for both medication and psychosocial interventions. Figure 5–1 shows responses from the APA Practice Research Network (PRN) Study of Psychiatric Patients and Treatments (American Psychiatric Association 1997, 1999). The PRN examines the practice characteristics of a large national, random sample of clinicians, including the impact of reimbursement on the provision of services. Because of the cost-containment policy of managed behavioral health care, it appears that many patients may receive a disjointed treatment experience. Finally, it is important to appreciate that although the predominant form of psychotherapy provided in the United States is undoubtedly supportive in nature, a large number of psychiatrists do utilize a psychodynamic framework as their overarching conceptualization (Misch 2000; Rockland 1989).

Psychoanalytic Psychotherapy and Medication: A Review of the Literature

Most studies examining the combination of psychotherapy and medication have examined this practice with CBT and interpersonal therapy. It is important to note that even with these treatments the literature is by no means in agreement; this is especially true regarding the treatment of depression, the disorder on which the majority of studies have focused (for more comprehensive reviews, see Kay 2001, 2005).

There have been some studies of the simultaneous provision of medication and psychoanalytic psychotherapy. More than 30 years ago, Luborsky

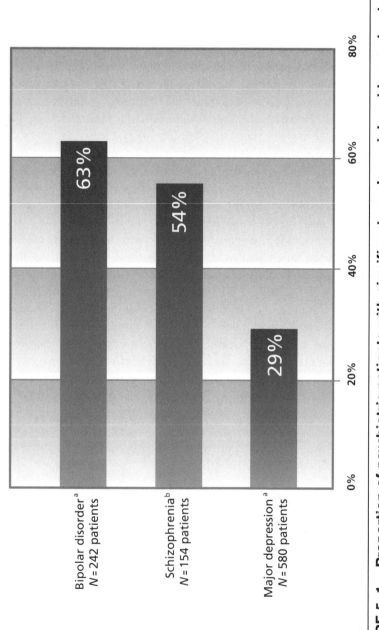

FIGURE 5–1. Proportion of psychiatric patients with significant psychosocial problems who do not receive psychotherapy consistent with American Psychiatric Association (APA) guideline recommendations.

[a]Data from the 1999 APA Practice Research Network Study of Psychiatric Patients and Treatments (American Psychiatric Association 1999).

[b]Data from the 1997 APA Practice Research Network Study of Psychiatric Patients and Treatments (American Psychiatric Association 1997)

and colleagues conducted a meta-analysis comparing the effectiveness of different types of psychodynamic therapies with or without medication (Luborsky et al. 1975). They found that all of the therapies appeared equally effective, but strong evidence indicated that combination therapy was superior to either psychotherapy or medication as monotherapy. Investigations undertaken since this analysis are discussed in more detail below.

As noted, most studies of combination therapy have focused on depression and have utilized either CBT or interpersonal therapy. However, Burnand et al. (2002) conducted a randomized controlled trial in which 74 outpatients with acute major depression were treated with medication alone (clomipramine) or combination therapy with psychodynamic psychotherapy. Marked improvement was noted in both groups, but subjects in the combination therapy group had lower rates of treatment failure, better work adjustment postdischarge, better global functioning, and lower hospitalization rates. Combination therapy with psychodynamic psychotherapy and clomipramine was also associated with lower direct costs and lower indirect costs as measured by the number of lost workdays. The cost savings per patient amounted to $2,311 in subjects who received both psychotherapy and medication.

A Dutch study compared brief (16-session) psychodynamic supportive psychotherapy plus medication versus medication monotherapy in the treatment of major depression (de Jonghe et al. 2001). The medication protocol allowed patients who experienced a poor response or significant side effects to try three different antidepressants (fluoxetine, amitriptyline, and moclobemide) in succession. Nearly one-third of the initial study subjects (84) refused pharmacotherapy, and 13% (11 of 83) refused combination therapy, leaving 72 subjects in the combination therapy group and 57 in the medication-only group. By the end of the 6-month study, 40% of subjects who began with pharmacotherapy only had stopped taking medication, whereas only 22% who were treated with combined therapy had discontinued medication. At 24 weeks, those who received combination therapy had a mean success rate of 59.2% compared with 40.7% in the medication-only group. The researchers noted that patients treated with medication and psychotherapy found their treatment significantly more acceptable, were less likely to drop out of treatment, and were more likely to recover.

Kool et al. (2003) further analyzed the data from this study and reported that combination therapy was superior to medication monotherapy only for patients with comorbid personality disorders. In patients with the diagnosis of depression alone, combination therapy was not superior. This finding is significant in light of the growing evidence that the treatment of affective disorders is more challenging when a comorbid personality disorder is not addressed as well (Oldham 2001).

TABLE 5–2. Patients' feelings about the psychiatrist in integrated treatment

Positive	Negative
Perceives that doctor genuinely acknowledges patient's pain	Senses doctor's discomfort with patient's plight
Perceives that doctor is interested in patient's feelings	Senses doctor's lack of interest in patient's feelings
Feels that doctor provides support and safety in treatment situation	Feels that doctor is attempting to control patient
Perceives that doctor is hopeful about symptom relief	Feels that doctor is attempting to minimize patient's problems
Appreciates doctor's skills	Fears that doctor has limited clinical skills
Feels comfortable with doctor's pharmacological approach and consistency of prescribing	Is angry over doctor's refusal to prescribe what patient desires or feels is needed

Source. Modified from Kay 2001.

A second Dutch study by de Jonghe et al. (2004) examined the helpfulness of combination therapy with psychodynamic supportive psychotherapy versus psychotherapy alone in patients with mild to moderate unipolar depression. More than 200 subjects participated in the study, with approximately equal numbers in each treatment group. Of interest is the fact that although patients reported experiencing the combination therapy as more efficacious, neither clinicians nor independent observers noted greater benefit from combination therapy.

Alliance, Compliance, and the Meaning of Medication

It is a clinical axiom that patients ascribe psychological meaning to the use of medication, even when they do so outside of their awareness. The resultant feelings often reflect their self-perception as well as their hopes and fears regarding their physician. Tables 5–2 and 5–3 list some of the feelings commonly encountered during integrated treatment.

The following vignette illustrates a frequent clinical situation. It highlights the need for patience and emphasizes the stance that must be adopted by the clinician in order to enhance the treatment process. One strength of

TABLE 5–3.　Patients' feelings about medication in integrated treatment

Positive	Negative
Is relieved that correct intervention is being offered	Experiences use of medication as evidence of his or her weakness
Perceives trustworthiness and efficacy of the intervention	Fears that medication is toxic or that using medication is a hurtful suggestion
Appreciates the integrative treatment plan	Becomes confused or resentful that the effective component of treatment is unclear

Source.　Modified from Kay 2001.

psychoanalytically oriented treatment is its commitment to understanding patients' behaviors and feelings as being the result of perceptual distortions that occur outside of their awareness (transference), and which become a central focus of treatment in all of its manifestations or derivatives.

> Mrs. H, a 33-year-old accountant, sought treatment for depression, which she attributed to her disappointing marriage. Over the previous year, her husband had begun drinking heavily, missed work often, was verbally abusive, and showed little sexual interest. She experienced early morning awakening, anhedonia, and frequent crying spells. The psychiatrist suggested that psychodynamic psychotherapy would be helpful in exploring her marital situation and the impact it had made on her life. In light of the patient's significant discomfort, the clinician also offered the patient an antidepressant.
>
> Although Mrs. H agreed to enter psychotherapy, she adamantly refused any medication. The psychiatrist was puzzled by her strong refusal to consider pharmacotherapy but assured the patient that he respected her feelings and that the subject could always be revisited. In the ensuing sessions, the patient described her chaotic and conflicted formative years with her mother, who suffered from severe bipolar disorder and frequently required hospitalization. The patient held intensely ambivalent feelings toward her mother and had had little contact with her after leaving home at the age of 18. Exploration of these feelings revealed that Mrs. H was frightened that she, too, might have a mood disorder and would become like her mother, whom she viewed as alienated, empty, and despondent. If she were to take medication, the patient feared she would end up like her mother. Complicating the medication issue was her husband's accusation that if she were to take medication, it would become a "crutch" because she was such a weak and dependent person. (Modified from Kay 2005, p. 464)

Yet another clinical example, although less common, illustrates the significant insight that can be achieved into a patient's characterological issues through the examination of responses and attitudes to medication:

> Mr. S, a 29-year-old married man, was referred by his endocrinologist for evaluation of a mood disorder despite effective treatment for a non-life-threatening tumor. It became apparent that this patient had suffered a long-standing dysthymic disorder (since adolescence) but that most of his emotional pain appeared to be secondary to self-defeating behavior. This finding prompted the psychiatrist to recommend psychoanalytically oriented psychotherapy and medication.
>
> Antidepressant medication was initiated, and the patient achieved improvement in his depressive symptoms. Seven weeks into the treatment, the psychiatrist inquired routinely about the need for a refill of the prescription; this revealed that the patient had let his prescription expire and that, as a result, he had not taken his medication for the previous week. Mr. S explained that his noncompliance was the result of his wife's failure to refill the prescription. Exploration of this unusual assignment of responsibility to the wife brought to light the fantasy that he had established the monitoring of his medication as a test of her caring for him. His wife, therefore, had disappointed him by failing to observe that Mr. S had run out of his medication. Despite an excellent response to medication, its discontinuation promoted a return of his irritability and increased argumentation in the marriage. Exploration of this behavior was remarkably productive in the psychotherapy, delineating the patient's passivity in his relationships with women and his inability to express his desires to others. With a greater appreciation of the meaning of his behavior regarding medication, the patient was able to resume pharmacotherapy, but assumed responsibility for his own medication. (Modified from Kay 2001, pp. 5–6)

It is important to note the provision of supportive dynamic psychotherapy in these two clinical vignettes. Regardless of the level of a patient's psychopathology, appreciation of the meaning that the patient attributes to medication is instrumental in effective treatment. In this regard, psychiatrists may become frustrated with adherence issues if they fail to clarify from the outset the meaning that patients attribute to, and the feelings they have toward, the use of medication.

Reasons for Medication Noncompliance

Problems with adherence to medication are ubiquitous. Some have argued that, until proven otherwise, clinicians should assume that noncompliance is a factor in each patient they treat (Rush 1988). Because as many as 60% of all patients, regardless of their diagnosis, fail to take their medications as prescribed, appreciating the reasons for noncompliance is a powerful tool in the therapeutic armamentarium (Basco and Rush 1996; Ellison and Harney 2000). Demyttenaere et al. (2001) studied depressed patients treated in primary care settings who dropped out of continuation treatment. They found that nearly 30% of patients had stopped treatment because they worried about becoming drug dependent, felt uncomfortable taking medications, or were concerned that they were relying inappropriately on medication to solve their problems. Similarly, a study of 155 depressed patients in primary care settings revealed that 28% had stopped taking their antidepressants by the end of the first month and 44% had done so by the end of the third month of treatment (Lin et al. 1995).

American and Canadian researchers studied why patients discontinue mental health care (Edlund et al. 2002). This study examined 1,200 patients from the United States and Ontario, Canada, in the early 1990s and found that treatment dropout rates were 19.2% and 16.9%, respectively. This difference was not statistically significant despite the fact that mental health insurance is a major problem for U.S. subjects, whereas Canadians have access to unlimited health care. Reasons for dropping out of treatment included a) the belief that mental health treatment is ineffective, b) embarrassment about seeking help, and c) being offered only medication or only psychotherapy instead of combination therapy. Only Americans cited not having insurance as an important reason for discontinuing treatment. Respondents who received combination therapy were less likely to leave treatment prematurely than their counterparts who were offered only monotherapy. In short, the unanticipated prevalence of stigma concerning mental health issues and the public's antimedication beliefs should not be underestimated (Benkert et al. 1997; Jorm et al. 1999).

Increasing the Likelihood of Medication Compliance

How should the clinician approach the initiation and continuing role of medication in treatment? The suggestions listed below, although not exhaustive, represent basic approaches to treatment with medication, be it integrated or split. It should be noted from the outset that all of these are predicated on the willingness of the clinician to recognize and explore a patient's expectable ambivalence about entering a treatment relationship. Ambivalence exists in the continuum of patients, from the most impaired to relatively high-functioning patients. In the former, for example, patients may have severe suspiciousness and delusional ideas about the meaning and effects of medication as well as an untrusting attitude toward the clinician. Above all, each clinician should be aware that the establishment of an empathic, nonjudgmental relationship, or therapeutic alliance, is the most potent predictor of outcome regardless of treatment modality.

An equally valid tenet is that the success of pharmacotherapy is intimately bound to the clinician's ability to establish a strong *pharmacothera-*

peutic relationship. Failure to implement such a relationship has relevance to malpractice issues as well, because most malpractice suits in the United States arise from the failure to intervene appropriately when treating suicidal patients and adverse drug responses. Without demonstrated interest by the clinician to address fundamental issues about symptoms and medication response within the context of a safe and secure relationship, communication is often much less effective. As Frank et al. (1995) have pointed out, a sound philosophy of care should focus on alliance, not compliance. Moreover, establishing a phenomenological diagnosis, even if accurate, does not guarantee the success of the therapeutic alliance.

Some Clinical Approaches to the Implementation of Pharmacotherapy

The following points characterize basic approaches to the use of pharmacotherapy:

- Within the context of traditional history taking, the clinician is obligated to inquire about the patient's satisfaction in previous treatment relationships with respect to both the general therapeutic alliance and medication experiences.
- The clinician must make clear to the patient that all effects of and responses to medication are worthy of examination and often provide helpful insights within treatment. Similarly, the patient's response to changes in medication, regardless of cause, is often of great importance.
- Given the complexity of treatment, the clinician should adopt a consistent method for addressing medication issues. To the degree that predictability can be instituted, deviation from a pattern often leads to the exploration of themes that can be an important indicator of countertransference issues. It is helpful to decide whether to address medication issues at the beginning or very end of a session. Each approach has its virtues. When medication is discussed at the beginning of a session, material may emerge reflecting important issues within the treatment relationship. Some clinicians prefer to address medication issues at the end of a session in order not to influence the content and process of the entire visit. However, this practice, some argue, may provide less opportunity for thematic exploration. Still others argue that medication issues should be attended to when they are raised by the patient.

  Beginning therapists often introduce medication issues in the middle of a session when they are uncomfortable with the unfolding of material or are anxious about understanding the process, as in the example below.

Introducing medication issues in this way invariably reflects a retreat to an exclusively medical treatment orientation, with which the therapist may be more comfortable:

> A beginning psychiatry resident was presenting to his supervisor a challenging and anxiety-provoking case in which a difficult patient had verbalized her strong sexual feelings for the resident. Immediately after the patient expressed these feelings, he asked her whether the medication she had been prescribed was helpful. With the supervisor's assistance, the trainee was able to appreciate that he had become anxious about the patient's expression of erotic longings and had switched the subject to medication as an attempt to combat his anxiety.

- The clinician should routinely ask the patient about his or her fears and fantasies about taking medication, to explore the possible meanings of medication and of the treatment in general. The discussion of a medication's indications, its potential side effects, and the advantages of taking one or more medications provides additional opportunities for exploration and can often foreshadow treatment issues to come. Obviously, the same may be said of the patient's feelings about requiring treatment for a mental disorder.

- The clinician should pay attention to questions that the patient asks about medication changes, be they the wish for new or additional medicines or the discontinuation of medicine. Such requests often reflect subtle resistance to the therapeutic process. Beginning clinicians may be more likely to institute medication changes as a sign of their growing frustration with a psychotherapeutic impasse.

- A major challenge for the psychiatrist conducting integrated treatment is learning to conduct two clinical tasks seamlessly, prescribing medication within the conduct of psychotherapy. Obviously the psychiatrist must continually elicit information regarding medication's effects, but he or she must also appreciate the need to approach the treatment process more globally. This approach is a healthy antidote to the prevailing view of a mind–body split that has so dominated modern Western medicine and often dichotomizes patients as having either brain-based disorders, which should be treated through medication, or disorders that have to do with the mind and should be addressed through psychosocial interventions. Kandel (1998, 1999) and others have emphasized that all mental processes are ultimately a product of brain activity and that psychotherapy, as noted earlier in this chapter in the discussion of the neurobiology of psychotherapy ("The Fallacy of Biology Versus Psychology"), changes brain structure and function in much the same fashion that medication does.

- The clinician must weigh the advantages of integrated as opposed to split treatment. The former may provide a better entrée into the central meaning that the patient assigns to medication. It may also provide a less intimidating venue for discussing troubling side effects, especially those having to do with sexual functioning. Many clinicians also believe that in integrated psychoanalytic psychotherapy, transference is less complicated and more readily available to inspection. Split treatment situations may be a quite different situation, as will be discussed shortly (see "Advantages of Conducting Split Treatment" and "Challenges of Providing Split Treatment"), in that simultaneous transferences, often of contrasting valences, arise with more than one clinician and can make treatment more complex.

- When treating patients with so-called primitive personality organizations (e.g., borderline and narcissistic personality disorders)—who tend to polarize treatment relationships, often indulge in self-harmful behavior, and may require hospitalization from time to time—some psychiatrists find integrated treatment more helpful than split treatment, which they feel complicates treatment needlessly. Integrated treatment may also be advantageous for patients with significant comorbid illness, the treatment of which requires the experience of a physician-therapist.

- The clinician should address the question of the return of symptoms at the conclusion of a successful treatment. The clinician should not assume in such cases that providing additional medication is the most helpful intervention. Exacerbation of symptoms can frequently be appreciated as a component of the patient's response to the ending of a significant, caring, and productive relationship. On the other hand, the psychiatrist's introduction of new medication at the termination may reflect ambivalence about stopping treatment.

The next vignette illustrates the helpfulness of addressing the meaning of medication side effects:

> Ms. R, a 24-year-old graduate student, was referred to a psychiatrist for twice-weekly psychoanalytic psychotherapy. Since the age of 13, this patient had experienced three episodes of major depression, the last of which occurred approximately 2 years earlier. In each case, she responded well to antidepressants. She had been euthymic for the past 2 years while on medication but expressed an interest in psychotherapy to explore her inhibitions with men as well as to monitor her medication use. As a child, the patient had grown up in a sexually stimulating and unsafe home. Ms. R was a striking woman who became quite anxious when, as frequently was the case, she was the object of inappropriate sexual remarks or rude glaring from men. The patient had never developed a serious relationship with a man, although she had many friendships. The patient acknowledged that because of her beginning work in psychotherapy, she was able to enter into a relationship with a young man.

After a month of intense and rewarding dating, Ms. R felt she could no longer resist her boyfriend's wish for a more intimate relationship. Her first sexual experience and subsequent sexual relations with this man were unsatisfying and she could not achieve orgasm. She did not speak about these experiences with her psychiatrist initially because she was uncomfortable discussing sexual topics. Shortly after beginning sexual relations, she became depressed again. After rather persistent exploration of her mood change by her psychiatrist, she finally admitted to discontinuing her medication because she attributed her sexual dysfunction to her antidepressant. A different medication, with fewer sexual side effects, was provided and her depression cleared.

In her therapy, she came to realize that her fear of discussing intimate matters with her psychiatrist was related to her experiences as a child and adolescent. She worried that to speak about her sexual relationship with her boyfriend, which she found very anxiety- and guilt-provoking, would overstimulate the psychiatrist, with the resultant loss of safety within the therapeutic dyad. (Kay 2005, pp. 465–466)

The final vignette in this section is presented because it summarizes common themes that can be exceptionally helpful in understanding the patient from the very beginning of treatment:

Ms. T, a 23-year-old graduate student, entered treatment because of numerous disappointing relationships with men and depression. Whenever she became close to a man, she sabotaged the relationship with numerous self-defeating behaviors. She was absolute in her conviction that her treatment should consist of medication only and idealized pharmacotherapy based on her reading on the Internet and direct pharmaceutical advertising.

During the initial diagnostic sessions, Ms. T acknowledged repeated sexual abuse at the hands of her father beginning when she was 12 years old. This history was shared with great reluctance and intense affect. Although the psychiatrist did not rule out the use of medication, he invited the patient to explore some of her reservations about psychotherapy as well. Fears of becoming overly dependent on the psychiatrist emerged. These were followed by concerns that if the psychiatrist understood her, he would come to dislike the patient in much the same fashion that she disliked herself. Shame and embarrassment from her sexual abuse were, not unexpectedly, at the forefront, but so was the fear that she would be taken advantage of by the physician. Further exploration of these concerns revealed that many of her male relationships became highly sexualized from the very beginning, much to her dismay. Discussion of this issue ultimately provided an appreciation that she was concerned about receiving psychotherapy from a man because the therapy could evoke strong erotic feelings toward the psychiatrist.

Needless to say, these themes became central to the therapy and foreshadowed critical transference issues having to do with Ms. T's father's betrayal. Exploration of medication issues from the very start hastened emergence of her concerns during treatment. Her depressive symptoms were acknowledged to be causing her significant emotional pain, so she was prescribed an antidepressant as an adjunct to her psychotherapy.

Split Treatment

Advantages of Conducting Split Treatment

As has been noted briefly, several important issues have led to significant growth in the practice of split treatment and include, but are not limited to, the following:

- Greater financial incentives for physicians because of low reimbursement rates for psychiatrists providing psychotherapy
- Diminishing choice of care options under managed care
- Decreasing number of psychiatrists participating in managed behavioral health care
- Adequate number of psychologists, social workers, and counselors
- De-emphasis on psychotherapy training in many residency programs
- Growing body of research supporting the efficacy and effectiveness of split treatment
- Limited availability of insurance coverage for mental health treatment

Proponents of split treatment have argued that it promotes the talents of more than one mental health professional and is therefore a more comprehensive and possibly more sophisticated approach. Some have advocated—although there are few data to support this—that it is less costly and permits greater access to care for more patients. Others have argued that split treatment may afford a greater opportunity for patients to be treated by clinicians of similar ethnicity. In the case of challenging patients, split treatment may afford greater emotional support to clinicians by protecting collaborators from very intense and taxing treatment relationships. It is also possible that continued professional development is more likely when two professionals learn from each other in a shared treatment arrangement. This is especially true when the result of a collaborative (i.e., split) treatment experience provides greater insight into the patient's fears and dynamics, thereby presenting a more comprehensive clinical understanding of the patient's plight. Also, the effectiveness of medication can illustrate the biological bases of some disorders for the psychotherapist and demonstrate the usefulness of medication in improving target symptoms in the areas of impulsivity, affective lability, and cognitive and perceptual limitations. Another advantage of conducting split treatment is that, according to some clinicians, intense transference reactions can be diluted and more readily addressed than in integrated treatment. It is also conceivable that collaborative treatment might curtail a patient's opportunity to spend too much time discussing medication issues at the expense of addressing psychological concerns.

Challenges of Providing Split Treatment

A common drawback to split treatment is that it is not always possible for each clinician to appreciate the qualifications of and ascertain the level of clinical sophistication of the collaborator. Under some conditions, collaborators may not have met each other. Anxiety about the reliability of a collaborator in this type of circumstance can be detrimental. It is naive to doubt that patients would comprehend this tension or, in some cases, that it would evoke splitting for patients vulnerable to such behavior. Other patients, who as children experienced significant conflict between parents, might attempt to neutralize tension between collaborators by adopting lifelong patterns of pacification and obsequiousness. The next vignette underscores the potential for complications in collaborative treatment:

> Dr. A, a psychoanalytically trained psychiatrist, had been treating a young woman for depression and fear of intimacy. During the first 4 months of weekly psychotherapy, it became clear that the patient was acting irresponsibly sexually and placing herself in harm's way. Neither increasing her antidepressant dose nor switching to a second agent appeared to be of significant help. The senior clinician requested a medication consultation with a newly relocated psychopharmacologist for suggestions about the resistant affective disorder and the patient's worrisome impulsivity.
>
> The consultant suggested an augmentation strategy for the depression and a low-dose antipsychotic medication for the patient's dangerous acting-out. However, during the consultation, the pharmacologist made some irresponsible comments about the value of psychotherapy, and the patient reacted strongly to the comments and became anxious and irritated with her psychotherapist. She questioned the helpfulness of the psychotherapy and the trustworthiness of her psychiatrist. The patient threatened to quit treatment, and it took considerable work in therapy to repair the rupture. Although this derailment ultimately assisted in the elucidation of important transference themes that centered on her abusive father, the patient nevertheless experienced unnecessary trauma.

By far the most common challenge to split treatment is insufficient communication between collaborators. This lack of communication typically has a negative impact on the patient's experience and may take multiple forms, including, but not limited to, the following examples:

- Prescribing of medication when the physician is unaware of the specifics of the psychotherapeutic treatment process with his or her colleague
- Unilateral initiation of medication by the prescribing physician to allay the physician's anxiety or discomfort with the patient, caused by concerns that the psychotherapy is not being helpful or an assumption that the patient is unable to handle the frustration of the psychotherapy

- Referring psychiatrist's subtle expression that the use of medication as prescribed by the second psychiatrist, while needed, is a violation of the former's clinical approach
- Inability of the psychiatrist to appreciate the impact of his or her competitive feelings toward the other clinician, which can cause the patient to engage in splitting. One source of this tension is envy about differential reimbursement for the services provided.
- Concern by one or both of the clinicians about liability issues
- Inability to appreciate that a patient is providing contradictory information to each clinician, which, in patients with significant characterological problems, often causes intense disruption of therapy
- Attempt by the psychopharmacologist to needlessly treat each of the patient's symptoms because of the lack of an overarching theoretical conceptualization of the treatment

The following clinical vignette illustrates the last point:

> Ms. F was being treated by an analyst for her enduring depression and anxiety, self-defeating and self-destructive behavior, and conflicts about achievement. The psychopharmacologist consultant prescribed multiple medications to address what he believed to be the patient's perceptual distortions, hopelessness, and affective instability. The consultant did not appreciate that these symptoms were reflections of the patient's complex PTSD, the genesis of which was early sexual and physical abuse at the hands of her older brother. Ms. F became needlessly upset by feelings that she was untreatable because she was too disturbed. This required her psychotherapist to address these issues with her, which reverberated throughout the treatment process.

Principles of Effective Split Treatment: Establishing Communication in Psychoanalytic Psychotherapy

As noted previously, accepting and understanding transference feelings within the therapeutic dyad is a central, and at times challenging, task in psychoanalytic psychotherapy. This task becomes enormously complicated when there are two clinicians about whom the patient has distinct transference reactions. Consider also that the patient is receiving medication about which he or she may have strong conscious and/or unconscious feelings. To this therapeutic relationship must be added the attendant countertransferences from each of the providers. It is not difficult to imagine that the treatment experience for all participants can become complicated and confusing. The following clinical vignette illustrates nearly every problem (including the failure to ascertain important transference issues and the meaningfulness of medication to the patient) that has been discussed. The frustrating experience for the collaborators, and undoubtedly for the patient as well, can be understood within the context of poorly defined clinical roles, expectations, and professional boundaries.

> Ms. D, a 27-year-old unmarried secretary, was referred by a recently relocated internist to a psychiatrist for assistance in managing the patient's depression and anxiety. According to her primary care practitioner, the patient did not respond to any of the various medications that he had prescribed over the last 6 months. She had a long-standing history of depressive episodes that began when she was a teenager. Work with the patient had been difficult for this physician, with the patient making frequent appointments for a multiplicity of symptoms and complaints. The internist was unable to ascertain any significant illness in the patient and all diagnostic tests proved normal. Because the psychiatrist had not worked previously with the referring doctor, she recommended that they meet to discuss the patient before treatment evaluation began. The physician put off the psychiatrist by saying he was pressed for time in his new practice and would prefer to send a summary of the patient's history. The psychiatrist, not willing to disappoint a new referral source, agreed reluctantly to see Ms. D.
>
> The patient told the psychiatrist that her doctor seemed disinterested in her and stated that she was instructed to see a mental health professional for counseling. She described her physician as very controlling, insisting that she take medication. The history indicated that the patient grew up in a household where both her mother and father were very demanding and rigid, always insisting that there was only one way to view life. Ms. D acknowledged that she had stopped taking the medications prescribed for her because of side effects, despite the fact that her doctor had reassured her that they would pass after the first week of treatment. She felt that he had been dishonest because some side effects, such as her sexual dysfunction, did not improve. The patient was effusive in her praise for the psychiatrist, who clearly was interested in her plight and gave her sufficient time to talk. This was not the case with her internist, whom she perceived as rigid.
>
> At the completion of the assessment, the psychiatrist summarized her thoughts about the possible ways in which to proceed and told the patient that she would be contacting the internist. She mentioned that the patient should discuss the medication's side effects with her physician and that there might be another medication that would be less problematic for her. The consultant tried to contact the referring physician, without success, to discuss her findings and the appropriateness of psychotherapy in addition to medication. Four days later she received a discouraging phone call from Ms. D's doctor, who felt he had been undermined in his treatment decisions because the patient refused to take any of the medications he wished to prescribe and had nothing but glowing words about her interaction with the psychiatrist. According to the physician, Ms. D explained that she was instructed to tell him that psychotherapy was indicated and not medication.

Some important tenets of effective collaboration can be garnered from the case of Ms. D:

- Collaborative treatment cases should be selected carefully and for well-thought-out reasons.
- Collaborators should meet to discuss the reasons for consultation when they have not worked together previously. Once a productive collaboration has been established and both parties feel comfortable, communication then may be by telephone or written reports.
- The psychiatrist and psychopharmacologist must agree on the responsibilities and boundaries of their collaboration. Is the latter a consultant only or are ongoing and regular patient visits expected?
- Confidentiality must be addressed with the patient by both collaborators. Likewise, if issues of suicidality or homicidality should arise, collaborators must be able to communicate freely about these matters.
- Both parties should agree on how to address medication side effects and their impact on the psychotherapy as well as on medication compliance.
- Collaborators should agree on the frequency of communication.
- Both parties should agree to solicit informed consent and Health Insurance Portability and Accountability Act (HIPAA) documents.
- Collaborators must never use the patient to convey information that should be discussed more appropriately between the providers.
- Sometimes the request for split treatment with a challenging referral can be a covert wish on the part of one clinician to either terminate treatment of or transfer a patient. It is difficult to overestimate the negative impact of such a situation on the patient as well as the collaborative relationship.
- When treatment is to be discontinued, the decision about termination and follow-up (if required) should be made jointly and explained to the patient by each collaborator.
- There is potential for detrimental effects on the patient when transfer to a new psychopharmacologist occurs. One study of psychiatry residents found that nearly 20% of patients being treated by senior residents experienced worsening of symptoms after being informed of such a decision, 32% required medication changes, and approximately10% became noncompliant (Mischoulon et al. 2000). Although the subjects in this study were psychopharmacologists' patients, this finding may be relevant in collaborative treatment as well.
- If a patient is not able to establish a therapeutic relationship with one of the collaborators, both have an obligation to support a change in the treatment relationship. An effective collaboration requires the willingness of both collaborators to identify a therapeutic impasse or plateau and jointly seek consultation.

Collaborators should also consider the following questions before treatment begins:

- If the need arises, which of the collaborators should speak with the patient's family members, and how?
- How will coverage be arranged in the absence of one or both collaborators?
- If problems arise, how should issues of the patient's insurance be addressed?
- If the need arises, how should a crisis or hospitalization be handled and by whom?

Conclusion

More comprehensive care and improved compliance are but two of the benefits in combining medication and psychotherapy. These benefits hold true in both the one-person and the two-person treatment model. Striking research in the neurobiology of psychotherapy, psychopharmacology, and the conduct of psychotherapy is diminishing the unproductive and anachronistic split mind-body argument. Further progress in this area can only provide more effective treatments and enhance the patient's experience.

Although there has been substantial research on combining medication and psychotherapy, several prominent questions have not been addressed. One of the foremost is, under what conditions is collaborative treatment more advantageous than integrated treatment? Other questions are: For what disorders should medication precede psychotherapy, and vice versa? For what disorders should medication use begin, whether via integrated or split treatment, at the start of psychotherapy? Finally, regarding cost-effectiveness, are some disorders best treated by a psychiatrist providing integrated treatment versus two clinicians providing split treatment?

Key Points

- Some of the benefits of adding medication to psychotherapeutic treatment include permitting the patient to express greater range of affect and troubling thoughts, enhancing the patient's self-esteem by decreasing passivity and the sense of helplessness through symptom improvement, and promoting more introspection through improving concentration and recall.
- When psychotherapy is added to ongoing pharmacotherapy, it may improve compliance, decrease relapse rates when medication is discontinued, provide a faster response to treatment, and improve long-term psychosocial functioning.
- Many medication compliance problems can be attributed to the psychiatrist's lack of appreciation of the meaning of medication to the patient.

- Some basic technical approaches to the use of pharmacotherapy include, but are not limited to, exploring the patient's previous psychotherapy and pharmacotherapy experiences, adopting a consistent approach to exploring medication once treatment has begun, and paying close attention to the possible meanings of the patient's request for medication changes as well as side effects.

- Caution is urged regarding the increasing of medication or switching to other medications during the termination stage of treatment, since there is often a return of symptoms during this critical phase of psychotherapy.

- The major challenge to implementing and maintaining effective split treatment is poor communication.

- Collaboration in split treatment must include agreement on the following topics: confidentiality, emergency issues (suicide, homicide, and hospitalization concerns) and coverage, frequency and form of communication, insurance matters, and attention to the patient's pitting the psychotherapist against the psychopharmacologist and vice versa.

References

American Psychiatric Association: Practice Research Network Study of Psychiatric Patients and Treatments (SPPT). Washington, DC, American Psychiatric Association, 1997

American Psychiatric Association: Practice Research Network Study of Psychiatric Patients and Treatments (SPPT). Washington, DC, American Psychiatric Association, 1999

Andreoli A, Burnand Y, Kolate E, et al: Combined treatment for major depression: does it save hospital days? in Syllabus and Proceedings Summary, American Psychiatric Association Annual Meeting, Chicago, IL, May 13–18, 2000. Washington, DC, American Psychiatric Association, 2000, p 14

Barlow DH, Gorman JM, Shear MK, et al: Cognitive-behavioral therapy, imipramine, or their combination for panic disorder: a randomized controlled trial. JAMA 283:2529–2536, 2000

Basco MR, Rush AJ: Cognitive-Behavioral Therapy for Bipolar Disorder. New York, Guilford, 1996

Bateman A, Fonagy P: Treatment of borderline personality disorder with psychoanalytically oriented partial hospitalization: an 18-month follow-up. Am J Psychiatry 158:36–42, 2001

Baxter LR Jr, Schwartz JM, Bergman KS, et al: Caudate glucose metabolic rate changes with both drug and behavior therapy for obsessive-compulsive disorder. Arch Gen Psychiatry 49:681–689, 1992

Benkert O, Graf-Morgenstern M, Hillert A, et al: Public opinion on psychotropic drugs: an analysis of the factors influencing acceptance or rejection. J Nerv Ment Dis 185:151–158, 1997

Bowers WA: Treatment of depressed in-patients: cognitive therapy plus medication, relaxation plus medication, and medication alone. Br J Psychiatry 156:73–78, 1990

Brody AL, Saxena S, Stoessel P, et al: Regional brain metabolic changes in patients with major depression treated with either paroxetine or interpersonal therapy: preliminary findings. Arch Gen Psychiatry 58:631–640, 2001

Burnand Y, Andreoli A, Kolatte E, et al: Psychodynamic psychotherapy and clomipramine in the treatment of major depression. Psychiatr Serv 53:585–590, 2002

de Jonghe F, Kool S, van Aalst G, et al: Combining psychotherapy and antidepressants in the treatment of depression. J Affect Disord 64:217–229, 2001

de Jonghe F, Hendricksen M, van Aalst G, et al: Psychotherapy alone and combined with pharmacotherapy in the treatment of depression. Br J Psychiatry 185:37–45, 2004

Demyttenaere K, Enzlin P, Dewé W, et al: Compliance with antidepressants in a primary care setting, 1: beyond lack of efficacy and adverse events. J Clin Psychiatry 62 (suppl 22):30–33, 2001

Dewan M: Are psychiatrists cost-effective? An analysis of integrated versus split treatment. Am J Psychiatry 156:324–326, 1999

Edlund MJ, Wang PS, Berglund PA, et al: Dropping out of mental health treatment: patterns and predictors among epidemiological survey respondents in the United States and Ontario. Am J Psychiatry 159:845–851, 2002

Ellison JM, Harney PA: Treatment-resistant depression and the collaborative treatment relationship. J Psychother Pract Res 9:7–17, 2000

Fava GA: Sequential treatment: a new way of integrating pharmacotherapy and psychotherapy. Psychother Psychosom 68:227–229, 1999

Fava GA, Rafanelli C, Grandi S, et al: Six-year outcome for cognitive behavioral treatment of residual symptoms in major depression. Am J Psychiatry 155:1443–1445, 1998

Fogel SP, Sneed JR, Roose SP: Survey of psychiatric treatment among psychiatric residents in Manhattan: evidence of stigma. J Clin Psychiatry 67:1591–1598, 2006

Frank E, Kupfer DJ, Siegel LR: Alliance not compliance: a philosophy of outpatient care. J Clin Psychiatry 56:11–16, 16–17 (discussion), 1995

Furmark T, Tillfors M, Marteinsdottir I, et al: Common changes in cerebral blood flow in patients with social phobia treated with citalopram or cognitive-behavioral therapy. Arch Gen Psychiatry 59:425–433, 2002

Gabbard GO, Kay J: The fate of integrated treatment: whatever happened to the biopsychosocial psychiatrist? Am J Psychiatry 158:1956–1963, 2001

Goldapple K, Segal Z, Garson C, et al: Modulation of cortical-limbic pathways in major depression: treatment-specific effects of cognitive behavior therapy. Arch Gen Psychiatry 61:34–41, 2004

Goldman W, McCulloch J, Cuffel B, et al: Outpatient utilization patterns of integrated and split psychotherapy and pharmacotherapy for depression. Psychiatr Serv 49:477–482, 1998

Joffe R, Segal Z, Singer W: Change in thyroid hormone levels following response to cognitive therapy for major depression. Am J Psychiatry 153:411–413, 1996

Jorm AF, Korten AE, Jacomb PA, et al: Attitudes towards people with a mental disorder: a survey of the Australian public and health professionals. Aust N Z J
Psychiatry 33:77–83, 1999

Kandel ER: A new intellectual framework for psychiatry. Am J Psychiatry 155:457–
469, 1998

Kandel ER: Biology and the future of psychoanalysis: a new intellectual framework
for psychiatry revisited. Am J Psychiatry 156:505–524, 1999

Kay J: Integrated treatment: an overview, in Integrated Treatment for Psychiatric
Disorders: Review of Psychiatry, Vol 20. Edited by Kay J. Washington, DC,
American Psychiatric Press, 2001, pp 1–29

Kay J: Psychotherapy and medication, in Oxford Textbook of Psychotherapy. Edited by Gabbard GO, Beck JS, Holmes J. New York, Oxford University Press,
2005, pp 463–476

Klerman GL, Dimascio A, Weissman M, et al: Treatment of depression by drugs
and psychotherapy. Am J Psychiatry 131:186–191, 1974

Kool S, Dekker J, de Jonghe F, et al: Efficacy of combined therapy and pharmacotherapy for depressed patients with or without personality disorders. Harv Rev
Psychiatry 11:133–141, 2003

Lin EH, Von Korff M, Katon W, et al: The role of the primary care physician in
patients' adherence to antidepressant therapy. Med Care 33:67–74, 1995

Luborsky L, Singer B, Luborsky L: Comparative studies of psychotherapies: is it
true that "everywon has one and all must have prizes"? Arch Gen Psychiatry
32:995–1008, 1975

Marks IM, Basoglu M, Noshirvani H, et al: Drug treatment of panic disorder: further comment. Br J Psychiatry 162:795–796, 1993

Martin SD, Martin E, Rai SS, et al: Brain blood flow changes in depressed patients
treated with interpersonal psychotherapy or venlafaxine hydrochloride: preliminary findings. Arch Gen Psychiatry 58:641–648, 2001

Mayberg HS: Defining neurocircuits in depression. Psychiatr Ann 36:258–267,
2006

Milrod B, Leon AC, Busch F, et al: A randomized controlled clinical trial of psychoanalytic psychotherapy for panic disorder. Am J Psychiatry 164:265–272,
2007

Misch DA: Basic strategies of dynamic supportive therapy. J Psychother Pract Res
9:173–189, 2000

Mischoulon D, Rosenbaum JF, Messner E: Transfer to a new psychopharmacologist: its effect on patients. Acad Psychiatry 24:156–163, 2000

Oldham J: Detection and treatment of depressive disorders (editorial). J Psychiatr
Pract 7:283, 2001

Pampallona S, Bollini P, Tibaldi G, et al: Combined pharmacotherapy and psychological treatment for depression: a systematic review. Arch Gen Psychiatry
61:714–719, 2004

Pava JA, Fava M, Levenson JA: Integrating cognitive therapy and pharmacotherapy
in the treatment and prophylaxis of depression: a novel approach. Psychother
Psychosom 61:211–219, 1994

Rockland LH: Psychoanalytically oriented supportive therapy: literature review and techniques. J Am Acad Psychoanal 17:451–462, 1989

Rush AJ: Clinical diagnosis of mood disorders. Clin Chem 34:813–821, 1988

Saarinen PI, Lehtonen J, Joensuu M, et al: An outcome of psychodynamic psychotherapy: a case study of the change in serotonin transporter binding and the activation of the dream screen. Am J Psychother 59:61–73, 2005

Schwartz JM, Stoessel PW, Baxter LR, et al: Systematic changes in cerebral glucose metabolic rate after successful behavior modification treatment of obsessive-compulsive disorder. Arch Gen Psychiatry 53:109–113, 1996

Seligman ME: The effectiveness of psychotherapy: the Consumer Reports study. Am Psychol 50:965–974, 1995

Teasdale JD, Scott J, Moore RG, et al: How does cognitive therapy prevent relapse in residual depression? Evidence from a controlled trial. J Consult Clin Psychol 69:347–357, 2001

Thase ME, Fasiczka AL, Berman SR, et al: Electroencephalographic sleep profiles before and after cognitive behavior therapy of depression. Arch Gen Psychiatry 55:138–144, 1998

Vergouwen AC, Bakker A, Katon WJ, et al: Improving adherence to antidepressants: a systematic review of interventions. J Clin Psychiatry 64:1414–1420, 2003

Viinamaki H, Kuikka J, Tiihonen J: Change in monoamine transporter density related to clinical recovery: a case control study. Nord J Psychiatry 52:39–44, 1998

Westra HA, Stewart SH, Conrad BE: Naturalistic manner of benzodiazepine use and cognitive behavioral therapy outcome in panic disorder with agoraphobia. J Anxiety Disord 16:233–246, 2002

Wiborg IM, Dahl AA: Does brief dynamic psychotherapy reduce the relapse rate of panic disorder? Arch Gen Psychiatry 53:689–694, 1996

Suggested Readings

Burnand Y, Andreoli A, Kolatte E, et al: Psychodynamic psychotherapy and clomipramine in the treatment of major depression. Psychiatr Serv 53:585–590, 2002

de Jonghe F, Hendricksen M, van Aalst G, et al: Psychotherapy alone and combined with pharmacotherapy in the treatment of depression. Br J Psychiatry 185:37–45, 2004

Gabbard GO, Kay J: The fate of integrated treatment: whatever happened to the biopsychosocial psychiatrist? Am J Psychiatry 158:1956–1963, 2001

Kandel ER: Biology and the future of psychoanalysis: a new intellectual framework for psychiatry revisited. Am J Psychiatry 156:505–524, 1999

Kay J: Integrated treatment: an overview, in Integrated Treatment for Psychiatric Disorders: Review of Psychiatry, Vol 20. Edited by Kay J. Washington, DC, American Psychiatric Press, 2001, pp 1–29

Roose S, Cabaniss DL, Rutherford B: Combined therapies: psychotherapy and pharmacotherapy, in Psychiatry, 3rd Edition. Edited by Tasman A, Kay J, Lieberman JA, et al. Chichester, UK, Wiley, 2008, pp 1807–1825

PART 2

Individual Cognitive-Behavioral Therapy

Section Editors
Jesse H. Wright, M.D., Ph.D.
Judith S. Beck, Ph.D.

Chapter 6

Theory of Cognitive Therapy

David A. Clark, Ph.D.
Michael Hollifield, M.D.
Robert Leahy, Ph.D.
Judith S. Beck, Ph.D.

Since its earliest days, cognitive therapy has been defined in terms of its theory of or perspective on psychopathology (A. T. Beck 1967). What makes a therapist's approach cognitive (or cognitive-behavioral) is not reliance on a defined set of intervention strategies but rather the theory of psychopathology and human change that guides the therapeutic enterprise. In this chapter, we provide an introductory overview of the tenets of cognitive theory for a variety of common psychiatric disorders. Our objective is to give readers a basic foundation in cognitive theory that will enable a better understanding of cognitive therapy.

Origins of Cognitive Therapy

Cognitive therapy emerged out of dissatisfaction with the strict behavioral therapy and traditional psychoanalytic psychotherapy that was dominant in the early to mid-1970s. Empirically oriented therapists were dissatisfied with the difficulty in operationally defining many of the central tenets of psychoanalysis as well as the limited empirical support in many key areas of theory and treatment. Behavioral approaches also proved disappointing for treating certain common psychiatric disorders, such as major depression, panic disorder, and generalized anxiety disorder (GAD), and again many key aspects of behavioral models were not confirmed by experiments (D.A. Clark et al. 1999; Dobson and Dozois 2001). This led to the *cognitive revolution* of the late 1970s and early 1980s, in which an increasing number of clinical researchers advocated a greater role for cognitive mediation in theory and treatment.

Basic Assumptions of Cognitive Theory

The basic proposition of cognitive theory is that information processing is a defining feature of what it means to be human, enabling individuals to make meaningful representations of themselves and their world. Humans are in a continual state of processing streams of information from their external and internal environments. They receive, encode, interpret, store, and retrieve information; this information processing plays a vital role in human adaptation and survival (D.A. Clark et al. 1999). Thus they respond to their *cognitive representations* of the environment rather than responding directly to the environment itself. These cognitive representations—thoughts, interpretations, beliefs, and attitudes—can be monitored, evaluated, and modified. Given the centrality of cognition and its malleability, change in cognition can have a significant influence on emotional and behavioral functioning (Dobson and Dozois 2001). In fact, the cognitive model considers cognitive change necessary in order to achieve enduring change in behavior or emotion.

Table 6–1 summarizes the key assumptions that define the cognitive perspective on psychopathology (see D.A. Clark et al. 1999 for elaboration).

Individuals are continually engaged in a personal construction of their reality. These perceptual-interpretive constructions direct affective, behavioral, and physiological responding either in a positive manner, indicative of adaptation, or in a negative fashion, which can lead to emotional disturbance and functional impairment. Our interpretations are a product not only of the sensory information we receive (e.g., seeing a figure lunging to-

TABLE 6–1. Basic assumptions of the cognitive theory of psychopathology

Information processing and meaning representation are essential functions for human survival and adaptation.

A basic function of the information-processing system is the personal construction of reality.

Information processing serves to guide emotional, behavioral, and physical aspects of human experience.

The interaction of bottom-up/stimulus-driven sensory information and top-down/higher-order semantic processes is evident in cognitive functioning.

The meaning-making structures of the information-processing system are characterized by different thresholds of activation.

Psychological disturbance is characterized by excessive and/or deficient activation of specific meaning-making structures (e.g., beliefs and attitudes).

Modification of meaning-making structures is central to the process of human change.

Source. D.A. Clark et al. 1999.

ward us) but also of long-term autobiographical memory and higher-order executive processes like reasoning and comprehension (e.g., remembering a recent assault and its implications). Which memory structures contribute most to the interpretation of an experience depends on their activation threshold. For example, semantic (i.e., meaning) representations of disease and death may be readily activated by a wide range of cues in those vulnerable to panic and health anxiety, whereas these representations have a much higher activation threshold in persons without that vulnerability.

According to the cognitive model, pathological disturbance in thought, feeling, and affect is characterized by a bias in the information-processing system in the form of excessive or deficient activation of particular meaning-making structures or schemas (A.T. Beck 1987). The goal of cognitive therapy, then, is to redress this bias in the information-processing system by damping down hypervalent negative or dysfunctional schemas (i.e., beliefs and attitudes) and strengthening access to more constructive modes of thinking (A.T. Beck 1996; D.A. Clark et al. 1999). The cognitive model assumes that change in maladaptive cognitions, processing strategies, and meaning-making structures is critical to symptomatic improvement in psychiatric and psychological disorders (A.T. Beck et al. 1979; Haaga et al. 1991).

Key Concepts of Cognitive Theory

Kendall and Ingram (1989) proposed a taxonomy to classify the various constructs that define cognitive theories of psychopathology. Table 6–2 provides a brief description of the four taxonomic elements: cognitive structure, propositions, operations, and products.

The cognitive basis of psychopathology involves each of these four conceptual levels. The biased thoughts, images, and interpretations that characterize psychiatric disorders are the end products of an information-processing system that is biased in the structures and processes that dominate during periods of emotional disturbance. The cognitive model offers a perspective on psychopathology at both a descriptive level and a vulnerability level (A.T. Beck 1987).

At the descriptive level of conceptualization, the cognitive model depicts the organization and function of various cognitive structures, processes, and products that characterize cognitive functioning during acute symptomatic episodes. Two hypotheses that are especially critical at this descriptive level are *cognitive content specificity* and *cognitive primacy* (D.A. Clark et al. 1999):

1. *Cognitive content specificity hypothesis:* Each psychiatric or psychological disorder has a distinct cognitive profile involving particular content or themes in the dysfunctional thoughts, images, beliefs, and appraisals that define the disorder.
2. *Cognitive primacy hypothesis:* Maladaptive thoughts and beliefs have a direct influence on the behavioral, emotional, somatic, and motivational symptoms of psychopathology.

The cognitive model also proposes certain constructs that have vulnerability or causal status in the etiology of psychopathology (A.T. Beck 1987, 1996; A.T. Beck et al. 2004; D.A. Clark et al. 1999; Haaga et al. 1991). Individual differences in susceptibility to various types of psychiatric disorders are viewed in terms of an underlying cognitive vulnerability, which remains latent and inactive until triggered by a relevant life experience. The cognitive model, then, takes a *diathesis-stress* perspective in which certain core maladaptive schemas, the product of negative developmental experiences, remain dormant until activated by a matching life event (A.T. Beck 1987). For example, a person predisposed to depression might possess core self-schemas of abandonment and rejection that remain latent until activated by an event such as the threat of losing a valued relationship. Once these maladaptive schemas are activated, they tend to dominate the information-processing system, leading to the well-recognized symptoms of depression.

TABLE 6–2.   Taxonomy for cognitive concepts

Conceptual level	Description
Cognitive structure	Concepts that refer to the storage and organization of information (e.g., schemas, semantic network, meaning representation)
Cognitive propositions	Concepts that focus on the content or information stored in memory structures (e.g., ideas, beliefs, attitudes)
Cognitive operations	Processes responsible for operation of the information-processing system (e.g., selective attention, encoding, retrieval)
Cognitive products	End result or output from the operation of the information-processing system (e.g., automatic thoughts, images, appraisals or interpretations)

Source.   Kendall and Ingram 1989.

Although empirical evidence for the descriptive predictions of the cognitive model has been supported by hundreds of studies on the cognitive basis of psychopathology (e.g., for reviews, see D.A. Clark and A.T. Beck, "Cognitive Therapy of Anxiety: Science and Practice," manuscript in preparation, 2008; D.A. Clark et al. 1999; and Gotlib and Neubauer 2000), it is only relatively recently that support for the vulnerability hypothesis has been forthcoming, with the advent of experimental procedures that involve mood-priming manipulations (Ingram et al. 1998; Scher et al. 2005).

The Cognitive Theory: A Definition

Over the years, the cognitive theory of psychopathology has been articulated in many publications (e.g., Alford and Beck 1997; A.T. Beck 1967, 1987, 1996; A.T. Beck et al. 1985, 2004; J.S. Beck 1995; D.A. Clark and A.T. Beck, "Cognitive Therapy of Anxiety: Science and Practice," manuscript in preparation, 2008; D.A. Clark et al. 1999; Leahy 2004b; Reinecke and Clark 2004; Riskind and Alloy 2006; Wells 1997). Although application of cognitive theory to various disorders has required some refinements and modifications, certain core assumptions and constructs are evident across all of the disorder-specific cognitive models. The following definition of the cognitive theory is applicable to the various disorder-specific models briefly described later in this chapter (see "The Cognitive Theory of Specific Clinical Disorders" section).

What Is the Cognitive Theory?

The cognitive theory of psychopathology explains psychological disturbance in terms of preexisting, idiosyncratic, maladaptive schematic representations of the self, others, and the personal world that are activated by
matching life experiences, resulting in a biased processing of self-referent
information, which leads to the maladaptive thoughts, affect, behavior, and
physiological responses that characterize specific psychopathological
states. According to this cognitive formulation, recovery from acute psychiatric episodes requires remediation of the biased information processing of
disorder-relevant experiences.

Although dysfunctional cognitive functioning contributes to the onset
and pathogenesis of disorders, it is neither necessary nor sufficient to cause
a disorder (Riskind and Alloy 2006). Rather, many factors at the genetic, developmental, biological, social, behavioral, and emotional levels contribute
to the development of and recovery from psychopathology (A.T. Beck
1987). Maladaptive cognition is one of many different types of contributors
to psychopathological states. The cognitive theory also notes that the biased information processing in psychopathology is not a general cognitive
deficit, but rather a feature that is highly specific to the personal concerns of
the target disorder. For example, a young man with panic disorder may exhibit biased processing of bodily sensations, which he misinterprets as a
possible heart attack, but show absolutely no concern about health habits
that increase the risk for cancer. Figure 6–1 illustrates the various interacting constructs of the cognitive model of psychopathology.

Maladaptive Cognitive Structures (Schemas)

Schemas are enduring internal semantic representations of stimuli, ideas,
or experience that organize and integrate new information in a meaningful
manner that determines how phenomena are perceived and conceptualized
(A.T. Beck 1967; D.A. Clark et al. 1999; Williams et al. 1997). As hypothetical structures containing the stored representations of meaning, schemas guide the selection, encoding, organization, storage, and retrieval of
information. Schematic content is evident in the beliefs, attitudes, and assumptions held by individuals. Because schematic content takes the form of
propositions that are abstracted from daily experience, schemas guide our
interpretation of life experiences. As a result, beliefs and attitudes determine the type and intensity of emotional response through their symbolic
representation of situations (D.A. Clark et al. 1999).

There are different types of schematic content. At the most basic level
are *simple schemas*, which represent knowledge about single objects or ideas
(the meaning of "chair," "shoe," etc.). At the next level are *intermediary be-*

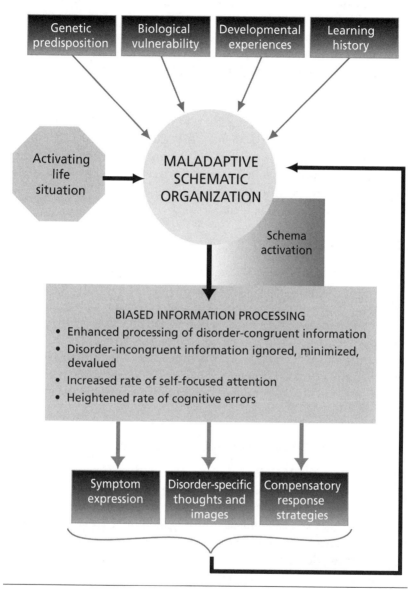

FIGURE 6–1. **The cognitive theory of psychopathology.**

liefs, which consist of rules, assumptions, and attitudes that we use to evaluate and guide ourselves as well as our interpretations of other people and personal experiences (A.T. Beck et al. 1985; J.S. Beck 1995; D.A. Clark et al. 1999). Examples of intermediary beliefs might be "I need to work harder than others in order to succeed," "It is important to ensure safety and avoid all risk," "Uncertainty needs to be minimized at all costs," "People cannot be trusted," and the like. A special class of intermediary beliefs is the *conditional rule*, which takes the form of "If…then" statements (e.g., "If I work hard, then I deserve to be rewarded," "If I am considerate of others, then they will be considerate of me," and "If I please others, then they will not abandon or exclude me"). The final type of schematic content that is central to cognitive theory and therapy is *core beliefs*. These beliefs are the most fundamental of schematic content and are often unarticulated, having their root in early childhood development (J. S. Beck 1995). Core beliefs are global, rigid, absolute, and overgeneralized convictions about the self, others, and the personal world that have powerful effects on how we perceive ourselves and our context. Examples of core beliefs are "I am unlovable," "I am weak and helpless," and "I'm incompetent."

Cognitive Errors

In psychopathological states, the activation of maladaptive schemas and biased information processing leads to inaccurate interpretations or appraisals of the self, personal experiences, and interpersonal relations. Although errors of inference and reasoning are common in psychiatrically healthy individuals, these errors become particularly salient during periods of emotional disturbance. Training patients in the identification and correction of their cognitive errors is an important component of cognitive therapy. Table 6–3 presents a list of common cognitive errors found in patients with psychiatric disorders.

Negative Automatic Thoughts and Images

Aaron T. Beck (1963, 1976) considered negative automatic thoughts a product of the biased information-processing system, which is of particular importance in understanding cognitive dysfunction in clinical states. He noted that automatic thoughts and images tend to be specific to current concerns and tend to be transient, involuntary, and highly plausible mentations reflecting the person's current affective state or personality disposition. Although automatic thoughts and images may not be readily apparent to the individual, with training the patient can learn to access this cognitive material. Cognitive theory postulates that the specific themes and content that characterize each clinical disorder will be evident in the patient's automatic thoughts and images (see, e.g., R. Beck and Perkins 2001).

Automatic thoughts and images play a central role in cognitive therapy because they are a primary subject matter for intervention. Correction of the biased information-processing system and modification of underlying

TABLE 6-3. Common cognitive errors found in psychopathological states

Cognitive error	Definition
Arbitrary inference	Drawing a specific conclusion in the absence of evidence or when the evidence is contrary to the conclusion
Selective abstraction	Focusing on a detail out of context while ignoring other, more salient features in the situation
Overgeneralization	Drawing a conclusion on the basis of one or more isolated incidents
Dichotomous thinking	The tendency to classify experience in one of two extreme categories, ignoring more moderate variations
Personalization	The tendency to relate external events to oneself
Magnification/ minimization	Exaggerating (i.e., catastrophizing) or belittling the significance or magnitude of an event

Source.   A.T. Beck 1963; A.T. Beck et al. 1979; D.A. Clark et al. 1999.

dysfunctional schemas occur when therapists repeatedly help patients identify and restructure the maladaptive thoughts and images associated with
personal experiences. Examples of negative automatic thoughts include the
student who goes into an exam thinking, "I don't know anything; I'm going
to fail," and the person at a business meeting who thinks, "Everyone is so
bored by my presentation." Cognitive-clinical researchers have also recognized other types of cognition that are important in psychopathology, such
as worry, rumination, and unwanted intrusive thoughts (D.A. Clark 2005;
Davey and Wells 2006; Leahy 2005; Papageorgiou and Wells 2004).

Compensatory Strategies

Judith Beck (1995) introduced the term *compensatory strategies* to refer to the
behavioral responses that individuals use to cope with maladaptive core beliefs. For example, a patient with a core belief such as "I am unlovable"
might go out of his or her way to please other people in an effort to gain
their favor. A person who believes "I am not very intelligent" might over-
prepare work assignments in order to compensate for perceived deficits in
intellectual ability. A.T. Beck et al. (2004) also noted that beliefs accompany
these compensatory strategies. A person who believes "I can't trust myself

to make the right decision" might develop the belief "If I get advice from others, I can ensure I've made the right decision," which makes the compensatory strategy of excessive reassurance-seeking understandable. The identification and modification of compensatory strategies and beliefs is an important component of cognitive therapy, especially in the treatment of individuals with Axis II disorders.

A Biopsychosocial Perspective

Research over the past 15 years has provided a web of evidence for the long-theorized relationships among biology, the social environment, and the psychological processes involving affect and cognition. Emerging evidence indicates that negative social experiences can affect aspects of neural development, and these effects in turn may increase the propensity to engage in the patterns of maladaptive cognition that characterize psychiatric disorders. Data indicate that an interaction exists among early life stress, a serotonin transporter gene polymorphism, and vulnerability to depression (Caspi et al. 2003; Vergne and Nemeroff 2006). Exposure to adverse experiences in childhood poses a major threat to the integrity of normal central nervous system functioning and a major risk for the development of mood and anxiety disorders (Bremner 2003; van der Kolk 2003). Chronic stress has its effects primarily in the amygdala, the hippocampus, and the prefrontal cortex—areas that are genetically determined to mediate memory, learning, and conditioning (McEwen 2004). Early adversity alters the glucocorticoid response to subsequent stress and leads to changes in glucocorticoid receptor numbers and sensitivity in brain areas responsible for cognition as well as other functions (Ladd et al. 1996; Levine et al. 1993; Stanton et al. 1988). Furthermore, adverse childhood experiences have lasting effects on multiple neurotransmitter systems and the hypothalamic-pituitary-adrenal (HPA) axis (Bremner 2003). Over time, the effects of chronic stress on the brain and the HPA axis increase the risk for maladaptive cognitions.

Neuroimaging research has suggested a neural model of cognitive therapy, in which ventral prefrontal and limbic areas generate stimulus-related negative affect, and dorsal prefrontal structures mediate cognitive reappraisal to dampen negative affect (Roffman et al. 2005). Various interventions have been shown to change cognition and the neurobiology associated with cognitive processes. Successful cognitive therapy for anxiety disorders has consistently been associated with attenuation of activity in ventral and limbic areas, and with activation in dorsal prefrontal areas (Roffman et al. 2005). Together with animal research on the neural basis of fear acquisition and inhibition, human neuroimaging research is elucidating the biological basis of cognition and emotion, highlighting the neural mechanisms that enable the higher cognitive processes emphasized in cognitive therapy to inhibit negative emotional responses, which are mediated in subcortical structures of the brain.

The Cognitive Theory of Specific Clinical Disorders

Major Depression and Dysthymia

The cognitive model was originally developed to account for depression, but over the years it has been significantly refined and elaborated (A.T. Beck 1967, 1987; A.T. Beck et al. 1979; D.A. Clark et al. 1999; Scher et al. 2004). The model assumes that the cognitive basis for depression is similar in major depression and dysthymia, although activation of depressogenic thinking styles may be more severe and generalized in major depression. In both major depression and dysthymia, the dominant theme is one of perceived loss or deprivation of valued resources. Aaron Beck (1967) coined the term *cognitive triad* to refer to the pervasive negativity in views of the self, the individual's personal world, and the future that is characteristic of episodic depression. The negative cognitive triad is evident in the automatic thoughts, beliefs, and assumptions of the depressed individual.

The maladaptive schemas activated during depression primarily reflect a negative evaluation of the self. Numerous studies have shown that the biased processing that characterizes depression is not a generalized cognitive deficit but rather one that is limited to the processing of information relevant to the self (i.e., self-referent thinking). Two sets of concerns are of particular importance in depression: those that deal with social relations and those that focus on mastery and achievement. A.T. Beck (1983, 1987) proposed two schematic organizations (i.e., cognitive personality predispositions) that might make a person susceptible to depression: sociotropy and autonomy. A highly *sociotropic* person possesses a constellation of beliefs centered on achieving self-worth through receiving love and acceptance from others, whereas the highly *autonomous* person has self-schemas that focus on attaining self-worth through experiencing a sense of control, mastery, and achievement. The cognitive model further posits that sociotropic individuals are more susceptible to the onset of depression when they experience a life event involving a loss of social resources, whereas autonomous persons are at higher risk for depression when they experience an event involving failure to achieve something of significant personal value.

Over the years numerous studies have generally supported the cognitive model of depression at the descriptive level (for reviews, see D.A. Clark et al. 1999; Haaga et al. 1991; Scher et al. 2004; Solomon and Haaga 2004).

During episodic depression, negative automatic thoughts of personal loss and failure predominate, with the frequency and plausibility of these negative thoughts closely linked to the severity of symptoms. Fairly consistent support exists for cognitive specificity in which self-referent thoughts of loss and failure are distinct to depression (e.g., R. Beck and Perkins 2001). Moreover, experimental information-processing studies have shown that depression is characterized by the following (D.A. Clark et al. 1999):

- Biased recall of negative self-referent material
- Selective encoding of negative self-referent material
- Biased perception of negative feedback
- A tendency to make negative causal attributions
- Negative expectancies for the future

In addition, empirical evidence has indicated that negative self-schemas may constitute a cognitive vulnerability to the onset of depression; this evidence comes from studies utilizing mood-priming manipulations or prospective high-risk behavioral designs (e.g., Alloy et al. 2006; Ingram et al. 2005; Scher et al. 2004, 2005; Zuroff et al. 2004). However, three issues remain unresolved:

1. Whether the cognitive dysfunction in depression primarily reflects enhanced processing of negative self-referent information or reduced processing of positive material
2. The extent to which the cognitive bias in depression involves preconscious, automatic versus conscious, effortful cognitive mechanisms
3. Whether cognitive dysfunction is a cause or consequence of depression

Bipolar Disorder

The cognitive model of bipolar disorder initially proposed that the manic episode is characterized by extreme positivity, with automatic thoughts reflecting an overly optimistic bias (e.g., "I can win no matter what" or "I am extremely attractive"), rigidity and impermeability of thought, and overly positive maladaptive assumptions ("If I simply want it, I can make it happen") (Leahy and Beck 1988). This cognitive formulation was extended to a general cognitive model of bipolar disorder that incorporates bipolar disorder within the case conceptualization model of automatic thoughts, conditional beliefs, and personal schemas (Newman et al. 2001).

Bipolar disorder is affected by life events, both positive and negative. Manic enthusiasm may be understood as increased self-esteem, energy, and goal-directed activities that result from the greater sensitivity of an individual's behavioral activation system (i.e., responsiveness to reward) when positive life events occur (Depue and Iacono 1989; Johnson 2005). In support, goal attainment is associated with subsequent increases in manic symptoms (Johnson et al. 2000), and bipolar individuals have greater reactivity to stimuli, perhaps accounting for their mood instability (Sutton and Johnson 2002).

Individuals with bipolar disorder in remission have overgeneralized autobiographical memory, similar to individuals with unipolar depression (Mansell and Lam 2004). Manic individuals recall more positive items—but also more negative items (Eich et al. 1997)—suggesting both polarized and overgeneralized memory. In some respects, bipolar individuals, even when manic, show both a heightened bias toward the positive in the present and a bias toward the negative in memory. These findings may lend some support to a *manic defense* hypothesis: the overly positive emphasis in mania may be a defensive coping strategy to compensate for the overly negative bias that also occurs. Another interpretation is that mania is often characterized by mixed states of both manic agitation and depressive pessimism.

Leahy (2004a) has proposed that manic individuals utilize a risk-loving style of thinking, often underestimating the probability, severity, and personal relevance of risk, and often discounting the difficulty of achieving goals. Mansell (2007) has proposed an integrative model of mania: when manic individuals experience intrusive thoughts and feelings, they appraise them in a manner that facilitates ascent of mood ("My mind is racing means I am creative") rather than attempting to control the mood (as would be the case in nonmanic individuals).

Studies of attributional style among bipolar individuals indicate a generally negative explanatory style, even when the disorder is in remission (Alloy et al. 1999). It may be that the generally negative explanatory style, coupled with unstable self-esteem, leads bipolar individuals to respond with overly positive (manic) cognitive styles—a cognitive model of the manic defense. In sum, a variety of dysfunctional cognitive processes characterize the manic phase, and the same negative, self-referent cognitive style that is evident in major depression predominates during the bipolar depressive phase.

Anxiety Disorders

Aaron Beck and colleagues (1985) theorized that selective biases in information processing lead anxiety-prone individuals to perceive certain internal or external situations as threatening, and to perceive themselves as unable to cope effectively with these threats. Cognitive components of anxiety include the following:

1. A tendency to generalize fearful thoughts beyond initially feared events
2. An overestimation of the degree of threat from the feared situation
3. An underestimation of one's ability to cope with or control the situation and the fear response
4. Resultant compensatory escape and avoidance behavior

People with pathological anxiety perceive threat where others do not, are unable to accurately evaluate safety, and reinforce their anxiety response by avoidance and escape.

Evidence for an underlying general cognitive vulnerability to *anxiety proneness* is based on findings that certain key cognitive constructs are common across specific anxiety disorders; these constructs include the following:

-   Anxiety sensitivity (a fear of the meaning and consequences of anxiety-related symptoms; Reiss and McNally 1985)
-   Pathological worry
-   Thought–action fusion (beliefs that thoughts and behaviors have reciprocal and equivalent effects; Shafran et al. 1996)
-   Intolerance of uncertainty (Starcevic and Berle 2006; Uhlenhuth et al. 1999)

The cognitive and behavioral precedents of anxiety may stem from anxiety sensitivity in childhood, coupled with separation anxiety and behavioral inhibition to novel stimuli, usually in social situations (Rosenbaum et al. 1993). The neural circuitry of learned anxiety involves both cortical and subcortical structures, and a significant portion of the pathology is likely to occur in interactions between prefrontal, temporal (amygdala and hippocampus), and medullary-limbic (thalamus, hypothalamus, and pituitary) structures (Cannistraro and Rauch 2003).

Panic Disorder

The key elements of the cognitive model of panic disorder are heightened anticipatory anxiety, a tendency to misinterpret certain bodily sensations in a catastrophic manner, hypervigilance for bodily sensations, and reliance on escape, avoidance, and other safety-seeking measures to reduce anxiety and the threat of panic (A. T. Beck et al. 1985; D.M. Clark 1986; Van den Hout and Griez 1984). For example, individuals with panic disorder who exhibit an attentional bias for chest pains or tightness immediately assume that an uncomfortable chest sensation might be indicative of a heart attack (i.e., they misinterpret the symptom in a catastrophic manner). They then experience a further elevation in anxiety that involves more physiological hyperarousal. Next, they engage in some safety-seeking behavior. For example, they may stop their physical activity, look to others for reassurance, and/or rush to the emergency room. Their erroneous misinterpretation of chest pain as signaling a possible heart attack is the critical variable in the cycle leading to the panic attack.

Studies in which panic attacks were induced with either carbon dioxide inhalation (van den Hout and Griez 1982) or hyperventilation (D.M. Clark and Hemsley 1982) lent support for this model. The degree to which patients experienced the procedures as aversive was influenced by cognitive variables such as the recall of previous experiences with the physical sensations and expectations of what was going to happen. More recent studies directly investigated some of the key predictions of the model. One study showed that panic disorder patients interpreted bodily sensations as being more threatening than non–panic disorder control subjects did, although they did not interpret the external events that evoked the bodily sensations as being more dangerous (Westling and Ost 1995). In another study, panic disorder patients demonstrated more sensitivity to physically threatening words but not to words representing an external social threat (van Niekerk et al. 1999). The bodily sensations that evoke fear (e.g., cardiovascular, cognitive, gastrointestinal, respiratory, and vestibular sensations; derealizations; and dizziness) are related to the type of catastrophe the individual anticipates (Hollifield et al. 2003).

Various cognitive errors such as errors in emotional reasoning and overgeneralization lead to more frequent and intense episodes of *apprehension* or anticipatory anxiety, and panic-prone individuals frequently try to avoid or escape from situations in which they predict they could experience panic symptoms. If avoidance is not possible, they may use safety behaviors such as insisting that others accompany them or taking anxiolytic medication. These behaviors then reinforce the fearful cognitions because they deprive individuals from discovering that the catastrophe they anticipated does not happen (Salkovskis et al. 1996).

Social Phobia

The cognitive model proposes that people with social phobia are unreasonably fearful that they will become the focus of attention. They are afraid that their physical manifestations of anxiety (blushing, trembling, sweating, etc.) will be readily apparent to others or that they will act in an embarrassing manner. They therefore predict that others will negatively evaluate or be critical of their physical appearance and/or social performance, and that they will feel humiliated (A.T. Beck et al. 1985). These persons engage in various safety behaviors such as avoiding eye contact or wearing heavy clothing to conceal sweating in an effort to avoid feared consequences (D.M. Clark 2001).

The schematic organization in social phobia has been well researched (D.M. Clark 2001; Rapee and Heimberg 1997; Wells and Clark 1997). Socially anxious individuals hold excessively high standards for their own social performance and believe that others hold the same excessive expectations. They have dysfunctional beliefs about the likelihood of negative consequences associated with their social performance—"People will judge me negatively"—as well as negative beliefs about their social self —"I'm boring" or "I'm a socially inadequate person" (D.M. Clark 2001). Socially anxious individuals form a schematic representation of the self as they believe others see them (Rapee and Heimberg 1997), which leads to excessive processing of the self as a social object (A.T. Beck et al. 1985; D.M. Clark 2001; Wells and Clark 1997). They automatically and excessively monitor their internal sensations, physical appearance, and personal performance (Wells and Clark 1997), paying more attention to how they feel and how they predict they are being perceived by others than to actual data from their social environment. Even when they do attend to others' reactions, they display a selective processing bias for negative evaluative information, which reinforces their negative core beliefs about themselves (Rapee and Heimberg 1997).

Schematic activation in social phobia frequently involves anticipatory as well as postevent processing that is dominated by negative self-evaluation and a focus on perceived negative feedback from the audience (D.M. Clark 2001). There is consistent empirical support for the following (for reviews, see Bögels and Mansell 2004; D.M. Clark 2001; Coles and Heimberg 2002; Hirsch and Clark 2004; and Ledley et al. 2005):

- Heightened self-focused attention
- Selective attentional bias for negative evaluative information
- Faulty subjective estimates of negative social events
- Excessive negative anticipatory and postevent processing (although there is little support for an explicit memory bias)

Generalized Anxiety Disorder

Pathological worry is the central feature of GAD (Roemer et al. 2002). The schematic basis of GAD involves activation of dysfunctional assumptions and beliefs about threats and danger across many domains (A.T. Beck et al. 1985; Sibrava and Borkovec 2006). When threat-related schemas are activated, individuals engage in an automatic attentional processing bias for threat-relevant information. Worry is viewed as a conscious, deliberate, cognitive response to a generalized future threat (A.T. Beck and Clark 1997; Borkovec 1994; D.A. Clark and A.T. Beck, "Cognitive Therapy of Anxiety: Science and Practice," manuscript in preparation, 2008; Mathews 1990).

In addition to the activation of generalized threat schemas, a number of other cognitive processes have been identified as responsible for the persistence of pathological worry (Leahy 2005). One view of worry is that it is a conceptually based cognitive avoidance response to underlying threat information (Borkovec 1994; Borkovec et al. 1991; Sibrava and Borkovec 2006). Because worry focuses on attempts to problem-solve for nonexistent future negative possibilities, it diverts attention away from a more disturbing immediate or future threat and one's perceived inability to cope with that threat (Roemer and Borkovec 1993). Worry is maintained by secondary avoidance functions such as the suppression of aversive images, the reduction of somatic activation, and a shift to abstract reasoning that results in reduced emotional processing (Sibrava and Borkovec 2006). From this perspective, then, worry is an avoidance strategy that paradoxically leads to continued activation of threat and danger schemas in GAD.

A metacognitive model of worry emphasizes positive as well as negative appraisals of and beliefs about worry (e.g., "worrying about worry"), which play a critical role in the persistence of excessive worry (Wells 1997, 2006). Positive beliefs about the utility of worry as a coping strategy (e.g., "Worry helps me find a resolution to problems") cause an individual to rely too much on worry to cope with life problems. This overreliance on worry increases the probability of experiencing the negative characteristics such as its uncontrollability. Activation of negative beliefs about the dangerousness and uncontrollability of worry increase anxiety and a sense of threat, causing the individual to engage in counterproductive coping strategies such as thought suppression or reassurance seeking. The net effect of these compensatory strategies is prevention of learning that the object of one's worry is harmless, and so the cycle of worry is perpetuated. Intolerance of uncertainty contributes to the persistence of worry and anxiety by causing a greater focus on uncertain events and biasing the application of problem-solving skills (Dugas et al. 1998; Koerner and Dugas 2006; Ladouceur et al. 1997).

There is considerable empirical support that individuals with GAD selectively attend to threatening information and generate biased interpretations of ambiguous situations; they also appear less able to reverse this automatic threat bias using corrective controlled processing techniques (MacLeod and Rutherford 2004). Emerging empirical evidence suggests that individuals with GAD endorse more positive and negative metacognitive beliefs (Wells 2006) and have greater intolerance of uncertainty (Koerner and Dugas 2006). Psychophysiological and other experimental research results also support the avoidance function of worry in GAD (Sibrava and Borkovec 2006).

Obsessive-Compulsive Disorder

In recent years a greater emphasis has been placed on the role of dysfunctional beliefs and appraisals in the etiology and persistence of obsessive-compulsive disorder (OCD). The central notion in cognitive models of OCD is that obsessions arise from a faulty appraisal of unwanted, threatening, and intrusive thoughts, images, or impulses (D.A. Clark 2004; Rachman 1997, 1998; Salkovskis 1985, 1999). Believing that the mental intrusion must be eliminated from conscious awareness in order to reduce anxiety and/ or the possibility of a dire consequence, the individual engages in various mental or behavioral strategies to neutralize the disturbing thought (i.e., compensatory strategies). In most cases of OCD, a person learns that a compulsive ritual is the quickest way to neutralize the obsession and its anticipated consequences. Although neutralization may temporarily relieve anxiety and seem to prevent some imagined threat, it has the unintended consequence of increasing the frequency and salience of the obsession by heightening attentional bias for the intrusion. This leads to an escalating cycle of obsessional intrusion, faulty appraisal, and dysfunctional control responses.

Having intrusive thoughts and images is a normal human experience in the stream of consciousness (e.g., Klinger 1978). Nonobsessional individuals consider unintended intrusive thoughts of doubt, sex, contamination, violence, and injury odd but rather benign. Obsession-prone individuals, however, attach exaggerated significance to these types of thoughts and images, believing they signify a dire threat to the self or others (Rachman 2003). Once a thought or image is considered a highly significant threat, obsessive thinkers make extraordinary efforts to control the thought and its associated distress, setting in motion an escalation in the frequency and severity of the obsession.

Several faulty appraisals have been identified as key in the pathogenesis of obsessions, including the following (D.A. Clark 2004; Obsessive Compulsive Cognitions Working Group 1997; Taylor 2002):

- *Inflated responsibility*—considering oneself as central to the prevention of some negative outcome
- *Overestimated threat*—an exaggerated evaluation of the probability and severity of harm
- *Overimportance of thought*—evaluating a thought as highly significant based on its mere occurrence

- *Excessive control*—overvaluing the need to exert complete control over a thought
- *Intolerance of uncertainty*—requiring absolute assurance of a desired outcome
- *Perfectionism*—intolerance of mistakes or any derivation from an ideal solution
- *Thought–action fusion*—belief that the mere presence of a thought increases the probability that a dreaded outcome will occur (Rachman and Shafran 1998)

These faulty appraisals are considered products of corresponding preexisting beliefs or schemas that constitute an increased cognitive vulnerability to OCD (Freeston et al. 1996). Various questionnaires and experimental studies have supported a significant role for these faulty appraisals and beliefs in the persistence of clinical obsessions, especially inflated responsibility, thought–action fusion, importance/control, and threat estimation (e.g., D.A. Clark 2004; Frost and Steketee 2002; Taylor et al. 2007).

Posttraumatic Stress Disorder

A cognitive model of posttraumatic stress disorder (PTSD) that unifies information from many theorists has been proposed by Ehlers and Clark (2000). The core feature of this model is that negative appraisals about a traumatic event and/or its sequelae and the nature of the trauma memory lead to a sense of a serious current threat. This sense of a threat, embodied in reexperiencing the event and hyperarousal symptoms of PTSD, leads to multiple compensatory strategies of avoidance and numbing that are intended to control the symptoms. As in other anxiety disorders, the compensatory strategies promote rather than diminish PTSD symptoms, in this case by preventing change in memories of the traumatic event, its appraisal, and other sequelae (Ehlers and Clark 2000). PTSD is unique among the anxiety disorders because anticipatory anxiety is related to an event that has already occurred. The anxiety that PTSD patients experience may be due to the high frequency of involuntary, intrusive recollections of the trauma, which occur because the patients have not adequately processed the trauma because of poor organization and temporal ordering in their memory of specific events that occurred during the trauma (Amir et al. 1998; Foa and Riggs 1993; Foa et al. 1995; Koss et al. 1996; van der Kolk and Fisler 1995), because they have poor retrieval of autobiographical memories (Kuyken and Brewin 1995; McNally et al. 1995), and/or because they use avoidance and numbing strategies. Other theorists note that conflicts between trauma-related information and beliefs about oneself and the world prior to traumatic experiences are at the heart of information-processing disturbances in PTSD (Resick and Schnicke 1992).

Research has demonstrated that the persistence of PTSD is predicted by the following:

1. Negative appraisals of the traumatic event(s) (Dunmore et al. 1998)
2. Negative interpretations of other people's responses after the event(s) (Dunmore et al. 1998)
3. Interpretations that initial PTSD symptoms are harbingers of worse things to come (Dunmore et al. 1998; Ehlers and Steil 1995)
4. Compensatory avoidance and numbing strategies (Dunmore et al. 1999, 2001; Ehlers et al. 1998)

Health Anxiety

Cognitive-behavioral models of health anxiety and/or hypochondriasis highlight dysfunctional assumptions and beliefs about the risk for illness and the meaning of bodily symptoms (Salkovskis and Warwick 2001); sensitivity to and awareness of bodily sensations, termed *somatosensory amplification* (Barsky 2001); and the inclusion of attentional factors in addition to cognitive and somatosensory concepts (Taylor and Asmundson 2004). People with high health anxiety demonstrate an exaggerated appraisal of health risks, health-related jeopardy, and vulnerability to disease (Barsky 2001). A key difference between persons with health anxiety and those with panic disorder is that the former fear eventual disease, disability, or death, whereas the latter fear an immediate physical or mental catastrophe.

An intervention study in which individuals with hypochondriasis displayed significant, treatment-related reductions of hypochondriacal symptoms, beliefs, and attitudes and health-related anxiety (Barsky and Ahern 2004) lent support for the cognitive model. Other support for the model is reviewed in a meta-analysis of 21 studies about cognitive appraisal variables in patients with health anxiety and 16 studies that assessed the relationship between health anxiety and scores on self-report measures of somatosensory amplification (Marcus et al. 2007). Data consistently show that people high in health anxiety tend to make misinterpretations of bodily sensations, view any physical symptom as a marker of illness, and believe they have low control over recurrence of illness. The cognitive basis of health anxiety is supported by studies indicating that people with health anxiety score high on scales of subjective perception of physical sensations, yet are not necessarily more aware of actual pain (Lautenbacher et al. 1998; Pauli et al. 1993) or their heart rate (Barsky et al. 1995). Somatosensory amplification, then, may be a mediator of the relationship between a perceived health threat and hypochondriacal concerns (Ferguson et al. 2000). People with high health anxiety may also be less extroverted and have more negative views about themselves than control subjects (Hollifield et al. 1999).

Schizophrenia and the Psychotic Disorders

The cognitive model of delusions and hallucinations stresses a model of continuity with "normal" functioning (e.g., Chapman and Chapman 1980), suggesting that a significant proportion of the nonclinical population also experiences these phenomena, and that a diathesis-stress vulnerability process underlies psychotic disorders.

Delusions and hallucinations may serve the function of providing some benefit to the individual, such as bolstering self-esteem or giving the individual the sense that he or she is important (e.g., delusions of grandeur). For example, a young man believed that the erotic spam e-mail that he received was directed toward him, which gave him a sense that he was desired by women throughout the world. Delusional thinking is often not open to *disconfirmation*—for example, "I know that you are hiding your hostile feelings from me"—and cannot be proven wrong for the paranoid individual. Many distortions of automatic thoughts, characteristic of depressed and anxious individuals, are exacerbated in psychosis—for example, mind reading, personalizing, labeling, and catastrophic thinking (Kingdon and Turkington 2005). Importantly, the confirmation bias in thinking—and the use of avoidance and withdrawal as safety strategies by psychotic individuals—may help maintain even the most distorted set of beliefs.

Similar to the metacognitive model of obsessive-compulsive intrusive thoughts, the cognitive model also suggests that psychotic individuals treat their delusional thoughts or images as actual facts or as predictive of specific outcomes. The concept of thought–action fusion (Rachman and Shafran 1998) is applicable to psychotic disorders in which thoughts are considered the same as reality. Individuals with these disorders view intrusive thoughts as personally relevant and as requiring them to respond in some way. Paranoid delusional individuals also display a tendency toward external attribution: "They are doing this to me" versus "It's my fault" (Bentall 1990). Psychotic individuals who have auditory hallucinations believe that the image or internal speech "in their head" has an external source ("They are talking about me"), despite the existence of subvocal "speech" (their tongue moves). In response, individuals employ a range of coping strategies, including active acceptance, passive coping, and resistance to dealing with the hallucinations (Farhall and Gehrke 1997).

An earlier model of delusional thought proposed that delusions develop as a way to "make sense" of unusual experiences—especially internal experiences (Maher 1974). Delusional thinking is an attempt to explain these unusual internal psychological states, and is often marked by a belief-confirmatory bias. The model has been expanded to incorporate the *threat anticipation model* of delusional thinking (Freeman and Garety 2004). In their search for meaning, paranoid individuals (who may have anomalous experiences or intense anxious arousal) are biased to select explanations based on an external threat (Freeman 2007).

The *theory of mind model* suggests that paranoid individuals have impairments and distortions in their understanding of the motivations and intentions of other people (Frith 2004). The delusional individual is more likely to infer intentions and motivations based on little evidence, thereby supporting a tendency to personalize the behavior of others (see also Morrison 2004).

Personality Disorders and Specific Schemas

A specific set of beliefs about the self, others, and the world, as well as a unique set of compensatory strategies, characterizes each Axis II disorder, as outlined in Table 6–4 (A.T. Beck et al. 2004).

Personality disorder schemas are overgeneralized, inflexible, imperative, and resistant to change. For example, individuals with a dependent personality disorder view themselves as helpless, incompetent, and weak and they view others as (potentially) nurturant, competent, and supportive. They develop strong coping strategies: encouraging others to protect and take care of them and subjugating their own desires to avoid abandonment. But their beliefs deter them from developing competence in making their own decisions and relying on themselves.

Similarly, individuals with obsessive-compulsive personality disorder view themselves as highly responsible, competent, and accountable; they become overly invested in working very hard, setting up rigid systems, holding high expectations, and attempting to control themselves and others, whom they see as irresponsible, casual, and self-indulgent. Unfortunately, they fail to develop behavioral patterns of spontaneity and playfulness.

Each personality disorder can be described in terms of belief structures as well as overdeveloped and underdeveloped strategies. Personality schemas affect attention, recall, and the value attached to information. The dependent individual attends to information related to signs of incompetence, abandonment, and loss ("I can't survive on my own"), and the avoidant individual attends to information about rejection and criticism ("Everyone thinks I'm a loser"). Spontaneous automatic thoughts reflect underlying beliefs. For example, the obsessive-compulsive individual thinks that anything less than perfect performance will lead to disaster (engages in fortune-telling and catastrophizing). The avoidant individual engages in mind reading ("They think I'm a loser"), labeling ("I am unlovable"), and discounting the positive ("She didn't really like me; she was just trying to be nice").

Each personality disorder is marked by conditional beliefs that follow from the core beliefs: "If I make sure everything is perfect, maybe things will turn out OK" (obsessive-compulsive); "If I maintain this relationship at all costs, I'll survive" (dependent); or "If I disguise my true self, I can avoid rejection" (avoidant). Furthermore, beliefs are often preserved, because individuals do not put themselves in situations in which their ideas could be disconfirmed. For example, avoidant individuals, fearing evaluation and rejection, tend to remain aloof, withdrawing or isolating themselves. Even when they do enter social situations, they selectively attend to negative (or even neutral) reactions from others and believe that they are being negatively evaluated. They also fail to notice or discount positive information that is contrary to their core beliefs.

The Personality Belief Questionnaire (A.T. Beck et al. 2001) contains 126 beliefs, pertaining to nine personality disorders, that were found to be consistent with an Axis II diagnosis based on clinical interviews (Butler et al. 2002). As an alternative cognitive perspective, a schema-focused model has been proposed (Young 1999) that describes a number of early maladaptive schemas as the cognitive basis for the personality disorders (Young et al. 2003). The evidence to date for both models supports the general categories of schemas. More research is needed to establish the relationship between early experience and the development of schemas and strategies.

Conclusion

In the last three decades the cognitive perspective on psychiatric and psychological disorders has become an established conceptual paradigm for research and treatment. Dysfunctional representations of the self, others, and personal experiences, as well as biased information processing and presence of disturbing, repetitive thoughts and images, are key elements in the persistence of psychopathological conditions. Over the years numerous correlational and experimental studies have supported many of the fundamental propositions of the cognitive theory, especially at the descriptive level of analysis. The cognitive basis of the major forms of mental illness has been well articulated and supported by decades of research and provides a solid theoretical basis for various cognitive therapy treatment protocols that have shown efficacy for a variety of psychiatric disorders.

Despite the significant advances made in elucidating the cognitive basis of psychopathology, progress has not been uniform across the disorders. A well-established research tradition on cognitive factors is evident

TABLE 6–4. Personality disorders (Axis II)

Personality disorder	View of self	View of others	Main beliefs	Main strategy
Avoidant	Vulnerable to depreciation/rejection	Critical	It's terrible to be rejected/put down.	Avoids evaluative situations
	Socially inept	Demeaning	If people know the real me, they will reject me.	
	Incompetent	Superior	I can't tolerate unpleasant feelings.	Avoids unpleasant feelings or thoughts
Dependent	Needy	Nurturant[a]	I need people to survive/be happy.	Cultivates dependent relationships
	Weak	Supportive[a]	I need a steady flow of support and encouragement.	
	Helpless	Competent[a]		
	Incompetent			

TABLE 6–4. Personality disorders (Axis II) *(continued)*

Personality disorder	View of self	View of others	Main beliefs	Main strategy
Passive-aggressive	Self-sufficient	Intrusive	Others interfere with my freedom of action.	Uses passive resistance
	Vulnerable to control/interference	Demanding	Control by others is intolerable.	Uses surface submissiveness
		Interfering Controlling Dominating	I have to do things my own way.	Evades/circumvents rules
Obsessive-compulsive	Responsible	Irresponsible	I know what's best.	Applies rules
	Accountable	Casual	Details are crucial.	Is a perfectionist
	Fastidious	Incompetent	People should be better/try harder.	Evaluates/controls
	Competent	Self-indulgent		Uses should's; criticizes/punishes
Paranoid	Righteous	Interfering	Motives are suspect.	Is wary
	Innocent/noble	Malicious	Be on guard.	Looks for hidden motives
	Vulnerable	Discriminatory	Don't trust.	Accuses
		Have abusive motives		Counterattacks

TABLE 6–4. Personality disorders (Axis II) *(continued)*

Personality disorder	View of self	View of others	Main beliefs	Main strategy
Antisocial	A loner Autonomous Strong	Vulnerable Exploitative	I'm entitled to break rules. Others are patsies/wimps. Others are exploitative.	Attacks/robs Deceives Manipulates
Narcissistic	Special/unique Deserving of special rules/superior Above the rules	Admirers Inferior	Because I'm special, I deserve special rules. I'm better than others. I'm above the rules.	Uses others Transcends rules Manipulates Is competitive
Histrionic	Glamorous Impressive	Seducible Receptive Admirers	People are there to serve or admire me. Others have no right to deny me my just deserts.	Uses dramatics/charm; temper tantrums/crying; suicide gestures
Schizoid	Self-sufficient A loner	Intrusive	Others are unrewarding. Relationships are messy/undesirable.	Stays away

[a]Idealized view.
Source. Reprinted from Beck AT, Freeman A, Davis DD, et al: *Cognitive Therapy of Personality Disorders,* 2nd Edition. New York, Guilford, 2004. Used with permission.

in major depression and the anxiety disorders. However, the cognitive theory of Beck and colleagues was only more recently applied to other conditions like bipolar disorder, schizophrenia, and the personality disorders, so progress in these areas is much more tentative. In some domains such as the personality disorders, cognitive theory led directly to the development of treatment protocols with only scanty research on the disorder-specific constructs proposed in cognitive theory. Thus, the scientific basis of the cognitive theory is unevenly represented across psychiatric conditions.

Another research question that is paramount in cognitive clinical research concerns the degree of commonality and specificity that characterize the various cognitive constructs of psychopathology. It is now clear that some cognitive structures and processes are transdiagnostic, whereas others are unique manifestations of particular disorders. The interaction and function of these common and specific cognitive processes are still a matter of continued investigation.

A final question that is a hotly debated topic among cognitive clinical researchers is that of causality. While few researchers would question the presence of maladaptive cognition in psychopathology, some continue to consider this a mere consequence of psychological disturbance. On the other hand, more recent experimental research using priming methodologies, as well as prospective studies that employ high-risk samples, is building a strong case that faulty information processing does have an etiological role in psychiatric conditions like major depression and the anxiety disorders. Whatever the case, given the heuristic value of cognitive theory and its expansion into many new domains of psychopathology, there is much that remains to be understood about the cognitive basis of mental health and well-being.

Key Points

- Psychiatric disorders are characterized by a biased information-processing system that contributes to disturbance in thought, emotions, and behavior.

- It is assumed that symptom improvement and remission of the clinical state are mediated by correction of the biased information-processing system.

- Each psychiatric disorder is characterized by a specific cognitive profile that is evident in the maladaptive thoughts, beliefs, and assumptions that define the specific disorder (e.g., personal loss and deprivation in depression, threat and danger in anxiety).

- Many individuals at risk for emotional disturbance have an underlying schematic vulnerability that contributes to disorder onset when activated by a matching life experience.

- The faulty information processing in psychopathology involves biased semantic-emotional internal meaning representations (i.e., schemas), certain cognitive-perceptual errors, negative automatic thoughts and images, and maladaptive compensatory coping strategies.

- The cognitive model embraces a biopsychosocial perspective, with recent findings from neuroscience demonstrating close connections among certain brain structures, their associated cognitive function, and their modulating effect on negative emotions.

- The cognitive dysfunction in depression is characterized by a pervasive self-oriented negativity, whereas mania reflects a heightened selectivity for the positive and a generally negative memory bias and attributional style suggestive of manic defense.

- The cognitive basis of the anxiety disorders consists of exaggerated appraisals of the likelihood and severity of threat, a heightened sense of personal vulnerability, maladaptive compensatory coping strategies (e.g., escape and avoidance), and a search for safety.

- A cognitive model for psychotic disorders stresses misattribution of intrusive thoughts and images, dominance of a belief-confirmation bias, the presence of self-serving functions, and the influence of cognitive errors in the persistence of delusions and auditory hallucinations.

- Each personality disorder is characterized by certain schemas and their associated compensatory strategies, which are overgeneralized, inflexible, and resistant to change.

References

Alford BA, Beck AT: The Integrative Power of Cognitive Therapy. New York, Guilford, 1997

Alloy LB, Reilly-Harrington N, Fresco DM, et al: Cognitive styles and life events in subsyndromal unipolar and bipolar disorders: stability and prospective prediction of depressive and hypomanic mood swings. Journal of Cognitive Psychotherapy: An International Quarterly 13:21–40, 1999

Alloy LB, Abramson LY, Whitehouse WG, et al: Prospective incidence of first onsets and recurrence of depression in individuals at high and low cognitive risk for depression. J Abnorm Psychol 115:145–156, 2006

Amir M, Weil G, Kaplan Z, et al: Debriefing with brief group psychotherapy in a homogenous group of non-injured victims of a terrorist attack: a prospective study. Acta Psychiatr Scand 98:237–242, 1998

Barsky AJ: Somatosensory amplification and hypochondriasis, in Hypochondriasis: Modern Perspectives on an Ancient Malady. Edited by Starcevic V, Lipsitt DR. New York, Oxford University Press, 2001, pp 223–248

Barsky AJ, Ahern DK: Cognitive behavior therapy for hypochondriasis: a randomized controlled trial. JAMA 291:1464–1470, 2004

Barsky AJ, Brener J, Coeytaux RR, et al: Accurate awareness of heartbeat in hypochondriacal and non-hypochondriacal patients. J Psychosom Res 39:489–497, 1995

Beck AT: Thinking and depression, 1: idiosyncratic content and cognitive distortions. Arch Gen Psychiatry 9:324–333, 1963

Beck AT: Depression: Causes and Treatment. Philadelphia, University of Pennsylvania Press, 1967

Beck AT: Cognitive Therapy of the Emotional Disorders. New York, New American Library, 1976

Beck AT: Cognitive therapy of depression: new perspectives, in Treatment of Depression: Old Controversies and New Approaches. Edited by Clayton PJ, Barrett JE. New York, Raven, 1983, pp 265–290

Beck AT: Cognitive models of depression. Journal of Cognitive Psychotherapy: An International Quarterly 1:5–37, 1987

Beck AT: Beyond belief: a theory of modes, personality, and psychopathology, in Frontiers of Cognitive Therapy. Edited by Salkovskis PM. New York, Guilford, 1996, pp 1–25

Beck AT, Clark DA: An information processing model of anxiety: automatic and strategic processes. Behav Res Ther 35:49–58, 1997

Beck AT, Rush AJ, Shaw BF, et al: Cognitive Therapy of Depression. New York, Guilford, 1979

Beck AT, Emery G, Greenberg RL: Anxiety Disorders and Phobias: A Cognitive Perspective. New York, Basic Books, 1985

Beck AT, Butler AC, Brown GK, et al: Dysfunctional beliefs discriminate personality disorders. Behav Res Ther 39:1213–1225, 2001

Beck AT, Freeman A, Davis DD, et al: Cognitive Therapy of Personality Disorders, 2nd Edition. New York, Guilford, 2004

Beck JS: Cognitive Therapy: Basics and Beyond. New York, Guilford, 1995

Beck R, Perkins TS: Cognitive content-specificity for anxiety and depression: a meta-analysis. Cognit Ther Res 25:651–663, 2001

Bentall RP: The illusion of reality: a psychological model of hallucinations. Psychol Bull 107:82–95, 1990

Bögels SM, Mansell W: Attention processes in the maintenance and treatment of social phobia: hypervigilance, avoidance and self-focused attention. Clin Psychol Rev 24:827–856, 2004

Borkovec TD: The nature, functions, and origins of worry, in Worrying: Perspectives on Theory, Assessment and Treatment. Edited by Davey GCL. Chichester, UK, Wiley, 1994, pp 5–33

Borkovec TD, Shadick RN, Hopkins M: The nature of normal and pathological worry, in Chronic Anxiety: Generalized Anxiety Disorder and Mixed Anxiety-Depression. Edited by Rapee RM, Barlow DH. New York, Guilford, 1991, pp 29–51

Bremner JD: Long-term effects of childhood abuse on brain and neurobiology. Child Adolesc Psychiatr Clin N Am 12:271–292, 2003

Butler AC, Brown GK, Beck AT, et al: Assessment of dysfunctional beliefs in borderline personality disorder. Behav Res Ther 40:1231–1240, 2002

Cannistraro PA, Rauch SL: Neural circuitry of anxiety: evidence from structural and functional neuroimaging studies. Psychopharmacol Bull 37:8–25, 2003

Caspi A, Sugden K, Moffitt TE, et al: Influence of life stress on depression: moderation by a polymorphism in the 5-HTT gene. Science 301:386–389, 2003

Chapman LJ, Chapman JP: Scales for rating psychotic and psychotic-like symptoms as continua. Schizophr Bull 6:476–489, 1980

Clark DA: Cognitive-Behavioral Therapy for OCD. New York, Guilford, 2004

Clark DA (ed): Intrusive Thoughts in Clinical Disorders: Theory, Research and Treatment. New York, Guilford, 2005

Clark DA, Beck AT, Alford BA: Scientific Foundations of Cognitive Theory and Therapy of Depression. New York, Wiley, 1999

Clark DM: A cognitive approach to panic. Behav Res Ther 24:461–470, 1986

Clark DM: A cognitive perspective on social phobia, in International Handbook of Social Anxiety: Concepts, Research, and Interventions Relating to the Self and Shyness. Edited by Crozier WR, Alden LY. Chichester, UK, Wiley, 2001, pp 405–430

Clark DM, Hemsley DR: The effects of hyperventilation; individual variability and its relation to personality. J Behav Ther Exp Psychiatry 13:41–47, 1982

Coles ME, Heimberg RG: Memory biases in the anxiety disorders: current status. Clin Psychol Rev 22:587–627, 2002

Davey GCL, Wells A (eds): Worry and Its Psychological Disorders: Theory, Assessment and Treatment. Chichester, UK, Wiley, 2006

Depue RA, Iacono WG: Neurobehavioral aspects of affective disorders. Annu Rev Psychol 40:457–492, 1989

Dobson KS, Dozois DJA: Historical and philosophical bases of the cognitive-behavioral therapies, in Handbook of Cognitive-Behavioral Therapies, 2nd Edition. Edited by Dobson KS. New York, Guilford, 2001, pp 3–39

Dugas MJ, Gagnon F, Ladouceur R, et al: Generalized anxiety disorder: a preliminary test of a conceptual model. Behav Res Ther 36:215–226, 1998

Dunmore E, Clark DM, Ehlers A: The role of cognitive factors in posttraumatic stress disorder following physical or sexual assault: findings from retrospective and prospective investigations. Paper presented at the Annual Conference of the British Association of Behavioural and Cognitive Therapies, Durham, UK, July 1998

Dunmore E, Clark DM, Ehlers A: Cognitive factors involved in the onset and maintenance of posttraumatic stress disorder (PTSD) after physical or sexual assault. Behav Res Ther 37:809–829, 1999

Dunmore E, Clark DM, Ehlers A: A prospective investigation of the role of cognitive factors involved in persistent posttraumatic stress disorder (PTSD) after physical or sexual assault. Behav Res Ther 39:1063–1084, 2001

Ehlers A, Clark DM: A cognitive model of posttraumatic stress disorder. Behav Res Ther 38:319–345, 2000

Ehlers A, Steil R: Maintenance of intrusive memories in posttraumatic stress disorder: a cognitive approach. Behavioural and Cognitive Psychotherapy 23:217–249, 1995

Ehlers A, Clark DM, Dunmore E, et al: Predicting response to exposure treatment in PTSD: the role of mental defeat and alienation. J Trauma Stress 11:457–471, 1998

Eich E, Macaulay D, Lam RW: Mania, depression, and mood dependent memory. Cogn Emot 11:607–616, 1997

Farhall J, Gehrke M: Coping with hallucinations: exploring stress and coping framework. Br J Clin Psychol 36:259–261, 1997

Ferguson E, Swairbrick R, Clare S, et al: Hypochondriacal concerns, somatosensory amplification, and primary and secondary cognitive appraisals. Br J Med Psychol 73:355–369, 2000

Foa EB, Riggs DS: Post-traumatic stress disorder in rape victims, in American Psychiatric Press Review of Psychiatry, Vol 12. Edited by Oldham JM, Riba MB, Tasman A. Washington, DC, American Psychiatric Press, 1993, pp 273–303

Foa EB, Riggs DS, Gershuny BS: Arousal, numbing, and intrusion: symptom structure of PTSD following assault. Am J Psychiatry 152:116–120, 1995

Freeman D: Suspicious minds: the psychology of persecutory delusions. Clin Psychol Rev 27:425–457, 2007

Freeman D, Garety PA: Paranoia: The Psychology of Persecutory Delusions. Hove, UK, Psychology Press, 2004

Freeston MH, Rhéaume J, Ladouceur R: Correcting faulty appraisals of obsessional thoughts. Behav Res Ther 34:433–446, 1996

Frith CD: Schizophrenia and theory of mind. Psychol Med 34:385–389, 2004

Frost RO, Steketee G (eds): Cognitive Approaches to Obsessions and Compulsions: Theory, Assessment, and Treatment. Amsterdam, Elsevier, 2002

Gotlib IH, Neubauer DL: Information-processing approaches to the study of cognitive biases in depression, in Stress, Coping and Depression. Edited by Johnson SL, McCabe PM. Mahwah, NJ, Erlbaum, 2000, pp 117–143

Haaga DAF, Dyck MJ, Ernst D: Empirical status of cognitive theory of depression. Psychol Bull 110:215–236, 1991

Hirsch CR, Clark DM: Information-processing bias in social phobia. Clin Psychol Rev 24:799–825, 2004

Hollifield M, Tuttle L, Paine S, et al: Hypochondriasis and somatization related to personality and attitudes toward self. Psychosomatics 40:387–395, 1999

Hollifield M, Finley MR, Skipper B: Panic disorder phenomenology in urban self-identified Caucasian-Non-Hispanics and Caucasian-Hispanics. Depress Anxiety 18:7–17, 2003

Ingram RE, Miranda J, Segal ZV: Cognitive Vulnerability to Depression. New York, Guilford, 1998

Ingram RE, Miranda J, Segal Z: Cognitive vulnerability to depression, in Cognitive Vulnerability to Emotional Disorders. Edited by Alloy LB, Riskind JH. Mahwah, NJ, Erlbaum, 2005, pp 63–91

Johnson SL: Mania and dysregulation in goal pursuit: a review. Clin Psychol Rev 25:241–262, 2005

Johnson SL, Sandrow D, Meyer B, et al: Increases in manic symptoms following life events involving goal-attainment. J Abnorm Psychol 109:721–727, 2000

Kendall PC, Ingram RE: Cognitive-behavioral perspectives: theory and research on depression and anxiety, in Anxiety and Depression: Distinctive and Overlapping Features. Edited by Kendall PC, Watson D. San Diego, CA, Academic Press, 1989, pp 27–53

Kingdon DG, Turkington D: Cognitive Therapy of Schizophrenia. New York, Guilford, 2005

Klinger E: Modes of normal conscious flow, in The Stream of Consciousness. Edited by Pope KS, Singer JL. New York, Plenum, 1978, pp 225–258

Koerner N, Dugas MJ: A cognitive model of generalized anxiety disorder: the role of intolerance of uncertainty, in Worry and Its Psychological Disorders: Theory, Assessment and Treatment. Edited by Davey GCL, Wells A. Chichester, UK, Wiley, 2006, pp 201–216

Koss MP, Figueredo AJ, Bell I, et al: Traumatic memory characteristics: a cross-validated mediational model of response to rape among employed women. J Abnorm Psychol 105:421–432, 1996

Kuyken W, Brewin CR: Autobiographical memory functioning in depression and reports of early abuse. J Abnorm Psychol 104:585–591, 1995

Ladd CO, Owens MJ, Nemeroff CB: Persistent changes in corticotropin-releasing factor neuronal systems induced by maternal deprivation. Endocrinology 137:1212–1218, 1996

Ladouceur R, Talbot F, Dugas MJ: Behavioral expressions of intolerance of uncertainty in worry: experimental findings. Behav Modif 21:355–371, 1997

Lautenbacher S, Pauli P, Zaudig M, et al: Attentional control of pain perception: the role of hypochondriasis. J Psychosom Res 44:251–259, 1998

Leahy RL: Cognitive therapy, in Psychological Treatment of Bipolar Disorder. Edited by Johnson SL, Leahy RL. New York, Guilford, 2004a, pp 139–161

Leahy RL (ed): Contemporary Cognitive Therapy: Theory, Research, and Practice. New York, Guilford, 2004b

Leahy RL: The Worry Cure: Seven Steps to Stop Worry From Stopping You. New York, Harmony Books, 2005

Leahy RL, Beck AT: Cognitive therapy of depression and mania, in Depression and Mania. Edited by Cancro R, Georgotas A. New York, Elsevier, 1988, pp 517–537

Ledley DR, Fresco DM, Heimberg RG: Cognitive vulnerability to social anxiety disorder, in Cognitive Vulnerability to Emotional Disorders. Edited by Alloy LB, Riskind JH. Mahwah, NJ, Erlbaum, 2005, pp 251–283

Levine S, Wiener SG, Coe CL: Temporal and social factors influencing behavioral and hormonal responses to separation in mother and infant squirrel monkeys. Psychoneuroendocrinology 18:297–306, 1993

MacLeod C, Rutherford E: Information-processing approaches: assessing the selective functioning of attention, interpretation, and retrieval, in Generalized Anxiety Disorder: Advances in Research and Practice. Edited by Heimberg RG, Turk CL, Mennin DS. New York, Guilford, 2004, pp 109–142

Maher BA: Delusional thinking and perceptual disorder. J Individ Psychol 30:98–113, 1974

Mansell W: An integrative formulation-based cognitive treatment of bipolar disorders: application and illustration. J Clin Psychol 63:447–461, 2007

Mansell W, Lam D: A preliminary study of autobiographical memory in remitted bipolar and unipolar depression and the role of imagery in the specificity of memory. Memory 12:437–446, 2004

Marcus DK, Gurley JR, Marchi MM, et al: Cognitive and perceptual variables in hypochondriasis and health anxiety: a systematic review. Clin Psychol Rev 27:127–139, 2007

Mathews A: Why worry? The cognitive function of anxiety. Behav Res Ther 28:455–468, 1990

McEwen BS: Protection and damage from acute and chronic stress: allostasis and allostatic overload and relevance to the pathophysiology of psychiatric disorders. Ann N Y Acad Sci 1032:1–7, 2004

McNally RJ, Lasko NB, Macklin ML, et al: Autobiographical memory disturbance in combat-related posttraumatic stress disorder. Behav Res Ther 33:619–630, 1995

Morrison A: Cognitive Therapy for Psychosis: A Formulation-Based Approach. London, Routledge & Kegan Paul, 2004

Newman CF, Leahy RL, Beck AT, et al: Bipolar Disorder: A Cognitive Therapy Approach. Washington, DC, American Psychological Association, 2001

Obsessive Compulsive Cognitions Working Group: Cognitive assessment of obsessive-compulsive disorder. Behav Res Ther 35:667–681, 1997

Papageorgiou C, Wells A (eds): Depressive Rumination: Nature, Theory and Treatment. Chichester, UK, Wiley, 2004

Pauli P, Schwenzer M, Brody S, et al: Hypochondriacal attitudes, pain sensitivity, and attentional bias. J Psychosom Res 37:745–752, 1993

Rachman SJ: A cognitive theory of obsessions. Behav Res Ther 35:793–802, 1997

Rachman SJ: A cognitive theory of obsessions: elaborations. Behav Res Ther 36:385–401, 1998

Rachman S: The Treatment of Obsessions. Oxford, UK, Oxford University Press, 2003

Rachman SJ, Shafran R: Cognitive and behavioral features of obsessive-compulsive disorder, in Obsessive-Compulsive Disorder: Theory, Research and Treatment. Edited by Swinson RP, Antony MM, Rachman S, et al. New York, Guilford, 1998, pp 51–78

Rapee RM, Heimberg RG: A cognitive-behavioral model of anxiety in social phobia. Behav Res Ther 35:741–756, 1997

Reinecke MA, Clark DA (eds): Cognitive Therapy Across the Lifespan: Evidence and Practice. Cambridge, UK, Cambridge University Press, 2004

Reiss S, McNally RJ: Expectancy model of fear, in Theoretical Issues in Behavior Therapy. Edited by Reiss S, Bootzin RR. New York, Academic Press, 1985, pp 107–121

Resick PA, Schnicke MK: Cognitive processing therapy for sexual assault victims. J Consult Clin Psychol 60:748–756, 1992

Riskind JH, Alloy LB: Cognitive vulnerability to emotional disorders: theory and research design/methodology, in Cognitive Vulnerability to Emotional Disorders. Edited by Alloy LB, Riskind JH. Mahwah, NJ, Erlbaum, 2006, pp 1–29

Roemer L, Borkovec TD: Worry: unwanted cognitive activity that controls unwanted somatic experience, in Handbook of Mental Control. Edited by Wegner DM, Pennebaker JW. Upper Saddle River, NJ, Prentice Hall, 1993, pp 220–238

Roemer L, Orsillo SM, Barlow DH: Generalized anxiety disorder, in Anxiety and Its Disorders: The Nature and Treatment of Anxiety and Panic. Edited by Barlow DH. New York, Guilford, 2002, pp 477–515

Roffman JL, Marci CD, Glick DM, et al: Neuroimaging and the functional neuroanatomy of psychotherapy. Psychol Med 35:1385–1398, 2005

Rosenbaum JF, Biederman J, Bolduc-Murphy EA, et al: Behavioral inhibition in childhood: a risk factor for anxiety disorders. Harv Rev Psychiatry 1:2–16, 1993

Salkovskis PM: Obsessional-compulsive problems: a cognitive-behavioural analysis. Behav Res Ther 23:571–583, 1985

Salkovskis PM: Understanding and treating obsessive-compulsive disorder. Behav Res Ther 37 (suppl 1):S29–S52, 1999

Salkovskis PM, Warwick HMC: Meaning, misinterpretations, and medicine: a cognitive-behavioral approach to understanding health anxiety and hypochondriasis, in Hypochondriasis: Modern Perspectives on an Ancient Malady. Edited by Starcevic V, Lipsitt DR. New York, Oxford University Press, 2001, pp 202–222

Salkovskis PM, Clark DM, Gelder MG: Cognition-behaviour links in the persistence of panic. Behav Res Ther 34:453–458, 1996

Scher CD, Segal ZV, Ingram RE: Beck's theory of depression: origins, empirical status, and future directions for cognitive vulnerability, in Contemporary Cognitive Therapy: Theory, Research, and Practice. Edited by Leahy RL. New York, Guilford, 2004, pp 27–44

Scher CD, Ingram RE, Segal ZV: Cognitive reactivity and vulnerability: empirical evaluation of construct activation and cognitive diatheses in unipolar depression. Clin Psychol Rev 25:487–510, 2005

Shafran R, Thordarson DS, Rachman S: Thought-action fusion in obsessive-compulsive disorder. J Anxiety Disord 10:379–391, 1996

Sibrava NJ, Borkovec TD: The cognitive avoidance theory of worry, in Worry and Its Psychological Disorders: Theory, Assessment and Treatment. Edited by Davey GCL, Wells A. Chichester, UK, Wiley, 2006, pp 239–256

Solomon A, Haaga DAF: Cognitive theory and therapy of depression, in Cognitive Therapy Across the Lifespan: Evidence and Practice. Edited by Reinecke MA, Clark DA. Cambridge, UK, Cambridge University Press, 2004, pp 12–39

Stanton ME, Gutierrez YR, Levine S: Maternal deprivation potentiates pituitary-adrenal stress responses in infant rats. Behav Neurosci 102:692–700, 1988

Starcevic V, Berle D: Cognitive specificity of anxiety disorders: a review of selected key constructs. Depress Anxiety 23:51–61, 2006

Sutton SK, Johnson SJ: Hypomanic tendencies predict lower startle magnitudes during pleasant pictures. Psychophysiology 39(suppl):S80, 2002

Taylor S: Cognition in obsessive-compulsive disorder: an overview, in Cognitive Approaches to Obsessions and Compulsions: Theory, Assessment, and Treatment. Edited by Frost RO, Steketee B. Oxford, UK, Elsevier, 2002, pp 1–12

Taylor S, Asmundson GJG (eds): Treating Health Anxiety: A Cognitive-Behavioral Approach. New York, Guilford, 2004

Taylor S, Abramowitz JS, McKay D: Cognitive-behavioral models of obsessive-compulsive disorder, in Psychological Treatment of Obsessive-Compulsive Disorder: Fundamentals and Beyond. Edited by Antony MM, Purdon C, Summerfeldt LJ. Washington, DC, American Psychological Association, 2007, pp 9–29

Uhlenhuth EH, McCarty T, Paine S, et al: The revised Anxious Thoughts and Tendencies (AT&T scale): a general measure of anxiety-prone cognitive style. J Affect Disord 52:51–58, 1999

van den Hout MA, Griez E: Cardiovascular and subjective responses to inhalation of carbon dioxide: a controlled test with anxious patients. Psychother Psychosom 37:75–82, 1982

Van den Hout MA, Griez E: Panic symptoms after inhalation of carbon dioxide. Br J Psychiatry 144:503–507, 1984

van der Kolk BA: The neurobiology of childhood trauma and abuse. Child Adolesc Psychiatr Clin N Am 12:293–317, 2003

van der Kolk BA, Fisler R: Dissociation and the fragmentary nature of traumatic memories: overview and exploratory study. J Trauma Stress 8:505–525, 1995

van Niekerk JK, Moller AT, Nortje C: Self-schemas in social phobia and panic disorder. Psychol Rep 84:843–854, 1999

Vergne DE, Nemeroff CB: The interaction of serotonin transporter gene polymorphisms and early adverse life events on vulnerability for major depression. Curr Psychiatry Rep 8:452–457, 2006

Wells A: Cognitive Therapy of Anxiety Disorders: A Practice Manual and Conceptual Guide. Chichester, UK, Wiley, 1997

Wells A: Metacognitive therapy for worry and generalized anxiety disorder, in Worry and Its Psychological Disorders: Theory, Assessment and Treatment. Edited by Davey GCL, Wells A. Chichester, UK, Wiley, 2006, pp 259–272

Wells A, Clark DM: Social phobia: a cognitive approach, in Phobias: A Handbook of Theory, Research and Treatment. Edited by Davey CGL. Chichester, UK, Wiley, 1997, pp 3–26

Westling BE, Ost LG: Cognitive bias in panic disorder patients and changes after cognitive-behavioral treatments. Behav Res Ther 33:585–588, 1995

Williams JMG, Watts FN, MacLeod C, et al: Cognitive Psychology and Emotional Disorders, 2nd Edition. Chichester, UK, Wiley, 1997

Young JE: Cognitive Therapy for Personality Disorders: A Schema-Focused Approach, 3rd Edition. Sarasota, FL, Professional Resource Press, 1999

Young JE, Klosko JS, Weishaar M: Schema Therapy: A Practitioner's Guide. New York, Guilford, 2003

Zuroff DC, Mongrain M, Santor DA: Conceptualizing and measuring personality vulnerability to depression: comment on Coyne and Whiffen (1995). Psychol Bull 130:489–511, 2004

Suggested Readings

Alloy LB, Riskind JH (eds): Cognitive Vulnerability to Emotional Disorders. Mahwah, NJ, Erlbaum, 2006

Beck AT: Depression: Causes and Treatment. Philadelphia, University of Pennsylvania Press, 1967

Beck AT: Cognitive models of depression. Journal of Cognitive Psychotherapy: An International Quarterly 1:5–37, 1987

Beck AT, Freeman A, Davis DD, et al: Cognitive Therapy of Personality Disorders, 2nd Edition. New York, Guilford, 2004

Clark DA: Cognitive-Behavioral Therapy for OCD. New York, Guilford, 2004

Clark DA, Beck AT, Alford BA: Scientific Foundations of Cognitive Theory and Therapy of Depression. New York, Wiley, 1999

Freeman D, Garety PA: Paranoia: The Psychology of Persecutory Delusions. Hove, UK, Psychology Press, 2004

Kingdon DG, Turkington D: Cognitive Therapy of Schizophrenia. New York, Guilford, 2005

Leahy RL (ed): Contemporary Cognitive Therapy: Theory, Research, and Practice. New York, Guilford, 2004

Rachman SJ: The Treatment of Obsessions. Oxford, UK, Oxford University Press, 2003

Scher CD, Segal ZV, Ingram RE: Beck's theory of depression: origins, empirical status, and future directions for cognitive vulnerability, in Contemporary Cognitive Therapy: Theory, Research, and Practice. Edited by Leahy RL. New York, Guilford, 2004, pp 27–44

Chapter 7

Techniques of Cognitive-Behavioral Therapy

Richard A. Bermudes, M.D.
Jesse H. Wright, M.D., Ph.D.
David Casey, M.D.

One of the distinguishing features of cognitive-behavioral therapy (CBT) is that it is a direct outgrowth of the basic theories and experimental findings on cognitive and behavioral pathology in specific psychiatric disorders (see Chapter 6, "Theory of Cognitive Therapy"). Thus, cognitive-behavioral therapists implement procedures that are wholly consistent with core theoretical constructs. For example, the cognitive restructuring and exposure and response prevention interventions used for panic disorder with agoraphobia are designed to reverse pathologies of 1) overestimates of risk or danger in situations; 2) underestimates of coping abilities; and 3) avoidance of feared situations. CBT methods are also distinguished by the large amount of empirical data that support their efficacy (see Chapter 8, "Applications of Individual Cognitive-Behavioral Therapy to Specific Disorders:

Efficacy and Indications"). Many outcome studies have found positive results for CBT for depression, anxiety disorders, eating disorders, psychosis, and a variety of other conditions.

In this chapter, we describe general CBT methods such as the collaborative-empirical therapeutic relationship, structuring procedures, and psychoeducation. Commonly used cognitive and behavioral interventions are then defined and illustrated. A therapy such as CBT that has highly detailed treatment techniques can be misapplied if the clinician puts too much emphasis on implementing specific methods without developing an effective case formulation or fully attending to the therapeutic relationship. We have observed this problem many times in trainees who rush to apply a technique such as a thought record or a behavioral intervention without developing a comprehensive treatment plan. Thus, we recommend that the techniques described in this chapter be used only when consistent with the case formulation and when coordinated with the overall plan for therapy.

After detailing basic methods, we then illustrate adaptations of CBT for specific disorders by briefly describing modifications for three common conditions: schizophrenia, eating disorders, and bipolar disorder. CBT interventions have been developed for a wide variety of other conditions, such as substance abuse (A.T. Beck et al. 1993), personality disorders (A.T. Beck and Freeman 1990), chronic pain (Morley et al. 1999), irritable bowel syndrome (Payne and Blanchard 1995), and fibromyalgia (K.P. White and Nielson 1995). Also, CBT methods have been detailed for group (J. White and Freeman 2000) and family (Epstein 2002) applications and for treating children and adolescents (Albano and Kearney 2000; Reinicke et al. 2003). Readers who are interested in a more thorough or comprehensive description of CBT procedures may wish to consult the references for the different disorders or applications. In addition, several CBT textbooks are available to help readers gain further knowledge on this topic. *Learning Cognitive-Behavior Therapy: An Illustrated Guide* (Wright et al. 2006) includes a DVD with video demonstrations of key CBT techniques, and *Cognitive Therapy: Basics and Beyond* (J.S. Beck 1995) describes how to use standard cognitive therapy interventions. A list of recommended books on CBT is provided at the end of the chapter.

General Cognitive-Behavioral Therapy Methods

Therapeutic Relationship

The therapeutic relationship in CBT is characterized by a high degree of collaboration between patient and therapist and an empirical tone to the work of therapy. The therapist and patient work together as an investigative

TABLE 7–1. Methods of enhancing collaborative empiricism

Work together as an investigative team.

Promote essential "nonspecific" therapist variables (e.g., warmth).

Encourage self-monitoring and self-help.

Obtain an accurate assessment of the validity of cognitions and the efficacy of behavior.

Develop coping strategies for real losses and actual deficits.

Provide and request feedback on a regular basis.

Be sensitive to sociocultural differences and issues.

Customize therapy interventions.

Use gentle humor.

Source. Adapted from Wright JH, Beck AT, Thase ME: "Cognitive Therapy," in *The American Psychiatric Publishing Textbook of Clinical Psychiatry*, 5th Edition. Edited by Hales RE, Yudofsky SC, Gabbard GO. Washington, DC, American Psychiatric Publishing, 2008, pp. 1211–1256. Used with permission.

team. They jointly develop hypotheses about the validity of automatic thoughts and schemas or, alternatively, about the effectiveness of patterns of behavior. A series of exercises or experiments is then designed to test the validity of the hypotheses and, subsequently, to modify cognitions or behavior. A. T. Beck et al. (1979) termed this form of therapeutic relationship *collaborative empiricism*. Methods for developing a collaborative and empirical relationship are listed in Table 7–1.

Basic counseling skills that promote a sound therapeutic alliance are also important in CBT. Therapists strive to build genuineness, warmth, trust, and acceptance into the treatment relationship, in addition to showing sensitivity to sociocultural and gender influences (Davis and Wright 1994; Wright et al. 2006). Accurate empathy is another important component of the collaborative relationship in CBT (Wright et al. 2006). From a cognitive-behavioral perspective, accurate empathy involves the capacity to place oneself in the position of the patient so that one can sense what he or she is feeling and thinking, while retaining objectivity for sorting out possible distortions, illogical reasoning, or maladaptive behavior that may be contributing to the patient's problems. Full expression of accurate empathy in CBT involves not only showing sensitive concern for patients but also actively searching for solutions and actions that reduce suffering and help the patient manage life problems.

TABLE 7–2. **Structuring procedures for cognitive therapy**

Set agenda for therapy sessions.

Give constructive feedback to direct the course of therapy.

Ask for feedback and summarization about the therapy from the patient.

Use common cognitive therapy techniques on a regular basis.

Assign homework to link sessions together.

Source. Adapted from Wright JH, Beck AT, Thase ME: "Cognitive Therapy," in *The American Psychiatric Publishing Textbook of Clinical Psychiatry*, 5th Edition. Edited by Hales RE, Yudofsky SC, Gabbard GO. Washington, DC, American Psychiatric Publishing, 2008, pp. 1211–1256. Used with permission.

Structuring of Cognitive Therapy Sessions

One of the most important techniques for CBT is the use of a therapy agenda (Table 7–2). At the beginning of each session, the therapist and patient work collaboratively to derive a short list of topics, usually consisting of two to four items, to be covered during the session. Generally, it is advisable to shape an agenda that 1) can be managed within the time frame of an individual session, 2) follows up on material from earlier sessions, 3) allows time to review any homework from the previous session and provides an opportunity for new homework assignments, and 4) contains specific items that are highly relevant to the patient but are not too global or abstract. Agenda setting facilitates problem solving and keeps the therapy efficient and focused on salient issues. It may also act to counteract hopelessness by reducing overwhelming problems into more manageable segments.

Cognitive-behavioral therapists provide and ask for feedback during each therapy session to build structure into the therapy session, enhance learning, and provide a forum for examining and correcting distortions about the content and process of the therapy. The following types of questions may be used to solicit feedback: What are the patient's reactions to the therapist? What things are going well? What would the patient like to change? Cognitive-behavioral therapists also are sensitive to nonverbal forms of feedback. Is the patient engaged in the therapeutic process? Has there been a change in mood? Cognitive-behavioral therapists monitor for these more covert forms of feedback and then inquire about the patient's thoughts when these clues are noted.

Cognitive-behavioral therapists also use summarization to enhance the patient's understanding of the main points of the therapy session. For example, patients are often asked to summarize key elements of the session or to explain what they understand about a specific intervention. Therapists may need to assist patients in this process if important information is not recalled or if patients have difficulty in providing summaries.

The use of standard cognitive and behavioral techniques in and between sessions adds an additional structural element to the therapy. Examples include activity scheduling, graded task assignments, and use of thought change records. These interventions, and others of similar nature, provide a clear and understandable method for reducing symptoms and changing behaviors. The repeated use of procedures such as recording, labeling, and modifying automatic thoughts helps to link sessions together, especially if they are introduced in therapy and then assigned as homework.

Psychoeducation

One of the core principles of CBT is that it relies heavily on psychoeducation to teach patients basic concepts and skills (Wright et al. 2006).

The educational process in sessions may be especially effective if it is woven into therapeutic work on recent, emotionally resonant situations and provides a "real life" demonstration of the value of CBT principles. For example, a 55-year-old businessman with depression and anger problems reported in his second session that he felt very guilty about "exploding" at his assistant earlier in the day. The therapist capitalized on this opportunity to educate the patient by detailing the triggering event (i.e., "She showed me a lot of new faxes that she thought were important, but I was busy doing something else"); identifying specific automatic thoughts (i.e., "I cannot deal with another single thing…She will drive me crazy…I'm on total overload"); and defining emotions that were experienced in the situation (i.e., anger, anxiety, and physical tension). In this first attempt to teach the patient about the basic CBT model, the therapist diagrammed the relation between events, cognitions, and emotions and then used this diagram to explain the nature of automatic thoughts. Because the situation was very important to the patient and it stimulated intense emotion, the lessons taught in the therapeutic interchange were likely to be remembered and used.

Several very useful educational methods can be assigned for homework outside sessions. Readings in self-help books, pamphlets, or handouts are used extensively in CBT (Table 7–3). We recommend that therapists read several of the commonly used books or pamphlets and be prepared to make customized recommendations that will best suit the needs and the cognitive capacities of the individual patient. Sometimes it can be more helpful to suggest reading a specific chapter or portion of a publication than to assign an entire book. When patients are deeply depressed or have high levels of anxiety, assigning too much reading can be overwhelming and lead to discouragement. Thus, we often suggest reading in a stepped fashion, with in-

TABLE 7–3.   Psychoeducational materials and programs for cognitive-behavioral therapy

Title	Authors	Description
Coping With Depression	A.T. Beck et al. 1974	Brief pamphlet
Feeling Good: The New Mood Therapy	Burns 1980, 1999	Book with self-help program
Getting Your Life Back: The Complete Guide to Recovery From Depression	Wright and Basco 2001	Book with self-help program; integrates cognitive therapy and biological approaches
Good Days Ahead: The Multimedia Program for Cognitive Therapy	Wright et al. 2004; see also Wright 2002, 2005	Computer-assisted therapy and self-help program; information available at http://www.mindstreet.com
Mastery of Your Anxiety and Panic	Barlow and Craske 2000	Self-help for anxiety
Mind Over Mood: Change How You Feel by Changing the Way You Think	Greenberger and Padesky 1996	Self-help workbook
Never Good Enough: How to Use Perfectionism to Your Advantage Without Letting It Ruin Your Life	Basco 2000	Book on perfectionism
Stop Obsessing: How to Overcome Your Obsessions and Compulsions	Foa and Wilson 2001	Self-help for obsessive-compulsive disorder
The Worry Cure: Seven Steps to Stop Worry From Stopping You	Leahy 2006	Book with self-help for anxiety and worry
The Bipolar Workbook: Tools for Controlling Your Mood Swings	Basco 2006	Self-help workbook

Source.   Adapted from Wright et al. 2008, pp. 1211–1256. Used with permission.

creases in volume or complexity based on the patient's grasp of previous material and the degree of cognitive and symptomatic improvement.

Computer programs for CBT are particularly valuable resources for providing psychoeducation, in addition to improving the efficiency of treatment by acting as a "therapist's assistant." Computer-assisted CBT can reinforce learning, deepen the patient's understanding of CBT principles, and promote the use of self-help methods. Wright et al. (1995, 2002, 2004, 2005) introduced a multimedia form of computer-assisted cognitive therapy that is designed to be user-friendly and to be suitable for a wide range of patients, including those with no previous computer or keyboard experience. This program (*Good Days Ahead: The Multimedia Program for Cognitive Therapy*) uses a DVD-ROM format and features large amounts of video and audio, along with interactive self-help exercises (Table 7–3).

Research on this program has indicated excellent acceptance by patients and substantial effects in reducing symptoms of depression (Wright et al. 2002, 2005). In a randomized controlled trial involving drug-free patients with major depression, computer-assisted CBT was equal in efficacy to standard CBT, despite the fact that therapist contact in computer-assisted CBT was reduced to about 4 hours (Wright et al. 2005). Also, patients who received the computer-assisted treatment learned significantly more about the basics of CBT and had lower scores on measures of cognitive distortions than did patients who received standard treatment. Several other computer programs for CBT have been developed and tested (Kenwright et al. 2001; Newman et al. 1997; Proudfoot et al. 2004).

Case Formulation

The case formulation is used as a road map for therapy. The patient's unique history is understood through the lens of cognitive-behavioral theory to select specific methods that match her or his problems, symptoms, assets, and potentials (Wright et al. 2006). The Academy of Cognitive Therapy (http://www.academyofct.org) recommends that the case conceptualization include the following:

1. An outline of the most salient aspects of the history and mental status examination
2. Detailing of at least three examples from the patient's life of the relation between events, automatic thoughts, emotions, and behaviors (illustrations of the cognitive model as it pertains to this patient)
3. Identification of important schemas
4. Listing of strengths
5. A working hypothesis that weaves together all of the information in numbers 1–4 with the cognitive and behavioral theories that most closely fit

TABLE 7–4. Working with automatic thoughts

Techniques to identify automatic thoughts	Techniques to modify automatic thoughts
Guided discovery	Examining the evidence
Recognizing mood shifts	Applying reattribution techniques
Imagery and role-play exercises	Identifying cognitive errors
Checklists for automatic thoughts	Using thought change records
Thought recording	

Source. Adapted from Wright JH, Beck AT, Thase ME: "Cognitive Therapy," in *The American Psychiatric Publishing Textbook of Clinical Psychiatry,* 5th Edition. Edited by Hales RE, Yudofsky SC, Gabbard GO. Washington, DC, American Psychiatric Publishing, 2008, pp. 1211–1256. Used with permission.

    the patient's diagnosis and symptoms (e.g., models for anxiety disorders, depression, eating disorders, psychoses, and other conditions)
6. A treatment plan that is based on the working hypothesis

    The book *Learning Cognitive-Behavior Therapy: An Illustrated Guide* (Wright et al. 2006) provides detailed methods, worksheets, and examples of use of this formulation method.

Cognitive Techniques

The cognitive interventions used in CBT are designed first to identify and then to modify dysfunctional thinking at two main levels of cognitive processing—automatic thoughts (Table 7–4) and core beliefs (schemas). We describe here some of the most commonly used procedures for recognizing and changing maladaptive cognitions.

Identifying Automatic Thoughts

Using Guided Discovery

Guided discovery is the most frequently used technique to help patients articulate automatic thoughts in sessions. This process involves gentle eliciting, exploring, and questioning of the patient's thinking. Instead of trying to debate, convince, or sell patients on an idea, therapists ask Socratic-type questions that encourage the patient to expand his or her perspective and become actively involved in the learning process.

Patient: My anxiety is off the chart this week. I just can't settle down.

Therapist: Did something happen this week that seemed to trigger it?

Patient: I just feel tense all of the time.

Therapist: In the last 24 hours, when was your anxiety the worst, and what were you doing at the time? (being specific)

Patient (*pauses*): I guess I was at my house alone watching television, and I started having that tingling and a weird sensation up here again. (*pointing all around his chest*)

Therapist: And what were you thinking at that point?

Patient: My chest feels strange.

Therapist: What did you think was going to happen next as a result of your discomfort? (probing for automatic thoughts)

Patient: I felt like, "Is this the big one?" "Is this my heart attack?" "I know that I am 25 and that I have been worked up a bunch of times at the emergency department, but I just can't help thinking this."

Therapist: Was the sensation bearable? (probing for more automatic thoughts)

Patient: No, it was terrible; I couldn't stand it. I felt that my chest was going to just open up and explode. (automatic image)

Therapist: So, it sounds as if you were thinking when this sensation occurred that you were going to die, you were having a heart attack, the sensation was terrible and unbearable, and you had an image of your chest actually opening up from the excruciating pain. Did I hear that right?

Patient: Yes, I hate it when these attacks come. I am never sure if it is the big one or not.

Recognizing Mood Shifts

One of the most powerful ways of teaching patients to detect automatic thoughts is to find a real-life example of how automatic thoughts influence their emotional responses. A shift in mood during the therapy session can be an opportune time for the therapist to facilitate the identification of automatic thoughts. When the therapist observes that a strong emotion such as sadness, anxiety, or anger has appeared, she or he can ask the patient to describe the thoughts that "went through your head" just prior to the mood shift. During periods of affective arousal, automatic thoughts and schemas may be especially potent and accessible. Hence cognitive therapists capitalize on spontaneously occurring mood shifts during sessions and also may pursue lines of questioning that are likely to produce intense emotional responses.

Imagery and Role-Play

Imagery and role-play are two methods for uncovering cognitions when direct questions are unsuccessful (or partially successful) in generating suspected automatic thinking (A. T. Beck et al. 1979). With some patients, this procedure can be introduced by simply asking the patient to imagine himself or herself back in the particularly troubling or emotion-provoking situation and then to describe the thoughts that occurred. Other patients may need facilitating questions that "set the scene." The therapist may ask the patient to describe the details of the setting. When and where did it take place? What happened immediately before the incident? How did the characters in the scene appear? What were the main physical features of the setting? These questions bring the scene alive in the patient's mind and facilitate recall of cognitive responses to the situation.

The objectives of role-play are similar. With this procedure, the therapist first asks a series of questions to try to understand an upsetting situation that involves an interpersonal relationship or other social interchange. With the permission of the patient, the therapist then briefly steps into the role of the individual in the scene and facilitates the playing out of a typical response set. Roles can be reversed if needed to further enhance recall of significant automatic thoughts.

Checklists for Automatic Thoughts

Checklists of thoughts provide an additional method to help patients identify their dysfunctional cognitions. The Automatic Thoughts Questionnaire (Hollon and Kendall 1980) is a comprehensive list of dysfunctional thoughts that has been used primarily in research studies. Similar lists can be used in clinical settings when patients are having difficulty detecting their automatic thoughts (see Wright et al. 2006 for an example). CBT computer programs also can be used to teach patients to develop their own customized list of negative automatic thoughts and other cognitions (Wright et al. 2004).

Thought Recording

Thought recording is a standard CBT procedure for identifying automatic thoughts (J.S. Beck 1995; Wright et al. 2006). Although patients can log their thoughts in several ways, most begin by using the two-column technique shown in Figure 7–1. In this example, the patient was asked to write down automatic thoughts that occurred in situations that he associated with his depressed mood. Alternatively, a three-column exercise could include a description of the situation, a list of automatic thoughts, and a list of associated emotions. Thought recording helps the patient recognize the effects of underlying automatic thoughts and understand how the basic CBT model (i.e., relation between situations, thoughts, feelings, and behaviors) applies to his or her own experiences.

Modifying Automatic Thoughts

Generally, no sharp distinction is seen between the processes of eliciting and modifying automatic thoughts. As patients begin to recognize the na-

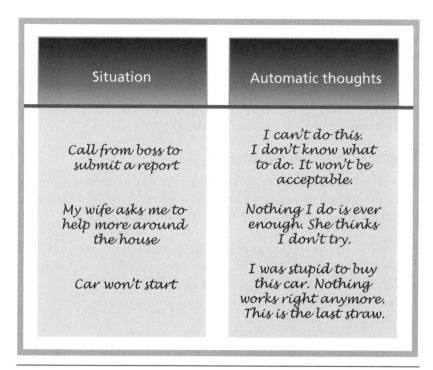

FIGURE 7–1. Two-column thought recording.

Source. Adapted from Wright JH, Beck AT, Thase ME: "Cognitive Therapy," in *The American Psychiatric Publishing Textbook of Clinical Psychiatry*, 5th Edition. Edited by Hales RE, Yudofsky SC, Gabbard GO. Washington, DC, American Psychiatric Publishing, 2008, pp. 1211–1256. Used with permission.

ture of their dysfunctional thinking, they typically have an increased degree of objectivity regarding the validity of their automatic thoughts and begin to question and revise their cognitive distortions. However, additional techniques are usually needed to promote changes in automatic thoughts. Methods discussed in this chapter for revising automatic thoughts include 1) examining the evidence, 2) applying reattribution techniques, 3) identifying cognitive errors, and 4) using thought change records (A.T. Beck et al. 1979; J.S. Beck 1995; Wright et al. 2006).

Examining the Evidence

Examining the evidence is a technique in which the therapist and patient collaboratively explore the evidence for and the evidence against a specific distorted thought or belief (Wright et al. 2006). When working through the exercise, the therapist typically writes the thought or belief at the top of a piece of paper and then labels two columns with "evidence for" and "evidence against." The patient is then guided to explore methodically and write down each piece of evidence. At the end of this procedure, the evidence for the cognition is quantified and estimated (e.g., 30%), as is the evidence against (e.g., 70%). Often cognitive errors can be identified in the evidence for maladaptive automatic thoughts or schemas. Typically, examining the evidence stimulates a rethinking of dysfunctional cognitions and the development of a more rational thinking style.

Applying Reattribution Techniques

The reattribution method is based on research that shows that depressed individuals often have negatively biased attributions (meanings attached to events) in three dimensions (Abramson et al. 1978):

1. Internal (excessive blame toward self for negative events) versus external
2. Global (circumscribed negative events are overgeneralized and are allowed to define one's entire self-concept) versus specific
3. Fixed (hopeless view of likelihood of positive change in future) versus variable

Cognitive-behavioral therapists use several different types of reattribution procedures, including psychoeducation about the attributional process, Socratic questioning to stimulate reattribution, scales or graphs to recognize and reinforce alternative attributions, and homework assignments to test the accuracy of attributions. The basic thrust of this work is to help patients make reasonable attributions about life events so that they do not blame themselves excessively or unnecessarily, give too much weight to negative events, or develop a sense of immutability about their lives. Actual flaws or negative events are recognized, but an accurate assessment of the meaning of these is encouraged.

Identifying Cognitive Errors

The thought processes of persons with emotional disorders are frequently characterized by a high frequency of errors in logic (LeFebvre 1981; Watkins and Rush 1983). A. T. Beck and others described six main categories of cognitive errors: 1) selective abstraction, 2) arbitrary inference, 3) absolutistic (dichotomous or all-or-nothing) thinking, 4) magnification and minimization, 5) personalization, and 6) catastrophic thinking (A. T. Beck et al. 1979; Clark et al. 1999). Definitions and examples of each of these cognitive errors are provided in Table 7–5.

Patients can be taught to spot characteristic cognitive errors to help in modifying their automatic thoughts. We find that most patients need a brief

TABLE 7–5. Cognitive errors

Selective abstraction (sometimes termed *mental filter*)	Drawing a conclusion based on only a small portion of the available data
Arbitrary inference	Coming to a conclusion without adequate supporting evidence or despite contradictory evidence
Absolutistic thinking (all-or-nothing thinking)	Categorizing oneself or personal experiences into rigid dichotomies (e.g., all good or all bad, perfect or completely flawed, success or total failure)
Magnification and minimization	Over- or undervaluing the significance of a personal attribute, a life event, or a future possibility
Personalization	Linking external occurrences to oneself (e.g., taking blame, assuming responsibility, criticizing oneself) when little or no basis exists for making these associations
Catastrophic thinking	Predicting the worst possible outcome while ignoring more likely eventualities

Source.   Adapted from Beck et al. 1979, p. 14.

period in session reviewing a basic handout on the definitions of cognitive errors as well as reading about cognitive errors in CBT books written for the general public (see Table 7–3 for a list of resources). Once patients have been exposed to these materials and have practiced spotting their errors in session, they often are able to recognize typical cognitive errors in their thinking. However, repeated practice may be needed before they can use this skill on a routine basis.

Using Thought Change Records

Self-monitoring with thought change records is a standard element of CBT for most emotional disorders (A.T. Beck et al. 1979; Wright et al. 2006). The thought change record helps patients 1) observe and recognize their automatic thoughts, 2) apply methods to modify their distorted thoughts, and 3) recognize positive outcomes in their emotions and behavior that result from changes in their thinking.

The thought change record (Figure 7–2) is a five-column table with the following headings: situation, automatic thoughts, emotions, rational re-

Situation	Automatic thoughts	Emotion(s)	Rational response	Outcome
Describe 1. Actual event leading to unpleasant emotion; or 2. Stream of thoughts, daydream, or recollection leading to unpleasant emotion; or 3. Unpleasant physiological sensations	1. Write automatic thought(s) that preceded emotion(s). 2. Rate belief in automatic thought(s), 0%–100%.	1. Specify sad, anxious, angry, etc. 2. Rate degree of emotion, 0%–100%.	1. Identify cognitive errors. 2. Write rational response to automatic thought(s). 3. Rate belief in rational response, 0%–100%.	1. Once again, rate belief in automatic thought(s), 0%–100%. 2. Specify and rate subsequent emotion(s), 0%–100%.

Tuesday				
I am reviewing policies and procedures at work, and I am immediately concerned about the amount of work.	1. I should have completed this weeks ago. 2. I always wait until the last minute to start things. 3. I'll never complete it.	Sad: 80% Anxious: 50%	1. Personalization. Although it is true that the project is overdue, I am not the only one assigned to this project. Two other people have been assigned to work on it and are just as responsible as I am. (80%) 2. All-or-nothing thinking. Although I wanted to start on this project earlier in the month, I was busy with other important duties that the company was asking me to complete. (90%) 3. Catastrophic thinking. Last year this was a big project, and I assisted in completing it. I have also completed other big projects for the company. The project is about 50% complete. (70%)	Sad: 80% Anxious: 50%

FIGURE 7–2. Thought change record: an example.

Source. Adapted from Wright JH, Beck AT, Thase ME: "Cognitive Therapy," in *The American Psychiatric Publishing Textbook of Clinical Psychiatry*, 5th Edition. Edited by Hales RE, Yudofsky SC, Gabbard GO. Washington, DC, American Psychiatric Publishing, 2008, pp. 1211–1256. Used with permission.

sponses, and outcome. Patients use the first two columns to write down an event, their associated automatic thoughts, and the degree (e.g., 0%–100%) of their belief in the automatic thoughts. The third column is used to identify the specific emotion linked with each automatic thought and the degree or level of each emotion (e.g., 0%–100%). The fourth column is used to record rational alternatives to distorted thoughts. This step is a critical element in the use of the thought change record because it stimulates patients to learn to assess the validity of their own thoughts. Several methods to modify automatic thoughts can be used to generate a list of alternative rational thoughts. For example, the technique of identifying cognitive errors can be used. Examining the evidence, applying reattribution, and a variety of other methods can be suggested as ways of generating rational thoughts for the thought change record. The fifth column—outcome—is used to record any changes that have occurred as a result of revising and modifying automatic thoughts. In the case example of a thought change record in Figure 7–2, the patient had a significant decrease in dysphoric mood. Although the use of the thought change record usually leads to the development of a more adaptive set of cognitions and a reduction in painful affect, sometimes the initial automatic thoughts will prove to be accurate. In such situations, the therapist helps the patient take a problem-solving approach, including the development of an action plan, to manage the stressful or upsetting event.

Identifying Schemas

The process of identifying and modifying schemas is usually more difficult than changing negative automatic thoughts because these core beliefs are more deeply embedded, may be largely out of the patient's awareness, and usually have been reinforced through years of life experience. Various cognitive techniques are used to work at the schema level (A. T. Beck et al. 1979; Wright et al. 2006), many of which overlap with the methods used by therapists to identify automatic thoughts (see Table 7–6). Two specific methods are discussed in this section: the downward arrow technique and identifying repetitive patterns of automatic thoughts. For a more detailed review of methods to identify and modify core beliefs, see *Learning Cognitive-Behavior Therapy: An Illustrated Guide* (Wright et al. 2006).

Downward Arrow Technique

The downward arrow technique is a powerful cognitive method to assist patients in uncovering negative core beliefs. The therapist asks a series of questions directed at exposing increasingly deeper levels of thinking. Questions are first aimed at automatic thoughts that are identified around an activating event. The therapist infers that an underlying schema is present

TABLE 7–6. Methods for identifying and modifying schemas

Techniques to identify schemas	Techniques to modify schemas
Using questioning methods[a]	Psychoeducation
Using imagery and role-play	Examining the evidence
Identifying repetitive patterns of automatic thoughts	Listing advantages and disadvantages
Using a schema checklist	Generating alternatives
	Using cognitive rehearsal

[a]Including the downward arrow technique.
Source.   Adapted from Wright JH, Beck AT, Thase ME: "Cognitive Therapy," in *The American Psychiatric Publishing Textbook of Clinical Psychiatry*, 5th Edition. Edited by Hales RE, Yudofsky SC, Gabbard GO. Washington, DC, American Psychiatric Publishing, 2008, pp. 1211–1256. Used with permission.

and constructs a chain of linked questions that builds on the supposition that the distorted cognitions are in fact true. Most questions take on the format of "If this thought were true, what would it mean about you (or about others or the future)?" This type of questioning needs to be done in a highly collaborative and supportive manner. In the following example, the therapist uses this technique to uncover a key schema in a patient with body dysmorphic disorder.

> **Therapist:** You mentioned that you had a plastic surgeon evaluate your nose for another surgery in the last week and that you are noticing a lot of the different imperfections. Did I get that right?
> **Patient:** Yes. I know we have talked about my concern about my body, but it just doesn't look right. There is big and rounded point here (*pointing to a place on his nose*).
> **Therapist:** Let's see if there is a larger meaning to these thoughts. If it were true that your nose was truly disfigured, what would that mean?
> **Patient:** I would be ugly and unattractive.
> **Therapist:** What if that were true?
> **Patient:** I don't think Julie or any other woman would be interested in dating me.
> **Therapist:** And if others were not interested in going out with you, what would that mean about you or your future?
> **Patient:** I would be alone, and I am not sure I could ever be happy without being in a relationship (*tearing up*).
> **Therapist:** So one thing that might be behind your multiple plastic surgeries is a belief that you are unattractive and that you are going to end

up alone and not in an intimate relationship. If this were true, what would this mean about you?

Patient: I'm unlovable.

Therapist: Am I hearing that you think you are ultimately unlovable?

Patient: I guess I have never thought of it in that way, but that is the way it feels now.

Identifying Repetitive Patterns of Automatic Thoughts

As the patient gains experience in recognizing automatic thoughts, repetitive patterns may begin to emerge that may suggest the presence of underlying schemas. Looking for patterns in automatic thoughts can be used as a specific therapy activity or homework assignment. Good sources for material for these reviews can be previous work with thought change records, examination of the evidence, or other CBT written exercises. Once a pattern is identified, patients are asked if the thoughts have a particular theme that suggests an underlying core belief.

Using Schema Checklists

In a manner similar to use of automatic thought checklists, patients can be asked to review lists of commonly endorsed core beliefs. An example of an inventory of maladaptive and adaptive schemas is provided in *Learning Cognitive-Behavior Therapy: An Illustrated Guide* (Wright et al. 2006). Use of a checklist can help patients recognize schemas that otherwise might have gone undetected. This type of exercise can be particularly useful for identifying positive or healthy core beliefs that have been obscured by depression, anxiety, or other symptoms of mental disorders. Recognition of adaptive schemas can provide good building blocks for enhancing self-esteem and self-efficacy.

Modifying Schemas

Interventions that are typically used to modify schemas include examining the evidence, generating alternatives, using cognitive rehearsal, and listing advantages and disadvantages. After a schema is identified, the therapist may ask the patient to use the double-column procedure described previously for examining the evidence for an automatic thought. This intervention is used to stimulate doubt in the validity of the schema and to start the patient thinking of alternative explanations.

An examining the evidence intervention is often combined with another step of schema modification, generating alternatives. The list of alternative schemas usually includes several different options, ranging from rather minor adjustments to extensive revisions in the schema. The therapist uses

Socratic questioning and other CBT techniques such as imagery and role-play to help the patient recognize potential alternative schemas. A "brainstorming" attitude is encouraged. Instead of trying to be sure that a revised schema is entirely accurate at first glance, the therapist usually suggests that they try to generate a variety of modified schemas without initially considering their validity or practicality. This approach stimulates creativity and gives the patient further encouragement to step aside from rigid long-standing schemas.

After alternatives are generated and discussed, the therapy turns toward examining the potential consequences of changing basic attitudes. Cognitive rehearsal can be used in the therapy session to test a schema modification. Homework may then be assigned to try out the revised schema in vivo. Usually specific behavior changes, consistent with the revised schema, need to be practiced repeatedly before modified core beliefs are fully accepted and put into action.

In addition to these techniques, patients can be taught to list the advantages and disadvantages of a schema. This procedure is designed to bring into awareness the hidden motivations that keep patients from fully accepting a more adaptive schema. Once these risks and benefits are clear, the patient can choose either to maintain the schema or to replace it with a more adaptive one.

Some schemas appear to have few, if any, advantages (e.g., "I'm stupid"; "I'll always lose in the end"), but many schemas have both positive and negative features (e.g., "If I decide to do something, I must succeed"; "I always have to work harder than others, or I'll fail"). The latter group of schemas may be maintained even in the face of their dysfunctional aspects because they encourage hard work, perseverance, or other adaptive behaviors. Yet the absolute and demanding nature of the schemas ultimately leads to excessive stress, failed expectations, low self-esteem, or other deleterious results. Listing advantages and disadvantages can help the patient to examine the full range of effects of a schema and often encourages modifications that can make the schema both more adaptive and less damaging. In Figure 7–3, Mr. A, a 43-year-old businessman, examined the advantages and disadvantages of a perfectionistic schema.

Behavioral Methods for Symptoms of Depression and Anxiety

Behavioral methods may be used to address many of the problems encountered in depression, anxiety, and other psychiatric conditions. Low energy, difficulty completing tasks, avoidance, lack of enjoyment of activities, and poor problem solving are among the issues that may be effectively addressed

Advantages	Disadvantages
I got my MBA.	I feel overburdened, depressed, and anxious. I can never relax.
My company knows they can count on me.	Everyone says, "He walks on water." With these expectations, I don't feel I can share my real self with others, and I feel lonely.
I am the "go-to-guy."	I never feel as if I can get away from work. They even call me when I am on vacation.
Life is predictable and controlled.	Everything is planned, and nothing ever is a surprise or spontaneous.
I can count on myself to get things done.	It prevents me from counting on others to get things done.

FIGURE 7–3. Mr. A's list of advantages and disadvantages for the belief "I must be perfect."

with the behavioral components of CBT. Several of the more commonly used behavioral methods are described here. Video illustrations and detailed instructions for using these methods are provided elsewhere by Wright and colleagues (2006).

Behavioral Activation

Behavioral activation is a technique in which patients are assisted in reversing patterns of inactivity, anhedonia, procrastination, and social withdrawal. Although some authors use the term *behavioral activation* to refer to any technique that mobilizes patients, we use the term to describe a rather straightforward or simple behavioral intervention in which patient and therapist agree on a plan for taking a single or low-complexity step toward reactivation. For patients who are in the early stages of therapy and are highly symptomatic, behavioral activation may involve the choice of a task or an activity that they may have been avoiding but that could stimulate increased activity and energy. Examples include making a commitment to walking for 20 minutes twice a week, agreeing to cook one meal in the next week, or accepting an invitation from a friend to go to the movies. More demanding activities can be used for behavioral activation later in therapy or for patients who are less symptomatic.

Choosing a problem to tackle for behavioral activation entails identifying a problem of sufficient magnitude to make the effort meaningful but also one for which the chances of success are high. Collaboration in choosing an activity is critical to success. Whenever possible, patients should take the lead in selecting the intervention target and giving an honest appraisal of their capabilities in completing the assignment. Therapists can often increase the chances of a good outcome by helping patients to identify barriers to completing the task. A good question to ask is, "What might get in the way of your following this plan?" If barriers or obstacles can be identified, then the therapist can help the patient develop solutions.

Activity Scheduling

Activity scheduling is frequently used in CBT when patients have low energy and anhedonia. It is a mainstay in the treatment of depression but also can be useful in any clinical condition in which patients have difficulty organizing their time. Activity scheduling includes an assessment of the patient's current activity and embodies an explicit goal of increasing mastery and pleasure. In this context, mastery ratings are used to measure the patient's sense of accomplishment in completing activities. Pleasure ratings are used to indicate the level of enjoyment experienced while participating in activities. Ratings may be made on 0- to 10-point scales in which 10 represents maximum mastery or pleasure and 0 represents no mastery or pleasure.

Typically, patients are introduced to an activity log during a therapy session and instructed how to complete it. (A template for an activity schedule log is provided by Wright et al. [2006].) Examples of specific activities from the recent past can be used to highlight the relation between participation in activities and the patient's experience of mastery and pleasure. To illustrate, a severely depressed man had earlier reported that he couldn't "enjoy anything." Yet when asked to rate his experiences while watching a son's soccer game, he noted a pleasure rating of 6 and a mastery rating of 7.

For some patients, a full week of activity scheduling can be a fruitful assignment. However, the exercise can be scaled down to only a day or part of a day for patients who are severely depressed or are having problems with concentration or very low energy.

After collecting baseline activity schedules with mastery and pleasure ratings, the therapist can help the patient to organize the daily schedule to enhance a sense of mastery and pleasure. The patient can try to increase activities that received higher ratings of mastery and pleasure and also brainstorm for ideas of stimulating or productive activities to add to the schedule. Problems or deficits in mastery or pleasure are discussed, and strategies are formulated to address these problems. The patient's management of time also may become a fruitful topic of discussion.

Review of an activity schedule can ascertain a host of opportunities to identify negative thoughts, cognitive distortions, or even schemas that may contribute to the behavioral manifestations of depression or anxiety. This interplay between the cognitive and behavioral aspects of treatment is an important element of CBT. For example, a 50-year-old salesman had a depressive episode after being fired from his job. He became withdrawn and lost interest in activities. The therapist introduced the concept of activity scheduling by asking him to keep a simple log of his current activities during the week between sessions. During the session, the log was reviewed, and the concept of rating activities was introduced. Maladaptive cognitions about behavioral activity became readily apparent as the patient reported thoughts such as "What's the use of doing anything...I'm too ashamed to go out in public...I'll never succeed." Thus, the therapist needed to help the patient reverse hopelessness to implement activity scheduling effectively.

Graded Task Assignments

Graded task assignments involve taking seemingly overwhelming tasks and breaking them down into manageable pieces. Developing a graded task assignment may require a cognitive analysis of the task to identify distortions prior to initiating a behavioral plan. Often, several iterations of the process are required as the patient and therapist work together to make each component of the task workable. The plan should begin with smaller tasks and gradually move toward larger, more difficult ones. Patients may need coaching on ways to complete steps in the assignment.

Use of a graded task assignment is illustrated in the treatment of a depressed woman who reported that her home was completely full of clutter, dirty dishes, and laundry. She felt overwhelmed and totally unable to tackle the task of cleaning up the mess. Her assessment of her incapacity was contributing to a downward spiral of depression in which negative cognitions were reinforcing maladaptive behavioral patterns, which were aggravating her low self-esteem. The patient and therapist agreed on a plan that divided the task into manageable segments with gradually building levels of effort. Successful progression through the steps appeared to be a catalyst in her overall recovery from depression.

Relaxation Training

Relaxation techniques are commonly used to treat anxiety symptoms, especially if the patient has muscle tension. A frequently used method is known as *progressive relaxation*. In this approach, the patient is instructed to relax muscle groups systematically throughout the body, one by one. This technique may be combined with imagery, meditation, or breathing techniques. During relaxation training, the patient may report emergence of cognitions that require further exploration. Relaxation techniques can be taught and practiced during sessions and then used by the patient between sessions.

Exposure and Response Prevention

Because avoidance is a central feature of anxiety disorders, exposure techniques are a major component of CBT for these conditions. Typically, exposure methods are graded so that the patient begins by facing stimuli that trigger lower levels of anxiety and then progressively experiences stimuli that may produce higher amounts of anxiety. A multiple-step hierarchy involving exposure to the stimulus is constructed in collaboration with the patient. Often a simple rating scale of 0–100 is used to rate the expected amount of anxiety associated with each progressive step. The exposure may be performed with imagery or in vivo. Virtual reality programs are available for simulating anxiety-producing situations (e.g., flying in the case of fear of flying, traumatic reminders in the case of posttraumatic stress disorder, social situations in the case of social anxiety disorder) in the therapist's office.

With these methods, therapist and patient work collaboratively to increase the patient's exposure to anxiety-provoking experiences that he or she is avoiding. This provides a context in which therapists can help patients test out their maladaptive beliefs about anxiety, their vulnerability, or their resources. The response prevention component of exposure therapy involves a detailed analysis of all avoidant behaviors, including misguided attempts to cope that actually reinforce avoidance (safety behaviors), and collaborative agreement to stop using these maladaptive behaviors. Although most exposure therapy is performed in a gradual manner, very rapid exposure protocols have been described and studied.

Cognitive-Behavioral Therapy Methods for Specific Disorders

Schizophrenia

The first reported case of CBT for schizophrenia occurred in 1952 when Aaron Beck described successful treatment of delusions in a patient with schizophrenia (A.T. Beck 1952). However, systematic exploration of the possible role of CBT in treatment of schizophrenia and other psychoses did not begin until the early 1990s (Kingdon and Turkington 1991, 1994; Tarrier et al. 1993). Over the past two decades, several books have been published that detail methods for performing CBT with psychotic patients (Chadwick et al. 1996; Kingdon and Turkington 1994, 2002, 2005); numerous outcome studies have been completed (reviewed in Chapter 8); and CBT applications for schizophrenia have been gaining increased acceptance. In the United Kingdom, where much of the research on CBT for psychoses has been conducted, the National Institute for Clinical Excellence (2002) guidelines for treatment of schizophrenia recommend a course of CBT for all patients who have this condition.

CBT methods for schizophrenia use the same basic strategies used in treatment of nonpsychotic Axis I disorders. However, modifications are made in the therapeutic relationship, the pace of therapy, targets for interventions, and implementation of techniques. Because patients with schizophrenia often have difficulty engaging in therapy and can be stigmatized by this illness, considerable effort is expended early in CBT on building a collaborative therapeutic relationship. The therapist uses a gentle, nonthreatening questioning style to try to set the patient at ease.

Psychoeducation and the "normalizing rationale" are key elements of the beginning stages of CBT for schizophrenia (Kingdon and Turkington 1991, 2005). One part of this process is for therapists to ask patients to give their explanations of symptoms. Often the responses reflect dysfunctional beliefs and thus offer useful opportunities for educating and destigmatizing (e.g., "The devil is talking to me," "I have done something terribly wrong and deserve to be punished," "Nobody else hears voices," "All doctors want to do is push pills—I won't take them").

The normalizing rationale can be a centerpiece of efforts to help patients understand their illnesses in more rational and affirming ways (Kingdon and Turkington 1991, 2005). The cognitive-behavioral therapist explains that experiences such as having paranoia or hearing voices are very common and can be induced by lack of sleep, sensory deprivation, medical illnesses, and other stresses. The discussion can then lead to presentation of a stress-vulnerability model for symptoms. The goal of this process is to help patients develop a conceptualization that has these core elements: 1) psychotic symptoms can occur in a wide range of people and thus can be a part of "normal" experience; 2) stress can interact with a biological vulnerability to produce or worsen symptoms; and 3) problems can be reduced or solved by learning ways to manage symptoms and cope with stress. If this conceptualization is understood and accepted, therapeutic work on reducing delusions and hallucinations and reversing negative symptoms is more likely to succeed.

CBT for delusions relies primarily on the use of Socratic questioning and guided discovery to gradually help patients see different perspectives. Examining the evidence can be a quite useful specific technique. For example, a patient might be asked to list the evidence for and against a belief that his food is being poisoned, people are following him, or microphones are hidden in the heating ducts. After the evidence is examined in a therapy session, homework assignments may be developed to test out the belief or to obtain further information. It is important for therapists to maintain an empirical stance when doing this type of work. Instead of trying to persuade the patient to give up a delusion, the therapist works with the patient to function as an investigative team. Together they explore evidence and attempt to draw the most rational conclusion.

An example of an examining the evidence exercise for a woman with paranoid schizophrenia is shown in Figure 7–4. As often happens in performing this type of exercise, the "evidence for" the delusional belief contains numerous cognitive errors that can be discussed in the therapy session. The intervention plan developed with this patient used graded exposure in a manner similar to the stepped approach used for anxiety disorders. This patient had been isolating herself in a darkened house with all of the shades drawn. Thus, a combined cognitive and behavioral intervention was used to decrease the intensity of her delusional belief and help her resume normal activities.

The CBT approach to hallucinations uses the educating and normalizing process outlined earlier to help patients understand these symptoms in the most adaptive way possible. The patient's attributions (explanation of causality) about these perceptions are elicited and discussed with the goal of developing an explanatory model that assists with coping. For example, a patient who first explained his auditory hallucinations as "coming from the devil" was eventually able to articulate and accept a much more adaptive construct: "I have an illness that affects my thinking and makes me hear voices...I don't need to pay attention to the voices or do what they say...The voices get softer and less bothersome when I pay less attention to them."

Therapeutic work with hallucinations also may involve developing lists of behaviors that either aggravate or reduce the intensity of the symptom. For example, a patient might note that lack of sleep, arguments with par-

Examining the evidence for a delusional belief:
people in red cars are trying to get me

Evidence For	Evidence Against
I see red cars going past my house every day.	There are so many red cars on the road; how could they all be after me?
It seems like people in red cars are staring at me.	No one in a red car has actually ever threatened me or hurt me.
A teacher who hated me drove a red car.	My chemical imbalance can make me afraid of things that won't harm me.
Someone in a red car slows down when she drives past my house.	I trust my sister, and she says that I don't need to be afraid of red cars.

My plan

I'll slowly check out this fear with these steps:
1. Take a walk in my neighborhood with my sister and walk past some red cars.
2. Take a drive with my sister and drive by some red cars on purpose.
3. If I am comfortable with the first two steps, I'll try to go to the mall. I'll walk through the parking lot and get used to seeing lots of red cars.

FIGURE 7–4. Examining the evidence for a delusional belief: people in red cars are trying to get me.

ents, and spending time alone with nothing to do may make her voices worse. Conversely, listening to soothing music, socializing with a friend, working on crafts projects, and going out to eat may reduce the hallucinations. Behavioral plans can be made to cope with aggravating influences and to use identified coping methods more frequently. If patients have difficulty finding ways to reduce hallucinations, it can be helpful to provide them with a list of commonly used strategies (see Kingdon and Turkington 2005, p. 123 for examples of coping methods).

Cognitive and behavioral interventions for negative symptoms are less direct than techniques for positive symptoms. Kingdon and Turkington (2005) recommend a "go slow" approach for negative symptoms. Instead of trying to aggressively push patients to break patterns of social isolation or apathy, therapists gradually build the therapeutic relationship and assist patients to meet their goals for change—even if these goals are rather modest. When patients are ready to begin changing negative symptoms, therapists may suggest techniques such as graded task assignments to help them take sequential steps toward improvement.

Eating Disorders

As noted in Chapter 8, CBT has been shown to be effective for bulimia and binge-eating disorder. Cognitive therapy for these conditions focuses on maladaptive beliefs about food, weight, body image, and self-worth and associated dysfunctional behaviors (Fairburn et al. 2003; Garner et al. 1997). Treatment plans typically start with behavioral interventions aimed at normalizing eating behavior, progresses to cognitive interventions aimed at underlying beliefs and maladaptive cognitions, and then concludes with relapse prevention strategies (Wonderlich et al. 2004).

Self-Monitoring and Meal Planning

In the first phase of treatment, patients create a self-monitoring form and use it to record everything they eat and any associated eating disorder symptoms. Patients record the time of day; the content of the meal; where the meal was consumed; whether it was a snack, binge, or meal; whether it was a planned or an unplanned meal; whether it led to associated purging, use of laxatives, or exercise; and associated thoughts and feelings.

A collaborative meal prescription can be used for some patients who require more structure (Garner and Bemis 1982). The eating prescription is a detailed written meal plan instructing patients when to eat, specifying the foods to be consumed, specifying where the meal is to be eaten, and indicating the duration of the meal. It temporarily takes "the decision" out of eating behavior. Meal planning can be implemented incrementally, with the initial focus on spacing meals throughout the day, lengthening the duration of eating within the meal, and eating foods the patient considers safe. After the early stages of meal planning are mastered, the therapist and patient can increase the quantity of food eaten and the range of food consumed.

Cognitive Restructuring

Individuals with eating disorders are taught to examine their cognitions carefully, identify instances of maladaptive thinking, and attempt to identify a more adaptive response to the cue or situation. For example, a person with an eating disorder may be trying on some clothes (stimulus) and have the thought "I look like an elephant." This thought is associated with disgust and sadness (emotional response) and may increase the likelihood of dieting or purging. Table 7–7 displays the five key cognitive constructs found in persons with eating disorders (Cooper et al. 2004).

If possible, the therapist helps the patient to move toward examining deeper self-schemas and their linked behavioral patterns (Garner et al. 1997). For example, patients with eating disorders often have poor self-esteem and devote a considerable amount of time to keeping a "balance sheet" of daily accomplishments and shortcomings. The technique of de-centering can be used to look at the patient's approach to self-worth and need to maintain perfection. Decentering involves asking patients if other individuals are considered less worthwhile if they make mistakes or do not perform well on a particular day. Would they consider the therapist "a loser" or less worthwhile if an appointment started 5 minutes late? Decen-tering and a variety of other cognitive restructuring techniques discussed earlier in this chapter can be used to help patients modify rigidly held sche-mas.

Bipolar Disorder

The primary emphasis of CBT for bipolar disorder is on helping patients learn to monitor symptoms effectively, identify potential triggers for relapse, and develop skills for halting escalation into depression or mania (Basco and Rush 2005). Because patients with this condition often downplay the sig-nificance of symptoms of hypomania or mania, or may completely deny that they have a problem, the opening phase of treatment is often devoted to de-veloping an effective working relationship and providing psychoeducation. Readings such as *An Unquiet Mind* (Jamison 1995) are typically suggested for both patients and family. Later, if patients have an improved under-standing of their illness and accept treatment, *The Bipolar Workbook: Tools for Controlling Your Mood Swings* (Basco 2006) can be a very useful tool for learning CBT skills for managing this disorder.

TABLE 7–7. Cognitive domains and cognitive-behavioral therapy methods for eating disorders

Cognitive domain	Typical automatic thoughts	Cognitive or behavioral methods
Overvaluation and overcontrol of eating, weight, and shape	"If I start eating that, I'll never stop."	Graded exposure experiment with analysis of feared outcome
		Meal prescription
		Decatastrophizing
		Thought change records
	"I have to be thin to be successful."	Survey others to gain more realistic view
	"If I don't exercise 2 hours a day, I'll get fat."	Gradually decrease safety behaviors and monitor frequency or effect of feared outcome; analysis of the advantages and disadvantages of change
Mood (emotion) intolerance	"I can't take this."	Gradual elimination of safety behaviors that allow patient to avoid mood states
		Graded exposure to distressful feelings
	"When I am upset, I have lost all control."	Thought change records (challenge dichotomous reasoning)
		Survey on the meaning of emotions or feelings

TABLE 7–7. Cognitive domains and cognitive-behavioral therapy methods for eating disorders (continued)

Cognitive domain	Typical automatic thoughts	Cognitive or behavioral methods
Low self-esteem	"If I am not perfect, I'm nothing."	Cognitive rehearsal (practice being not perfect and monitor for feared outcome)
	"I'm no good…stupid…ugly."	Thought change records (distill vague statements about self into specific beliefs to make the distortion highly apparent)
		Practice tasks or situations in which belief will be challenged
Perfectionism	"I must do things perfectly."	Activity scheduling/planning (reduce checking of performance with specific activities or increase activities with the specific purpose of pleasure)
Interpersonal difficulties	"I can't let anyone down (they are counting on me)."	Exposure to putting own needs first, with analysis of feared consequences
	"I will upset them if I tell them what I really think."	Role-playing/assertiveness training in sessions; graded practice of expressing emotions and feelings

Source. Adapted from Cooper M, Whitehead L, Boughton N: "Eating Disorders," in *Oxford Guide to Behavioural Experiments in Cognitive Therapy.* Edited by Bennett-Levy J, Butler G, Fennell M, et al. New York, Oxford University Press, 2004, pp. 269–272. Used with permission.

Mood graphs are a frequently used tool for increasing patient awareness (Basco and Rush 2005). Another helpful method suggested by Basco and Rush (2005) is a symptom summary worksheet. This exercise assists patients with identifying early warning signs of impending mood shifts, in addition to the more pronounced signs of full episodes of depression or mania. In the example provided in Figure 7–5, a middle-aged man with bipolar disorder was able to spot several indicators of possible switches to hypomania or depression. His worksheet could be used to plan interventions to decrease the risk for an escalation of symptoms. He could agree to curtail his Internet research to no more than 30 minutes on weeknights and 1 hour during the day on weekends. Another intervention could be a CBT exercise to list advantages and disadvantages of trying again to start a home-based business. During past episodes of hypomania, he had made unwise financial decisions about starting businesses that ultimately failed. A fully developed relapse prevention plan for this patient would include various coping strategies for limiting the development of both hypomanic and depressive symptoms.

Other common targets for CBT interventions in bipolar disorder are 1) sleep disruption, 2) pharmacotherapy nonadherence, 3) cognitive distortions and automatic thoughts in mania, 4) stress, and 5) lack of a daily routine. CBT methods for insomnia have proven to be quite effective (Edinger et al. 2001; Sivertsen et al. 2006) and are used routinely in the treatment of bipolar disorder (Basco and Rush 2005). Adherence is promoted by use of behavioral reminder systems and by eliciting and modifying dysfunctional attitudes about taking medication. Therapists may help patients identify barriers to adherence and then design plans to overcome these obstacles. CBT for automatic thoughts and cognitive errors in hypomania or mania can use standard interventions such as thought change records and examining the evidence exercises. However, the focus is on positively distorted cognitions, underestimates of risk, and externalization of blame.

The importance of following a daily routine has been confirmed in research on social rhythm therapy for bipolar disorder (Frank et al. 2005). In CBT, therapists inquire about habits of sleep and wake times, mealtimes, work schedules, and other activities that define patients' daily schedules. If significant irregularity occurs in the daily schedule, changes are recommended to reduce this variability. CBT methods for bipolar disorder also may include work on building stress management skills. For example, relaxation training, breathing exercises, or imagery could be applied to reduce tension; pleasant event scheduling could be used to provide healthy distractions from stressful situations; or efforts could be made to enhance problem-solving capacity.

A symptom summary worksheet: early warning signs of hypomania and depression

Hypomania	Depression
I stay up 1–2 hours late to do Internet research on home-based business opportunities.	I'm more likely to procrastinate about projects at work and home.
I start to talk more at work about movies, sports, jokes, etc. This interrupts others in their work and distracts me from getting my work done.	I start to turn down invitations to do things. I'd prefer to stay to myself and avoid being around others.
I drive faster.	The fun or excitement goes out of my work. I feel like I'm just going through the motions.
I'm more irritable with my wife and children.	
I feel more creative at work. More ideas and plans are going through my head.	I start having more self-critical thoughts.
	My confidence drops.
This is mostly good if it doesn't get out of control.	I feel like I'm more distant from my wife and children.

FIGURE 7–5. A symptom summary worksheet: early warning signs of hypomania and depression.

Conclusion

CBT methods are based directly on core theories of altered information processing and associated maladaptive behavior in psychiatric disorders. Therapists select techniques on the basis of an individualized CBT formulation, the patient's diagnosis, and the objectives or agenda that is collaboratively set during each session. General or nonspecific features of all effective psychotherapies are also important in CBT. Thus, therapists work to promote understanding, trust, genuineness, and accurate empathy. The CBT relationship is highly collaborative and active. Specific emphasis is placed on psychoeducation, structuring sessions, and enhancing learning and skill acquisition. A variety of cognitive techniques such as thought recording, examining the evidence, and rehearsal are used to modify dysfunctional automatic thoughts and schemas. Also, behavioral methods such as activity scheduling, graded task assignments, and exposure and response prevention are used routinely in CBT sessions.

CBT has been studied extensively in randomized controlled trials, and detailed treatment guidelines and techniques have been described for most psychiatric conditions. Future challenges for CBT include the study of methods to further enhance treatment results, detailed examination of predictors for outcome, incorporation of new developments in computer-assisted learning or other technologies, and research on best practices for dissemination of CBT methods to trainees across health care disciplines and in various health care settings.

Key Points

- Cognitive-behavioral therapy (CBT) methods are constructed from the basic theories and experimental findings on cognitive and behavioral pathology in specific psychiatric disorders.

- Prior to the selection and implementation of specific CBT methods, the patient's unique history is understood through the lens of cognitive and behavioral theory. Specific methods are then selected that match the patient's problems, symptoms, assets, and potential.

- General CBT methods such as the collaborative-empirical therapeutic relationship and structuring procedures are used across sessions and are incorporated into the treatment of all disorders.

- All CBT treatment plans aim to modify patients' maladaptive automatic thoughts and schemas. Various cognitive methods enable patients to engage in this process.

- Several methods target problematic behaviors associated with depression and anxiety. These methods include activity monitoring, behavioral activation, and exposure and response prevention and are also incorporated into the treatments of other disorders.

- CBT methods for schizophrenia include many of the typical procedures for depression and anxiety conditions. However, the "normalizing rationale" is central to assisting patients to understand their illness in a more rational and affirming way.

- CBT methods for eating disorders focus on maladaptive beliefs about food, weight, body image, and self-worth and on dysfunctional behaviors.

- The primary emphasis of CBT for bipolar disorder is on helping patients learn to monitor symptoms effectively, identify triggers for relapse, and develop skills for halting escalation into depression or mania.

References

Abramson LY, Seligman MEP, Teasdale J: Learned helplessness in humans: critique and reformulation. J Abnorm Psychol 87:49–74, 1978

Albano AM, Kearney CA: When Children Refuse School: A Cognitive-Behavioral Therapy Approach: Therapist Guide. San Antonio, TX, Psychological Corporation, 2000

Basco MR: Never Good Enough: How to Use Perfectionism to Your Advantage Without Letting It Ruin Your Life. New York, Free Press, 2000

Basco MR: The Bipolar Workbook: Tools for Controlling Your Mood Swings. New York, Guilford, 2006

Basco MR, Rush AJ: Cognitive-Behavioral Therapy for Bipolar Disorder, 2nd Edition. New York, Guilford, 2005

Beck AT: Successful outpatient psychotherapy of a chronic schizophrenic with a delusion based on borrowed guilt. Psychiatry 15:305–312, 1952

Beck AT, Freeman A: Cognitive Therapy of Personality Disorders. New York, Guilford, 1990

Beck AT, Greenberg RL: Coping With Depression. Philadelphia, PA, Beck Institute for Cognitive Therapy and Research, 1974

Beck AT, Rush AJ, Shaw BF, et al: Cognitive Therapy of Depression. New York, Guilford, 1979

Beck AT, Wright FW, Newman CF, et al: Cognitive Therapy of Substance Abuse. New York, Guilford, 1993

Beck JS: Cognitive Therapy: Basics and Beyond. New York, Guilford, 1995

Burns DD: Feeling Good: The New Mood Therapy. New York, Signet, 1980

Burns DD: Feeling Good: The New Therapy, Revised Edition. New York, Avon, 1999

Chadwick P, Birchwood M, Trower P: Cognitive Therapy of Voices, Delusions, and Paranoia. Chichester, UK, Wiley, 1996

Clark DA, Beck AT, Alford BA: Scientific Foundations of Cognitive Theory and Therapy of Depression. New York, Wiley, 1999

Cooper M, Whitehead L, Boughton N: Eating disorders, in Oxford Guide to Behavioural Experiments in Cognitive Therapy. Edited by Bennett-Levy J, Butler G, Fennell M, et al. New York, Oxford University Press, 2004, pp 269–272

Craske MG, Barlow DH: Mastery of Your Anxiety and Panic, 3rd Edition. San Antonio, TX, Psychological Corporation, 2000

Davis D, Wright JH: The therapeutic relationship in cognitive-behavioral therapy: patient perceptions and therapist responses. Cogn Behav Pract 1:25–45, 1994

Edinger JD, Wohlgemuth WK, Redtke RA, et al: Cognitive behavioral therapy for treatment of chronic primary insomnia: a randomized controlled trial. JAMA 285:1856–1864, 2001

Epstein N: Couple and family therapy, in Comparative Treatments of Depression. Edited by Reinicke MA, Davison MR. New York, Springer, 2002, pp 358–396

Fairburn CG, Cooper Z, Shafran R: Cognitive behaviour therapy for eating disorders: a "transdiagnostic" theory and treatment. Behav Res Ther 41:509–528, 2003

Foa EB, Wilson R: Stop Obsessing! How to Overcome Your Obsessions and Compulsions, Revised Edition. New York, Bantam Books, 2001

Frank E, Kupfer DJ, Thase ME, et al: Two-year outcomes for interpersonal and social rhythm therapy in individuals with bipolar I disorder. Arch Gen Psychiatry 62:996–1004, 2005

Garner DM, Bemis KM: A cognitive-behavioral approach to anorexia nervosa. Cognit Ther Res 6:123–150, 1982

Garner DM, Vitousek KM, Pike KM: Cognitive behavioral therapy for anorexia nervosa, in Handbook of Treatment for Eating Disorders, 2nd Edition. Edited by Garner DM, Garfinkel PE. New York, Guilford, 1997, pp 94–144

Greenberger D, Padesky CA: Mind Over Mood: Change How You Feel by Changing the Way You Thin. New York, Guilford, 1996

Hollon SD, Kendall PC: Cognitive self-statements in depression: development of an automatic thoughts questionnaire. Cognitive Therapy and Research 4:383–395, 1980

Jamison K: An Unquiet Mind. New York, Alfred A Knopf and Random House, 1995

Kenwright M, Liness S, Marks I: Reducing demands on clinicians by offering computer-aided self-help for phobia/panic: feasibility study. Br J Psychiatry 179:456–459, 2001

Kingdon D, Turkington D: The use of cognitive behavior therapy with a normalizing rationale in schizophrenia: preliminary report. J Nerv Ment Dis 179:207–211, 1991

Kingdon D, Turkington D: Cognitive Behavior Therapy of Schizophrenia. New York, Guilford, 1994

Kingdon DG, Turkington D: A Case Study Guide to Cognitive Therapy of Psychosis. Chichester, UK, Wiley, 2002

Kingdon D, Turkington D: Cognitive Therapy for Schizophrenia. New York, Guilford, 2005

Leahy RL: The Worry Cure: Seven Steps to Stop Worry From Stopping You. New York, Harmony Press, 2006

LeFebvre MF: Cognitive distortion and cognitive errors in depressed psychiatric and low back pain patients. J Consult Clin Psychol 49:517–525, 1981

Morley S, Eccleston C, Williams A: Systematic review and meta-analysis of randomized controlled trials of cognitive behaviour therapy and behaviour therapy for chronic pain in adults, excluding headache. Pain 80:1–13, 1999

National Institute for Clinical Excellence: Schizophrenia: core interventions in the treatment and management of schizophrenia in primary and secondary care (Clinical Guideline 1). London, National Institute for Health and Clinical Excellence, December 2002. Available at: http://www.nice.org.uk/nicemedia/pdf/CG1NICEguideline.pdf. Accessed March 20, 2008.

Newman MG, Kenardy J, Herman S, et al: Comparison of palmtop-computer-assisted brief cognitive-behavioral treatment to cognitive-behavioral treatment for panic disorder. J Consult Clin Psychol 65:178–183, 1997

Payne A, Blanchard EB: A controlled comparison of cognitive therapy and self-help support groups in the treatment of irritable bowel syndrome. J Consult Clin Psychol 63:779–786, 1995

Proudfoot J, Ryden C, Everitt B, et al: Clinical efficacy of computerised cognitive-behavioural therapy for anxiety and depression in primary care: randomised controlled trial. Br J Psychiatry 185:46–54, 2004

Reinicke MA, Dattilio FM, Freeman A (eds): Cognitive Therapy With Children and Adolescents: A Casebook for Clinical Practice, 2nd Edition. New York, Guilford, 2003

Sivertsen B, Omvik S, Pallesen S, et al: Cognitive behavioral therapy vs zopiclone for treatment of chronic primary insomnia in older adults: a randomized controlled trial. JAMA 295:2851–2858, 2006

Tarrier N, Beckett R, Harwood S, et al: A trial of two cognitive-behavioural methods of treating drug-resistant residual psychotic symptoms in schizophrenic patients, I: outcome. Br J Psychiatry 162:524–532, 1993

Watkins JT, Rush AJ: Cognitive response test. Cognit Ther Res 7:125–126, 1983

White J, Freeman A: Cognitive-Behavioral Group Therapy for Specific Problems and Populations. Washington, DC, American Psychological Association, 2000

White KP, Nielson WR: Cognitive behavioral treatment of fibromyalgia syndrome: a follow-up assessment. J Rheumatol 22:717–721, 1995

Wonderlich SA, Mitchell JE, Swan-Kremier L, et al: An overview of cognitive-behavioral approaches to eating disorders, in Clinical Handbook of Eating Disorders: An Integrated Approach. Edited by Brewerton TD. New York, Marcel Dekker, 2004, pp 403–424

Wright JH, Basco MR: Getting Your Life Back: The Complete Guide to Recovery From Depression. New York, Free Press, 2001

Wright JH, Salmon P, Wright AS, et al: Cognitive Therapy: A Multimedia Learning Program. Louisville, KY, MindStreet, 1995

Wright JH, Wright AS, Salmon P, et al: Development and initial testing of a multimedia program for computer-assisted cognitive therapy. Am J Psychother 56:76–86, 2002

Wright JH, Wright AS, Beck AT: Good Days Ahead: The Multimedia Program for Cognitive Therapy. Louisville, KY, MindStreet, 2004

Wright JH, Wright AS, Albano AM, et al: Computer-assisted cognitive therapy for depression: maintaining efficacy while reducing therapist time. Am J Psychiatry 162:1158–1164, 2005

Wright JH, Basco MR, Thase ME: Learning Cognitive-Behavior Therapy: An Illustrated Guide. Washington, DC, American Psychiatric Publishing, 2006

Suggested Readings

Barlow DH, Cerney JA: Psychological Treatment of Panic. New York, Guilford, 1988

Basco MR, Rush AJ: Cognitive-Behavioral Therapy for Bipolar Disorder, 2nd Edition. New York, Guilford, 2005

Beck AT, Freeman A: Cognitive Therapy of Personality Disorders. New York, Guilford, 1990

Beck AT, Rush AJ, Shaw BF, et al: Cognitive Therapy of Depression. New York, Guilford, 1979

Beck AT, Emery GD, Greenberg RL: Anxiety Disorders and Phobias: A Cognitive Perspective. New York, Basic Books, 1985

Beck AT, Wright FD, Newman CF, et al: Cognitive Therapy of Substance Abuse. New York, Guilford, 1993

Beck JS: Cognitive Therapy: Basics and Beyond. New York, Guilford, 1995

Clark DA, Beck AT, Alford BA: Scientific Foundations of Cognitive Theory and Therapy of Depression. New York, Wiley, 1999

Fairburn C, Brownell K (eds): Eating Disorders and Obesity: A Comprehensive Handbook, 2nd Edition. New York, Guilford, 2002

Kingdon D, Turkington D: Cognitive Therapy for Schizophrenia. New York, Guilford, 2005

Leahy RL: Contemporary Cognitive Therapy: Theory, Research, and Practice. New York, Guilford, 2004

Linehan MM: Cognitive-Behavioral Treatment of Borderline Personality Disorder. New York, Guilford, 1993

Meichenbaum DB: Cognitive-Behavior Modification: An Integrative Approach. New York, Plenum, 1977

Reinicke MA, Dattilio FM, Freeman A (eds): Cognitive Therapy With Children and Adolescents: A Casebook for Clinical Practice, 2nd Edition. New York, Guilford, 2003

Salkovskis PM (ed): Frontiers of Cognitive Therapy. New York, Guilford, 1996

Wilkes TCR, Belsher G, Rush AJ, et al: Cognitive Therapy for Depressed Adolescents. New York, Guilford, 1994

Wright JH, Basco MR, Thase ME: Learning Cognitive-Behavior Therapy: An Illustrated Guide. Washington, DC, American Psychiatric Publishing, 2006

Chapter 8

Applications of Individual Cognitive-Behavioral Therapy to Specific Disorders

Efficacy and Indications

Amanda M. Epp, B.A.
Keith S. Dobson, Ph.D.
Jean Cottraux, M.D., Ph.D.

Cognitive-behavioral therapy (CBT) has received an enormous amount of research attention (Butler et al. 2006) and has been identified as an empirically supported therapy for numerous psychiatric disorders and medical conditions with psychological components. It is one of the most commonly used psychotherapeutic treatments in adults (Leichsenring et al. 2006). Surveys indicate that CBT is expected to remain among the foremost foci of psychotherapy training in the coming years, and its importance in the field of psychotherapy is likely to increase (Norcross et al. 2002). In this chapter we review applications of individual CBT to a variety of psychiatric disorders and review their efficacy and indications. We also discuss the limitations of and knowledge gaps within the current empirical literature, and present suggestions for future research and applications.

Brief Review of Cognitive-Behavioral Therapy

CBT was developed in the early 1970s because of a growing dissatisfaction with traditional behavioral therapy and the psychodynamic model of personality and therapy. CBT is based on scientific models of human behavior, cognition, and emotion. CBT proposes the following (Dobson 2001):

- That cognitive activity affects behavior and emotion
- That cognitive activity may be monitored and altered
- That desired emotional and behavior change may be obtained through cognitive change

Thus, the main indices of change in CBT are cognition and behavior.

All the various forms of CBT adhere to the mediational position, in which it is postulated that internal covert processes (thinking or cognition) mediate the individual's behavioral and emotional responses to his or her environment and determine to some extent the individual's adjustment or maladjustment. Thus, although there are technical differences among CBTs in how they combine cognitive and behavioral techniques, they share a theoretical model distinct from that of the strictly behavioral therapies (for an extensive description of the theory of CBT, see Chapter 6, "Theory of Cognitive Therapy").

The term *cognitive-behavioral therapy* is often used to refer to a variety of approaches in which both cognitive and behavioral strategies are used. It refers to both standard cognitive therapy (Beck et al. 1979) and an atheoretical combination of cognitive and behavioral therapies. Thus, in this chapter, we consider all forms of CBT and cognitive therapy in reviewing the efficacy of and indications for CBT.

Applications of Cognitive-Behavioral Therapy

CBT is a general model that can be applied to a wide variety of specific problems (see Chapter 7, "Techniques of Cognitive-Behavioral Therapy," for a description of the CBT techniques for specific problems). The efficacy of CBT has been studied with regard to a broad range of psychiatric disorders and other problems, including mood disorders, anxiety disorders, psychotic disorders, eating disorders, personality disorders, somatoform disorders (e.g., irritable bowel syndrome), alcohol abuse, sleep disorders, fibromyalgia, chronic fatigue syndrome, hypochondria, sexual dysfunction, couples' problems, anger, stress, and suicide. CBT has also been studied as an adjunctive treatment for problems related to medical conditions such as incontinence in women, arthritis (both to reduce pain and to improve function), chronic pain, procedural distress, diabetes, sickle cell disease, dementia, obesity, chronic prostatitis subsequent to sexually transmitted diseases, health anxiety in cancer patients, and children's behavior and social competence following brain injury. Finally, CBT has been studied both in direct comparison to, and as a combination treatment with, medications for a number of disorders.

Given the vast assortment of disorders and problems to which CBT has been applied, the scope of this chapter does not allow for a comprehensive review. In the chapter we focus only on those psychiatric disorders that have received the most attention in the literature. CBT has been adapted for and used with geriatric and pediatric/adolescent populations. For most disorders, however, the majority of the literature refers to adult populations, and they are therefore the focus of this chapter.

Efficacy Versus Effectiveness

The clinical efficacy of a given treatment can be determined through various methods (Chambless and Ollendick 2001; Institut National de la Santé et de la Recherche Médicale 2004), but the "gold standard" in psychotherapy research has become the randomized controlled trial (RCT). RCTs can evaluate whether the therapeutic effects of a particular intervention are at least as good as other available interventions and better than no intervention at all. The advantage to conducting efficacy research is that it is well controlled and the results are relatively comparable across studies. Efficacy differs from effectiveness: the former refers to the outcomes of a treatment within an experimental setting; the latter refers to the outcomes of a treatment in the real world of actual clinical practice (Kazdin 2003).

There are three types of CBT efficacy studies for psychiatric disorders:

1. Most of the literature gauges the efficacy of an active CBT treatment versus a no-treatment alternative or standard care. These trials have established that CBT has a clinical effect and are referred to as demonstrating *absolute efficacy*.
2. *Relative efficacy* studies contrast the outcomes of active psychotherapies. Much debate exists in the literature as to whether there are meaningful

differences in efficacy among psychotherapies, however. Proponents of the *dodo bird hypothesis* argue that the differences among treatments are small to none, because the efficacy of psychotherapy is largely attributable to the pervasive common factors that are shared by all psychotherapies, rather than to a specific technique (e.g., Hansen 2005). Many other authors argue that the dodo bird hypothesis is false or at least premature (e.g., Beutler 2002), having found that although these common factors are essential, specific interventions account for the greater efficacy of empirically validated treatments for specific disorders.

3. A specific type of relative efficacy can involve comparisons between CBT and pharmacotherapy (see Chapter 9, "Combining Cognitive-Behavioral Therapy With Medication," for a description of studies examining the combined efficacy of CBT and pharmacotherapy). In this chapter, the question of relative efficacy compared with pharmacotherapy is addressed for each disorder for which data are available.

Because of the wealth of efficacy literature for CBT, several studies have employed meta-analysis in an attempt to aggregate the available data (Kazdin 2003). Although meta-analysis tends to minimize the variable methodological details across studies, its strong advantage is that it takes into account the sample size and the magnitude of the effect size for the interventions compared in each study (Rosenthal 1998). The following précis relies predominantly on the results of meta-analyses. Findings from recent single RCTs are also reported where appropriate. When findings from RCTs are lacking, controlled outcome studies are described.

Efficacy of Individual Cognitive-Behavioral Therapy

Mood Disorders

Unipolar Depression

Absolute efficacy.   CBT for adult unipolar depression has been extensively studied in the literature. The first meta-analysis on cognitive therapy for adult depression revealed strong evidence for the superiority of cognitive therapy relative to no treatment or a waiting-list control condition (Dobson 1989). A more recent meta-analysis corroborated this finding, indicating that outcomes were superior in patients treated with cognitive therapy compared with waiting-list or placebo control groups (Gloaguen et al. 1998). A recent RCT that compared standard cognitive therapy, computer-assisted cognitive therapy, and a waiting-list control condition found that both forms of cognitive therapy were superior to the waiting-list condition and equivalent to each other (Wright et al. 2005). Treatment gains with both the standard and the computer-assisted cognitive therapies were maintained at 3 and 6 months posttreatment.

Relative efficacy. Dobson (1989) and Gloaguen et al. (1998) also compared cognitive therapy with pharmacotherapy, behavioral therapy, and a mixed group of "other" psychotherapies. Dobson (1989) found that cognitive therapy was significantly superior in all comparisons (and that the advantages were unrelated to length of therapy or gender ratio), whereas Gloaguen et al. (1998) found that cognitive therapy was significantly superior to pharmacotherapy and other psychotherapies but was not significantly better than behavior therapy. In addition, at 1-year follow-up Gloaguen et al. (1998) found that approximately twice as many individuals who had received pharmacotherapy had relapsed into depression compared with those who had received cognitive therapy (see Hollon et al. 2006 for a similar conclusion).

It is commonly found that psychotherapy and pharmacotherapy result in comparable outcomes for the acute treatment of mild and moderately depressed patients (Hansen 2005). DeRubeis et al. (2005) compared the efficacy of pharmacotherapy with that of cognitive therapy or a placebo in patients with moderate to severe depression. They found that 24 sessions of cognitive therapy, when it was delivered by experienced therapists, was as efficacious as pharmacotherapy. Hollon et al. (2005) conducted a follow-up to this study to examine long-term effects. Participants from the original study who had responded to the medications were followed while either maintaining the same dosage of medication or receiving a placebo. Those who had responded to cognitive therapy were followed after discontinuing treatment, although they were allowed up to three booster sessions. Patients who had received cognitive therapy were significantly less likely to relapse over a period of 12 months than those who discontinued medication, and had relapse rates comparable to those in patients who continued medication (see Dimidjian et al. 2006 for comparable results).

Bipolar Disorder

Few studies have investigated the efficacy of psychotherapy for bipolar disorder (Colom and Vieta 2004). Although absolute efficacy of CBT has not yet been demonstrated for treating this disorder, there is evidence for the efficacy of CBT in combination with pharmacotherapy (Colom and Vieta 2004; Lam et al. 2003; Scott et al. 2001). Scott et al. (2001) found that individuals who had received 6 months of CBT, combined with treatment as usual (TAU) (including medication, outpatient services, and other services), demonstrated greater improvement in their symptoms at 6-month follow-up compared with waiting-list control subjects (who also received TAU), and a reduction in relapse rates at 12-month follow-up. Lam et al. (2003) investigated the potential of CBT to reduce relapse rates in patients with bipolar disorder. The treatment group received, on average, 14 sessions of CBT over the first 6 months followed by 2 booster sessions in the next 6 months. When treated with CBT in conjunction with mood stabilizers and regular psychiatric follow-up, subjects at risk for relapse had better social functioning, fewer symptoms, and fewer relapses over a 12-month period, compared with those who received TAU (mood stabilizers and psychiatric follow-up). In a subsequent study with the same patient group, Lam et al. (2005) found that CBT led to less robust results as therapy became more distant over the course of an additional 18 months. However, they did not investigate the possible effects of maintenance therapy, such as booster sessions, beyond the first 12 months. In addition, they found improvements on other outcome measures, including the number of days in bipolar episodes, mood ratings, social functioning, coping with bipolar prodromal signs, and dysfunctional goal-attainment cognitions.

Summary: Mood Disorders

There is ample and strong evidence that CBT is an efficacious treatment for unipolar depression. CBT has demonstrated some superiority over other psychotherapies in the treatment of unipolar depression. CBT is as efficacious as pharmacotherapy in the acute treatment of unipolar depression but has an enduring effect beyond the end of treatment, stronger than that observed for pharmacotherapy. Though little research has been done on the absolute or relative efficacy of CBT for bipolar disorder, recent research suggests that in conjunction with pharmacotherapy, CBT can reduce relapse rates for bipolar disorder in the short term, and improve symptoms and social functioning acutely and in the longer term.

Anxiety Disorders

CBT has been evaluated as a treatment for a broad range of anxiety disorders and typically includes psychoeducation, cognitive restructuring, and exposure to the anxiety-provoking stimulus, situation, memory, or physiological experience (Barlow 2004).

Panic Disorder With or Without Agoraphobia

Absolute efficacy. Several meta-analytic reviews of the treatment outcome literature for panic disorder with or without agoraphobia have been conducted in the past decade, although some meta-analyses have exclusively examined behavioral treatments. Oei et al. (1999) conducted both a qualitative and a quantitative review of the literature. They found that CBT was efficacious at reducing self-reported agoraphobic symptoms and that its clinical efficacy was substantially demonstrated with community norms. They did not draw any definitive conclusions about the long-term efficacy of CBT, although they noted that different forms of CBT may vary in the minimum periods of time necessary for change. Results of their qualitative review demonstrated that CBT is associated with significant and positive changes on several measures (e.g., panic, fear, avoidance, anxiety, and depression) immediately posttreatment and at follow-up periods of up to 16 months. Gould et al. (1995) conducted a standard meta-analysis comparing pharmacotherapy, CBT, their combination, and a control (no treatment, waiting list, a placebo pill, or psychological placebo), for panic disorder with or without agoraphobia. All three types of active treatment were superior, in acute treatment, to control conditions. Long-term treatment effects were roughly equal to acute treatment effects, although assessment times were not reported.

Relative efficacy. CBT, including cognitive restructuring and exposure elements, is the standard approach in treating panic disorder (Butler et al. 2006). Gould et al. (1995) found this combination to be the most efficacious of the treatments they investigated. They also found that pharmacotherapy combined with CBT was not as efficacious as CBT alone. They noted, however, that selective serotonin reuptake inhibitors (SSRIs) are more efficacious at treating panic disorder than benzodiazepines and other commonly used antidepressants. Thus, the efficacy of the combination of SSRIs and CBT needs to be studied. Gould et al. (1995) also found that patients treated with pharmacotherapy alone experienced the greatest reduction of treatment effects over time. In contrast, the combination of CBT plus pharmacotherapy as well as CBT alone typically resulted in maintenance of treatment gains. Two more recent meta-analyses (van Balkom et al. 1997 and, in a later analysis of the same studies, Bakker et al. 1998) demonstrated that although CBT was superior to pill placebo, attention placebo, and waiting list, the most efficacious acute treatment method was the combination of antidepressants and in vivo exposure. The psychotherapeutic and pharmacotherapeutic treatment gains for panic disorder patients with and without agoraphobia, over an average follow-up of 62 weeks, tended to be stable.

Specific Phobias

There is little research on the efficacy of CBT for specific phobias. A recent RCT found that cognitive restructuring (cognitive therapy) and in vivo exposure (behavior therapy) were equally efficacious at improving self-reported fear of snakes and decreasing behavioral avoidance in nondiagnosed university students (Hunt et al. 2006). However, cognitive restructuring outperformed exposure for those individuals who were highly fearful. Both treatments were significantly superior to the minimal exposure: relaxation control. Another study found that single-session behavior therapy and CBT were similarly efficacious at reducing symptoms in students with small animal phobias (Koch et al. 2004). In both studies, participants found the active treatment with cognitive components less aversive and/or less intrusive than the treatment based solely on exposure.

Social Phobia

Absolute efficacy. Treatments for social phobia frequently include exposure, social skills training, cognitive restructuring, or a combination of these strategies (Deacon and Abramowitz 2004). Gould et al. (1997a) conducted a meta-analytic review of the efficacy of CBT and pharmacotherapy for social phobia. They examined how treatment improved social anxiety or avoidance, cognition, and depression. All forms of both group and individual CBT were superior to no treatment, a waiting-list condition, or psychological placebo. Analyses based on the within-group changes from posttreatment to follow-up indicated that modest improvements were still present 3 months after treatment only in the CBT group. These findings replicated those of Feske and Chambless (1995), whose meta-analytic review of treatment outcome studies (group and individual treatment) suggested that exposure alone and exposure plus cognitive restructuring are superior to one of several control conditions, usually a waiting-list condition.

Relative efficacy. Exposure therapies alone and in combination with cognitive restructuring have been found to be equally efficacious in the treatment of social phobia (Feske and Chambless 1995; Gould et al. 1997a). In addition, Gould et al. (1997a) found that exposure therapies alone and in combination with cognitive restructuring were more efficacious than cognitive restructuring alone. Fedoroff and Taylor (2001), whose meta-analytic review was more recent than that of Feske and Chambless, concluded that although exposure therapy demonstrated the largest treatment effects at posttreatment compared with cognitive therapy alone or exposure plus cognitive therapy, these effects were not significantly different from zero. It is likely that small sample sizes masked the effects of exposure alone in this study (Deacon and Abramowitz 2004). Furthermore, Gould et al. (1997a) found that CBT alone, pharmacotherapy alone, and CBT and pharmacotherapy in combination were equally efficacious. Few studies have compared CBT with other psychotherapies in the treatment of social phobia. In an exception, Cottraux et al. (2000) found that CBT was superior to supportive therapy. Treatment effects for CBT were sustained at 36- and 60-week follow-ups, but the long-term effects of supportive therapy were not assessed.

Obsessive-Compulsive Disorder

Absolute efficacy.   The efficacy of CBT for obsessive-compulsive disorder (OCD) has been extensively studied in both adult and pediatric populations. Exposure and response prevention (ERP) is the most widely studied treatment for OCD (Abramowitz 1997). Although ERP is typically categorized as a behavioral procedure, it involves cognitive elements and overlapping procedures (Allen 2006). It is possible that cognitive therapy and ERP utilize similar mechanisms of change (Abramowitz 1997).

In an early meta-analysis, van Balkom et al. (1994) found that both cognitive therapy and CBT were more efficacious than placebo therapy on self- and assessor-rated obsessive-compulsive symptoms, and that treatment effects persisted at 6 and 12 months. Abramowitz (1997) examined the relative efficacies of ERP and cognitive therapy and the absolute efficacy of ERP in a more recent meta-analysis of RCTs. Compared with a control treatment (progressive muscle relaxation), ERP was considerably more efficacious at reducing obsessive-compulsive symptoms posttreatment. In addition, increased time spent in therapist-guided exposure improved the efficacy of the treatment.

Relative efficacy.   Abramowitz (1997) found small and nonsignificant differences in treatment outcomes between cognitive therapy and ERP. Whittal et al. (2005) also failed to find significant differences between ERP and CBT in their randomized trial. Compared with ERP, CBT resulted in a nonsignificantly higher percentage of participants who had recovered from OCD posttreatment and at 3-month follow-up. Cottraux et al. (2001), in an RCT comparing cognitive therapy and intensive ERP, found that while both groups improved significantly, and the rate of response was similar in the two groups, cognitive therapy demonstrated a greater effect at reducing depressive symptoms in posttreatment testing. Improvements were retained at 1-year follow-up, but the intent-to-treat analysis (using the last-analysis-carried-forward approach) found no between-group differences in the prevalence of obsessions, rituals, or depression.

Kobak et al. (1998) performed a meta-analysis comparing CBT, pharmacotherapy (SSRIs), and their combination in the treatment of OCD. Although CBT was reported to be superior to the use of SSRIs, this difference disappeared when the outcomes were controlled by the year of publication of the studies and the CBT methods that were used. More recently, Foa et al. (2005) categorized ERP as a form of CBT in their RCT comparing CBT, pharmacotherapy, and the combination of CBT plus pharmacotherapy. They found that intensive CBT alone and the combination of CBT plus clomipramine had comparable short-term effects, and that both were more efficacious than clomipramine alone.

Posttraumatic Stress Disorder

Absolute efficacy. Posttraumatic stress disorder (PTSD) is most commonly treated with behavioral and cognitive techniques (Deacon and Abramowitz 2004). The National Institute for Health and Clinical Excellence (NICE; formerly National Institute for Clinical Excellence) in the United Kingdom has developed a set of guidelines for the treatment and management of PTSD (National Institute for Clinical Excellence 2005). As part of the guideline development process, they conducted a meticulous meta-analytic review of psychological and pharmacological treatments for PTSD. For the purposes of their review, they divided the psychotherapies into four categories: 1) trauma-focused CBT (e.g., exposure, biofeedback-assisted desensitization treatment, and cognitive reprocessing therapy); 2) eye movement desensitization and reprocessing, stress management, and relaxation (stress inoculation training and progressive muscle relaxation); 3) other therapies (supportive therapy/nondirective counseling, psychodynamic therapies, and hypnotherapy); and 4) group CBT. All studies included in the meta-analysis were RCTs.

Trauma-focused CBT demonstrated a short-term treatment advantage over the waiting-list control condition, on all measures, for reducing PTSD symptoms. Individuals in the trauma-focused CBT groups included a mixed assortment of trauma survivors, and the effectiveness with this group strongly suggests that CBT is a broadly applicable treatment for PTSD. Unfortunately, long-term outcomes were not reported for this study. Blanchard and colleagues (2003, 2004) compared an active form of supportive therapy, encompassing psychodynamic principles, with CBT and a waiting-list control group in patients with PTSD following motor vehicle accidents. At 3-month follow-up, both CBT and supportive therapy were found to be superior to the waiting-list condition. In another RCT, Ehlers et al. (2004) found that cognitive therapy was superior to being on a waiting list at 3 months posttreatment on measures of PTSD symptoms, disability, and associated symptoms of anxiety and depression. These treatment gains were maintained at 6-month follow-up.

Relative efficacy. The NICE study found that neither eye movement desensitization and reprocessing nor trauma-focused CBT demonstrated an advantage over the other (National Institute for Clinical Excellence 2005). In addition, no differences were found among the various versions of trauma-focused CBT; all appeared to be equally efficacious. However, there was some evidence that trauma-focused CBT was superior to the supportive/nondirective therapies, indicating that the efficacy of trauma-focused CBT is not due to nonspecific factors. In their controlled comparison, Marks et al. (1998) found that cognitive therapy and behavior therapy showed equivalent outcomes, but no additive effects when combined. In addition, both treatments were superior to relaxation on testing posttreatment and at 6 months posttreatment.

A follow-up to another RCT reported favorable outcomes for cognitive therapy compared with imaginal exposure after 5 years (Tarrier and Sommerfeld 2004). Blanchard and colleagues (2003, 2004) found that CBT was more efficacious than supportive therapy at 3-month follow-up; at 2-year follow-up, CBT remained statistically superior to supportive therapy, although the differences were less significant, in part because fewer patients who had completed 1 year of the study were evaluated. The improvement from posttest to follow-up was modest. Finally, in a 4-year follow-up of a comparison between CBT and supportive counseling (education, support, and problem solving) in patients with acute stress disorder, CBT was found to provide better outcomes (Bryant et al. 2003). No large, well-designed study has directly compared the relative and combined efficacy of pharmacotherapy and (trauma-focused) CBT (National Institute for Clinical Excellence 2005).

Generalized Anxiety Disorder

Absolute efficacy.   Because of the obscure nature of external triggers for the anxiety associated with generalized anxiety disorder (GAD), this disorder has not been amenable to the same exposure methods that have been efficacious with the other anxiety disorders (Deacon and Abramowitz 2004). Although the number of studies is small, the meta-analytic literature supports the efficacy of CBT for GAD. Gould et al. (1997b) compared CBT with no-treatment, waiting-list, placebo pill, or psychological placebo control groups. Short-term (maximum, 16-week) treatment outcomes indicated that CBT is highly efficacious at reducing symptoms of anxiety and depression. No significant differences were found between group and individual therapy formats, and longer duration of treatment was not associated with better outcomes. Gould et al. (1997b) also found some limited evidence for the long-term (minimum, 6-month) maintenance of treatment gains, in terms of reduced anxiety symptoms.

Relative efficacy.   Gould et al. (1997b) found that CBT provided superior outcomes compared with relaxation training with biofeedback. Their meta-analysis also compared CBT with pharmacotherapy and found no differences between the two on measures of change in anxiety severity, but CBT showed advantages over pharmacotherapy in improving depressive symptoms. Earlier, in a controlled study, Borkovec and Costello (1993) compared the efficacy of nondirective therapy, applied relaxation, and CBT for the treatment of GAD. Acute treatment findings indicated that applied relaxation and CBT were generally equally efficacious, and superior to nondirective therapy. Evidence indicated stronger long-term effects for CBT than for nondirective therapy and applied relaxation. More recently, Durham et al. (2003) examined the long-term efficacy of CBT in a follow-up of two clinical RCTs. Individuals who had received CBT demonstrated less severe symptoms at follow-up (8–14 years) than individuals who received pharmacotherapy, placebo, or analytic psychotherapy.

Summary: Anxiety Disorders

Recent meta-analyses have demonstrated strong acute treatment effects for combined cognitive-behavioral procedures, and some evidence indicates that CBT has long-term efficacy in treating anxiety disorders. CBT is also frequently found to be at least as efficacious as behavioral interventions, including exposure-based procedures. In addition, some studies have found that therapies incorporating a combination of behavioral and cognitive components are perceived as less aversive to participants (e.g., for the treatment of specific phobias) and drop-out rates are lower (e.g., for the treatment of OCD) than for behavioral treatments alone. Despite these findings, there remains some debate in the literature as to whether combining cognitive and behavioral techniques provides an advantage over behavior therapy alone. Part of the problem is that behavioral therapies, and ERP in particular, are sometimes classified as behavioral and sometimes as cognitive-behavioral, thus obfuscating comparisons between the two. Few studies have compared CBT with other forms of therapy, aside from behavior therapy, and few studies have examined the relative efficacy of cognitive therapy alone. It is difficult to draw a firm conclusion about the efficacy of CBT relative to pharmacotherapy, because many studies did not make this direct comparison. Evidence indicates that pharmacotherapy and CBT are equally efficacious for short-term treatment of some anxiety disorders (e.g., social phobia or GAD) but that CBT reduces the risk of relapse relative to pharmacotherapy alone.

Other Disorders

Schizophrenia

CBT has only been studied as an adjunctive treatment to pharmacotherapy for schizophrenia. Gould et al. (2001) conducted a meta-analysis of the effects of cognitive therapy (combined with pharmacotherapy) on decreasing psychotic symptoms (hallucinations and delusions) and modifying core dysfunctional beliefs in patients with schizophrenia, schizoaffective disorder, or delusional disorder. They found large acute treatment effects for cognitive therapy across seven controlled studies, and these effects were maintained, and even increased in some cases, over time. When compared with a control condition (waiting list, TAU, or psychological placebo), cognitive therapy was superior in five of the seven studies, but no significant differences between cognitive therapy and control conditions were seen in two of these studies.

Rector and Beck (2001) performed a meta-analysis of seven RCTs and found that CBT plus routine care (pharmacotherapy and active case management) significantly improved positive and negative symptoms of schizophrenia, both at the time of acute care and at follow-up. They also found that CBT plus routine care outperformed supportive therapy plus routine care, while the latter combination improved outcomes compared with routine care alone. These results held long-term.

More recently, Temple and Ho (2005) conducted a case-controlled outcome study comparing CBT with routine care for patients with medication-resistant psychotic symptoms. (In addition to medication management, routine care consisted of a variety of services, such as case management and community-based psychotherapy, but not CBT.) CBT resulted in improved adaptive functioning and greater reductions in the severity of psychotic symptoms, psychotic symptoms overall, and the severity of delusions.

Bulimia Nervosa

Although very few controlled studies have examined the use of CBT to treat anorexia nervosa (Butler et al. 2006), substantial literature exists on the efficacy of CBT for the treatment of bulimia nervosa (Leichsenring et al. 2006). Whittal et al. (1999) compared nine double-blind, placebo-controlled medication trials with 26 randomized psychosocial studies and found that CBT was more efficacious in the short term than medication on all measures of treatment outcomes (binge and purge frequency, depression, and eating attitudes). In addition, they found evidence suggesting that a combination of CBT plus medication is better than CBT alone for reducing binge frequency, but not purge frequency. They also reported the results of one study that found that, although almost half of the patients still had a diagnosable eating disorder at extended follow-up (average, 5.8 years), the majority remained in remission from posttreatment to follow-up. An earlier meta-analysis by Lewandowski et al. (1997) provided preliminary support for the above findings.

Personality Disorders

The efficacy of CBT for personality disorders has not been widely studied; of these disorders, borderline personality disorder (BPD) has likely received the most attention. Dialectical behavioral therapy (DBT), a particular form of CBT geared specifically toward the treatment of BPD, has been shown to be efficacious for many symptoms of the disorder (Linehan 1993). Bohus et al. (2004) found that a sample of female inpatients who underwent 3 months of DBT demonstrated significant reductions in the frequency of self-mutilation, and significant improvements in dissociation, depression, anxiety, interpersonal functioning, social adjustment, and global psychopathology at 1 month postdischarge. They also found that those inpatients who received DBT had greater clinical improvement on all but two outcome measures, compared with a waiting-list control group. Long-term effects, however, were not assessed. Linehan et al. (2006) have presented results of a controlled comparison between CBT and community treatment of female BPD patients. The treatments lasted 12 months and the follow-up period was 12 months. DBT was found to be superior to community treatment in the intent-to-treat analysis because it led to greater reductions in suicidal behavior, suicidal ideation, emergency visits, hospitalization, self-injuries, and medical risk, and there were fewer dropouts among DBT recipients.

Davidson et al. (2006) compared CBT+TAU versus TAU alone. They did not find significant differences in outcomes between the two groups at 12 or 24 months in terms of scores assessing depression, trait anxiety, other psychiatric symptoms, interpersonal functioning, or quality of life. In addition, although all patients demonstrated gradual and sustained improvement, levels of distress and dysfunction remained relatively high over the course of the 2-year study. However, at 12 months the CBT+TAU group showed greater improvement than the treatment-as-usual group in symptom distress, and at 24 months showed greater improvement in dysfunctional core beliefs and state anxiety. The mean number of suicidal acts over the course of the study was also significantly reduced in the CBT+TAU group. Although the findings of Davidson et al. (2006) were mixed, a smaller, uncontrolled trial (Brown et al. 2004) found that cognitive therapy for BPD was associated with significant and clinically important improvements on measures of suicidal ideation, hopelessness, and depression, and in the number of borderline symptoms and dysfunctional beliefs, at the end of treatment and at 6-month follow-up.

Giesen-Bloo et al. (2006) recently compared the efficacy of Young's schema-focused therapy (SFT; Young et al. 2003) with the psychodynamically based transference-focused psychotherapy (TFP) in patients with BPD. They conducted a randomized study with a two-group design in four general community mental health centers in the Netherlands over a 3-year period. Results revealed that significantly more SFT patients recovered or showed reliable clinical improvements on the Borderline Personality Disorder Severity Index, on levels of general psychopathological dysfunction, and on quality-of-life measures. In addition, there was a higher drop-out rate with TFP than with SFT.

Svartberg et al. (2004) randomly assigned patients with a diagnosis of one or more Cluster C personality disorders to either short-term dynamic psychotherapy or cognitive therapy. Overall, both psychotherapies were associated with significant patient improvements on all measures (assessing symptom distress, interpersonal problems, and core personality pathology) during treatment, and these improvements were maintained after treatment. The measures were administered at baseline, midtherapy, termination, 6-month follow-up, 12-month follow-up, and 24-month follow-up. No significant differences were seen between groups on any of the measures, during any of the time periods. However, significant changes were seen in symptom distress posttreatment for those patients who received dynamic psychotherapy, but not for those who received cognitive therapy.

Conclusion

The empirical literature on CBT has proliferated in recent decades, and new developments have led to the use of CBT in a wide variety of contexts. Broadly speaking, CBT is an efficacious treatment across a range of psychiatric disorders. Findings differ within and between disorders regarding the relative efficacy of CBT compared with other psychotherapies and pharmacotherapy. Although there is still a paucity of research on the efficacy of CBT for patients with bipolar disorder, preliminary evidence indicates that cognitive therapy, in conjunction with pharmacotherapy, can reduce relapse rates in the short term and improve symptoms and social functioning both acutely and in the longer term. The evidence for the efficacy of CBT in the treatment of unipolar depression is far greater, demonstrating that CBT can be highly efficacious. Notably, although pharmacotherapy and CBT are equally efficacious for acute treatment of depression, CBT treatment effects are maintained at follow-up. In contrast, the effects of pharmacotherapy attenuate following medication discontinuation. Also, CBT often reduces comorbid depressive symptoms across a variety of disorders (e.g., GAD), even if treatment did not target comorbid symptoms associated with the disorder.

The literature indicates that CBT is highly superior in efficacy to control conditions in the treatment of anxiety disorders and is roughly comparable to behavior therapy. However, a particular source of confusion in the literature is that interventions involving the same procedures are sometimes referred to as behavioral and sometimes as cognitive-behavioral (Deacon and Abramowitz 2004). It is difficult to make conclusive statements about the relative efficacy of CBT compared with pharmacotherapy in the treatment of anxiety disorders and about long-term outcomes in general. Further research in these domains is needed.

CBT for the treatment of schizophrenia has recently generated increased interest as an adjunct to pharmacotherapy and case management. Meta-analyses have focused primarily on the efficacy of cognitive therapy—cognitive restructuring in particular—in decreasing hallucinations and delusions. CBT has demonstrated superiority over other psychotherapies such as supportive therapy and has also been shown to have lasting effects.

The bulimia literature suggests that CBT is more efficacious than medication, and a combination of CBT and medication may be more effective than CBT alone. Follow-up analyses indicate that although CBT may not result in lifetime recovery, it may promote remission of bulimia.

Although CBT has not been investigated for treating all of the personality disorders, the cluster C personality disorders have received some attention. The evidence indicates that some forms of CBT can reduce symptoms and increase quality of life for individuals with BPD. The relative efficacy of cognitive therapy and short-term dynamic psychotherapy for the cluster C personality disorders requires further study.

In addition to being highly efficacious in the treatment of a wide assortment of psychiatric disorders, CBT has numerous other strengths. For example, CBT has lower drop-out rates than pharmacotherapy in the treatment of panic disorder (Gould et al. 1995) and bulimia nervosa (Whittal et al. 1999) and lower drop-out rates than ERP in the treatment of OCD (Abramowitz et al. 2005). CBT is also perceived as less aversive or intrusive by individuals being treated for specific phobias, compared with exposure-based interventions. Thus, research indicates that CBT is both a highly efficacious and an acceptable treatment choice. Although the research base for CBT is quite extensive, there are nonetheless limitations and knowledge gaps that need to be addressed. The following section outlines issues associated with research on the efficacy of CBT and provides suggestions for future directions and applications.

Limitations, Knowledge Gaps, and Future Directions

Well-conducted RCTs employ an elegant research design that allows the researcher to make reasonable conclusions about the treatment(s) under investigation. Nonetheless, this form of research has some limitations. For example, the generalizability of RCT results to routine clinical practice is sometimes limited by the level of control exerted over the experimental situation (Leichsenring et al. 2006). The therapists involved in RCTs typically have substantial skill in delivering the treatment(s), and patients may or may not be representative of the general population of people with the disorder under study because of exclusion criteria. Another concern about efficacy research is researcher allegiance, or the tendency of the authors of a comparative treatment study to prefer one treatment over another, introducing bias in favor of the preferred treatment (Butler et al. 2006). Difficulties in conducting long-term outcome assessments include ethical restrictions on maintaining participants in control conditions for extended periods of time.

In this chapter we relied predominantly on meta-analyses to reach broad conclusions about the efficacy of CBT across psychiatric disorders. Meta-analysis has itself been critiqued as a method, for the following reasons:

- The outcome measures employed across different studies often differ. The choice of outcome measures (e.g., self-reporting vs. clinician ratings) can bias the relative strength of a treatment effect. Thus, the total effect size for a particular treatment calculated by meta-analysis will be biased by the inclusion of various dependent measures (Clum et al. 1993), as cited in Gould et al. 1997a, 1997b).
- The number of treatment sessions and length per session can vary across studies, systematically bolstering or weakening effect sizes depending on the studies included in the analysis.
- Meta-analysis tends to collapse treatment effects across divergent patient samples, potentially reducing the attention to interactions between various treatments and patient characteristics.
- The computational formulae and procedures for meta-analysis have evolved over time, and such issues as the use of unweighted or weighted effect size estimates, and within-study or community comparisons for the computation of effect size, can affect the conclusions of different meta-analyses within a given treatment area.

In addition to the limitations to efficacy research in general, and to meta-analysis as a statistical tool, the extant research on the efficacy of CBT also has specific limitations. In particular, there is still very little literature on the comparison of other psychotherapies with CBT, especially for the anxiety disorders. The lack of long-term evidence for the majority of psychiatric disorders constitutes another knowledge gap in the literature on the efficacy of CBT. Many studies do not assess long-term outcomes at all, some provide only relatively short-term outcomes, and others do not explicitly report the time points at which follow-ups were conducted. Most studies that incorporate waiting-list controls provide treatment to control participants after a certain period of time, thereby rendering the comparative assessment of long-term outcomes between treatment groups and controls impossible. Some studies have resolved this issue by conducting within-group analyses, thus providing the long-term outcome for the treatment group without comparison to a control group (e.g., Gould et al. 1995, 1997a, 1997b). However, findings calculated by this method are not as informative as the alternative. Further research comparing the long-term efficacy of different active treatments is indicated.

Parker et al. (2003) raised some concerns about the Dobson (1989) and Gloaguen et al. (1998) meta-analyses, asserting that amalgamating placebo controls and wait-listed participants into a composite control condition provides confounding results. Control subjects receiving placebo may have a hopeful reaction to "treatment" because they are under the assumption that they are being treated, whereas waiting-list control subjects may be discouraged because they are not yet undergoing any treatment. Parker et al. recommended that future research compare active treatments to each of these control conditions separately. In the same vein, Gould and colleagues (1995, 1997a, 1997b, 2001) have argued that CBT is favored in comparisons with pharmacotherapy, because CBT is frequently compared with a waiting-list control condition, whereas drug trials typically involve placebo pill controls. In this regard, nondirective therapy has been recommended as a psychological placebo, because it has greater credibility than waiting-list or no-treatment control conditions. In addition, placebo pills and nondirective therapy are similar to each other in terms of resulting positive treatment effects.

The issue of treatment labeling stands out as a significant concern in the literature. Behavioral therapies are sometimes classified as behavioral and sometimes as cognitive-behavioral, even when they use highly similar treatment elements, and comparisons between studies are therefore confounded. Moreover, the comparison between cognitive therapy and other kinds of psychotherapy may be blurred in some trials. As one notable example, analysis of the videotaped therapy sessions of the National Institute of Mental Health collaborative project comparing interpersonal therapy, cognitive therapy, placebo, and pharmacotherapy demonstrated that therapists in the interpersonal therapy group adhered more to the cognitive therapy protocol than to the interpersonal therapy protocol (Ablon and Jones 2002). This example underscores the importance of adherence to treatment manuals in research trials, and assessment of therapist fidelity to treatment conditions, to ensure a fair test of the treatments under investigation (McGlinchey and Dobson 2003).

Several other knowledge gaps exist. For example, although the depression literature has examined the efficacy of CBT in geriatric populations, and the PTSD literature has looked at minority populations, there is generally insufficient empirical research with diverse populations. More research is needed to assess the efficacy of CBT in preventing relapses across disorders. Comorbidities are frequent among psychiatric disorders but may be either controlled for in RCTs through exclusionary criteria or simply not addressed. The exclusionary approach to comorbid diagnoses makes RCT results less generalizable, increasing the discrepancy between efficacy and effectiveness research findings. Finally, aside from research on ERP, research on the efficacy of specific forms of CBT for specific disorders is still largely lacking. Such efficacy research could provide better insight into the mechanisms of change that are most beneficial for each disorder.

In summary, a considerable and growing body of evidence generally supports the continued use of CBT as a treatment for a wide variety of disorders. Additional research is needed comparing the efficacy of CBT with and without the use of pharmacotherapy. Also, the relative efficacy of CBT versus other bona fide psychological treatments has not been extensively examined. The long-term benefits of CBT have been studied considerably less than its short-term and acute treatment effects. Finally, firm conclusions about the generalizability of CBT to a broad range of patient groups with a large set of patient characteristics must await further study. The design of randomized trials, in which treatment interactions can be studied by patient type or characteristics, will help to advance the field in the direction of treatment guidelines, a necessary step in maximizing the successful treatment of the broad range of mental health disorders.

Key Points

- Cognitive-behavioral therapy (CBT) is prefaced on the theory that cognition mediates the individual's behavioral and emotional responses to his or her environment and thus influences individuals' adjustment or maladjustment to their environment.

- CBT has been extensively studied and found to be efficacious for a wide range of psychiatric disorders and problems—mood, anxiety, psychotic, eating, personality, somatoform, and sleep disorders; alcohol abuse, fibromyalgia, chronic fatigue syndrome, hypochondria, sexual dysfunctions, couples' problems, anger, stress, and suicide—and as an adjunctive treatment for problems related to some medical conditions (e.g., incontinence, arthritis, chronic pain, procedural distress, diabetes, sickle cell disease, dementia, obesity, chronic prostatitis, cancer, pediatric brain injury).

- CBT has been demonstrated to be highly efficacious for mild, moderate, and severe depression. Although pharmacotherapy and CBT are equally efficacious as acute treatment, CBT maintains treatment effects at follow-up; the effects of pharmacotherapy attenuate following medication discontinuation.

- Preliminary evidence for bipolar disorder indicates that as an adjunctive treatment with pharmacotherapy, CBT can reduce relapse rates in the short term and improve symptoms acutely and in the longer term.

- CBT is an efficacious treatment for anxiety disorders; more research is needed comparing its efficacy with that of pharmacotherapy.

- As an adjunct to pharmacotherapy for the treatment of schizophrenia, CBT has been found to be superior to other psychotherapies and has shown lasting effects.

- CBT promotes remission in bulimia nervosa and has demonstrated superiority over medication, though a combination of CBT and medication may be more effective than CBT alone.

- Literature on the efficacy of CBT to treat personality disorders is scarce. However, the available evidence indicates that some forms of CBT can reduce symptoms and increase quality of life for individuals with borderline personality disorder.

- For some disorders, CBT has lower drop-out rates than pharmacotherapy, and for others it is perceived as less aversive or intrusive than some behavioral interventions. Thus, CBT has been found to be both a highly efficacious and an acceptable treatment choice.

References

Ablon J, Jones E: Validity of controlled clinical trials of psychotherapy: findings from the NIMH Treatment of Depression Collaborative Research Program. Am J Psychiatry 159:775–783, 2002

Abramowitz JS: Effectiveness of psychological and pharmacological treatments for obsessive-compulsive disorder: a quantitative review. J Consult Clin Psychol 65:44–52, 1997

Abramowitz JS, Taylor S, McKay D: Potentials and limitations of cognitive treatments for obsessive-compulsive disorder. Cogn Behav Ther 34:140–147, 2005

Allen A: Cognitive-behavior therapy and other psychosocial interventions in the treatment of obsessive-compulsive disorder. Psychiatr Ann 36:474–479, 2006

Bakker A, van Balkom A, Spinhoven P, et al: Follow-up on the treatment of panic disorder with or without agoraphobia: a quantitative review. J Nerv Ment Dis 186:414–419, 1998

Barlow DH: Psychological treatments. Am Psychol 59:869–878, 2004

Beck AT, Rush AJ, Shaw BF, et al: Cognitive Therapy of Depression. New York, Guilford, 1979

Beutler LE: The dodo bird is extinct. Clinical Psychology: Science and Practice 9:30–34, 2002

Blanchard EB, Hickling EJ, Devineni T, et al: A controlled evaluation of cognitive behavioural therapy for posttraumatic stress in motor vehicle accident survivors. Behav Res Ther 41:79–96, 2003

Blanchard EB, Hickling EJ, Malta LS, et al: One- and two-year prospective follow-up of cognitive behaviour therapy or supportive psychotherapy. Behav Res Ther 42:745–759, 2004

Bohus M, Haaf B, Simms T, et al: Effectiveness of inpatient dialectical behavioral therapy for borderline personality disorder: a controlled trial. Behav Res Ther 42:487–499, 2004

Borkovec TD, Costello E: Efficacy of applied relaxation and cognitive-behavioral therapy in the treatment of generalized anxiety disorder. J Consult Clin Psychol 61:611–619, 1993

Brown GK, Newman CF, Charlesworth SE, et al: An open clinical trial of cognitive therapy for borderline personality disorder. J Personal Disord 18:257–271, 2004

Bryant RA, Moulds ML, Nixon RV: Cognitive behaviour therapy of acute stress disorder: a four-year follow-up. Behav Res Ther 41:489–494, 2003

Butler AC, Chapman JE, Forman EM, et al: The empirical status of cognitive-behavioral therapy: a review of meta-analyses. Clin Psychol Rev 26:17–31, 2006

Chambless DL, Ollendick TH: Empirically supported psychological interventions: controversies and evidence. Annu Rev Psychol 52:685–716, 2001

Clum GA, Clum GA, Surls R: A meta-analysis for panic disorder. J Consult Clin Psychol 61:317–326, 1993

Colom F, Vieta E: A perspective on the use of psychoeducation, cognitive-behavioral therapy and interpersonal therapy for bipolar patients. Bipolar Disord 6:480–486, 2004

Cottraux J, Note I, Albuisson E, et al: Cognitive behavior therapy versus supportive therapy in social phobia: a randomized controlled trial. Psychother Psychosom 69:137–146, 2000

Cottraux J, Ivan NI, Yao SN, et al: A randomized controlled trial of cognitive therapy versus intensive behavior therapy in obsessive compulsive disorder. Psychother Psychosom 70:288–297, 2001

Davidson K, Norrie J, Tyrer P, et al: The effectiveness of cognitive behavior therapy for borderline personality disorder: results from the borderline personality disorder study of cognitive therapy (BOSCOT) trial. J Personal Disord 20:450–465, 2006

Deacon BJ, Abramowitz JS: Cognitive and behavioral treatments for anxiety disorders: a review of meta-analytic findings. J Clin Psychol 60:429–441, 2004

DeRubeis RJ, Hollon SD, Amsterdam JD, et al: Cognitive therapy vs medications in the treatment of moderate to severe depression. Arch Gen Psychiatry 62:409–416, 2005

Dimidjian S, Hollon SD, Dobson KS, et al: Randomized trial of behavioral activation, cognitive therapy, and antidepressant medication in the acute treatment of adults with major depression. J Consult Clin Psychol 74:658–670, 2006

Dobson KS: A meta-analysis of the efficacy of cognitive therapy for depression. J Consult Clin Psychol 57:414–419, 1989

Dobson KS (ed): Handbook of Cognitive-Behavioral Therapies, 2nd Edition. New York, Guilford, 2001

Durham RC, Chambers JA, MacDonald RR, et al: Does cognitive-behavioral therapy influence the long-term outcome of generalized anxiety disorder? An 8–14 year follow-up of two clinical trials. Psychol Med 33:499–509, 2003

Ehlers A, Clark DM, Hackmann A, et al: Cognitive therapy for post-traumatic stress disorder: development and evaluation. Behav Res Ther 43:413–431, 2004

Fedoroff IC, Taylor S: Psychological and pharmacological treatments of social phobia: a meta-analysis. J Clin Psychopharmacol 21:311–324, 2001

Feske U, Chambless DL: Cognitive behavioral versus exposure only treatment for social phobia: a meta-analysis. Behav Ther 26:695–720, 1995

Foa EB, Liebowitz MR, Kozak MJ, et al: Randomized, placebo-controlled trial of exposure and ritual prevention, clomipramine, and their combination in the treatment of obsessive-compulsive disorder. Am J Psychiatry 162:151–161, 2005

Giesen-Bloo J, van Dyck R, Spinhoven P, et al: Outpatient psychotherapy for borderline personality disorder: randomized trial of schema-focused therapy vs transference-focused psychotherapy. Arch Gen Psychiatry 63:649–658, 2006

Gloaguen V, Cottraux J, Cucherat M, et al: A meta-analysis of the effects of cognitive therapy in depressed patients. J Affect Disord 49:59–72, 1998

Gould RA, Otto MW, Pollack MH: A meta-analysis of treatment outcome for panic disorder. Clin Psychol Rev 15:819–844, 1995

Gould RA, Buckminster S, Pollack MH, et al: Cognitive-behavioral and pharmacological treatment for social phobia: a meta-analysis. Clinical Psychology: Science and Practice 4:291–306, 1997a

Gould RA, Otto MW, Pollack MH, et al: Cognitive behavioral and pharmacological treatment of generalized anxiety disorder: a preliminary meta-analysis. Behav Ther 28:285–305, 1997b

Gould RA, Mueser KT, Bolton E, et al: Cognitive therapy for psychosis in schizophrenia: an effect size analysis. Schizophr Res 48:335–342, 2001

Hansen B: The dodo manifesto. Australian and New Zealand Journal of Family Therapy 26:210–218, 2005

Hollon SD, DeRubeis RJ, Shelton RC, et al: Prevention of relapse following cognitive therapy vs medications in moderate to severe depression. Arch Gen Psychiatry 62:417–422, 2005

Hollon SD, Stewart MO, Strunk D: Enduring effects for cognitive behavior therapy in the treatment of depression and anxiety. Annu Rev Psychol 57:285–315, 2006

Hunt M, Bylsma L, Brock J, et al: The role of imagery in the maintenance and treatment of snake fear. J Behav Ther Exp Psychiatry 37:283–298, 2006

Institut National de la Santé et de la Recherche Médicale: Psychothérapie: Trois Approches Évaluées, une Expertise Collective de l'INSERM. Paris, France, INSERM, 2004

Kazdin AE: Research Design in Clinical Psychology, 4th Edition. Boston, MA, Allyn & Bacon, 2003

Kobak KA, Greist JH, Jefferson JW, et al: Behavioral versus pharmacological treatments of obsessive compulsive disorder: a meta-analysis. Psychopharmacology (Berl) 136:205–216, 1998

Koch EI, Spates CR, Himle JA: Comparison of behavioral and cognitive-behavioral one-session exposure treatments for small animal phobias. Behav Res Ther 42:1483–1504, 2004

Lam DH, Watkins ER, Hayward P, et al: A randomized controlled study of cognitive therapy for relapse prevention for bipolar affective disorders: outcome of the first year. Arch Gen Psychiatry 60:145–152, 2003

Lam DH, Hayward P, Watkins ER, et al: Relapse prevention in patients with bipolar disorder: cognitive therapy outcome after 2 years. Am J Psychiatry 162:324–329, 2005

Leichsenring F, Hiller W, Weissberg M, et al: Cognitive behavioral therapy and psychodynamic psychotherapy: techniques, efficacy, and indications. Am J Psychother 60:233–259, 2006

Lewandowski LM, Gebing TA, Anthony JL, et al: Meta-analysis of cognitive-behavioral treatment studies for bulimia. Clin Psychol Rev 17:703–718, 1997

Linehan MM: Cognitive-Behavioral Treatment of Borderline Personality Disorder. New York, Guilford, 1993

Linehan MM, Comtois KA, Murray AM, et al: Two-year randomized controlled trial and follow-up of dialectical behavioral therapy versus therapy by experts for suicidal behaviors and borderline personality disorder. Arch Gen Psychiatry 63:757–766, 2006

Marks I, Lovell K, Noshirvani H, et al: Treatment of posttraumatic stress disorder by exposure and/or cognitive restructuring: a controlled study. Arch Gen Psychiatry 55:317–325, 1998

McGlinchey J, Dobson KS: Treatment integrity concerns in cognitive therapy for depression. Journal of Cognitive Psychotherapy: An International Quarterly 17:299–318, 2003

National Institute for Clinical Excellence: Post-Traumatic Stress Disorder: The Management of PTSD in Adults and Children in Primary and Secondary Care (National Clinical Practice Guideline 26). London, National Institute for Clinical Excellence, 2005. Available at: http://www.nice.org.uk/nicemedia/pdf/CG026fullguideline.pdf. Accessed March 24, 2008.

Norcross JC, Hedges M, Prochaska JO: The face of 2010: a Delphi poll on the future of psychotherapy. Prof Psychol Res Pract 33:316–322, 2002

Oei TPS, Llamas M, Devilly GJ: The efficacy and cognitive processes of cognitive behaviour therapy in the treatment of panic disorder with agoraphobia. Behavioural and Cognitive Psychotherapy 27:63–88, 1999

Parker G, Roy K, Eyers K: Cognitive behavior therapy for depression? Choose horses for courses. Am J Psychiatry 160:825–834, 2003

Rector NA, Beck AT: Cognitive behavioral therapy for schizophrenia: an empirical review. J Nerv Ment Dis 189:278–287, 2001

Rosenthal R: Meta-analysis: concepts, corollaries and controversies, in Advances in Psychological Science: Social, Personal and Cultural Aspects, Vol 1. Edited by Adair J, Belanger D. Hove, UK, Psychology Press, 1998, pp 371–384

Scott J, Garland A, Moorhead S: A pilot study of cognitive therapy in bipolar disorders. Psychol Med 31:459–467, 2001

Svartberg M, Stiles TC, Seltzer MH: Randomized, controlled trial of the effectiveness of short-term dynamic psychotherapy and cognitive therapy for cluster C personality disorders. Am J Psychiatry 161:810–817, 2004

Tarrier N, Sommerfeld C: Treatment of chronic PTSD by cognitive therapy and exposure: a 5-year follow-up. Behav Ther 35:231–246, 2004

Temple S, Ho BC: Cognitive therapy for persistent psychosis in schizophrenia: a case-controlled clinical trial. Schizophr Res 74:195–199, 2005

van Balkom AJLM, van Oppen P, Vermeulen AWA, et al: A meta-analysis on the treatment of obsessive-compulsive disorder: a comparison of antidepressants, behavior, and cognitive therapy. Clin Psychol Rev 14:359–381, 1994

van Balkom AJ, Bakker A, Spinhoven P, et al: A meta-analysis of the treatment of panic disorder with or without agoraphobia: a comparison of psychopharmacological, cognitive-behavioral, and combination treatments. J Nerv Ment Dis 185:510–516, 1997

Whittal ML, Agras WS, Gould RA: Bulimia nervosa: a meta-analysis of psychosocial and pharmacological treatments. Behav Ther 30:117–135, 1999

Whittal ML, Thordarson DS, McLean PD: Treatment of obsessive-compulsive disorder: cognitive behavior therapy vs. exposure and response prevention. Behav Res Ther 43:1559–1576, 2005

Wright JH, Wright AS, Albano AM, et al: Computer-assisted cognitive therapy for depression: maintaining efficacy while reducing therapist time. Am J Psychiatry 162:1158–1164, 2005

Young JE, Klosko JS, Weishaar M: Schema Therapy: A Practitioner's Guide. New York, Guilford, 2003

Suggested Readings

Butler AC, Chapman JE, Forman EM, et al: The empirical status of cognitive-behavioral therapy: a review of meta-analyses. Clin Psychol Rev 26:17–31, 2006

Chambless DL, Ollendick TH: Empirically supported psychological interventions: controversies and evidence. Annu Rev Psychol 52:685–716, 2001

Deacon BJ, Abramowitz JS: Cognitive and behavioral treatments for anxiety disorders: a review of meta-analytic findings. J Clin Psychol 60:429–441, 2004

Roth A, Fonagy P (eds): What Works for Whom? A Critical Review of Psychotherapy Research, 2nd Edition. New York, Guilford, 2005

Chapter 9

Combining Cognitive-Behavioral Therapy With Medication

Edward S. Friedman, M.D.
Michael E. Thase, M.D.

Although it may seem intuitively correct to routinely combine cognitive-behavioral therapy (CBT) and medications for treatment of a wide range of disorders, the advantage of this therapeutic approach is not strongly supported by the results of randomized controlled trials (RCTs). In this chapter we briefly review the issue of combining medications and CBT in the major categories of psychiatric disorders: schizophrenia, anxiety disorders, and mood disorders. Because of the dearth of data on the combination of med-

This research was supported in part by grants MH-71799, MH-58356, and MH-69618 from the National Institute of Mental Health.

ication and CBT in the treatment of schizophrenia and the anxiety disorders, we focus on the mood disorders. We also examine the methodological problems inherent in combination treatment studies and, using the example of major depressive disorder, present another model to better understand the effects of combining CBT and medication therapy.

We then describe a clinical model for combining pharmacotherapy and CBT. Finally, we review ways of integrating and implementing combination treatment with CBT and medications for the treatment of major depression. We refer the readers to Chapter 8 ("Applications of Individual Cognitive-Behavioral Therapy to Specific Disorders: Efficacy and Indications") by Drs. Epp, Dobson, and Cottraux for a review of the efficacy, indications, and applications of CBT for the psychiatric disorders discussed in this chapter.

Historical Background

In the early 1980s, Klerman and Schechter contributed a chapter to Paykel's classic text *Handbook of Affective Disorders*, titled "Drugs and Psychotherapy" (Klerman and Schechter 1982). It is instructive to briefly review some aspects of that chapter because it is written from the perspective of psychotherapists confronting the growing dominance of psychopharmacology in psychiatry at that time. First, Klerman and Schechter noted the paucity of evidence for the efficacy of combining psychotherapy and drug therapy. They next reviewed ideological issues involved in combining drugs and psychotherapy. They discussed possible negative effects of drug therapy on psychotherapy: that introducing drug therapy into the psychotherapeutic process might engender transference reactions, and that drugs may alleviate symptoms, undercut defenses, and alter therapy expectations, thereby reducing the efficacy of therapy. They noted possible positive effects of drug therapy on psychotherapy, including the possibilities that drugs may facilitate psychotherapy; that drugs may stabilize ego functions and enable better participation in psychotherapy; and that drug therapy may be abreactive in itself and exert a positive placebo effect.

Thus we can see that the introduction of pharmacotherapy into a field dominated by psychotherapy required a new and radically different paradigm. Klerman (1991) subsequently observed that the ideologies of competing schools of thought in American psychiatry (e.g., the psychoanalytic, the biological, and the psychosocial schools) had competing concepts of the etiology, diagnosis, and treatment of mental illness that profoundly shaped practitioners' reactions to the introduction of pharmacotherapy. By the 1990s, within the context of increasing evidence from RCTs that both pharmacotherapy and targeted forms of psychotherapy were efficacious as monotherapies, the use of combination therapy was gaining wider acceptance (Friedman 1997). For example, the Agency for Health Care Policy and Research, in its clinical practice guideline "Depression in Primary Care" (1993, p. 41), advised the following:

> [A]lthough the routine use of both medications and a formal psychotherapy is not recommended as the initial treatment for most patients...combined treatment may be specifically useful in the following instances:
>
> - Either treatment alone, optimally given, is only partially effective.
> - The clinical circumstances suggest two discrete targets of therapy (e.g., symptom reduction addressed by medication and psychological/social/occupational problems addressed by psychotherapy).
> - A more chronic history or poor interepisodal recovery.

The American Psychiatric Association (1993), in its practice guideline for major depressive disorder (which was based on systematic review of the literature and expert consensus), likewise recommended combination therapy. By 1995, as represented by a *Consumer Reports* survey (Seligman 1995), consumers were rating combination therapy very positively—particularly in comparison with pharmacotherapy alone—despite very limited empirical validation (Friedman 1997).

By the middle of this first decade of the twenty-first century, the evidence base for combining psychotherapy and pharmacotherapy had grown sufficiently that the efficacy of CBT and pharmacotherapy as monotherapies was well established (Friedman and Thase 2006). With respect to health care trends, the pendulum has swung to the opposite position: pharmacotherapy is the most common treatment modality for both mood and anxiety disorders, and insurance providers often limit the intensity and duration of psychotherapy. Certainly the cost of treatment has become an important concern, and—all other things being equal—it is generally more costly to treat an episode of depression or one of the anxiety disorders with the combination of psychotherapy and pharmacotherapy. Thus the routine prescription of combination therapy without evidence of clear benefits can no longer be justified. Furthermore, what constitutes combined pharmacotherapy and psychotherapy remains unclear because treatment can be delivered as an integrated treatment by a psychiatrist or, more commonly, as a split treatment by a pharmacotherapist and psychotherapist team, with treatment delivered either simultaneously or sequentially.

So, in summary, despite the intuitive sense that combination treatment helps our patients get well faster, much remains to be studied and proven in this area.

Review of the Empirical Evidence for Combining CBT With Medication to Treat Psychiatric Disorders

Schizophrenia

Kingdon et al. (2007) recently reviewed the subject of combining CBT[1] and medication to treat patients with schizophrenia. These authors noted that empirical studies of CBT for schizophrenia have been conducted only in patients receiving medications, and that typically CBT is utilized to enhance collaboration, especially medication compliance, and to improve insight. Kingdon et al. also reviewed the interactions between pharmacotherapy and CBT. A number of studies have been completed that have compared the combination of CBT plus pharmacotherapy versus treatment as usual (pharmacotherapy plus medication management). The overall results of these studies suggest an additive effect of CBT when used with medication (Kingdon et al. 2007).

Eating Disorders

Only a few studies combining CBT with medications to treat patients with eating disorders have been performed. Bowers and Andersen (2007) summarized the small number of studies and concluded that it appears that the combination of medication plus CBT is superior to medication alone and that CBT alone is superior to drug therapy alone. Similar to two earlier studies using tricyclic antidepressants, a more recent RCT of CBT and fluoxetine (Walsh et al. 1997), in which combination therapy was compared with control psychotherapy and with placebo pills, suggested that a combination of CBT and fluoxetine may provide the optimal treatment. Of note, in all three of these trials, CBT alone performed better than did medication alone (Walsh et al. 1997).

Reviews of research on combining CBT and pharmacotherapy to treat bulimia have found that CBT has an additive effect with antidepressant medication (Ricca et al. 2000; Wilson 1999). On the other hand, with no RCTs available, data on the use of combination CBT and pharmacotherapy for the treatment of anorexia nervosa remain scarce. Some tentative guide-

---

[1]The term *cognitive-behavioral therapy*, as noted by Epp et al. in Chapter 8 ("Applications of Individual Cognitive-Behavioral Therapy to Specific Disorders: Efficacy and Indications"), "is often used to refer to a variety of approaches in which both cognitive and behavioral strategies are used. It refers to both standard cognitive therapy...and an atheoretical combination of cognitive and behavioral therapies."

lines for combining psychotherapy and medications are available (see Mitchell et al. 2001).

Anxiety Disorders

Although both CBT and medication have demonstrated efficacy in treating a wide variety of anxiety disorders, as Epp and coauthors describe in Chapter 8, only limited evidence exists about the efficacy or effectiveness of CBT in combination with medication versus medication therapy alone. We briefly review those randomized controlled studies combining medication and CBT for patients with social phobia or obsessive-compulsive disorder (OCD). There are no controlled trials of combination CBT and medication therapy for posttraumatic stress disorder or for generalized anxiety disorder. Although no adequate large-scale, controlled studies have compared CBT and medication alone and in combination to treat social phobia, one early, small study ($N=34$, with subjects divided into four cells) by Clark and Agras (1991) reported that CBT plus buspirone was better than buspirone therapy alone for treating performance anxiety in musicians. Few RCTs have examined combining CBT and medication for the treatment of OCD. Despite this, in a review, Hollifield et al. (2006) argued that combination therapies are often justified due to the partial response to each of the monotherapies. An important trial ($N=122$) that confirmed this opinion was performed by Foa et al. (2005). They found that CBT alone (which included exposure and ritual prevention behavioral techniques) and CBT plus clomipramine had comparable effects and that both were superior to the serotonin-norepinephrine reuptake inhibitor clomipramine alone.

Chronic Depression

The Cognitive-Behavioral Analysis System of Psychotherapy (CBASP) was developed by McCullough (2000) specifically to address the problems encountered in the treatment of patients with chronic depression and dysthymia. It provides additional therapeutic techniques adapted to these difficult-to-treat patients. CBASP and CBT adapted for treatment-resistant and chronic depression are usually provided in the context of optimized pharmacotherapy. Traditional CBT modified for patients with treatment-resistant and chronic depression addresses the prolonged hopelessness and helplessness, the persistent anhedonia and anergia, the strongly entrenched dysfunctional beliefs, the consequences of interpersonal ineffectiveness, the need to treat comorbid anxiety symptoms, and the necessity of maintaining pharmacotherapy (Antonuccio et al. 1984; Cole et al. 1994; Fava et al. 1997; Thase and Howland 1994; Wright et al. 2006). Similarly, McCullough

(2000) conceptualizes chronic depression to be the product of dysfunctional cognitions of helplessness, hopelessness, and failure that are linked to a detached and maladaptive interpersonal style, which is reinforced by habitually poor social problem solving. Crucially, patients' history of medication failure reinforces their belief in the inevitability of their remaining ill. These patients' perceptual distortions lead to behaviors that are incompatible with their desired outcomes (such as giving up on medication adherence, which reduces the likelihood of achieving or sustaining a prolonged remission of symptoms). CBASP helps such patients to establish, or reestablish, interpersonal connections and to learn new and adaptive coping styles.

Keller and colleagues (2000) compared CBASP with the serotonin-norepinephrine reuptake inhibitor nefazodone alone and in combination with CBASP. They found that each monotherapy yielded a response rate of 55%, compared with an 85% response rate for combination treatment, at the end of 12 weeks of treatment. This study most impressively supports the concept of using combination treatment in a difficult-to-treat population. Currently, CBASP augmentation for the treatment of chronic depression is being compared with brief supportive therapy in a study sponsored by the National Institute of Mental Health; the intention is to determine whether the results of the Keller et al. (2000) study can be replicated. Because all patients will be receiving medication according to an algorithm with both forms of psychotherapy, these results may enhance our understanding of the role of combination treatment for complex and chronic depression and whether CBASP (a problem-solving, CBT-based therapy) provides a specific psychotherapeutic benefit over and above supportive psychotherapy. Table 9–1 describes the psychotherapeutic techniques developed by McCullough (2000) to treat patients with treatment-resistant depression.

Bipolar Disorder

As there have been modifications of CBT to treat chronically depressed patients, so too have there been modifications of traditional CBT to treat patients with bipolar disorder. Using CBT for bipolar disorder, as when used for chronic depression, augments optimized pharmacological treatment. Basco and Rush (2005), Basco et al. (2007), and Newman and coworkers (2002) have described the basic principles of using CBT for bipolar disorder. The first goal of combination treatment is to stabilize the acute mood symptoms. A key component of CBT in treating bipolar disorder is an increased emphasis on preventing progression of the disease. This is accomplished by a focus on basic CBT techniques as well as additional relapse prevention techniques, such as the following:

TABLE 9–1. Cognitive-Behavioral Analysis System of Psychotherapy (CBASP) treatment modifications for chronic depression

---

Situational analysis

Teaches patients to identify negative affects.

Helps patients compare and contrast their typical problem-solving style with an alternative solution.

Highlights the relief patients have experienced and the specific cognitive and behavioral processes that precipitated that relief.

Models behavioral change and helps to motivate the individual to continue in a process of change.

Interpersonal discrimination exercise

Teaches new cognitive/behavioral strategies for interpersonal interactions.

- Therapist uses data about the patient's intimate relationships to generate a cognitive-behavioral conceptualization of the patient.

- Therapist explores areas where the patient believes his or her needs are not being met, situations that elicit thoughts of failure, or situations associated with the generation of negative affects.

- Therapist–patient relationship serves as a model for appropriate interpersonal interaction.

- McCullough observed that patients with chronic depression impose past behavioral patterns on the therapeutic relationship. Patients are taught to identify, compare, and contrast actual vs. expected outcomes of in-session behavior. Patients can then begin to perceive, and enact, new ways of behaving with other important people in their lives based on what they have learned through CBASP analysis of transference relationships.

Interpersonal transference hypothesis exercise

Generates and tests hypotheses about the patient's interpersonal style.

- Issues relating to problems with intimacy, failure experiences, unmet emotional needs, ridicule and punishment, and fears of expressing negative affects are explored in a methodical manner.

Significant-other list

Helps the therapist learn about the major persons who have influenced the patient either positively or negatively.

- The patient creates a list of significant others, whose relationships with the patient are examined to clarify the consequences of each relationship on the patient's belief system.

Source.   Reprinted, with permission, from McCullough 2000.

- Acceptance of and psychoeducation about bipolar disorder
- Symptom monitoring to help patients monitor their illness so they can better identify and initiate treatment changes with the onset of new episodes
- A focus on sleep hygiene and daily activity scheduling
- Development of better coping skills to reduce interpersonal stressors

Cognitive interventions are used to treat depressive symptoms in a manner similar to that of standard CBT for depression (Beck et al. 1979), and techniques such as thought monitoring and identification of cognitive errors are employed to counter expansiveness in hypomania and mania. Additionally, attention is paid to medication adherence. Overall, the increased use of behavioral strategies aims to decrease the risk of symptom recurrence or worsening. Newman et al. (2002) recommended more extensive use of cognitive methods for both phases of the disorder.

Combining CBT and pharmacotherapy to treat bipolar disorder involves many of the methods used for the treatment of depression, such as the use of structuring, psychoeducation, and adherence interventions and tailoring the treatment plan to meet the needs of each patient. However, greater effort is usually spent on helping the patient and his or her family understand the disorder and recognize early signs of relapse. One commonly used strategy is to develop a Symptom Summary Worksheet in which the patient (and family, if possible) develops a customized list of the cognitive, behavioral, physiological, interpersonal, and other changes that occur when he or she begins to shift into a depressive or hypomanic phase. This worksheet is also used to record symptoms that are experienced during more severe mood swings. After symptoms are identified with this method, the clinician helps the patient learn specific strategies to manage symptoms and stop the escalation into depression or mania. For example, a behavioral intervention could be designed to curtail excessive spending; an exercise of examining the evidence could be used to reduce grandiose thinking; and CBT methods could be employed to promote healthy sleeping habits.

Several RCTs have studied the combination of CBT with pharmacotherapy for treating bipolar disorder. In a small, early trial ($N=28$), Cochran (1984) studied whether a 6-week course of CBT improved lithium compliance at 6 and 12 months after treatment compared with control subjects who only received pharmacotherapy. No difference was found in lithium compliance on the self-reports, on the informant reports, or in serum levels, although on the basis of composite scores, the combination group had better compliance. Lam and colleagues (2003) examined whether adding CBT (14 sessions during the first 6 months and 2 booster sessions in the subsequent 6 months) prevented relapse in patients ($N=103$) taking mood stabilizer medication. Outcomes were measured at 6 and 12 months posttreatment. The authors reported that patients in the combination CBT plus mood stabilizer group had significantly fewer bipolar episodes, fewer days per episode, and fewer hospitalizations. When Lam et al. examined the outcomes after 2 years, they reported that the combination treatment group had fewer bipolar episodes, better mood ratings, better psychosocial function, and better management of prodromal symptoms (Lam et al. 2005a). They also determined that CBT plus mood stabilizer medication was superior to mood stabilizer treatment alone in terms of cost-effectiveness for patients with frequent relapses of bipolar disorder (Lam et al. 2005b).

Ball and coworkers (2006) randomly assigned 52 bipolar patients to receive either 6 months of CBT plus treatment as usual, or treatment as usual (mood stabilizers). Posttreatment scores on rating scales indicated that depression was less severe and attitudes less dysfunctional in the CBT-added group. The authors stated that this study corroborates previous bipolar disorder research demonstrating the value of CBT in combination with treatment as usual. They also reported that the continuation of benefit appears to diminish over time, suggesting that booster CBT sessions may be necessary to maintain the beneficial effects of CBT added to treatment as usual (Ball et al. 2006).

In summary, research on CBT used combined with medication in patients with bipolar disorder suggests that combination treatment increases medication adherence, improves symptom management and episode stability, and may augment relapse prevention.

Methodological Problems in Combination Psychotherapy and Pharmacotherapy Studies in Major Depressive Disorder

In this section we examine the evidence supporting the idea that combination treatment provides additional benefit beyond the effect of either monotherapy alone. It has long been assumed that because psychotherapy and pharmacotherapy target different aspects of major depression, they are likely to have additive or even synergistic effects (American Psychiatric Association 1993). In this regard, *additive effect* refers to the two treatments together resulting in a better outcome than would be expected from either treatment alone and *synergistic effect* refers to an outcome that is over and above a simple summation of the effects of the monotherapies. After three decades of research on this topic, two conclusions can be drawn: 1) psychotherapy and pharmacotherapy have at best only partially additive effects (i.e., $1.0 + 1.0 = 1.5$) and 2) there is no credible evidence that combining these treatments can actually have synergistic effects (Thase 2000).

To better understand the phenomenon of partial summation of effects, we must examine how these trials are performed. Most of the studies examining the efficacy of treatments are relatively short-term or acute-phase therapy trials (Frank et al. 1991), and, given the heterogeneity of major depressive disorder, the sample compositions of particular studies can vary remarkably with respect to the proportions of participants with severe, chronic, recurrent, comorbid, or treatment-resistant depressive episodes. Thus, a study with a population of patients who have relatively acute, milder, and less complicated forms of the disorder is unlikely to yield the same results as an RCT involving patients with more severe and complex forms of depression.

Another problem stems from overestimation of the likely effects of treatment. It is now known that the so-called nonspecific effects of treatment are generally larger than the specific effects of antidepressants and focused forms of psychotherapy in contemporary clinical trials (Thase 2000). Moreover, after the magnitude of placebo expectancy effects is taken into account, the specific effects of treatment are relatively modest (e.g., Cohen's d effect size values range between 0.2 and 0.5; Thase 2000), so studies need to be relatively large in order to have the statistical power to reliably detect between-group differences. Thus, although it is true that most early studies that compared cognitive therapy and pharmacotherapy, singly and in combination, indicated that combining these modalities did not result in statistically significant additive effects (Friedman 1997), it is also true that these studies only had the power to detect relatively large additive effects. Examination of the average differences between the respective monotherapies and their combinations almost always reveals at least some numeric advantage for combination therapy, albeit with relatively small effect sizes. Whereas most studies comparing psychotherapy and pharmacotherapy singly and in combination have had 30 or fewer patients in each arm of the experiment, a study designed to reliably detect a small additive effect would need more than 250 patients in each treatment arm (e.g., see Kraemer and Thiemann 1987). To our knowledge, only one such large study with adequate power has ever been conducted, that of Keller et al. (2000).

It is also true that a small overall additive effect in a study of a heterogeneous group of patients may conceal a mixture of outcomes, ranging from no additive effect among patients with less severe or less complicated disorders to a large additive effect in particular subgroups (Jindal and Thase 2003; Pampallona et al. 2004), and more recent studies provide data to support this position (Friedman et al. 2006; Hollon et al. 2005).

In Table 9–2 we review the relevant RCTs of combination CBT and medication for major depressive disorder that we are examining as an example of the difficulties in performing combination therapy studies. After a thorough search of the published (English language) literature, we identi-

TABLE 9–2. Meta-analysis of response to pharmacotherapy alone versus combination therapy with cognitive-behavioral therapy and pharmacotherapy in randomized controlled trials for major depressive disorder

Study	N	Response, %		P
		Drug	Combination	
Blackburn et al. 1981	58	39	60	0.11
Hollon et al. 1992	82	30	48	0.11
Keller et al. 2000	453	16	33	0.0001
Miller et al. 1989	46	24	48	0.10
Murphy et al. 1984	46	38	55	0.25

Favoring Drug   Favoring Combination

Note. This analysis is of patients achieving remission and completing the study; these data are used to be most similar to the outcomes of the other studies. Methodology adapted from Pampallona et al. 2004. All randomized clinical trials used Beck's model of cognitive-behavioral therapy (Beck et al. 1979) except the study by Keller et al., which used McCullough's Cognitive-Behavioral Analysis System of Psychotherapy (McCullough 2000).
In plot on right, odds ratios of 1.0 and higher indicate the superiority of combination therapy; horizontal lines depict 95% confidence intervals.

fied only four RCTs that utilized Beck's model of CBT (Beck et al. 1979) in outpatients with major depressive disorder and reported a comparison between pharmacotherapy alone and in combination with CBT. These studies suggest that the conventional idea that the severity of symptoms signals when combination treatment is needed may be inaccurate. Instead, other moderators or predictors, such as a history of chronic depression, psychological trauma, or comorbid insomnia, anxiety, and/or medical disorders, may indicate the need for combination treatment. Table 9–2 summarizes the response rates observed in each of the combination CBT plus pharmacotherapy studies and presents odds ratios and confidence intervals.

For the purpose of comparison, we also included the study by Keller et al. (2000). This RCT is not just the only study to show a statistically significant advantage for combination therapy. It is also unique because it was larger than all the other studies put together (i.e., it had adequate statistical power to detect a difference between treatments) and because this study used a modified form of CBT developed to treat chronic depression (it enrolled only patients with chronic forms of major depressive disorder, a population that is more difficult to treat).

To help to sort out whether the differences between the findings of Keller et al. (2000) and the remainder of the studies are the result of the Keller et al. study's greater statistical power or the study's focus on a higher-risk patient subgroup, we performed a meta-analysis of the effect of adding CBT to pharmacotherapy in the five studies reviewed in Table 9–2 (Friedman et al. 2006). The table presents a forest plot summarizing the meta-analysis of response to combination therapy compared with the response to medication alone. In this meta-analysis, the lack of an effect is represented by an odds ratio of 1.0 or less, indicating there is no difference between a pair of treatments, and values higher than 1.0 represent advantages favoring combination therapy. Statistical significance is determined by the 95% confidence intervals, depicted as horizontal lines extending from both sides of each odds ratio. Inspection of Table 9–2 indicates that although only the Keller et al. (2000) study observed a significant advantage favoring combination therapy, each of the other studies yielded odds ratios that were quite similar to that of Keller et al.; the major difference was not the magnitude of the advantage for combination therapy but rather the wider confidence intervals of the smaller studies. It is likely that the Keller et al. study forecasts the primary finding of the meta-analysis because of its size, rather than because the patients were chronically depressed or treated with CBASP rather than Beck's model of CBT.

Despite the fact that this meta-analysis is limited by a very small set of available and relevant studies, it is nonetheless consistent with the larger analysis by Pampallona et al. (2004), who came to similar conclusions and included all combination psychotherapy and pharmacotherapy studies. Those investigators examined almost 1,000 patients in each of the two treatment groups and found that patients receiving combination therapy improved significantly compared with those receiving drug treatment alone (odds ratio = 1.86; 95% confidence interval = 1.38–2.52). These meta-analytic findings suggest that adding CBT to pharmacotherapy definitely increases the likelihood of response in depressed patients. Moreover, this effect is clinically meaningful and is at least as large as the average difference between an antidepressant and placebo in contemporary RCTs (Thase 2000).

Combining CBT With Medication to Treat Major Depression: The CBT–Biological Therapy Model Expanded

The CBT–biological therapy model (Wright and Thase 1992) provides a theoretical basis for combining pharmacotherapy and psychotherapy. The CBT-biological model takes a systems approach, reflecting the view that multiple influences—for example, cognitive, behavioral, interpersonal, social, cultural, and biological—contribute to the development and expression of mental disorders. In theory, the efficacy of combination treatment results from the targeting of different vulnerability factors. From this point of view, interventions designed to improve a problem in one system may also contribute to improvement in other areas in mutually reinforcing ways. For example, a cognitive intervention to ensure medication compliance intervenes in both the cognitive and biological systems in a synergistic manner: a positive behavioral outcome results in improved pill taking, which leads to a greater degree of biological stabilization of the illness, making it more likely that the patient will continue taking the medication on into the future.

Compelling support for the need to combine biological models of understanding depression with cognitive and behavioral models of psychopathology and behavioral change, comes from functional imaging studies in depression. Drevets (2003) examined patients with mood disorders and identified a region in the subgenual prefrontal cortex that was 40% decreased in volume in patients with depression. Mayberg (2003) also identified that region as being a common target of pharmacotherapy, being the area of the highest concentration of serotonin in the brain. When this research group analyzed patients treated with a selective serotonin reuptake inhibitor (paroxetine) and CBT, they demonstrated that CBT was associated with characteristic metabolic changes in the frontal cortex, cingulate, and hippocampal regions of the brain as opposed to the characteristic changes in the prefrontal cortex, hippocampal, and subgenual cingulate regions that result from treatment with selective serotonin reuptake inhibitors (Goldapple et al. 2004). Mayberg and colleagues interpreted these findings as indicating that

CBT and medications have different primary targets of action, with cortical top-down effects characterizing a psychotherapy effect and a subcortical bottom-up effect accounting for the effect of medication.

These imaging data lend support to a theoretical position that suggests combination treatment may be synergistic in its benefit, given that the different modalities affect different brain centers. This suggestion becomes even more intriguing if we consider the possibility that genomics might also aid in determining whether different treatments may be more beneficial to different patients. For example, Lesch and colleagues (1996) reported that there is an insertion-deletion polymorphism of the serotonin transporter gene that affects transcriptional activity and accounts for differences in serotonin transporter density among individuals. Of the 27 variants of this gene, one polymorphism in the promoter region (5-HTTLPR) has a long and short allele variation. Caspi and coworkers (2003) studied the genetic profiles of individuals in 1,057 consecutive births in New Zealand who were followed over a period of 26 years. At age 26, 17% of this cohort reported a major depressive episode. Neither life stress nor 5-HTT transporter genotype predicted the onset of depression. However, subjects with the short form of the alleles had more depressive episodes in the context of increased stressful life events, whereas those with the long form of the alleles had low rates of depression in the context of steady levels of life stress. In a study that combined neurobiological and genomic observations, Pezawas and colleagues (2005) identified the cingulate–amygdala pathway as the structural and functional site for the differences produced by the 5-HTTLPR polymorphisms. They suggested that variation in this system provides a susceptibility mechanism for depression. Individuals with this genetic vulnerability demonstrate biased processing of emotionally laden stimuli. Other studies have correlated this polymorphic variation with antidepressant response (Kugaya et al. 2004; Yu et al. 2002). Thus, the genomic and functional brain imaging data demonstrate CBT–biological therapy interactions that may be amenable to combination treatment strategies.

Other studies suggest common areas of improvement from CBT and medication interventions (Wright 2004). Researchers (Baxter et al. 1992; Schwartz et al. 1996) have reported that behavioral interventions for OCD have the same effects on brain positron emission tomography (PET) scans that fluoxetine does. The same group of researchers (Brody et al. 1998) also demonstrated that normalization of metabolism in the orbitofrontal cortex shown on PET scans was a predictor of response to behavioral treatment and fluoxetine. A similar result for patients with social phobia has been demonstrated: Furmark et al. (2002) studied patients with social phobia and found that CBT and citalopram responders demonstrated similar changes on PET scans (decreased regional blood flow in the amygdala and hippocampus).

Wright and Thase (1992) elaborated on several assumptions that derive from the CBT–biological therapy model and can be used to inform treatment:

1. Cognitive processes modulate the effects of the external environment on central nervous system processes involved in emotion and behavior. For example, stressful life events can modulate neurotransmitter function, activation of central nervous system pathways, and neuroendocrine tone.
2. Dysfunctional cognitions are the product of both psychological and physiological influences.
3. Biological treatments can alter cognitions.
4. Cognitive and behavioral interventions can modulate biological processes.
5. Environmental, cognitive, behavioral, emotional, and biological processes should be conceptualized as components of a whole system.

As a consequence of these assumptions, a clinician combining CBT and pharmacotherapy must attempt to integrate as many of these system components as possible into a comprehensive case conceptualization. From this wider perspective, the clinician can adapt interventions derived from these multiple areas to promote therapeutic change.

Combining CBT and Pharmacotherapy for the Treatment of Mood Disorders: A Clinical Perspective

CBT and pharmacotherapy share many features that facilitate the development of an integrated treatment approach. Both treatments are empirically based, pragmatic psychiatric treatments. Structure and psychoeducation are critical to the treatment processes. Adherence to the therapeutic plan is also critical to the success of both forms of treatment. Using a comprehensive model that incorporates biological, cognitive, interpersonal, and behavioral elements of understanding and treating illness, clinicians can utilize a cohesive blend of useful interventions. Key methods for integrating CBT with pharmacotherapy for depression are discussed below (see also Table 9–3).

In research studies, CBT and pharmacotherapy are compared against each other in order to examine the relative efficacy of different interventions. Separate clinicians deliver the two treatments (split treatment), and defined protocols are followed to reduce variation in therapy methods. To our knowledge, there are no studies of combination therapy in which the same psychophar-

---

TABLE 9–3.   Methods for combining cognitive-behavioral therapy (CBT) with antidepressant medication

---

Develop a comprehensive treatment model.

Individualize treatment plans.

Address cognitive-behavioral features of depression.

Recognize effects of medication on cognition and behavior.

Unite therapies through session structure and psychoeducation.

Use CBT methods to enhance adherence.

---

macotherapist (integrated treatment) delivered both interventions, or in which, despite splitting the functions, pharmacotherapists worked as part of an integrated team alongside a nonprescribing cognitive therapist, both of whom used a flexible approach. Pharmacotherapy protocols in controlled, comparative studies are handicapped by the requirement that patients remain on the initial medication for 12 or even 16 weeks regardless of the level of response. In practice, a medication switch or augmentation strategy could be implemented over this same time frame. In practice, combination therapy benefits from the strengths of each treatment and is flexible enough to customize methods to meet the particular needs of the patient (Wright 2004; Wright and Thase 1992). For example, CBT might be used to target anhedonia, concomitant anxiety, or procrastination in a patient with anxious depression that is complicated by socially isolating avoidance behaviors. Pharmacotherapy can be tailored to the individual and—although the first treatment may not be effective—following a reasonable medication algorithm, a realistic appraisal of positive medication effects on individual depressive symptoms can highlight a process of gradual improvement. Simultaneously, the therapist can help the patient examine the belief that "Because my last med trial didn't help, no med will help," therein helping the patient to modify the unrealistic expectation of an immediate and complete response to a single modality of treatment.

For patients with severe, complex, or high-risk depression, acute-phase pharmacotherapy can be augmented with CBT to help modify thoughts of helplessness and hopelessness and to introduce alternative behaviors in response to suicidal ideation before the onset of a medication's effect. Brown and colleagues (2005) have demonstrated that CBT lowers the risk of recurrent suicide attempts in patients treated with antidepressants. Pharmacotherapy options that can enhance the patient's ability to respond to CBT include 1) selecting medications that improve concentration, sleep, energy, and other functions needed for obtaining full benefit from psychotherapy; 2) minimizing drug side effects that might interfere with the implementation of CBT; and 3) being aware of negative medication–therapy interactions, such as the potential interference of the simultaneous use of high-potency benzodiazepines with the effects of CBT (e.g., using alprazolam when attempting exposure therapy; Marks et al. 1993).

Pharmacotherapy and CBT both incorporate structuring techniques and psychoeducation. Thus, the pharmacotherapy session can be structured using standard CBT techniques such as the following:

- Setting an agenda
- Checking the status of symptoms
- Pacing sessions to enhance the efficiency of treatment
- Targeting specific problems for intervention (in particular, therapy-blocking behaviors that lead to medication noncompliance)
- Maintaining a collaborative empirical position
- Using feedback to promote patients' understanding

Psychoeducational materials such as readings, videos, and computer-assisted learning can be employed to convey information about both pharmacotherapy and CBT. For example, clinicians, or clinician pairs who are trained in both CBT and pharmacotherapy, can do the following:

1. Present a brief overview of how medications and therapy can work effectively as partners in treatment, then offer more specific education on pharmacotherapy strategies and side effects.
2. Present the CBT model.
3. Demonstrate ways to record and modify automatic thoughts.
4. Identify dysfunctional attitudes and beliefs.
5. Initiate alternative behaviors.
6. Monitor for relapse.

(See Wright et al. 2006 for greater detail on CBT techniques for structuring sessions and educating patients.)

A straightforward mechanism by which CBT helps to improve the outcome of pharmacotherapy is improving patients' adherence to medication. Studies assessing medication adherence have documented favorable effects of adding CBT to standard drug treatment for various disorders, such as bipolar disorder (Cochran 1984), schizophrenia (Lecompte 1995), and psychosis (Kemp et al. 1996, 1998). Typical CBT interventions to improve adherence include eliciting and modifying maladaptive cognitions about treatment (e.g., "If I take a drug, it means I'm weak"; "I'm always the one to get side effects"; "Doctors who prescribe medications don't really want to listen to you"). Also, behavioral methods such as using reminder systems, pairing medication ingestion with routine activities, and developing specific plans to overcome identified barriers to adherence may be helpful in promoting follow-through with the treatment plan (Wright et al. 2006).

The issue of potential negative consequences of adding medication to CBT has received little attention. In one of the few controlled clinical trials in this area, Curran et al. (1994) reported the negative impact of benzodiazepines on learning and/or memory such that the efficacy of exposure therapy for agoraphobia in patients with panic disorder was diminished. Furthermore, Otto and coworkers (1996) found that panic disorder patients who achieved remission with combination CBT plus benzodiazepine medication relapsed sooner than patients who achieved remission with CBT alone. Beyond the issue of benzodiazepine use, however, there is scant information supporting the hypothesis that medications have a negative interaction with the CBT process. In fact, quite to the contrary, Otto and Deckersbach (1998) reported that stepwise exposure therapy added to pharmacotherapy has consistently shown benefit in extending the gains made from the pharmacological treatment of panic disorder.

Application of Combination Therapy for Mood Disorders

Whether combination CBT and medication is delivered as split treatment or provided by a single psychiatrist (an ideal that is impractical because there are not enough psychiatrists to adequately address the public health need for depression treatment), it is neither practical nor always necessary nor cost-effective to offer every patient combination therapy. And as we have seen, there is only limited evidence (which needs replication) supporting the use of combination therapy. So one outstanding goal remains: to develop usable methods of identifying subgroups of depressed patients who are most likely to benefit from medication alone, CBT alone, or the two in combination. Although this call to research has been made for the past 25 years, the practical question of which treatment to use when remains unanswered. Until definitive prospective data are available in studies with adequate power and diverse samples, or new technology (e.g., scanning techniques, as discussed by Mayberg [2003] and summarized in section "Combining CBT With Medication to Treat Major Depression") becomes available, we suggest that practitioners do the following:

- Focus on variables that are associated with lower rates of response to pharmacotherapy alone (such as chronicity, inpatient status, and other indicators of marked severity; comorbid anxiety; or a history of early sexual or physical abuse or neglect).

• Monitor the response of each patient receiving monotherapy, using symptom severity measures to identify those patients who require a swift change from monotherapy to combination therapy.

Conclusion

Because of the dearth of data on the combination of medication and CBT in the other major categories of psychiatric disorders, we focused this review on the mood disorders. Studies of CBT in combination with medication for depression demonstrate a benefit for combination treatment over pharmacotherapy alone. It appears that combination pharmacotherapy plus CBT will become the treatment of choice for patients with bipolar illness. Long-range outcomes for patients with major depressive disorder are better when CBT is included, regardless of whether CBT is concurrent with or follows pharmacotherapy. The research challenge ahead is to determine which patients will benefit most from combination therapy and what is the optimal sequencing of treatments to achieve remission of symptoms, to prevent relapse, to produce recovery, and to avoid recurrence. As in the Keller et al. (2000) study, moderators of therapeutic response are beginning to be identified and point the way to a more sophisticated model of treatment. As research identifies these moderators of responses to CBT and medication, our preceding speculations should be replaced with and be continuously updated by more refined, evidence-based recommendations for, guidelines for, and pathways of treatment.

Key Points

• The efficacy of combination therapy with cognitive-behavioral therapy (CBT) and pharmacotherapy has not yet been established because of a lack of studies.

• CBT and medication in combination for depression appears to be efficacious.

• CBT has been demonstrated to improve medication compliance and treatment adherence in the context of several psychiatric disorders.

References

Agency for Health Care Policy and Research, Depression Guideline Panel: Depression in Primary Care, Vol 1: Detection and Diagnosis. Clinical Practice Guideline Number 5 (AHCPR Publ No 93-0550). Rockville, MD, U.S. Department of Health and Human Services, April 1993

American Psychiatric Association: Practice guideline for major depressive disorder in adults. Am J Psychiatry 150 (suppl 4):1–26, 1993

Antonuccio DO, Atkins WT, Chatam PM, et al: An exploratory study: the pycho-educational group treatment of drug-refractory unipolar depression. J Behav Ther Exp Psychiatry 15:309–313, 1984

Ball JR, Mitchell PB, Corry JC, et al: A randomized controlled trial of cognitive therapy for bipolar disorder: focus on long-term change. J Clin Psychiatry 67:277–286, 2006

Basco MR, Rush AJ: Cognitive-Behavioral Therapy for Bipolar Disorder, 2nd Edition. New York, Guilford, 2005

Basco MR, Ladd G, Myers DS, et al: Combining medication treatment and cognitive-behavior therapy for bipolar disorder. Journal of Cognitive Psychotherapy: An International Quarterly 21:7–15, 2007

Baxter LR, Schwartz JM, Bergman KS, et al: Caudate glucose metabolic rate changes with both drug and behavioral therapy for obsessive-compulsive disorder. Arch Gen Psychiatry 49:681–689, 1992

Beck AT, Rush AJ, Shaw BF, et al: Cognitive Therapy of Depression. New York, Guilford, 1979

Blackburn IM, Bishop S, Glen AI, et al: The efficacy of cognitive therapy in depression: a treatment trial using cognitive therapy and pharmacotherapy, each alone and in combination. Br J Psychiatry 139:181–189, 1981

Bowers WA, Andersen AE: Cognitive-behavior therapy with eating disorders: the role of medications in treatment. Journal of Cognitive Psychotherapy: An International Quarterly 21:16–27, 2007

Brody AL, Saxena S, Schwartz JM, et al: FDG-PET predictors of response to behavioral therapy and pharmacotherapy in obsessive compulsive disorder. Psychiatry Res 84:1–6, 1998

Brown GK, Ten Have T, Henriques GR, et al: Cognitive therapy for the prevention of suicide attempts: a randomized controlled trial. JAMA 294:563–570, 2005

Caspi A, Sugden K, Moffitt TE, et al: Influence of life stress on depression: moderation by a polymorphism in the 5-HTT gene. Science 301:386–389, 2003

Clark DB, Agras WS: The assessment and treatment of performance anxiety in musicians. Am J Psychiatry 148:598–605, 1991

Cochran SD: Preventing medication noncompliance in the outpatient treatment of bipolar affective disorders. J Consult Clin Psychol 52:873–878, 1984

Cole AJ, Brittlebank AD, Scott J: The role of cognitive therapy in refractory depression, in Refractory Depression: Current Strategies and Future Directions. Edited by Nolen WA, Zohar J, Roose SP, et al. Chichester, UK, Wiley, 1994, pp 117–120

Curran HV, Bond A, O'Sullivan G, et al: Memory functions, alprazolam and exposure therapy: a controlled longitudinal study of agoraphobia with panic disorder. Psychol Med 24:969–976, 1994

Drevets WC: Neuroimaging abnormalities in the amygdala in mood disorders. Ann N Y Acad Sci 985:420–444, 2003

Fava GA, Savron G, Grandi S, et al: Cognitive-behavioral management of drug-resistant major depressive disorder. J Clin Psychiatry 58:278–282, 1997

Foa EB, Liebowitz MR, Kozak MJ, et al: Randomized, placebo-controlled trial of exposure and ritual prevention, clomipramine, and their combination in the treatment of obsessive-compulsive disorder. Am J Psychiatry 162:151–161, 2005

Frank E, Prien RF, Jarrett RB, et al: Conceptualization and rationale for consensus definitions of terms in major depressive disorder: remission, recovery, relapse, and recurrence. Arch Gen Psychiatry 48:851–855, 1991

Friedman ES: Combined therapy for depression. Journal of Practical Psychiatry and Behavioral Health 3:211–222, 1997

Friedman ES, Thase ME: Cognitive-behavioral therapy for depression and dysthymia, in Textbook of Mood Disorders. Edited by Stein DJ, Kupfer DJ, Schatzberg AF. Washington, DC, American Psychiatric Publishing, 2006, pp 353–371

Friedman ES, Wright JH, Jarrett RB, et al: Combining cognitive behavior therapy and medication for mood disorders. Psychiatr Ann 36:321–328, 2006

Furmark T, Tillfors M, Marteinsdottir I: Common changes in cerebral blood flow in patients with social phobia treated with citalopram or cognitive-behavior therapy. Arch Gen Psychiatry 59:425–433, 2002

Goldapple K, Segal Z, Carson C, et al: Modulation of cortical-limbic pathways in major depression: treatment-specific effects of cognitive behavior therapy. Arch Gen Psychiatry 61:34–42, 2004

Hollifield M, Mackey A, Davidson J: Integrating therapies for anxiety disorders. Psychiatr Ann 36:329–338, 2006

Hollon SD, DeRubeis RJ, Evans MD, et al: Cognitive therapy and pharmacotherapy for depression: singly and in combination. Arch Gen Psychiatry 49:774–781, 1992

Hollon SD, Jarrett RB, Nierenberg AA, et al: Psychotherapy and medication in the treatment of adult and geriatric depression: which monotherapy or combined treatment? J Clin Psychiatry 66:455–468, 2005

Jindal RD, Thase ME: Integrating psychotherapy and pharmacotherapy to improve outcomes among patients with mood disorders. Psychiatr Serv 54:1484–1490, 2003

Keller MB, McCullough JP, Klein DN, et al: A comparison of nefazodone, the cognitive behavioral-analysis system of psychotherapy, and their combination for the treatment of chronic depression. N Engl J Med 342:1462–1470, 2000

Kemp R, Hayward P, Applewhaite G, et al: Compliance therapy in psychotic patients: randomised controlled trial. BMJ 312:345–349, 1996

Kemp R, Kirov G, Everitt B, et al: Randomised controlled trial of compliance therapy: 18-month follow-up. Br J Psychiatry 172:412–419, 1998

Kingdon D, Rathod S, Hansen L, et al: Combining cognitive therapy and pharmacotherapy for schizophrenia. Journal of Cognitive Psychotherapy: An International Quarterly 21:28–36, 2007

Klerman G: Ideologic conflicts in integrating pharmacotherapy and psychotherapy, in Integrating Pharmacotherapy and Psychotherapy. Edited by Breitman B, Klerman G. Washington, DC, American Psychiatric Press, 1991, pp 3–19

Klerman GL, Schechter GS: Drugs and psychotherapy, in Handbook of Affective Disorders. Edited by Paykel ES. New York, Guilford, 1982, pp 329–337

Kraemer HC, Thiemann S: How Many Subjects? Statistical Power Analysis in Research. Newbury Park, CA, Sage, 1987

Kugaya A, Sanacora G, Staley JK, et al: Brain serotonin transporter availability predicts response to selective serotonin reuptake inhibitors. Biol Psychiatry 56:497–502, 2004

Lam DH, Watkins ER, Hayward P, et al: A randomized controlled study of cognitive therapy for relapse prevention for bipolar affective disorders: outcome of the first year. Arch Gen Psychiatry 60:145–152, 2003

Lam DH, Hayward P, Watkins ER, et al: Relapse prevention in patients with bipolar disorder: cognitive therapy outcome after 2 years. Am J Psychiatry 162:324–329, 2005a

Lam DH, McCrone P, Wright K, et al: Cost-effectiveness of relapse-prevention cognitive therapy for bipolar disorder: 30-month study. Br J Psychiatry 186:500–506, 2005b

Lecompte D: Drug compliance and cognitive-behavioral therapy in schizophrenia. Acta Psychiatr Belg 95:91–100, 1995

Lesch KP, Bengel D, Heils A, et al: Association of anxiety-related traits with a polymorphism in the serotonin receptor gene regulatory system. Science 274:1527–1531, 1996

Marks IM, Swinson RP, Basoglu M, et al: Alprazolam and exposure alone and combined in panic disorder with agoraphobia: a controlled study in London and Toronto. Br J Psychiatry 162:776–787, 1993

Mayberg HS: Modulating dysfunctional limbic-cortical circuits in depression: towards development of brain-based algorithms for diagnosis and optimised treatment. Br Med Bull 65:193–207, 2003

McCullough JP: Cognitive Behavioral Analysis System of Psychotherapy: Treatment of Chronic Depression. New York, Guilford, 2000

Miller IW, Norman WH, Keitner GI, et al: Cognitive-behavioral treatment of depressed inpatients. Behav Ther 20:25–47, 1989

Mitchell JE, Peterson CB, Myers T, et al: Combining pharmacotherapy and psychotherapy in the treatment of patients with eating disorders. Psychiatr Clin North Am 24:315–323, 2001

Murphy GE, Simons AD Wetzel RD, et al: Cognitive therapy and pharmacotherapy: singly and together in the treatment of depression. Arch Gen Psychiatry 41:33–41, 1984

Newman CF, Leahy RL, Beck AT, et al: Bipolar Disorder: A Cognitive Therapy Approach. Washington, DC, American Psychological Association, 2002

Otto MW, Deckersbach T: Cognitive-behavioral therapy for panic disorder, in Panic Disorder and Its Treatment. Edited by Rosenbaum JF, Pollack MH. New York, Marcel Dekker, 1998, pp 181–203

Otto MW, Pollack MH, Sabatino SA: Maintenance of remission following cognitive-behavioral therapy for panic disorder: possible deleterious effects of concurrent medication treatment. Behav Ther 27:473–482, 1996

Pampallona S, Bollini P, Tibaldi G, et al: Combined pharmacotherapy and psychological treatment for depression: a systematic review. Arch Gen Psychiatry 61:714–719, 2004

Pezawas L, Meyer-Lindenberg A, Drabant EM, et al: 5-HTTLPR polymorphism impacts human cingulate-amygdala interactions: a genetic susceptibility mechanism for depression. Nat Neurosci 8:828–834, 2005

Ricca V, Mannucci E, Succhi T, et al: Cognitive-behavioural therapy for bulimia nervosa and binge eating disorder: a review. Psychother Psychosom 69:287–295, 2000

Schwartz JM, Stoessel PW, Baxter LR Jr, et al: Systematic changes in cerebral glucose metabolic rate after successful behavior modification treatment of obsessive-compulsive disorder. Arch Gen Psychiatry 53:109–113, 1996

Seligman ME: The effectiveness of psychotherapy: the Consumer Reports study. Am Psychol 50:965–974, 1995

Thase ME: Recent developments in the pharmacotherapy of depression, in Psychiatric Clinics of North America Annual of Drug Therapy, Vol 7. Philadelphia, PA, WB Saunders, 2000, pp 151–171

Thase ME, Howland RH: Refractory depression: relevance of psychosocial factors and therapies. Psychiatr Ann 24:232–240, 1994

Walsh BT, Wilson GT, Loeb KL, et al: Medication and psychotherapy in the treatment of bulimia nervosa. Am J Psychiatry 154:523–531, 1997

Wilson GT: Cognitive behavior therapy for eating disorders: progress and problems. Behav Res Ther 37 (suppl 1):S79–S95, 1999

Wright JH: Combined cognitive therapy and pharmacotherapy, in Contemporary Cognitive Therapy. Edited by Leahy R. New York, Guilford, 2004, pp 341–366

Wright JH, Thase ME: Cognitive and biological theories: a synthesis. Psychiatr Ann 22:451–458, 1992

Wright J, Basco MR, Thase ME: Learning Cognitive-Behavior Therapy: An Illustrated Guide. Washington, DC, American Psychiatric Publishing, 2006

Yu YW, Tsai SJ, Chen TJ, et al: Association study of the serotonin transporter promoter polymorphism and symptomatology and antidepressant response in major depressive disorders. Mol Psychiatry 7:1115–1119, 2002

Suggested Readings

Friedman ES, Wright JH, Jarrett RB, et al: Combined cognitive therapy and medication for mood disorders. Psychiatric Annals 36:320–329, 2006

Gabbard GO: The rationale for combining medication and psychotherapy. Psychiatric Annals 36:314–319, 2006

Hollifield M, Mackey A, Davidson J: Integrating therapies for anxiety disorders. Psychiatric Annals 36:329–340, 2006

Lipsitt DR, Starcevic V: Psychotherapy and pharmacotherapy in the treatment of somatoform disorders. Psychiatric Annals 36:341–353, 2006

Oldham JM: Integrated treatment for borderline personality disorder. Psychiatric Annals 36:361, 2006

Riba MB, Tasman A: Psychodynamic perspective on combining therapies. Psychiatric Annals 36:353–361, 2006

PART 3

Individual Interpersonal Psychotherapy

Section Editor
John C. Markowitz, M.D.

Chapter 10

Theory of Interpersonal Psychotherapy

Joshua D. Lipsitz, Ph.D.

Since the publication of the original interpersonal therapy (IPT) text (Klerman et al. 1984), little attention has been paid to clarifying the unique conceptual approach of IPT. This is no accident. IPT was devised with a clear emphasis on clinical utility and practical efficacy rather than theory (Weissman 2006). Its advocates have tried to retain focus on IPT technique and on efficacy research. However, inattention to theoretical issues has led to some confusion about the conceptual boundaries of IPT and how this treatment contrasts with other commonly used psychotherapies (Markowitz et al. 1998). It has also been suggested that lack of elaboration on IPT's conceptual approach may impede broader dissemination—as practitioners are unsure what distinguishes IPT from other approaches (Stuart 2006).

In this chapter I trace the theoretical roots of IPT. In the first section I review interpersonal theory. I then attempt, in the second section, to clarify how the interpersonal approach evolved into IPT. A common source of confusion is that IPT is contrasted with psychodynamic therapies of a more classic Freudian approach. However, IPT also differs in important ways from other forms of interpersonally oriented therapy, such as those that fall within the psychoanalytic tradition, and in the third section I specify these distinctions.

Interpersonal Theory of Psychopathology

The Psychobiology of Adolf Meyer

Although interpersonal theory is most commonly identified with the work of Harry Stack Sullivan, IPT's pluralistic approach traces its lineage more directly to the work of Adolf Meyer. One of Sullivan's strongest influences, Meyer was a leading figure in American psychiatry in the first half of the twentieth century. He was steeped in the Kraepelinian medical-nosological approach, which was the predominant orientation of American psychiatry in the 1920s. However, he was also influenced by the American philosophical school of pragmatism, which emphasized observable behavior, and by the emerging field of social science.

Meyer espoused an integrative approach to psychopathology, which he called *psychobiology*, also referred to as the *genetic-dynamic approach* (Winters 1951). This approach combined the traditional medical psychiatry of Emil Kraepelin with the broader perspectives of psychology and social science. For example, the psychologist William James (1890) saw the human being as having a wide range of instincts, including playfulness, curiosity, and sociability. George Herbert Mead (1934) had posited that the individual is a product of the social environment. Charles Cooley's theory of social subjectivity went even further in seeing society and the individual as virtually inseparable (Cooley 1902).

Meyer's integrative approach contrasted with both the narrowly biological approach of Kraepelin and the purely intrapsychic emphasis of Freud. Meyer insisted that he was interested in "the function of the total person" (Winters 1951). Meyer accepted Kraepelin's notion that psychopathology occurs within the biological organism. However, he dramatically broadened the field of view by emphasizing how the organism adapts to its environment. Taking a page from social Darwinism, Meyer saw the social-interpersonal environment as the most important locus of the individual's adaptation.

Meyer's clinical approach also showed the influences of the pragmatist school. Meyer attached great importance to detailed empirical observation. In his observations, he attended with equal energy to psychosocial and biological factors. Meyer devised a system using a detailed chronological life chart, which incorporated both biological and psychosocial components of the patient's history. Another important contribution from Meyer was his focus on the *here and now* of the therapeutic interview. Finally, he explicitly described the importance of the human aspect of contact between the patient and therapist (Sullivan 1954), anticipating the concept of the therapeutic alliance.

Harry Stack Sullivan and Interpersonal Psychoanalysis

Harry Stack Sullivan, the most influential figure in the development of the interpersonal theory of psychopathology, is often credited with bridging the gap between psychiatry and social science. Sullivan was influenced by the thinking of Meyer and by another interpersonally minded psychiatrist, William Alanson White. Completing his medical education in Chicago, Sullivan had close contact with members of the Chicago school of philosophy and social science, and his thinking was deeply influenced by the work of such individuals as George Herbert Mead, Charles Cooley, and Edward Sapir. Whereas Meyer presented an interpersonally informed alternative to the psychoanalysis of Freud, Sullivan revolutionized psychoanalysis itself by creating an entirely new interpersonal approach to psychoanalytic work. This approach, which remains an influential strain within psychoanalysis to this day, focuses on relationships rather than drives as the most basic and important aspect of human experience.

Sullivan saw the human being as intrinsically and unavoidably interpersonal. "The field of psychiatry is the field of interpersonal relations; a person can never be isolated from the complex of interpersonal relations in which the person lives and has his being" (Sullivan 1940, p. 10). According to Sullivan, the need for interpersonal relations is not secondary to more basic biological needs: it is itself the individual's most basic and important need. Mental health thus depends on healthy connections to other people. Psychopathology is also, at its core, the study of human relationships. The journal that Sullivan helped found was named the *Journal of the Biology and Pathology of Interpersonal Relations* (later retitled *Psychiatry*).

Consistent with psychoanalytic theory, Sullivan's approach viewed psychopathology as inseparable from personality. Psychopathology occurs when there is a problem with optimal personality development. Thus Sullivan developed an interpersonal theory of development, emphasizing the importance of interpersonal experience in infancy and childhood. According to Sullivan, the developing infant has two sets of needs. The first set includes the need for satisfaction, which relates initially to basic biological needs such as hunger. As the infant develops, however, satisfaction pertains with equal valence to emotional-relational needs. Sullivan saw the developmental phases as organized around specific emotional needs of each phase:

from 1 year to 4 years of age the youngster needs adults to witness and approve of his or her activities; from 4 years to 8 years of age the youngster needs playmates with whom to compete and cooperate; from age 8 to adolescence the youngster looks for a "chum," a close friend of the same sex; and from adolescence onward, the individual seeks an intimate heterosexual relationship (Sullivan 1972).

Psychopathology, according to Sullivan, is more closely tied to a second type of need, the need for security. The individual requires a sense of safety and competence in the interpersonal sphere, especially in response to the looming threat of interpersonal anxiety. Sullivan's view was that anxiety does not stem from frustration of biological needs but is introduced through the interpersonal relationship—namely through the mother's (contagious) experience of anxiety. The mother's anxiety may be a response to the infant's behavior but may also be unrelated to the infant and his or her needs. Because of the infant's intense investment in this relationship, the mother's anxiety is passed to the infant and assumes great importance. According to Sullivan, this contagious anxiety lies at the core of psychopathological development. Psychopathology's derivative negative emotions are thus caused by the emotional atmosphere in the person's earliest interactions (Sullivan 1953).

In response to the need for security, the individual implements *security operations*, a concept loosely related to Freud's *defense mechanisms*. When behavior receives a positive response from the mother, associated feelings are experienced as a desirable part of the self ("good me"). An anxious reaction from the mother may lead to internal feelings being experienced as undesirable ("bad me") or even untenable ("not me"). These feelings are dissociated, leading to personality dysfunction. Common security operations include selective inattention (the tendency to avoid noticing certain things to avoid experiencing anxiety), sublimation, and obsessionalism (Sullivan 1953, pp. 161–164).

Importance of Social Roles

Influenced by the work of Mead and Cooley, Sullivan emphasized the importance of social roles and reactions of others in shaping the individual. Sullivan wrote that the self is made up of *reflected appraisals* (Sullivan 1940, p. 22). Thus it is not only interpersonal behavior per se but also the person's place within the social environment that is important. In contrast with social psychology, which emphasizes the impact of society in general and social institutions, Sullivan's approach focuses mostly on close individual relationships, such as those in the nuclear family, the extended family, the peer group, and the workplace.

Schizophrenia and the Therapeutic Community

Sullivan's own clinical work focused largely on schizophrenia. For many years, he ran a schizophrenia ward in the Sheppard and Enoch Pratt Hospital in Baltimore, Maryland. Sullivan saw schizophrenia as essentially a disorder in the ability to relate to other people. He believed schizophrenia could be reversed with proper psychotherapy aimed at integrating cut-off aspects of the patient's internal life. Sullivan (1929) argued that even the most bizarre psychotic content makes sense when considered within the interpersonal context of the patient's life. If schizophrenia is viewed as an interpersonal disorder, it follows that the patient's condition would be influenced by social factors, including those of the patient's current hospital surroundings. Therefore, Sullivan paid attention to many details in the overall social milieu for patients. This later came to be called the *therapeutic community*.

The goal of therapy, according to Sullivan, is to help the patient improve negative interpersonal patterns and integrate dissociated aspects of personality. Primary goals are to identify and elucidate interpersonal patterns in which distortions occur and to explore their origins in interactions with significant people in the patient's past. Identifying negative patterns involves analyzing patterns of communication and subtleties of language. Clinical observation most keenly focuses on interpersonal patterns as they emerge, and the patterns are analyzed within the therapeutic relationship.

Therapist Stance

An essential component of Sullivan's theory concerns the therapist's role within therapy or the psychiatric interview. On one hand, Sullivan felt it was important for the therapist to assume the role of expert. This would inspire the patient's respect in the clinician's competence and confidence, and motivate the patient to continue the therapeutic process. However, this expert role did not imply aloofness on the part of the therapist. The therapist was to be a *participant-observer* in the relationship (Sullivan 1954, pp. 18–24). Sullivan saw the therapeutic relationship as not unlike any other relationship, in which all interactions are reciprocal and in which the therapist's own personal qualities, unconscious material, and so forth necessarily influence interactions. This perspective contrasted with the then-prevailing psychoanalytic view that the therapist should try to remain objective (a "blank screen") by not letting his or her own personal psychological baggage influence therapy. Sullivan also challenged the passive therapist stance commonly used to facilitate free association. Because Sullivan was interested in real events and real interactions (in addition to unconscious processes), he advocated the use of direct inquiry (Sullivan 1954).

The Interpersonal School of Psychoanalysis

Sullivan spawned the interpersonal school of psychoanalysis, which remains an influential approach to this day. Three of the most prominent figures in this school of thought were Frieda Fromm-Reichmann, Karen Horney, and Erich Fromm. Following Sullivan's lead, Frieda Fromm-Reichmann practiced and taught interpersonal psychoanalysis to treat patients with schizophrenia at the famed Chestnut Lodge in Rockville, Maryland (Fromm-Reichmann 1960). Karen Horney focused on the interpersonal understanding of prevalent neurotic reactions (Horney 1950). She emphasized the oppressive cost to the individual of forced, artificial social roles, which people embrace in order to maintain approval and acceptance. Erich Fromm focused on interpersonal relationships within the broader culture, seeing pathological interpersonal relationships as pervasive in modern society. According to Fromm (1941), individuals become stuck in infantile, often destructive, interpersonal patterns and cling to these patterns for fear of facing being alone and to avoid the existential burden of independence.

Object Relations

The British school of object relations, another influential strain within psychoanalysis, also identifies human relationships as the most important arena of human experience and the primary focus of psychotherapy. However, as the term *object* suggests, this approach involves a more abstract view of the patient's internal representations of the other person in a relationship and of the self.

Early theorists of this school, such as Melanie Klein (1935), tied their thinking closely to Freud's drive theory and focused predominantly on imagined representative relationships within fantasy rather than on real relationships. However, some later adherents gave greater emphasis to real relationships. W.R.D. Fairbairn, for example, suggested that personality problems arise when the infant's needs for attachment meet with absent, intrusive, or chaotic parents (Fairbairn 1952). Not unlike interpersonal psychoanalysis, object relations therapy might examine both external relationships and the therapeutic relationship to uncover faulty internal templates and eventually ameliorate problematic interpersonal patterns. Given the understanding that detrimental effects are caused by deficiencies in early nurturing, D.W. Winnicott (1965) proposed that psychotherapy may also serve as a "corrective emotional experience" in which the therapist, through a caring, empathic relationship, helps compensate for lack of nurturance in earlier relationships.

Attachment and Loss

John Bowlby, whose background was in psychoanalytic object relations, is most responsible for bringing the concept of attachment in normal and abnormal development into prominence. Bowlby (1969) saw attachment as a complex, biologically determined system designed to keep the caregiver in close proximity. He observed that youngsters often seek out parents as a safe haven in times of distress and that attachment serves as a base from which to launch goal-oriented behaviors. Thus a secure attachment early in life forms a foundation for later success in interpersonal relationships. Although the survival function of attachment is most acute in infancy, the system remains essential throughout life, providing individuals with warmth, nurturance, and protection through relationships. In the object relations tradition, Bowlby emphasized "internal working models" that the child develops based on early experiences. These models guide expectations, and thus interpersonal behaviors, in future relationships.

One insight into the importance of attachment came from observing what happens when an infant is separated from his or her caregiver. Building on observations of René Spitz and Katherine Wolf (1946) and their own systematic observations of youngsters separated from caregivers, Bowlby and James Robertson described a predictable sequence of strong emotional responses. First the separated infant *protests*, a stage characterized by overt distress and increased motor activity; then *despairs*, which involves crying and reduced motor activity; and finally shows *detachment*, withdrawing and seeming to lose interest in other people (Bowlby 1969).

Bowlby saw emotional difficulties as originating from early disturbances in attachment: all anxiety is, at its core, anxiety about separation. Bowlby's work was later expanded by Mary Ainsworth (1979) and others, who conceptualized different *attachment styles* with which individuals approach and negotiate relationships. These internal templates are determined by the success or failure of early attachment experiences. They include *secure*, *anxious-ambivalent*, and *avoidant* attachment styles, which help determine the quality of later adult relationships.

Real Relationships Versus Intrapsychic Factors

Sullivan's interpersonal psychoanalysis and the object relations approaches firmly established interpersonal relationships as the primary subject matter for psychotherapeutic work. To varying degrees these approaches focus attention on the patient's real relationships outside of therapy. They all see internal factors—in the form of experiential residue, object representations, internal working models, attachment styles, and so forth—as determinants of real interpersonal problems. Thus the patient's internal life and early childhood experiences that determined the internal life become the foci of the therapeutic work.

An individual may meet a new colleague and perceive himself or herself as helpless and flawed and the colleague as unrealistically powerful. This perception is due to the individual's internal experiences and may have originated in early contacts with a controlling parent. The internal template creates expectations and causes the individual to attend to some features of the interaction and not to others. Such internal factors also contribute to the real relationship's unfolding in a certain way. For example, this individual might be overly deferential to the new colleague. The colleague, influenced by this behavior and also by his or her own internal experiences, may respond by acting more like a supervisor than a colleague. Sullivan's interpersonal psychoanalysis and the object relations approaches dismiss the superficial handling of an interpersonal predicament as unlikely to have any lasting benefit for the patient.

From Interpersonal Theory to Interpersonal Psychotherapy

Interpersonal Theory of Depression

Because IPT was initially developed for the treatment of depression, its unique interpersonal approach was developed with the backdrop of important theoretical developments in the understanding of depression and the impact of interpersonal factors on this disorder. Interpersonal and object relations psychoanalytic approaches conceptualized depression as a fluid outgrowth of (dysfunctional) personality development. Sullivan himself related depression to repetitive patterns and internal vulnerabilities and rejected the depressed patient's attempts to tie the depression to a contemporaneous external event (Sullivan 1940). Cohen and colleagues (1954), of the interpersonal school, suggested that severe depression stems from having had a parent who resisted the child's move to independence and put excessive pressure on the child to achieve. They suggested that this led to dependency on the parent and alienation from peers, who were seen as competitors. Others (Fairbairn 1952; Klein 1935) theorized that depression results from early experiences of intense anger toward the frustrating but all-important internalized representation of the mother, and that this anger engendered feelings of ambivalence, guilt, helplessness, and ultimately depression.

Interpersonal Problem Areas in Interpersonal Therapy

The therapeutic work of IPT is organized around one (or possibly two) central interpersonal problem area in the patient's life. In acute treatment for depression, the problem areas can be classified as *role transitions* (associated with stressful life events), *grief*, *role disputes* (e.g., in marriage), or *interpersonal deficits* (lack of social support). In this section I briefly examine the conceptual basis for linking depression to these overall areas of interpersonal life.

Stressful Life Events and Depression

By the time of IPT's conception, a growing body of evidence indicated that recent stressful life events are associated with the onset of depression. Thus it is not necessary to trace the origins of internal distress and vulnerability to adverse experiences in infancy as in interpersonal psychoanalysis. A patient's distress could be caused by painful or challenging experiences in adulthood. Paykel et al. (1969), for example, noted that certain types of events were more frequently reported prior to onset of depression—particularly "exit events," such as death of a loved one or separation from a spouse, and "negative" events such as physical illness, work-related problems, or sexual difficulties. Brown and Harris (1978), in their study of women working outside the home, also observed that stressful life events were associated with depression.

A great deal of research on stressful life events and depression has been conducted since IPT was first formulated (Hammen 2005). In this time, the challenges and limitations of life-events research have become more evident. Some research indicates that a significant proportion of life events are caused by genetic (Kendler and Karkowski-Shuman 1997) or other personal (Hammen 2006) factors. Furthermore, stressful life events seem to be more prominent in the first episode of depression than in subsequent episodes (Kendler et al. 2000). However, the overall evidence from this now-extensive body of research indicates that life events are associated with the onset of depression, and this is particularly so for events of loss and separation (Paykel 2003). In IPT this complexity is not particularly troubling because stressful events are not presumed to "cause" depression; it is merely posited that illness episodes and life events are linked.

IPT Problem Area: Role Transition

Although specific stressful experiences are relevant to other IPT problem areas (shown below) in the broadest sense, adjusting to stress and change in the social context requires a role transition. This might be the case in depression following college graduation, the birth of a child, retirement, medical illness, divorce, and so forth.

Bereavement and Depression

Freud's "Mourning and Melancholia" (1917[1915]) highlighted specific differences between grief reactions and clinical depression in the context of other obvious similarities. Lindemann's (1944) careful description of a large sample of bereaved individuals as having somatic distress, preoccupation with the deceased, guilt, and anger (all common symptoms of depression) reinforced the association between bereavement and clinical depression. Years later, Paykel et al.'s (1969) study showed that although bereavement was a common stressor prior to depression, the majority of people who experienced bereavement did not subsequently become depressed. Similarly, Clayton (1982) found that a large majority of bereaved women did not go on to develop clinical depression. However, specific factors (e.g., younger age) make clinical depression more likely to occur in those who are bereaved. Depression may also be more likely to occur among bereaved individuals with poor social support (Maddison and Walker 1967).

IPT Problem Area: Grief

IPT's developers reasoned that bereavement is a potential precursor of clinical depression. Development of clinical depression following a death is evidence that the normal grief process did not take place and that the individual has had an abnormal (i.e., delayed or prolonged) grief reaction. In such cases the work of IPT is to help the patient experience the normal grief process. IPT for treating grief differs from IPT for treating other problem areas in its substantially internal focus, at least in the initial stages. The goal is to resolve a problem in a real relationship. However, the relationship is with the deceased, and resolution means working through the grief reactions, letting go, and learning to move on.

Marriage and Depression

Weissman and Paykel (1974) identified interpersonal factors that characterized depressed women. They found marital and family difficulties were the most prominent feature among depressed women. Furthermore, they found that these difficulties often persisted after the depression improved, suggesting that the problems were not simply a result of the patient's depressed mood. Marital difficulties were also associated with depression in the study by Brown and Harris (1978). Subsequent research has supported the association of marital discord and depression (Downey and Coyne 1990; Hammen 2003; Hooley and Teasdale 1989). The negative effects of marital conflict on mood may result from the direct emotional impact of negative emotions such as anger, resentment, guilt, and distrust. However, increased vulnerability to depression may also be a result of the lack of a supportive, cohesive relationship and the buffering role such a relationship would provide. Although there is some evidence that depression may engender marital problems, evidence also suggests that external factors (e.g., the depressed individual's spouse's own personality issues) contribute to marital difficulties.

IPT Problem Area: Role Dispute

A role dispute can occur in any important relationship. However, the relationship that is most commonly the focus of treatment is the patient's relationship with his or her spouse or significant other. Disputes with life partners provide a compelling and clinically ubiquitous model of the potentially devastating and pervasive effects of a role dispute.

Depression and Social Support

One of the important contributions of Brown and Harris (1978) was their consideration of lasting features of the social context, including positive, potentially buffering features, in determining whether depression would occur. In their study of working women, lack of a close confidant was a strong risk factor for later depression. Around this time, Henderson and colleagues' pioneering work identified the association between weak social bonds or a poor social support network and neurosis (much of which was depression) (Henderson et al. 1978). Since then, numerous studies have documented a link between poor social support and depressive symptoms (Duer et al. 1988; Monroe et al. 1986). However, there are methodological challenges in these studies, and causal pathways are not entirely clear. Social supports may serve to buffer the effects of adversity, or they may serve as an independent positive factor that is important to psychological health (Overholser and Adam 1997). Conversely, loneliness itself may be a risk factor for depression (Dill and Anderson 1999; Green et al. 1992).

IPT Problem Area: Interpersonal Deficits

In interpersonal deficits, the patient's primary problem is seen as a paucity of social connections. Relationships buffer the individual against stressful life events and are essential to psychological well-being. As such, the primary goal is to enhance the level of social connection through concrete positive changes in the patient's social activities (e.g., joining a club, taking a class). Attention to social support and a positive social network is also a component of work in the other IPT problem areas. In a role transition, the individual may need to renegotiate or start new relationships in order to obtain needed support within the new role. In a role dispute, the individual may need to reach out positively to others—aside from the other person in the dispute—to navigate and successfully resolve the dispute.

Impact of Depression on Interpersonal Relationships

Many clinicians have recognized that interacting with depressed patients often affects other people, including the therapist. Although depression initially may evoke sympathy, its excessive dependency and helplessness sometimes leaves others frustrated or angry, which may cause them to withdraw from the depressed person. Some commentators have taken a decidedly unsympathetic view of the depressive mode of interacting, interpreting it as evidence of veiled hostility (Bonime 1976).

Coyne (1976) proposed an interactional theory of depression in which the depressed individual seeks reassurance from others close to him or her but is unable to accept the reassurance. This creates a cycle of excessive reassurance-seeking by the depressed person and increased frustration and irritation in the other person, ultimately leading the other to avoid the depressed individual. The depressed individual thereby experiences increased isolation and decreased social connections, which together contribute to maintaining the depressive state. A more behavioral theory by Lewinsohn (1974) proposes that depressed individuals lack the necessary social skills to meet their needs for social warmth and approval. Therapy then involves helping patients develop social skills sufficient to meet their interpersonal needs.

Interpersonal Psychotherapy Versus Interpersonal Psychoanalytic Therapy

How does IPT differ from interpersonal and relational models of psychoanalytic therapy? IPT embraces Sullivan's overall focus on human relationships as essential to understanding psychopathology. It incorporates many important innovations from the interpersonal approach such as attention to the here and now, acknowledgment of the importance of the real relationship between therapist and patient, and analysis of communication as one part of the therapeutic process. In IPT it is appreciated that earlier relationships may color current experiences—for example, as Freud (1917[1915]) noted, earlier losses may predispose a person to complicated bereavement following later loss of a significant other—and that it is important to consider them in addressing the interpersonal problems in the here and now of a patient's life. However, IPT differs from the interpersonal psychoanalytic approach in several key respects, as described below. We are presenting these points with regard to depression, but most apply equally to other Axis I disorders for which IPT is used.

1. **Salience of the current interpersonal context.** In IPT it is presumed that current/recent interpersonal events, experiences, and pre-

dicaments are important and meaningful at face value and may cause distress regardless of the patient's early history, personality, or vulnerabilities. The IPT therapist takes an initial inventory of past experiences and considers interpersonal patterns to gain a deeper understanding of current problems. However, the work of IPT is largely about helping patients "fix the problem," which includes their emotional feelings about the current problem. The interpersonal work in IPT is not aimed at unconscious or characterological problems. IPT does not address potent representations of past important figures (Sullivan 1953), internal object relations (Fairbairn 1952; Klein 1935), attachment style (Ainsworth 1979), attributional style (Seligman et al. 1984), or interpersonal schemas (Young 1990).

It is hoped that for some patients, successfully negotiating the current interpersonal problem may help change their interpersonal trajectory and that this may impact positively on lasting internal feelings and patterns. In fact, there is some evidence that longer (maintenance) IPT may ameliorate some personality problems (Cyranowski et al. 2004). However, this is neither an explicit goal nor a necessary criterion for the success of IPT.

2. **Amelioration of symptoms of depression as an explicit goal of the therapy.** In IPT, improving interpersonal functioning is a goal, but also a means to achieving another, perhaps more urgent, goal: decreasing symptoms of depression. If the patient resolves the interpersonal problem but the depression does not resolve, the therapy is not considered successful, and the therapist proposes another antidepressant treatment option.

3. **Depression as a clinical disorder.** In IPT, depression is conceptualized as a clinical syndrome, which is distinct from the patient's overall personality. IPT's development coincided with the growth of psychiatric epidemiology and the development of the systematic diagnostic criteria of DSM-III (American Psychiatric Association 1980).

> One of the major characteristics of IPT for depression is that it approaches depression as a clinical disorder. The justification for this is not only the widespread prevalence of depression but also the therapeutic importance of providing patients with a diagnostic label and legitimizing their assumption of the "sick role." Since this approach places IPT within the broad definition of the medical model, it is thus a different approach from that of many psychotherapists. In the psychotherapeutic community there has been an anti-diagnostic bias and a tendency to depreciate symptoms. We feel this approach is in error, both theoretically and therapeutically. (Klerman et al. 1984, p. 37)

4. **Giving the patient the sick role.** If depression is a disorder that is not under the patient's control and leads to negative effects on relationships, then it is appropriate to "blame" the disorder rather than the patient for some of the patient's current difficulties, to validate the patient's feelings of helplessness and disability—but not self-blame—and to sympathize with the challenges of this difficult predicament. This approach contrasts with psychoanalytic and, often, cognitive approaches, which seek to identify the patient's role in bringing about current difficulties.

5. **Pragmatic connection between life events and mood regardless of the temporal direction of the link.** In IPT the focus is on the link between the depressive mood episode as an illness and current life events, but the connection is a two-way street. Life events may trigger depression in susceptible individuals, a temporal relationship as recognized in earlier interpersonal theory. But IPT therapists also recognize that negative life events may arise as a consequence of the depressive illness: depressed individuals have more negative life events once they are depressed. The IPT therapist makes a pragmatic connection between life events and mood regardless of the temporal direction of the link.

6. **The multiple causes of depression.** Within the broader context of the medical model, it is presumed in IPT that depression arises from a variety of causes. It is not presumed that IPT undoes or corrects the problem that initially "caused" the disorder. Indeed, the assumption is that there is no single cause, that the problem is multifactorial.

> With regard to etiology, the pluralistic point of view maintains that no single cause in itself can explain depression. Genetics, early life experience, environmental stress, and personality combine in complex ways to produce the etiology and pathogenesis of depression. These factors will operate in different degrees for individual patients. (Klerman et al. 1984, p. 38)

7. **Importance of explaining the diagnosis and treatment.** In IPT it is maintained that diagnosing and explaining the disorder provide reassurance and encouragement to the patient and help enlist his or her motivation and collaboration in the treatment plan. Instilling hope and mobilizing the patient's positive expectations have been found to be a powerful predictor of psychotherapy's success (Frank 1973). This approach is indeed consistent with Sullivan's overall recommendations regarding the expert role of the therapist (Sullivan 1954). However, it is avoided in other psychodynamic approaches because it focuses too much on symptoms and requires too active a stance from the therapist, interfering with the unfolding of transference.

8. **Influence of depression on both the interpersonal environment and patterns associated with personality.** Once we accept that depression is a clinical disorder and not merely an expression of dysfunctional personality, it becomes important to consider the interactive and reciprocal relationship between depression and interpersonal relationships. One reason the focus in IPT is not on personality is because it is difficult to determine during a depressive episode which aspects of the patient's current functioning are part of the patient's personality and which are associated with depression.

9. **Time-limited therapy.** In IPT the time-limited approach is seen not as a concession or limitation but as the most appropriate and ethical approach for patients with an acute debilitating disorder. In order for the therapist to enlist motivation and instill hope, it is helpful for patients to see the light at the end of the tunnel. In light of the efficacy of antidepressant medications in the 1950s and 1960s, some clinicians began to question the propriety of keeping patients in psychotherapy for long periods of time with no evidence of improvement.

10. **Limiting of goals of therapy.** Within the limited time frame, it is necessary to limit the goals of therapy. Although goal-oriented therapy is now more common, IPT was a major departure from the type of therapy practiced by most therapists in the 1970s. The eminent interpersonally oriented psychiatrists Silvano Arieti and Jules Bemporad (1978) went so far as to object to IPT's use of the term *psychotherapy:* "Although literally correct, the therapy did not consist of an analysis of character defenses, unconscious cognitive contents, or transference manifestations" (p. 291). In psychoanalysis and much of psychodynamic therapy, the array of symptoms that constitute the patient's syndrome may be the presenting problem, but they are seen as related to deeper, persistent problems that need to be addressed. In IPT the value of broader therapy specifically aimed at modifying lasting maladaptive patterns is not discounted. The patient may be inclined to enter this kind of therapy once the acute disorder has improved. As mentioned above, maintenance forms of IPT may hold promise for these broader benefits.

11. **Limiting of the interpersonal problems that must be addressed for the patient's condition and disorder to improve.** In IPT the focus of therapy is limited to the most salient interpersonal problem areas. Therapists are sometimes struck by the pervasiveness of their patients' interpersonal problems and struggle to decide where to begin. In IPT the therapist is required to make a tactical decision to limit the focus to a problem that can be addressed and potentially improved within the brief (e.g., 12-week) course of acute therapy. It is hoped that this work may also lead to other improvements, by inspiring the pa-

tient to take further positive steps in other areas, for example. However, many patients who successfully complete IPT will continue to have interpersonal problems.

12. **Avoidance of interpreting transference.** One of the most obvious distinctions of IPT within the broader interpersonal approach is that it avoids addressing transference during therapy. This is more out of respect for the compelling power of transference than out of ignorance of its importance. To achieve the goals of therapy, the IPT therapist vigorously maintains the focus on the current interpersonal problem—in the patient's life outside of therapy. Because the emphasis is more on the actual interpersonal problem than on the patient's interpersonal style or propensities, interpretation of transference has only secondary importance. Given the time limitations of IPT, the development, analysis, and working through of transference and bringing interpretations to bear on real life are seen as an ambitious and insurmountable task. Practically, there are situations in IPT in which the therapeutic relationship is used to help elucidate a current problem, but such use of the therapeutic relationship is generally kept to a minimum and does not become the central focus of the therapy.

Conclusion

Interpersonal psychotherapy traces its theoretical and clinical origins to the interpersonal approach of Adolf Meyer and the interpersonal psychoanalytic theory of Harry Stack Sullivan. IPT theory builds on other relational theories, including object relations theory, particularly with regard to the centrality of attachment. However, the theory of IPT is applied within a conceptual and clinical framework that differs significantly from that of Sullivan and much of relational theory. The goal of IPT is to treat depression and other disorders, and IPT theory conceptualizes the disorders as clinical entities that are distinct from the patient's overall personality. Acknowledging the importance of the patient's personality and early life experience, IPT pragmatically opts to narrow its focus to address one or two areas of interpersonal life that seem to require the most attention.

Key Points

- Interpersonal psychotherapy (IPT) is based on the interpersonal tradition of Adolf Meyer and Harry Stack Sullivan.

- IPT incorporates the medical model of psychopathology, which sees depression and other psychiatric disorders as illnesses distinct from the patient's personality.

- Partly because of the medical model, IPT's approach differs from that of interpersonal psychoanalytic therapy in several important ways.
- Research findings support IPT's linking of depression with current interpersonal problems (difficulties in marriage, inadequate social support, bereavement) rather than with problems exclusively related to early childhood.
- In IPT, psychopathology is viewed as arising from multiple causes, and not all of them need be addressed to achieve symptomatic improvement.

References

Ainsworth MDS: Attachment as related to mother-infant interaction, in Advances in the Study of Behavior, Vol 9. Edited by Rosenblatt JS, Hinde RA, Beer C, et al. New York, Academic Press, 1979, pp 1–51

American Psychiatric Association: Diagnostic and Statistical Manual of Mental Disorders, 3rd Edition. Washington, DC, American Psychiatric Association, 1980

Arieti S, Bemporad J: Severe and Mild Depression: The Psychotherapeutic Approach. New York, Basic Books, 1978

Bonime W: The psychodynamics of neurotic depression. J Am Acad Psychoanal 4:301–326, 1976

Bowlby J: Attachment and Loss, Vol 1: Attachment. New York, Basic Books, 1969

Brown GW, Harris T: Social Origins of Depression: A Study of Psychiatric Disorder in Women. New York, Free Press, 1978

Clayton PJ: Bereavement, in Handbook of Affective Disorders. Edited by Paykel ES. New York, Guilford, 1982, pp 403–415

Cohen MB, Blake G, Cohen RA, et al: An intensive study of twelve cases of manic-depressive psychosis. Psychiatry 17:103–138, 1954

Cooley CH: Human Nature and the Social Order (1902). New York, Schocken, 1964

Coyne JC: Toward an interactional description of depression. Psychiatry 39:28–40, 1976

Cyranowski JM, Frank E, Winter E, et al: Personality pathology and outcome in recurrently depressed women over 2 years of maintenance interpersonal psychotherapy. Psychol Med 34:659–669, 2004

Dill JC, Anderson CA: Loneliness, shyness, and depression: the etiology and interrelationships of everyday problems in living, in The Interactional Nature of Depression. Edited by Joiner T, Coyne JC. Washington, DC, American Psychological Association, 1999

Downey G, Coyne JC: Children of depressed parents: an integrative review. Psychol Bull 108:50–76, 1990

Duer S, Schwenk TL, Coyne JC: Medical and psychosocial correlates of self-reported depressive symptoms in family practice. J Fam Pract 27:609–614, 1988

Fairbairn WRD: An Object Relations Theory of the Personality. New York, Basic Books, 1952

Frank JD: Persuasion and Healing: A Comparative Study of Psychotherapy. Baltimore, MD, Johns Hopkins University Press, 1973

Freud S: Mourning and melancholia (1917[1915]), in The Standard Edition of the Complete Psychological Works of Sigmund Freud, Vol 14. Translated and edited by Strachey J. London, Hogarth Press, 1957, pp 237–260

Fromm E: Escape From Freedom. New York, Farrar & Rinehart, 1941

Fromm-Reichmann F: Principles of Intensive Psychotherapy. Chicago, IL, University of Chicago Press, 1960

Green BH, Copeland JR, Dewey ME, et al: Risk factors for depression in elderly people: a prospective study. Acta Psychiatr Scand 86:213–217, 1992

Hammen C: Interpersonal stress and depression in women. J Affect Disord 74:49–57, 2003

Hammen C: Stress and depression. Annu Rev Clin Psychol 1:293–319, 2005

Hammen C: Stress generation in depression: reflections on origins, research, and future directions. J Clin Psychol 62:1065–1082, 2006

Henderson S, Byrne DG, Duncan-Jones P, et al: Social bonds in the epidemiology of neurosis: a preliminary communication. Br J Psychiatry 132:463–466, 1978

Hooley JM, Teasdale JD: Predictors of relapse in unipolar depressives: expressed emotion, marital distress and perceived criticism. J Abnorm Psychol 98:229–235, 1989

Horney K: Neurosis and Human Growth. New York, WW Norton, 1950

James W: The Principles of Psychology (1890). New York, Dover, 1950

Kendler KS, Karkowski-Shuman L: Stressful life events and genetic liability to major depression: genetic control of exposure to the environment? Psychol Med 27:539–547, 1997

Kendler KS, Thornton LM, Garner CO: Stressful life events and previous episodes in the etiology of major depression in women: an evaluation of the "kindling" hypothesis. Am J Psychiatry 157:1243–1251, 2000

Klein M. A contribution to the psychogenesis of manic-depressive states (1935), in Contributions to Psychoanalysis, 1921–1945. New York, McGraw-Hill, 1964

Klerman GL, Weissman MM, Rounsaville BJ, et al: Interpersonal Psychotherapy of Depression. New York, Basic Books, 1984

Lewinsohn PM: A behavioral approach to depression, in The Psychology of Depression: Contemporary Theory and Research. Edited by Friedman RM, Katz MM. New York, Wiley, 1974, pp 157–185

Lindemann E: Symptomatology and management of acute grief. Am J Psychiatry 101:141–148, 1944

Maddison D, Walker WL: Factors affecting the outcome of conjugal bereavement. Br J Psychiatry 113:1057–1067, 1967

Markowitz JC, Svartberg M, Swartz HA: Is IPT time-limited psychodynamic psychotherapy? J Psychother Pract Res 7:185–195, 1998

Mead GH: Mind, Self and Society. Chicago, IL, University of Chicago Press, 1934

Monroe S, Bromet E, Connel M, et al: Social support, life events, and depressive symptoms: a one-year prospective study. J Consult Clin Psychol 54:424–431, 1986

Overholser JC, Adam DM: Stressful life events and social support in depressed psychiatric inpatients, in Clinical Disorders and Stressful Life Events. Edited by Miller TW. Madison, CT, International Universities Press, 1997

Paykel ES: Life events and affective disorders. Acta Psychiatr Scand 108:61–66, 2003

Paykel ES, Myers JK, Dienelt MN, et al: Life events and depression: a controlled study. Arch Gen Psychiatry 21:753–760, 1969

Seligman ME, Peterson C, Kaszlow NJ, et al: Attributional style and depressive symptoms among children. J Abnorm Psychol 93:235–238, 1984

Spitz RA, Wolf KM: The smiling response: a contribution to the ontogenesis of social relations. Genet Psychol Monogr 34:57–125, 1946

Stuart S: Interpersonal psychotherapy. Psychiatr Ann 36:526–529, 2006

Sullivan HS: Research in schizophrenia. Am J Psychiatry 9:553–567, 1929

Sullivan HS: Conceptions of Modern Psychiatry (1940). New York, WW Norton, 1953

Sullivan HS: The Interpersonal Theory of Psychiatry. Edited by Perry HS, Gawel ML. New York, WW Norton, 1953

Sullivan HS: The Psychiatric Interview. Edited by Perry HS, Gawel ML. New York, WW Norton, 1954

Sullivan HS: Personal Psychopathology: Early Formulations. New York, WW Norton, 1972

Weissman MM: A brief history of interpersonal psychotherapy. Psychiatr Ann 36:553–557, 2006

Weissman MM, Paykel ES: The Depressed Woman: A Study of Social Relationships. Chicago, IL, University of Chicago Press, 1974

Winnicott DW: The Maturational Processes and the Facilitating Environment: Studies in the Theory of Emotional Development (1965). Madison, CT, International Universities Press, 1987

Winters EE (ed): The Collected Papers of Adolf Meyer. Baltimore, MD, Johns Hopkins University Press, 1951

Young JE: Cognitive Therapy for Personality Disorders: A Schema-Focused Approach, 3rd Edition. Sarasota, FL, Professional Resource Exchange, 1990

Suggested Readings

Bowlby J: Attachment and Loss, Vol 1: Attachment. New York, Basic Books, 1969

Brown GW, Harris T: Social Origins of Depression: A Study of Psychiatric Disorder in Women. New York, Free Press, 1978

Greenberg JR, Mitchell SA: Object Relations in Psychoanalytic Theory. Cambridge, MA, Harvard University Press, 1983

Joiner T, Coyne JC (eds): The Interactional Nature of Depression. Washington, DC, American Psychological Association, 1999

Klerman GL, Weissman MM, Rounsaville BJ, et al: Interpersonal Psychotherapy of Depression. New York, Basic Books, 1984

Sullivan HS: The Psychiatric Interview. Edited by Perry HS, Gawel ML. New York, WW Norton, 1954

Chapter 11

Techniques of Individual Interpersonal Psychotherapy

Holly A. Swartz, M.D.
John C. Markowitz, M.D.

Interpersonal psychotherapy (IPT) is a practical, intuitively reasonable treatment for depression that incorporates strategies used in general psychiatric practice and thus has face validity for practicing clinicians (Weissman et al. 2000, 2007). Readers new to IPT will find that much of what we describe below sounds familiar and overlaps with other psychotherapies. Therefore, on one level, IPT demands few novel skills from therapists and is relatively easy to learn.

This work was supported in part by grants from the National Institute of Mental Health (MH-64518 and MH-30915) and by a NARSAD Young Investigator Award (to Dr. Swartz).

The challenges of IPT lie not in any individual technique or strategy, but in organizing these approaches to establish and maintain a coherent primary treatment focus. Therapists comfortable with less structured approaches may initially find it difficult to organize sessions around a specific IPT focus and to eschew the temptations of digressing into extraneous clinical material. Moreover, therapists accustomed to more prescriptive treatments may struggle to balance the exploratory aspects of IPT with the need to stay focused. Additional challenges arise from "unlearning" reflexive responses from prior training experiences, such as transference-focused interventions (for psychodynamic therapists) or identification of automatic cognitions and schemas (for cognitive therapists).

In this chapter we focus on the basic strategies and techniques of IPT, highlighting aspects of treatment that, in our experience, challenge clinicians learning IPT. Beyond identifying common "IPT pitfalls" that therapists encounter, this chapter also clarifies, from a practical standpoint, the relationship of IPT to other psychotherapies described in this textbook. We focus on major depression, the first and still best-tested indication for IPT, though the same principles may apply to other disorders (see Chapter 12, "Applications of Individual Interpersonal Psychotherapy to Specific Disorders: Efficacy and Indications"). For additional information about IPT, readers are referred to the IPT manuals (Weissman et al. 2000, 2007).

Common Therapeutic Factors

The concepts and techniques of IPT are straightforward but require sophisticated application. IPT therapists take a warm, supportive, understanding, and encouraging stance. They pull for affect, focusing on patients' feelings in the context of discrete recent life events; they cheer patients' successes and commiserate with patients when there are setbacks. The therapist leans forward (unless the patient finds this intrusive), avoids abstractions, focuses on particulars, and fosters hope. Thus, IPT shares with many other psychotherapies so-called nonspecific factors that contribute to its efficacy (Frank 1971). For instance, IPT techniques may facilitate the therapeutic alliance that is crucial to good outcome (Krupnick et al. 1996), but it takes a caring and competent therapist to develop that alliance. The mechanical use of any psychotherapeutic technique is futile (Frank 1971).

Link Between Mood and Life Events

IPT spans two primary domains: the patient's current mood state and recent interpersonal experiences. IPT helps patients understand the connection between the two. Upsetting life events trigger depressive episodes in vulnerable individuals, and negative interpersonal encounters lower mood;

conversely, depressed mood impairs social functioning. The putative mechanism of IPT works so that as patients manage interpersonal experiences more effectively, mood improves (Markowitz et al. 2006). In an iterative fashion, improved mood then allows patients to manage interpersonal stressors more effectively. Thus, the sine qua non of IPT is constant attention to the link between mood and interpersonal life events. This theme recurs throughout treatment.

In the initial phase (see Table 11–1 later in this chapter), IPT serves to identify an interpersonal relationship or life event linked to the onset or maintenance of the patient's mood episode. In the intermediate phase (see Table 11–2), the therapist connects changes the patient is making in his or her life circumstances to their impact on mood, and vice versa. In IPT, *life events* refers to events taking place in the here and now (in contrast to the "there and then"). Unlike psychodynamic psychotherapy, IPT is not focused on early childhood experiences and long-standing familial dynamics. Thus, the patient's current mood state is linked to recent experiences rather than those rooted in the distant past. Nor does IPT focus on transferential events *within the office*, except in the relatively rare instance when problems arise in the therapeutic alliance. Consequently, the therapy highlights recent experiences *outside the office*.

Blame the Depression

Unlike most psychotherapies, the roots of IPT are in the medical tradition. Although many patients who receive IPT demonstrate marked improvements in interpersonal functioning (Weissman et al. 1979), self-efficacy (Grote et al. 2004), and maladaptive personality traits (Cyranowski et al. 2004), the fundamental goal of IPT is to resolve depressive episodes. Klerman and colleagues (1984) made the crucial observation that depression is an illness comparable with any other medical condition, such as hypertension, asthma, or the flu. Whereas patients with other medical diagnoses generally recognize that they are ill, depressed patients blame themselves. One therapeutic goal of IPT is to shift excessive guilt from the patient to the illness (or, alternatively, to the patient's environment). Without being disingenuous, the therapist seeks to "blame the depression" whenever the patient falters and credit the patient whenever he or she succeeds.

Therapists who employ IPT provide psychoeducation about depression, stressing its biological underpinnings and the fact that it is a very treatable illness—by medication, empirically validated psychotherapies, or their combination. IPT is likened to a "verbal pill" for depression, much as penicillin treats a bacterial infection. Using a stress-diathesis model to explain the interaction between biological vulnerability and stressful life events, therapists help patients to understand that they are not responsible (or to blame) for their illness but that they are in an excellent position to help themselves recover from depression. Statements such as those that follow serve to emphasize this perspective:

> It's very difficult to complete tasks and maintain relationships when you are depressed.
>
> Your depression makes it difficult for you to function as well as you would when you are feeling well.
>
> I am impressed that despite your depressive symptoms, you were able to confront your boss about your work schedule. And even though it didn't go as well as you would have liked—no doubt because the depression was interfering—it sounds like your mood did improve because you risked taking this important step.

Because guilt and low self-esteem are characteristic of depression, patients frequently blame themselves and think of themselves as "bad" when problems arise. Although many depressed patients report these negative cognitions, the therapist *does not* systematically question and evaluate the automatic negative thoughts. Unlike cognitive therapists, interpersonal therapists neither employ thought records nor weigh the evidence to help patients reevaluate negative cognitions. Instead, therapists shift blame to the illness, which often provides patients with an immediate feeling of relief. Therapists then capitalize on this transient mood improvement by encouraging patients to take positive steps toward resolving interpersonal problems.

Phases of Interpersonal Psychotherapy

IPT is a time-limited psychotherapy. As with any acute antidepressant treatment, its goal is to treat depression in a short time frame (typically, 12–16 sessions, depending on patient preference, insurance constraints, and the complexity of therapeutic issues, with subsequent transition to maintenance treatment or no treatment, depending on psychiatric history and post-IPT treatment needs). Thus, the patient and therapist understand from the outset that therapy will last for a predetermined interval and that its goal is symptomatic relief, to be achieved by resolving an interpersonal crisis. The time limit places pressure on both patient and therapist to act.

To keep treatment on track, the therapist must manage time strategically. Unlike open-ended therapy, IPT denies the therapist the luxury of allowing treatment to unfold spontaneously or over an indefinite duration. The therapist is obliged to watch the clock and redirect the patient, as necessary, to accomplish specified IPT goals within the allotted time frame. For the purposes of organizing the treatment, IPT is divided into three

TABLE 11–1.   Techniques of initial phase of interpersonal psychotherapy (IPT)

Goal	Technique
Make diagnosis.	Use psychiatric interview and assessment.
Systematically review depressive symptoms.	Assess with a standardized depression rating scale.
Induct the patient into the sick role and the medical model of depression.	Provide psychoeducation.
Evaluate interpersonal relationships.	Take an interpersonal inventory.
Select IPT problem area.	Construct an illness time line and take an interpersonal inventory.
Develop a treatment contract.	Make an IPT case formulation.
Provide hope.	Provide psychoeducation and maintain an optimistic therapeutic stance.

parts: initial phase, middle phase, and termination. Each phase has specific goals and a specific duration. The initial phase lasts up to 3 sessions; the middle phase occurs in 9–11 sessions, and the termination phase takes place over 2–3 sessions. The IPT therapist remains aware of the current phase of treatment—indeed, the exact session number—at every session.

Initial Phase

In the initial phase of treatment, a specific treatment focus is identified, IPT principles are outlined, and the time limit is established. Many novice IPT therapists find the numerous tasks of the initial phase the most difficult part of conducting IPT (see Table 11–1).

Making the Diagnosis

The first, most important step is to determine the patient's diagnosis. Using the medical model, the IPT therapist conducts a careful diagnostic interview to evaluate DSM-IV-TR (American Psychiatric Association 2000) or ICD-10 (World Health Organization 1992) syndromal illness. This process is both good clinical practice and familiar to mental health professionals who are comfortable eliciting a medical history, probing for psychiatric symptoms, ruling out medical confounds, and establishing diagnoses. We often tell psychiatry trainees that the first IPT session resembles an intake interview in the emergency room or on an inpatient unit. Much as a clinician would conduct a thorough psychiatric history in an intake setting, the IPT clinician asks about prior episodes of mood disorders, prior treatment experiences, medical history, history of manic symptoms, recent substance abuse, and the like. A family history, beyond assisting with diagnostic accuracy, helps the therapist build the argument for depression as a biological illness with a genetic component—demonstrated in the patient's own family.

Using a Standardized Rating Scale

A standardized rating scale is useful for evaluating the severity of a patient's depressive symptoms. The therapist readministers the same rating scale at regular intervals, providing an assessment of baseline severity against which to measure improvement.

> When you came in, you scored a 23; now you are at 10, which is almost in the "not depressed" range.

Standardized ratings help to educate patients about the symptoms of depression and confer validity to the construct of depression as a "real" illness that can be reliably assessed and quantified. Any standardized patient- or therapist-rated measure is acceptable. Examples include the Hamilton Rating Scale for Depression (Hamilton 1960), the Beck Depression Inventory–II (Beck 1996), and the Quick Inventory for Depressive Symptomatology (Rush et al. 2003).

Inducting the Patient Into the Sick Role

Parsons (1951) defined the *sick role* as a social role that absolves the patient from responsibilities that the illness precludes while presenting new responsibilities related to the illness. Following the medical model, the IPT therapist inducts the patient into the sick role by explaining that he or she is suffering from a medical illness—like influenza or diabetes—that may interfere with fulfilling social obligations such as entertaining friends, working every day (if the illness is very severe), or caring for an ailing relative. While offering a respite from these responsibilities, the therapist simultaneously confers upon the patient responsibility for self-care and illness management. The therapist uses psychoeducation to help the patient understand that depression is a "real" illness with clear biologic underpinnings and that, as with other medical illnesses, treatment is needed for recovery. The patient is responsible for regaining his or her health: attending therapy appointments, taking medications (if prescribed), and addressing the identified IPT problem area. This double-sided message not only relieves patients of unmanageable obligations but also serves to prioritize treatment.

The cornerstone of IPT case formulation is the interpersonal inventory. Conducted over the course of one or two sessions, the inventory is a careful review of the important people currently in the patient's life and the quality of his or her relationships. The goal is to determine available social supports and relationship difficulties that may be a cause or consequence of the depressive episode, and to understand the patient's handling of intimacy, self-assertion, and anger.

Taking an Interpersonal Inventory

Beginning with open-ended questions, the therapist asks progressively more directive questions, as needed, to obtain a complete picture of the patient's social relationships:

> Tell me about the important people in your life.
>
> In whom do you confide?
>
> How well do you get along with your coworkers?
>
> Tell me about your romantic partner(s).

Although IPT does not focus on early childhood experiences and relationships, the therapist asks about the family of origin and current relationships with family members as part of the interpersonal inventory.

The concept of nonreciprocal role expectations is important to IPT. This notion underscores that it is not expectations themselves that are problematic in relationships; rather, conflict arises when two individuals disagree about their expectations of one another. For instance, when a couple inhabits traditional gender roles in a marriage, conflict is unlikely if both agree on these social roles. Yet, conflict is very likely if expectations are nonreciprocal: for example, the husband wants a stay-at-home wife and the wife plans to pursue her career outside of the home. Thus, beyond understanding who is central to the patient's life, it is important to explore the nature of expectations within relationships. Therapists elicit this information by asking questions such as

> Are you satisfied in your relationship with your wife?
>
> Do you and your boss agree on job expectations?
>
> How do you and your partner handle financial decisions?
>
> What are sources of friction in your relationship? What happens when you disagree?

Providing Psychoeducation

The therapist initiates a process of psychoeducation that will continue throughout therapy. Psychoeducation provides information about the causes, course, and prevalence of unipolar depression. In IPT, psychoeducation also helps the patient to understand how the depressive episode interferes with interpersonal functioning and complicates the patient's efforts to resolve interpersonal problems.

Psychoeducation can have tremendous impact. It removes blame, conveys hope, and identifies the problem as time-limited. Given that depression is so widespread, psychoeducation also helps normalize and contextualize the patient's distress. The following are statements that could be offered to inform the patient about the prevalence of depression:

> This is a common problem [illness], and it is very treatable.
>
> One out of every five women will develop a depressive episode in her lifetime. You're in good company!

Like the assignment of the sick role, psychoeducation helps patients to understand the expectations and requirements for achieving improvement.

Constructing a Time Line

To determine the treatment focus, the therapist links the onset or maintenance of the depressive episode to events in the patient's interpersonal life. Sometimes this is straightforward (e.g., "I became depressed after my husband left me for another woman"). In more complex cases, it may be helpful to construct an illness time line with the patient. The time line charts the temporal sequence of mood changes and symptoms against changing relationships or life events, allowing therapist and patient to identify the links between them. The therapist may ask the patient to rate his or her mood at each time point on a scale of 1–10 (where 1 is the depths of depression and 10 is a normal or euthymic mood) to gauge the severity of mood symptoms over time. Figure 11–1 illustrates a time line showing that the patient's mood relates less to her pregnancy than to the relationship with her husband. Figure 11–2 is a blank time line that can be completed with a patient.

Selecting the IPT Problem Area and Making a Case Formulation

In IPT, the therapist selects one of four possible problem areas as the treatment focus: *grief, role transition, role dispute,* or *interpersonal deficits.* Using the information gathered in the interpersonal inventory and time line, the therapist selects a problem area that encompasses an event or relationship change temporally linked to the onset or persistence of the mood symptoms. When there is more than one reasonable option, the therapist suggests the problem area with maximal emotional valence for the patient. Occasionally, the therapist may opt to focus on two problem areas; however, every effort is made to choose a single problem area if possible.

The case formulation formally synthesizes the elements covered in the initial phase (Markowitz and Swartz 2007). The therapist reviews the patient's diagnosis, explicitly links the interpersonal problem area to the onset of the depressive episode, and obtains explicit agreement from the patient to focus on this problem area for the remainder of treatment:

> You began to experience financial problems 2 years ago, but your mood did not deteriorate until these problems forced you and your children to move back home with your parents. Although you continued to view yourself as an independent adult who sets the rules for your own children, your mother believes that while you live in her house, she has ultimate authority over your children. Because you feel indebted to your parents in this time of crisis, you are reluctant to argue with your mother about the rules she is setting for your kids. Yet, you disagree with her decisions, like her allowing them to watch a lot of TV and using candy treats to discipline them. You have been keeping these thoughts to yourself but feel very angry inside.
>
> Although the financial issues were very stressful, you were managing okay until the problems with your mother started. We call this struggle between you a role dispute. You and your mother disagree about how to handle your children and who's in charge where they're concerned. This dispute is clearly connected to your depression: the more your mother undermines your parental authority, the worse your mood gets.
>
> I suggest that we spend the next nine sessions focusing on this dispute. My bet is that as your relationship with your mother improves, so will your mood. How does that sound to you?

Providing Hope and Agreeing on a Treatment Contract

The initial phase ends with agreement on a formal treatment contract and the therapist's provision of hope. The therapist affirms the agreement to focus on the problem area identified in the case formulation and reviews the time frame of treatment. The therapist explicitly states, *"We will meet weekly an additional 12 times over the next 3 months to work through the role transition that you are experiencing."* In addition, the therapist reviews practical issues regarding treatment such as scheduling, fees, and policies about missed sessions.

Another component of IPT is to provide hope. Throughout treatment, the therapist reminds the patient that depression is a treatable illness and that although it may be hard to believe right now, he or she will, in all likelihood, get better. As the patient responds to IPT (and virtually all patients improve),

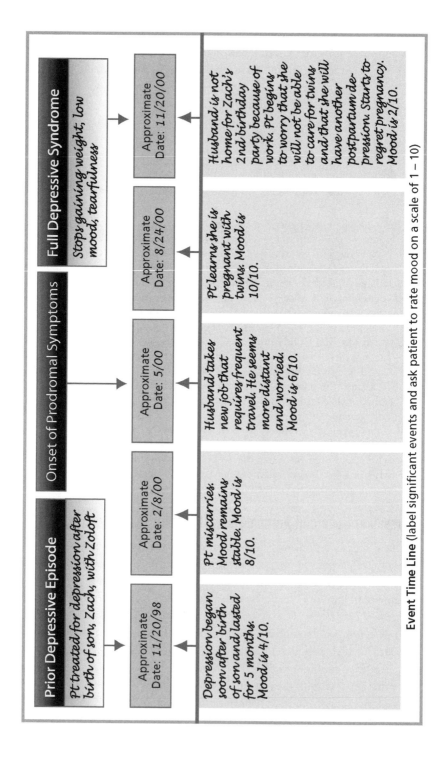

Prior Depressive Episode

Pt treated for depression after birth of son, Zach, with Zoloft

Onset of Prodromal Symptoms

Full Depressive Syndrome

Stops gaining weight; low mood, tearfulness

Approximate Date: 11/20/98

Approximate Date: 2/8/00

Approximate Date: 5/00

Approximate Date: 8/24/00

Approximate Date: 11/20/00

Depression began soon after birth of son and lasted for 5 months. Mood is 4/10.

Pt miscarries. Mood remains stable. Mood is 8/10.

Husband takes new job that requires frequent travel. He seems more distant and worried. Mood is 6/10.

Pt learns she is pregnant with twins. Mood is 10/10.

Husband is not home for Zach's 2nd birthday party because of work. Pt begins to worry that she will not be able to care for twins and that she will have another postpartum depression. Starts to regret pregnancy. Mood is 2/10.

Event Time Line (label significant events and ask patient to rate mood on a scale of 1–10)

FIGURE 11–1. Completed depression time line.

Based on the time line, the therapist suggests that although the patient is anxious about the possibility of another postpartum depression, she is not unhappy about the pregnancy per se. Rather, it seems that her mood worsened in May in the context of her husband's emotional withdrawal and increased absences from the house. In fact, the patient was initially quite happy about the pregnancy. But as her husband's absences (physical and emotional) continued, her mood worsened. These feelings were magnified when her husband was not home for their son's second birthday. Although the patient attributes low mood to worries about pregnancy, it seems that she is experiencing a covert role dispute with her husband around his job travel and emotional withdrawal. Rather than focusing on role transition (from parent of one child to pregnant with twins), the therapist suggests they focus on a role dispute with the husband. This decision is based on temporal sequence of mood changes and concurrent life events.

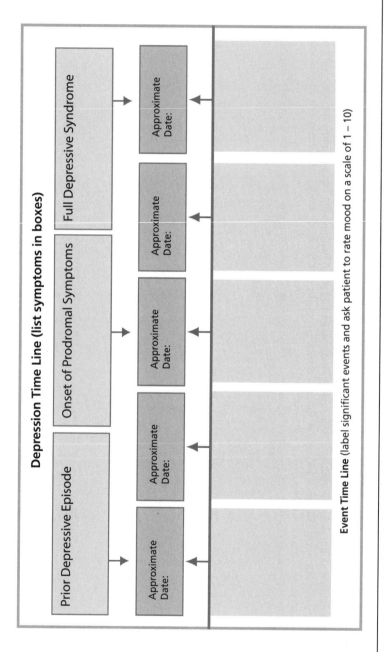

FIGURE 11–2. **Blank time line that can be completed with patient.**

the therapist can say with certainty, "You are very likely to feel better in a few weeks." If the patient is skeptical and asks, "What if I am the one person who doesn't respond to IPT?" (as depressed patients are wont to do), the therapist reminds him or her that hopelessness is a symptom of depression and suggests that in the unlikely event that IPT fails, many other effective antidepressant treatment options exist and can be discussed, if needed.

Middle Phase

The middle phase is the working portion of IPT. During these sessions (typically, sessions 4–13), the therapist actively engages the patient in the process of resolving the central interpersonal problem area and further exploring the links between the patient's mood and interpersonal focus. A more intensive focus on interpersonal issues has been associated with better outcomes for patients receiving IPT (Frank et al.1991). Below we describe general IPT techniques of the middle phase and specific techniques associated with each of the four problem areas (see Table 11–2), illustrated by the hypothetical case of Ms. A:

> Ms. A is a 31-year-old mother of two children, whose husband, Jeff, works as director of sales for a small health care technology company. Ms. A's depression began when Jeff's work responsibilities shifted, requiring him to travel frequently to solicit out-of-state customers. Ms. A described feeling sad and lonely during his absences, but also angry that he was spending less time with her and the children. Jeff, on the other hand, seemed to think that Ms. A should feel grateful because his increased responsibilities meant better compensation, which, in turn, helped the family financially.

"How have you been since we last met?" This seemingly prosaic phrase opens all IPT sessions after the first session. By invoking the temporal frame "since we last met," the therapist focuses the patient on recent (as opposed to past) events and mood states. "How have you been?" elicits a response with either mood-related content:

> I've been sad.
>
> I've been fine.
>
> I've been so-so.

or life-event-related content:

> Jeff and I have been fighting nonstop.
>
> Jeff was gone all week.
>
> I tried to get the kids to listen to me, but it was hopeless.

TABLE 11–2. Techniques of middle phase of interpersonal psychotherapy (IPT)

Goal	Technique
Focus on mood and recent life events.	Inquire about mood and recent life events—"How have you been since we last met?"
Systematically review depressive symptoms.	Assess with a standardized depression rating scale.
Improve capacity for communication.	Use communication analysis and role-play.
Explore options.	Use decision analysis.
Focus on IPT problem area.	Relate change in depressive symptoms to changes in interpersonal problem area.
Enhance understanding of depression as medical illness.	Provide psychoeducation.
Protect the therapeutic relationship.	Use reflective listening, empathic statements, and attention to affect within the session.
Enhance activation.	Encourage increased socialization in a graded fashion; reinforce even small steps toward increased activity levels.

During sessions, the therapist encourages the patient to expand on both mood and recent interpersonal experiences, helping him or her to see links between the two over the past week. If the patient responds with mood-related content, the therapist encourages the patient to elaborate on mood and depressive symptoms:

Tell me what you mean by "so-so."

Can you rate your mood on a scale of 1 to 10?

And how has your sleep been?

After obtaining a clear understanding of the patient's depressive symptoms over the past week, the therapist then links the mood state to the interpersonal problem area:

> It sounds like your depression has been worse this week. Tell me what's been going on in your role dispute with Jeff.

If the therapist chooses wisely in the initial phase, the patient's life events will connect to the problem area selected as the treatment focus. The therapist can then encourage the patient to elaborate on the interpersonal context of these events:

> Tell me more about what has been happening between you and Jeff.
>
> Tell me about how much contact you had with Jeff while he was away.

After exploring these interpersonal issues, the therapist helps the patient to connect the events to his or her mood:

> Tell me how all this fighting has affected your mood.

Alternatively, if the patient responds to the opening question by describing an event, the therapist asks:

> How did that make you feel?

Thus, after two questions, the therapist has elicited a recent, affectively charged event. Therapist and patient can then work on understanding what happened, the relationship of the event to the patient's mood, and potential solutions to the problematic situation.

If the content of the patient's response is *not* related to the treatment focus, the therapist listens politely and looks for an opening to redirect the patient. For instance, if the treatment focus is a role dispute and Ms. A starts the session by telling the therapist about her recent high school reunion, the therapist may make a general comment about the reunion but then reframe the discussion in terms of the dispute:

> It sounds like it was nice to connect with old friends. Did Jeff go to the reunion with you? What's been going on between the two of you?

Usually, the patient responds to gentle redirection. On occasion, however, the therapist may need to firmly invoke the treatment contract made in the initial phase:

> You and I agreed to focus on your role dispute with Jeff because we both saw that your role dispute with him seemed inextricably connected to your mood symptoms. I think it's important for us to return to this because we still have a lot of work to do in this area. If we have extra time at the end of the session, we can spend a few minutes talking about your high school re-

union, as social supports from friends certainly can be helpful when you're feeling depressed. But we should put most of our energy into figuring out what's been happening between you and Jeff. How does that sound to you?

Using a Standardized Rating Instrument

The IPT therapist completes (or asks the patient to complete) a standardized depression rating scale every few sessions and uses the rating to track the patient's progress. The therapist reminds the patient of his or her score at treatment onset and contrasts the original score with the current score, linking symptomatic improvement to interpersonal improvement in the problem area:

> Your BDI score is half of what it was when we started IPT. This seems to reflect about a 50% improvement in your relationship with Jeff. You've made real progress! Let's think about other issues we need to address in your dispute with Jeff to get you to 100% better in the next few sessions.

A standardized instrument allows evaluation of treatment response. Although most patients will, at a minimum, partially respond to IPT, some may not. Others may even worsen. Rating scores that remain flat or deteriorate over time are a signal either to change directions in IPT (i.e., consider a different approach to the problem area, or an alternative problem area) or to consider a different treatment altogether.

Therapists without research experience may initially feel uncomfortable rating patients. They may lack appreciation for the meaning of the scores or feel that rating creates distance in the therapeutic relationship. Over time, however, most therapists accommodate. Patients typically find ratings helpful from the outset, given that they clarify the symptoms of depression and provide an objective metric of their progress. The use of a scientific measure adds credibility to the concept of depression as a medical condition that can be systematically quantified and evaluated.

Using Communication Analysis

Depressed individuals tend not to communicate well. When angry, they make irritable comments and find themselves being short with significant others, but rarely feel capable of expressing the anger directly in the service of resolving interpersonal conflict. Anger feels like a "bad" feeling. Alternatively, many depressed people are withdrawn or feel slowed down, which also impairs communication. Some individuals' impairment is long-standing; for others, it is acute and clearly related to the current depressive episode. IPT almost always addresses patients' capacity to communicate more effectively.

Communication analysis, the primary IPT technique of enhancing communication skills, dissects in detail the communication between two individuals. The exploration includes the patient's inner feelings, which the therapist tries to validate; what was said and not said, how it was said, where it was said, and what speaking or not speaking one's feelings meant in the context of the interchange. The therapist also explores changes in the patient's feelings during and following the encounter. The IPT therapist works to clarify the interaction by asking for details:

> Where were the two of you when this discussion took place?
>
> Was the television on?
>
> Had he been drinking?
>
> Where were the kids while you were talking?
>
> What exactly did you say?
>
> What exactly did he say?
>
> How did you feel then?
>
> Can you say it to me using the same tone of voice that you used then?
>
> What was his frame of mind at the time you initiated the discussion?

Having obtained a detailed account, the therapist reinforces the patient's successful interventions and/or helps the patient understand maladaptive aspects of the interaction and how to remediate the situation. At first, the therapist explores with Ms. A the effect of her communication on her partner:

> What impact do you think having the kids in the room had on your ability to speak freely with Jeff?
>
> How did you feel telling Jeff how angry you've been feeling?
>
> How did Jeff react when you said that?

The therapist asks leading questions, hoping that the patient (in this case, Ms. A) will recognize errors herself and spontaneously offer suggestions for improvement. If the patient is too depressed or too interpersonally impaired to "get it," the therapist makes more directive statements:

> I imagine that Jeff would feel attacked if you started the conversation with a string of insults.
>
> If the kids are in the room with the two of you, you will edit your comments, making it more difficult for you to say to Jeff what you really feel.
>
> It seems like your mood was a little better after telling him how you felt.

After identifying problems in communication, the dyad works to identify more adaptive means of interacting. The therapist asks, "What do you really want to say to him?" and then explores options, asking the patient for suggestions on how to get that idea or feeling across. The therapist can use role-play (i.e., the therapist enacts Jeff and Ms. A plays herself) or coaching to help the patient learn more adaptive means of communicating. This process is usually framed as a rehearsal for an interaction the patient is encouraged to try out with the significant other between sessions. The therapist may also offer the patient general suggestions such as

> It's often helpful to make "I" statements in these situations.

> Maybe you can try having this kind of conversation with Jeff this week and we can discuss what happened during our next session.

Exploring Options and Using Decision Analysis

Although it may seem simplistic, it is important to ask *what the patient wants* in a given situation. Depressed patients often neglect their own needs and desires because they lack energy, motivation, or interest, or because they feel that doing so is "selfish." Thus, when faced with an interpersonal problem, the therapist asks the patient how she would like to resolve the issue:

> Given Jeff's reluctance to take a different kind of job—one that would let him be home more often—what would you like him to do so that you feel less alone? Are there specific things that you would want him to say? Are there things that you'd like him to do when he's home? Could he communicate with you more often while he is on the road?

Depressed patients may initially have difficulty envisioning solutions. Therefore, therapists may have to be relatively active at first, helping patients generate a list of options. Ms. A viewed Jeff's absence as absolute and had difficulty imagining that he could become more involved with the family, even if he was often absent because of work. After generating options, the patient and therapist evaluate the alternatives to assess how realistic they are. They discuss resources the patient needs to achieve the desired outcome and develop a plan to execute necessary changes. If the patient's desire is not feasible (e.g., Jeff getting a new job), the therapist helps the patient mourn the loss of that potential outcome.

Providing Psychoeducation

In the middle phase, the therapist continues to point out how depression has hampered effective interpersonal relationships and communication. As always, the therapist tries to appropriately blame failures in these arenas on the depression rather than the individual, and offers reassurance that symptomatic improvement will restore capacity to manage these processes. If difficulties arise, the therapist acknowledges the disappointment, credits the patient for risking the effort, explores the roles of depression and of the significant other in the outcome, and encouragingly helps the patient to consider other options to resolve the conflict:

> It's wonderful that you tried to talk to Jeff about your disappointment and anger over his lack of attention to you and the children. Depression makes it hard to take risks like this, but you did it despite significant depressive symptoms. It's disappointing that it didn't work out better, but the fact that it didn't go as well as you would have liked is in large part related to the depression. As we've discussed, depression makes it difficult to be assertive, to remain calm in the face of an argument, and to think as clearly as you would when not depressed. And Jeff was not particularly cooperative. We can work on figuring out what went wrong and how to make it go right next time.

As always, the therapist reminds the patient that depression is a medical illness and that as he or she continues to access treatment, these symptoms will likely improve and the interpersonal interactions will proceed more easily. And, conversely, as the relationship improves, his or her mood is likely to lift as well.

Encouraging Socialization and Activity

Socialization and pleasurable activities are inherently antidepressant. Indeed, behavioral activation is a key active ingredient in cognitive-behavioral therapy (Jacobson et al. 2001). In middle-phase IPT, the therapist gently encourages the patient to increase activity and decrease social isolation. Increasing activity is graduated so that the patient does not feel overwhelmed. The therapist presents social encounters as providing crucial interpersonal information and as win-win situations: if the patient succeeds, he or she will feel better; even if the encounter is disappointing, it will provide data to discuss in sessions that will generate alternative approaches. The therapist provides emotional support and practical skills to help achieve these goals. Unlike in behavior therapy, however, the IPT therapist does not specifically assign homework.

Attending to Affect and the Therapeutic Relationship

Therapists continue to apply the "common factors" of psychotherapy in the middle phase of IPT. They facilitate expression of affect, remain attentive to the emotional significance of the therapeutic experience for patients, and maintain a supportive, encouraging stance. When patients discuss emotionally laden therapeutic material, therapists allow time in the session for crying or expression of anger. Therapists can encourage this process with empathic comments:

> That sounds very upsetting.
>
> This must be difficult to talk about.
>
> I can see how painful these feelings are for you.

As in any psychotherapy, the IPT therapist must address therapeutic rifts such as recurrent lateness to appointments, direct complaints from the patient, or concern that the patient is withholding important information. In general, the IPT therapist initially blames the depression:

> When you are depressed, it's very hard to get to places on time or feel motivated to talk about painful subjects.

If that approach fails, the therapist may address issues in the context of the therapeutic relationship, using the time constraints as leverage:

> I know the depression makes it hard to get here on time, but it's really important to do so in order to fight those very symptoms. And unfortunately we only have seven sessions left to work on this.

The IPT therapist does not interpret transference. Nevertheless, transference reactions may arise. IPT therapists tacitly note this process and may use the information to inform their treatment approach, but they do not discuss it explicitly with the patient. The same is true for countertransference. If countertransference feelings seem to interfere with the conduct of IPT, it should be addressed with a supervisor, colleague, or one's own therapist.

Techniques and Strategies Associated With Specific Problem Areas

Grief or complicated bereavement. When the onset or maintenance of the depressive episode is associated with the death of someone important to the patient, the therapist employs specific techniques to treat grief and complicated bereavement. IPT defines other losses (e.g., loss of physical health, ending a relationship) as role transitions. The goals of treatment are to help the patient work through the grief, ultimately helping him or her reestablish social contacts and activities. Specifically, the therapist relates the depressive symptoms to the death or to reactivation of emotions around the anniversary of the death. This process takes place through a careful reevaluation of the relationship with the deceased and clarification of the circumstances of the death.

In nonjudgmental fashion, the therapist explores the events leading up to the death, the death itself, and the events immediately following the death. The therapist encourages the patient to relate how the death unfolded and his or her role in the events. Although it may be painful or frightening for the patient to discuss these memories, it is crucial to grief work. The therapist gently elicits the story by asking the following kinds of questions:

How did you first find out that your mother was ill?

How did you find out that your mother had died? Were you present? Who gave you the news?

Were you able to say everything you wanted to say to your mother before she died? Were there things left unsaid?

Did you attend the funeral? Did you go to the grave? What did you do with her possessions?

Because many patients fear and avoid the intense feelings associated with grief, the therapist should reassure the patient that the emotions are normal and, once tolerated, are likely to subside over time. The therapist tries to pace the session so that the patient has time to pull himself or herself together before its end.

An individual who experiences complicated bereavement often idealizes his or her relationship with the deceased. It may be too painful to remember fights with or shortcomings of the deceased. Often beginning by eliciting positive reminiscences with questions such as "What did you love about him? and What did you love about your relationship?" the therapist helps the patient reconstruct a more realistic view of the relationship, which includes both positive and negative aspects:

What wasn't so great between you?

Every relationship has some friction.

To accomplish this goal, it is often useful for the patient to visit places that stir memories and to look at photos or mementos of the deceased. These tangible items may spur the patient to remember additional events and forgotten aspects of the relationship.

As the patient achieves some catharsis, therapy helps him or her to accept and move beyond the loss. The therapist encourages actions to advance the mourning process such as visiting the grave, reconnecting with family and friends of the deceased, making a scrapbook, or writing a letter to the deceased. Toward the end of treatment, the therapist encourages the patient to reestablish interests and relationships outside of those specifically associated with the deceased.

Role transition.   The problem area of role transition links the onset or maintenance of the depressive episode to difficulty coping with recent or impending life changes in relationships, vocational functioning, financial situation, physical health status, and the like. The transition is conceptualized as difficulty moving from one role to another (e.g., from stay-at-home mother to working mother or from medical student to doctor). Examples of role transitions include being hired or fired, becoming a parent, getting married or divorced, graduating from school, moving to a new city, and being diagnosed with a serious medical condition. Goals of treatment resemble the goals in addressing bereavement: to establish a more realistic view of the old role (which is typically idealized) and the new role (which is typically devalued), and to help patients acquire skills and resources needed to improve functioning in the new role. Thus, patients mourn the lost status but also gain appreciation for and mastery of the new role.

Therapists initially encourage patients to review the positive and negative aspects of the old social role, to mourn its loss, and to explore the feelings associated with the change (anger, sadness, fear, etc). The interpersonal therapist might ask the following questions to encourage the patient to review the important change:

> What was life like before you immigrated to the United States?
>
> What were your goals/dreams/hopes for your marriage before the divorce?
>
> How did you feel when you learned about your promotion?
>
> What are the good and bad things about being at college and away from home?

As therapy progresses, focus shifts toward greater attention to the new role. The patient is encouraged to think about new opportunities afforded by the new role, as well as new skills that will be needed in order to more successfully cope:

> Although you didn't want to be single again, are there any opportunities that being single offers to you?
>
> It sounds like being diagnosed with cancer is helping you to think about what is really important to you. This may be the "silver lining" of the diagnosis.
>
> What's especially challenging about being a new parent? What can you do to learn more about parenting a newborn?

As always, the IPT therapist links changes in the patient's ability to manage the new role to changes in depressive symptoms. The therapist anticipates for the patient that as the depression improves, the patient will cope better with the new role, and that as he or she becomes more comfortable in the new role, the depression will improve.

Role dispute.   The role dispute problem area links onset or maintenance of the depressive episode to an unsatisfying interpersonal relationship characterized by nonreciprocal role expectations. As discussed earlier (see "Taking an Interpersonal Inventory"), having expectations within relationships is inevitable; role disputes arise when two individuals disagree about these expectations and cannot negotiate a compromise. Examples include:

- A college student who expects to be treated as an adult by parents who view him as an adolescent requiring guidance and limits
- An employer who expects her employees to work independently with little supervision but whose employee wants frequent suggestions and reassurance
- A man who expects his girlfriend to devote all her free time to him, whereas she wants to spend time with her friends as well

The therapist's first task is to determine the stage of the dispute. In IPT parlance, there are three stages:

1. *Renegotiation:* an active dispute in which the two parties are trying to work things out—albeit unsuccessfully.
2. *Impasse:* a stalemate— when the two parties are locked in opposing positions, not actively negotiating their differences.
3. *Dissolution:* the end of the dispute, beyond hope of resolution, when the parties are poised to end the relationship.

Disputes require objective staging, as depressed patients tend to see hopeless impasses even where negotiation is possible.

In renegotiation, the therapist may intervene to calm overt hostilities while encouraging improved communication. If the relationship is at an impasse, the therapist attempts to move the individuals toward renegotiation so that they can begin to work through their differences. It is often helpful to offer the caveat "things may get worse before they get better," when the dispute moves from impasse to renegotiation. Typically, the therapist uses communication analysis and role-play to help the patient learn new ways of communicating. If the relationship is in the dissolution phase, the therapeutic task becomes a role transition: to help the patient mourn the loss of the relationship and focus on new activities or relationships.

Role dispute work is sometimes likened to "unilateral couples therapy." In working on this problem area, it may be helpful to bring the other party in the dispute into a session. The purpose of this one session for the couple is to educate the other party about depression, and for the therapist to gain a better understanding of the relationship. Aside from one pilot study (Foley et al. 1989), however, IPT has not been conceptualized as couples therapy.

IPT techniques used to identify and resolve role disputes include expression of affect, relationship appraisal to identify nonreciprocal role expectations, communication analysis, role-play, and problem solving. As in other IPT problem areas, the therapist continually links the patient's mood to the role dispute, expecting to see improvement as the dispute resolves.

Interpersonal deficits. Interpersonal deficits constitute the poorly named IPT category of last resort. Although many patients seeking IPT treatment have notable deficits in interpersonal functioning, the deficits category is reserved for cases in which no other potential foci exist: that is, for patients who lack life events. Such patients tend to have chronic impairments in relationships and may have comorbid dysthymic disorder (Markowitz 1998), social phobia (Lipsitz et al. 1999), and/or traits of DSM Cluster A or C personality disorders. Not surprisingly, patients with chronic impairment in social functioning who lack the life events on which IPT focuses fare worse in IPT (Sotsky et al. 1991) and their treatments are more difficult to conduct.

The goals of treatment for acutely depressed individuals in the interpersonal deficits focus include reducing the patient's isolation and encouraging new social relationships. Although this may sound like an agenda for a longer therapy, the IPT therapist focuses on the patient's isolation in the context of the current depressive episode rather than its historical origins. The therapist reviews depressive symptoms and relates depressive symptoms to the problems of social isolation or unfulfillment. The therapist explores past significant relationships, asking the patient to discuss both their positive and negative aspects. The therapist attempts to determine any evident maladaptive patterns in these relationships and to help the patient understand them. In a departure from the general IPT stance, the therapist may explicitly discuss the patient's feelings about the therapist—using an interpersonal, here-and-now focus—and seek parallels in other relationships.

In other problem areas, the therapist uses the IPT label to explain the problem area to the patient, as in, "We call this a role transition." Because the word *deficits* has disparaging connotations, the therapist explains the problem using more appropriate terms such as *interpersonal sensitivity* or *social isolation.*

Termination

The final phase comprises the last two or three sessions of treatment. IPT likens termination to a graduation: the patient has usually made meaningful gains, feels better, and is now ready for something different (i.e., a new treatment, maintenance treatment, or no treatment). Thus, termination is a role transition from acute therapy. Table 11–3 summarizes the tasks associated with termination.

TABLE 11–3. **Techniques of termination phase of interpersonal psychotherapy (IPT)**

Goal	Technique
Determine remaining treatment needs.	Review depressive symptoms, current interpersonal functioning, and persistent difficulties.
Reinforce treatment gains.	Review treatment gains; review changes in standardized depression assessment over time; explicitly discuss new skills that were acquired.
Manage feelings associated with termination.	Normalize feelings of sadness and loss; differentiate sadness from depression; probe for other feelings associated with termination.
Confer mastery.	Draw analogies with graduation and congratulate patient on gains made in treatment.
Avoid blaming the patient.	Blame the therapy rather than the patient for unmet treatment needs and treatment "failures."
Provide for continuity of care.	Arrange for follow-up care (maintenance treatment, additional treatment), as needed.
Relapse prevention/ planning.	Identify potential triggers for recurrence; provide psychoeducation about risk of recurrence; discuss use of IPT strategies to manage stressors; establish plan for seeking treatment in the future, if needed.

Therapist and patient review the course of treatment, relating improvement in depressive symptoms to interpersonal changes that the patient made in the focal problem area. The therapist credits the patient for making these changes, emphasizing his or her independent competence as acute therapy draws to a close. The therapist continues to offer psychoeducation by reviewing depressive symptoms and instructing the patient to seek appropriate treatment should these symptoms reemerge in the future. The therapist reminds the patient that depression is often a recurrent illness and that recurrence is treatable, and not the patient's fault. If the patient has not improved, the therapist attributes this to IPT (much as one would in a failed pharmacotherapy trial), gives the patient credit for making the effort, and encourages the patient to consider the alternative available treatment options.

In addition to reviewing gains, the dyad explores areas that have not been adequately addressed in IPT. If the depression has not fully remitted, the therapist, following a psychopharmacology model, blames the treatment rather than the patient and suggests alternative or adjunctive treatments that might address remaining symptoms. The therapist may also identify interpersonal issues that have not been adequately addressed in IPT, such as ongoing marital discord or job dissatisfaction, and perhaps recommend follow-up care for help in working on those difficulties:

> You've done a great job, and your depression has remitted. But you and Jeff still have issues to work out. What options do you have to deal with those problems?

Throughout the termination phase, therapists attend to patients' feelings about ending therapy, encouraging patients to verbalize the range of feelings experienced as IPT comes to an end, including anger, relief, worry, and curiosity. Feelings of sadness or loss are normalized in the context of ending a relationship that has been supportive and helpful. It is critical to differentiate normal feelings of sadness about separation, from the pathological symptoms of depression the patient experienced at the outset of treatment:

> We all feel sad at times. Ending therapy is a time when many people feel a little sad. But sadness is a useful signal of social separation, and very different from the numbness and despair that you felt when you were depressed. Remember that depression usually involves changes in sleep and appetite in addition to changes in mood. That may help you figure out whether you are lapsing into depression again or not.

Because the therapeutic relationship in IPT is more collaborative than paternalistic, IPT therapists may acknowledge they will miss and have enjoyed working with the patient (if accurate). Both therapist and patient can voice shared regret about breaking up a good team, while the therapist simultaneously indicates confidence in the patient's ability to continue to do well on his or her own.

The final component of the termination phase is addressing relapse prevention. Patients are encouraged to continue to monitor mood, perhaps using a depression screen intermittently. Therapists point out new skills patients have acquired, review opportunities to implement these skills, identify future interpersonal difficulties or high-risk scenarios that might trigger another episode, and discuss strategies to use in those circumstances. Patients should know how to reach a mental health professional in the event of a future episode. When possible, IPT therapists leave the door open for future consultation, if needed.

Conclusion

Interpersonal psychotherapy is a time-limited treatment for depression that focuses on the link between mood and interpersonal relationships. Working within the medical model, IPT assumes the patient has an underlying genetic/biologic vulnerability to mood disorders. It also assumes the environment interacts with biology such that stressful interpersonal relationships or events can precipitate episodes of depression in biologically vulnerable individuals (a "stress-diathesis" model). By identifying a precipitating interpersonal problem area—grief, role transition, role dispute, or interpersonal deficits—the therapist focuses the treatment on a discrete issue that is directly linked to the current depressive episode whose reolution is likely to lead to improvement in mood.

As we stated at the outset of this chapter, the individual elements of IPT are not novel. Rather, its innovation rests in the way the elements are organized to provide therapists with a coherent strategy to treat patients who suffer from major depressive disorder. The intuitively reasonable idea that mood is connected to life events appeals to therapist and patients, and the empirical evidence base clearly supports the efficacy of the IPT approach (Weissman et al. 2000). The International Society for Interpersonal Psychotherapy (www.interpersonalpsychotherapy.org) serves as an online forum for therapists interested in IPT and provides information about training opportunities for individuals who may be interested in gaining further experience with this modality.

Key Points

- Interpersonal psychotherapy (IPT) explores the link between mood and interpersonal relationships.

- Depression, like diabetes or cancer, is a medical illness in which environmental factors can increase or mitigate genetic vulnerability to the disorder.

- Depression is treatable (hopelessness notwithstanding) and not the patient's fault (guilt notwithstanding).

- The therapist must choose and maintain focus on one of four possible IPT problem areas: grief, role transition, role dispute, or (as a last resort) interpersonal deficits.

- The time limit accelerates and intensifies acute IPT.

- IPT techniques build upon the foundation of nonspecific "common factors" of psychotherapy.

References

American Psychiatric Association: Diagnostic and Statistical Manual of Mental Disorders, 4th Edition, Text Revision. Washington, DC, American Psychiatric Association, 2000

Beck AT: BDI-II: Beck Depression Inventory: Manual. New York, Harcourt Brace, 1996

Cyranowski JM, Frank E, Winter E, et al: Personality pathology and outcome in recurrently depressed women over 2 years of maintenance interpersonal psychotherapy. Psychol Med 34:659–669, 2004

Foley SH, Rounsaville BJ, Weissman MM, et al: Individual versus conjoint interpersonal psychotherapy for depressed patients with marital disputes. International Journal of Family Psychiatry 10:29–42, 1989

Frank E, Kupfer DJ, Wagner EF, et al: Efficacy of interpersonal therapy as a maintenance treatment of recurrent depression: contributing factors. Arch Gen Psychiatry 48:1053–1059, 1991

Frank JD: Therapeutic factors in psychotherapy. Am J Psychother 25:350–361, 1971

Grote NK, Bledsoe SE, Swartz HA, et al: Culturally relevant psychotherapy for perinatal depression in low-income ob/gyn patients. Clin Soc Work J 32:327–347, 2004

Hamilton M: A rating scale for depression. J Neurol Neurosurg Psychiatry 23:56–62, 1960

Jacobson NS, Martell CR, Dimidjian S: Behavioral activation treatment for depression: returning to contextual roots. Clinical Psychology: Science and Practice 8:255–270, 2001

Klerman GL, Weissman MM, Rounsaville BJ, et al: Interpersonal Psychotherapy of Depression. New York, Basic Books, 1984

Krupnick JL, Sotsky SM, Simmens S, et al: The role of the therapeutic alliance in psychotherapy and pharmacotherapy outcome: findings in the National Institute of Mental Health Treatment of Depression Collaborative Research Program. J Consult Clin Psychol 64:532–539, 1996

Lipsitz JD, Markowitz JC, Cherry S, et al: Open trial of interpersonal psychotherapy for the treatment of social phobia. Am J Psychiatry 156:1814–1816, 1999

Markowitz JC: Interpersonal Psychotherapy for Dysthymic Disorder. Washington, DC, American Psychiatric Press, 1998

Markowitz JC, Swartz HA: Case formulation in interpersonal psychotherapy of depression, in Handbook of Psychotherapy Case Formulation, 2nd Edition. Edited by Eells TD. New York, Guilford, 2007, pp 221–250

Markowitz JC, Bleiberg KL, Christos P, et al: Solving interpersonal problems correlates with symptom improvement in interpersonal psychotherapy: preliminary findings. J Nerv Ment Dis 194:15–20, 2006

Parsons T: Illness and the role of the physician: a sociological perspective. Am J Orthopsychiatry 21:452–460, 1951

Rush AJ, Trivedi MH, Ibrahim HM, et al: The 16-item Quick Inventory of Depressive Symptomatology (QIDS) Clinician Rating (QIDS-C) and Self-Report (QIDS-SR): a psychometric evaluation in patients with chronic major depression. Biol Psychiatry 54:573–583, 2003

Sotsky SM, Glass DR, Shea MT, et al: Patient predictors of response to psychotherapy and pharmacotherapy: findings in the NIMH Treatment of Depression Collaborative Research Program. Am J Psychiatry 148:997–1008, 1991

Weissman MM, Prusoff BA, Dimascio A, et al: The efficacy of drugs and psychotherapy in the treatment of acute depressive episodes. Am J Psychiatry 136:555–558, 1979

Weissman MM, Markowitz JC, Klerman GL: Comprehensive Guide to Interpersonal Psychotherapy. New York, Basic Books, 2000

Weissman MM, Markowitz JC, Klerman GL: Clinician's Quick Guide to Interpersonal Psychotherapy. New York, Oxford University Press, 2007

World Health Organization: The ICD-10 Classification of Mental and Behavioural Disorders: Clinical Descriptions and Diagnostic Guidelines. Geneva, World Health Organization, 1992

Suggested Readings

Elkin I, Shea MT, Watkins JT, et al: National Institute of Mental Health Treatment of Depression Collaborative Research Program: general effectiveness of treatments. Arch Gen Psychiatry 46:971–982, 1989

Frank E: Interpersonal psychotherapy as a maintenance treatment for patients with recurrent depression. Psychotherapy 28:259–266, 1991

Frank E: Treating Bipolar Disorder: A Clinician's Guide to Interpersonal and Social Rhythm Therapy. New York, Guilford, 2005

International Society for Interpersonal Psychotherapy (Web site: http://www.interpersonalpsychotherapy.org/)

Markowitz JC: The future of interpersonal psychotherapy. J Psychother Pract Res 6:294–299, 1997

Markowitz JC: Interpersonal Psychotherapy for Dysthymic Disorder. Washington, DC, American Psychiatric Press, 1998

Markowitz JC, Swartz HA: Case formulation in interpersonal psychotherapy of depression, in Handbook of Psychotherapy Case Formulation, 2nd Edition. Edited by Eells TD. New York, Guilford, 2007, pp 221–250

Mufson L, Moreau D: Interpersonal psychotherapy for adolescent depression, in Interpersonal Psychotherapy. Edited by Markowitz JC (Review of Psychiatry Series, Vol 17; Oldham JM and Riba MB, series eds). Washington, DC, American Psychiatric Press, 1998, pp 35–66

O'Hara MW, Stuart S, Gorman LL, et al: Efficacy of interpersonal psychotherapy for postpartum depression. Arch Gen Psychiatry 57:1039–1045, 2000

Reynolds CF 3rd, Perel JM, Frank E, et al: Three-year outcomes of maintenance nortriptyline treatment in late-life depression: a study of two fixed plasma levels. Am J Psychiatry 156:1177–1181, 1999

Swartz HA, Markowitz JC, Frank E: Interpersonal psychotherapy for unipolar and bipolar disorders, in Treating Chronic and Severe Mental Disorders: A Handbook of Empirically Supported Interventions. Edited by Hofmann SG, Tompson MC. New York, Guilford, 2002, pp 131–158

Weissman MM, Markowitz JC, Klerman GL: Clinician's Quick Guide to Interpersonal Psychotherapy. New York, Oxford University Press, 2007

Wilfley DE, MacKenzie KR, Welch RR, et al: Interpersonal Psychotherapy for Group. New York, Basic Books, 2000

Chapter 12

Applications of Individual Interpersonal Psychotherapy to Specific Disorders

Efficacy and Indications

John C. Markowitz, M.D.
Myrna M. Weissman, Ph.D.

Interpersonal psychotherapy (IPT) was developed in the 1970s by the late Gerald L. Klerman, M.D., Myrna M. Weissman, Ph.D., and their colleagues at Harvard and Yale universities (Weissman 2006). From its inception, IPT was a research therapy. Moreover, whereas much of psycho-

Material for this chapter has been adapted, with permission, from Markowitz JC: "Interpersonal Psychotherapy," in *Psychiatry*, Third Edition. Edited by Tasman A, Kay J, Lieberman JA, et al. Chichester, UK, Wiley, 2008.

therapy research before IPT was on the process of psychotherapy, IPT research has focused on the outcome of treatment. As Gerald Klerman would remark, "Who cares why a therapy works if we don't know *that* it works?" IPT has been tested in a series of randomized controlled trials (RCTs), generally with success. Indeed, for many years IPT was essentially *only* a research treatment, with few practitioners in the community. Now, because of its success in research studies, IPT has been included as an indicated treatment in numerous guidelines for mood and eating disorders (Agency for Health Care Policy and Research 1993; American Psychiatric Association 2006; "Practice Guideline for Major Depressive Disorder in Adults" 1993). Clinicians are increasingly seeking training because of its empirically demonstrated efficacy. A new manual geared to clinicians describes how to conduct IPT (Weissman et al. 2007). Older manuals describe the efficacy and empirical basis in greater detail (Klerman et al. 1984; Weissman et al. 2000).

In this chapter we address the applications of IPT as an individual psychotherapy for psychiatric disorders and review their efficacy and indications. Although IPT was developed as an individual psychotherapy, it has been adapted for other formats, including group (Wilfley et al. 2000), couples (Foley et al. 1989), and telephone treatment (Miller and Weissman 2002; Neugebauer et al. 2006, 2007). (For a discussion of IPT in combination with pharmacotherapy, see Chapter 13, "Combining Interpersonal Psychotherapy With Medication.")

Efficacy and Effectiveness

Efficacy research refers to testing a treatment under highly controlled conditions, with experienced therapists, rating instruments, and treatment monitoring in RCTs. Therapists become trained by reading a treatment manual, videotaping or audiotaping their treatment sessions, and receiving intensive case supervision from IPT experts during the pilot study and subsequent studies (Rounsaville et al. 1986). Patients in these trials meet careful inclusion and exclusion criteria to limit heterogeneity. Demonstrating efficacy answers the question Does the treatment work? and indicates that a treatment is superior to a control condition in these structured circumstances. Once a treatment has demonstrated efficacy for patients with a particular diagnosis, the next step is to test its *effectiveness* under less rigorously monitored conditions in the community setting. The question becomes: Does it work in a real-life setting? Both questions are important.

IPT research has demonstrated the efficacy of IPT for treating patients with major depressive disorder across a range of ages and contexts, and for treating patients with bulimia nervosa (Table 12–1). One large trial indicated that it is efficacious (modified as *interpersonal and social rhythm therapy*, or IPSRT) as an adjunctive treatment for bipolar disorder (Frank et al. 2005). Less strong evidence suggests the potential benefits of IPT in treating several anxiety disorders. IPT has shown no advantages over control psychotherapies for dysthymic disorder or substance abuse disorders. For depressed adolescents, IPT has shown not only efficacy (Mufson et al. 1999) but also effectiveness in a school-based program (Mufson et al. 2004a).

Because IPT focuses clinically on the social context of the depressive episode, researchers have sometimes adapted IPT when applying it to different treatment populations, developing manuals for different age groups or subpopulations (e.g., Frank 2005; Markowitz 1998; Mufson et al. 2004b) and occasionally adding focal problem areas. IPT has also been used at different lengths, and in different formats, as well as in one pilot couples adaptation (Foley et al. 1989), and as a telephone intervention (Donnelly et al. 2000; Miller and Weissman 2002; Neugebauer et al. 2006, 2007). Nonetheless, all these adaptations retain the basic principles of IPT: a no-fault definition of the patient's problem as a medical illness, excusing the patient from blame for his or her symptoms, and a continual focus on the relationship between the patient's moods and life situation (Weissman et al. 2000, 2007). Thus IPT remains consistent across conditions and adaptations.

The continuing growth of IPT research precludes an exhaustive description of studies. In this chapter we present a selection of key research trials of IPT for mood and other disorders.

Major Depressive Disorder

Major depressive disorder is the target diagnosis for which IPT was developed and for which its efficacy remains best demonstrated.

Acute Treatment

IPT was first tested as an acute antidepressant treatment in a four-cell, 16-week randomized trial. This study compared IPT, amitriptyline, the combination of IPT and amitriptyline, and a nonscheduled control treatment for 81 outpatients with major depression (DiMascio et al. 1979; Weissman et al. 1979). Although amitriptyline alleviated symptoms faster than IPT did, no significant difference in symptom reduction was seen with amitriptyline versus IPT at 16 weeks. The active treatments all reduced symptoms significantly more than the nonscheduled control treatment did, and the amitriptyline-IPT combination was more efficacious than either active monotherapy. Unsurprisingly, IPT did not help patients with delusional depression. At 1-year follow-up, many patients who had received the brief IPT intervention had sustained improvement. Moreover, IPT patients had developed significantly better psychosocial functioning, whether or not

TABLE 12–1. Empirically based indications for interpersonal psychotherapy (IPT)

Major depression

    Acute

    Recurrent (prophylaxis)

    Geriatric patients

    Adolescent patients

    HIV-positive patients

    Primary care patients

    Conjoint therapy for depressed married women

    Postpartum and antepartum patients

Bipolar disorder (adjunctive treatment)

Subsyndromal depression (interpersonal counseling)

Bulimia (individual or group format)

Social phobia[a]

Posttraumatic stress disorder[a]

[a]Preliminary results encouraging.

they had received medication. This effect on social functioning was not found in patients treated with amitriptyline alone and had not been evident in IPT recipients at 16 weeks (Weissman et al. 1981).

    A landmark trial in the history of antidepressant psychotherapy was the multisite National Institute of Mental Health Treatment of Depression Collaborative Research Program (NIMH TDCRP; Elkin et al. 1989). Investigators randomly assigned 250 outpatients with major depression to receive 16 weeks of IPT, cognitive-behavioral therapy (CBT; Beck et al. 1979), imipramine plus clinical management, or placebo pills plus clinical management. This study was the first comparison of IPT and CBT, each of which had demonstrated efficacy in separate trials, and the first trial to use treatment manuals and monitor the psychotherapeutic input of pharmacotherapists. Most patients completed at least 12 once-weekly treatment sessions or 15 weeks of therapy. Those with milder depression (defined as a score of <20 on the 17-item Hamilton Rating Scale for Depression [Ham-D; Hamilton 1960]) improved equally regardless of which treatment was used. For more severely depressed patients (those with a Ham-D score of ≥20), imipramine worked fastest and was most consistently superior to placebo. IPT and imipramine had comparable effects on Ham-D scores and several other outcome measures, and were superior to placebo for more severely depressed patients. CBT was not superior to placebo among the more depressed patients.

A reanalysis of NIMH TDCRP data by Klein and Ross using the Johnson-Neyman technique reported the order of treatment efficacy as "medication superior to psychotherapy, [and] the psychotherapies somewhat superior to placebo...particularly among the symptomatic and impaired patients" (Klein and Ross 1993, p. 241). Klein and Ross found that "CBT [was] relatively inferior to IPT for patients with BDI [Beck Depression Inventory] scores greater than approximately 30, generally considered the boundary between moderate and severe depression" (p. 247). The reanalysis sharpens the differences seen among treatments.

In a follow-up of NIMH TDCRP subjects 18 months later, Shea et al. (1992) found no significant differences in terms of recovery among remitters (those with minimal or no symptoms when treatment ended, with remission sustained during follow-up) among the four treatments. Thirty percent of CBT, 26% of IPT, 19% of imipramine, and 20% of placebo subjects who had achieved remission with acute treatment maintained remission during the 18 months. Among acute remitters, relapse rates over the 18-month follow-up were 36% for CBT, 33% for IPT, 50% for imipramine (even though medication had been stopped at 16 weeks!), and 33% for placebo. Shea and colleagues concluded that 16 weeks of therapy with these specific treatments was insufficient to achieve full and lasting recovery for many patients.

Maintenance Treatment

IPT was first tested in an 8-month, six-cell trial of maintenance therapy (Klerman et al. 1974; Paykel et al. 1975). This study today would be considered a *continuation* treatment, as the concept of long-term maintenance antidepressant treatment has lengthened. Acutely depressed female outpatients were first treated with amitriptyline for 4–6 weeks. Those who responded to amitriptyline ($n=150$) were randomly assigned to receive 8 months of treatment with either 1) weekly IPT, 2) amitriptyline, 3) a pill placebo, 4) IPT plus amitriptyline, 5) IPT plus a pill placebo, or 6) no pill (low contact). Randomization to IPT or a low-contact psychotherapy occurred at entry into the continuation phase, whereas randomization to medication, placebo, or no pill occurred at the end of the second month of the continuation phase. Continuation pharmacotherapy prevented relapse and symptom exacerbation, whereas IPT improved social functioning (Weissman et al. 1974). The effects of IPT on social functioning did not appear for 6–8 months. Patients who received psychotherapy combined with pharmacotherapy had the best outcomes.

Longer antidepressant maintenance trials of IPT have been conducted at the Western Psychiatric Institute and Clinic. Frank, Kupfer, and their colleagues treated 128 outpatients with multiply and rapidly recurrent depression (Frank et al. 1990, 1991). These patients initially received combination therapy with high-dose (mean dosage>200 mg/day) imipramine plus weekly sessions of IPT. Responders continued to take high-dose medication while IPT was tapered to a monthly frequency during a 4-month continuation phase. Patients who remained in remission were then randomly assigned to receive 3 years of either 1) ongoing high-dose imipramine plus clinical management, 2) high-dose imipramine plus monthly IPT, 3) monthly IPT alone, 4) monthly IPT plus a placebo pill, or 5) placebo pill plus clinical management. High-dose imipramine proved the most efficacious treatment, protecting more than 80% of patients against relapse for 3 years. In contrast, most placebo recipients relapsed within the first few months. In maintenance IPT, therapists were permitted to switch interpersonal foci in order to deal with patients' current life problems. Once-monthly IPT, although less efficacious than medication, was statistically and clinically superior to placebo in this high-risk patient population. Reynolds and colleagues (1999) at the University of Pittsburgh Medical Center replicated the superiority of IPT over placebo but found advantages for combined treatment over both monotherapies in a maintenance study comparing IPT, nortriptyline, their combination, and placebo in 187 elderly patients with recurrent major depression (average age, 67 years; see "Geriatric Patients" section for further description of this study, and for further discussion of the Frank et al. study results).

The typical depressed patient is a woman of childbearing age. Frank and colleagues (1991) found that depressed patients who received IPT were recurrence free for an average of 82 weeks, which would suffice to protect many women with recurrent depression throughout pregnancy and nursing, without medication. Further study is required to determine the efficacy of IPT relative to newer medications (e.g., selective serotonin reuptake inhibitors), and at different dosages (i.e., frequency of sessions other than once monthly). In a study of differing dosages of maintenance IPT for depressed patients in Pittsburgh, Frank et al. (2007) did not find differences in outcomes based on frequency of sessions. This study found that Cluster C Axis II pathology receded over the course of 2 years of maintenance IPT (Cyranowski et al. 2004). Perhaps optimal dosing of maintenance IPT depends on individual patients' needs.

Geriatric Patients

The first geriatric depression study involving IPT used it as augmentation to pharmacotherapy in a small (N=18) 6-week trial in order to enhance compliance and to provide some treatment for the placebo control subjects (Rothblum et al. 1982; Sholomskas et al. 1983). Grief and role transition specific to life changes were the prime treatment foci. The investigators suggested modifications to IPT for older patients, including a more flexible duration of sessions and greater use of practical advice and support (e.g., arranging transportation, calling the physician). They also noted that major role changes may be impractical and detrimental in this patient population (e.g., divorce at age 75). Another 6-week trial compared standard IPT versus nortriptyline in 30 depressed geriatric patients. Results showed some advantages for IPT, largely due to a higher attrition rate in the medication group caused by nortriptyline side effects (Sloane et al. 1985).

Using a study design similar to that of the study by Frank et al. (1990), Reynolds et al. (1999) conducted a 3-year maintenance study for geriatric patients with recurrent major depression, using IPT and/or nortriptyline. The IPT manual was modified to allow more flexibility in the length of sessions, under the assumption that some elderly patients might not tolerate 50-minute sessions (as recommended earlier by Rothblum, Sholomskas, and colleagues; see Rothblum et al. 1982; Sholomskas et al. 1983). Reynolds et al. found that older patients needed to address early life relationships in their psychotherapy, a distinction from the typical *here-and-now* focus of IPT. The investigators felt, as Rothblum and Sholomskas et al. had, that therapists need to help patients solve practical problems and to acknowledge that some problems may not be amenable to resolution, such as existential late-life issues or lifelong psychopathology.

In Reynold et al.'s study, 187 geriatric patients (60 years and older) with recurrent major depression received acute combined treatment with IPT and nortriptyline; 107 patients experienced remission of symptoms and then achieved recovery with continuation therapy. These patients were then randomly assigned to one of four 3-year maintenance groups: 1) nortriptyline, with monthly medication clinic visits maintaining steady-state nortriptyline plasma levels within a therapeutic window of 80–120 ng/mL; 2) placebo with monthly medication clinic visits; 3) monthly IPT plus placebo; or 4) monthly IPT plus nortriptyline (combined treatment). Elderly depressed patients whose sleep quality normalized by the early continuation phase had an 80% chance of remaining euthymic during the first year of maintenance treatment. Depression recurrence rates were 20% with combined treatment, 43% with nortriptyline, 64% with IPT plus placebo, and 90% with placebo alone. Each monotherapy was statistically superior to placebo, whereas combined therapy was superior to IPT alone and showed a trend toward superiority compared with medication alone (Reynolds et al. 1999). Patients in their 70s were more likely to have a recurrence and were likely to have depression recur more quickly than patients in their 60s.

The Reynolds et al. (1999) study corroborates Frank et al.'s (1990, 1991) original maintenance study in showing a maintenance effect for monthly maintenance IPT, with the difference that combined treatment had advantages compared with pharmacotherapy alone for geriatric patients. In a similar, subsequent study of 116 depressed patients 70 years or older who had responded to the combination of IPT and paroxetine, Reynolds and colleagues (2006) again found that once-monthly maintenance IPT was not efficacious in preventing relapse.

It is easy to misinterpret the comparison of high-dose tricyclic antidepressants to low-dosage maintenance IPT in both the Frank et al. (1990, 1991) and the Reynolds et al. (1999) studies. These first tests of psychotherapy as a maintenance treatment compared the lowest-ever dosages of psychotherapy and the highest-ever maintenance doses of medication. Had the tricyclic doses been lower, recurrence of depression in the medication groups might well have been greater; had psychotherapy been more frequent, perhaps relapse rates would have been lower. Yet this was unprecedented research. Under the circumstances, the choice of monthly dosing for maintenance IPT, although the lowest ever prescribed in a psychotherapy trial, was reasonable, and indeed patients benefited from monthly IPT. In a new maintenance study by Frank et al. (2007), increasing the maintenance dosage of IPT did not increase the efficacy of the therapy.

Adolescent Patients

Mufson et al. (2004a) modified IPT to incorporate adolescent developmental issues (IPT for adolescents, or IPT-A). They first conducted an open feasibility and follow-up trial, then a controlled 12-week clinical trial comparing IPT-A versus clinical monitoring in 48 clinic-referred adolescents, ages 12–18 years, who met DSM-III-R criteria for major depressive disorder (American Psychiatric Association 1987). Patients were seen fortnightly by independent evaluators, blinded to the treatments administered, so that symptoms, social functioning, and social problem-solving skills could be assessed. Thirty-two of the 48 patients completed the protocol (21 IPT-A recipients and 11 control subjects).

Patients receiving IPT-A showed significantly greater improvement in depressive symptoms and overall social functioning, including functioning with friends and problem-solving skills. In the intention-to-treat sample, 75% of IPT-A patients met the criterion for remission (a Ham-D score of ≤ 6), compared with 46% of control patients. These findings support the feasibility, patient acceptance, and efficacy of 12 weeks of IPT-A in acutely depressed adolescents to reduce depressive symptoms and improve social functioning and interpersonal problem-solving skills (Mufson et al. 1999).

Mufson and her colleagues (2004b) subsequently tested IPT-A in an effectiveness study of depressed adolescents ($N=63$) in school-based clinics, a common site for adolescent treatment, yet one where empirically based therapies have been nearly absent. The investigators found that IPT-A, delivered by school social workers, was markedly superior to treatment as usual. The same research group is now studying IPT-A in a group format for depressed adolescents (Mufson et al. 2004c) and training therapists in the use of IPT-A in larger health care systems.

Rosselló, Bernal, and Rivera at the University of Puerto Rico randomly assigned adolescents ages 13–18 years who met DSM-III-R criteria for major depression, dysthymia, or both to 12 weeks of IPT ($n=22$), CBT ($n=25$), or a waiting-list control condition ($n=24$). The investigators found both IPT (effect size >0.73) and CBT (effect size >0.43) more efficacious than the control condition in reducing adolescents' self-rated depressive symptoms. IPT increased self-esteem and social adaptation more effectively than CBT (Rosselló and Bernal 1999).

HIV-Positive Patients

Markowitz et al. (1992, 1998) modified IPT (IPT-HIV) for depressed HIV-positive patients to emphasize issues that this population faces, including concerns about illness and death, grief, and role transitions. In a pilot open trial, 20 of 23 depressed adults with HIV recovered from depression after a mean of 16 sessions (Markowitz et al. 1992). In a later, 16-week study, 101 subjects were randomly assigned to receive IPT-HIV, CBT, brief supportive psychotherapy, or imipramine plus brief supportive psychotherapy (Markowitz et al. 1998). Echoing the outcomes in the more severely depressed subjects in the NIMH TDCRP study (Elkin et al. 1989), all treatments were associated with symptom reduction, but IPT-HIV and imipramine plus brief supportive therapy produced significantly greater improvements in symptoms and functioning than CBT or supportive therapy alone. Many patients reported improvement in depressive physical symptoms that they had mistakenly attributed to HIV infection.

Primary Care Patients

Schulberg and colleagues compared IPT and nortriptyline for depressed ambulatory medical patients in a primary care setting (Schulberg and Scott 1991; Schulberg et al. 1993, 1996). They did not modify the IPT manual, but they did integrate IPT into the routine of the primary care center: nurses took vital signs before each session, and therapists saw patients at the medical clinic. If patients were hospitalized (for a nonpsychiatric condition), IPT was continued in the hospital when possible.

Patients with current major depression ($n=276$) were randomly assigned to receive IPT, nortriptyline, or their primary care physician's usual care. IPT sessions were held weekly for 16 weeks and monthly thereafter for 4 months (Schulberg et al. 1996). Depressive symptom severity declined more rapidly with either nortriptyline or IPT than with usual care. Approximately 70% of treatment completers who received nortriptyline or IPT had recovered after 8 months, versus only 20% of those who received usual care.

In a secondary analysis on Schulberg et al.'s sample, Brown et al. (1996) found that depressed subjects who had a lifetime history of comorbid panic disorder had a poorer response across treatments than subjects with major depression alone. Frank and colleagues (2000a) reported a similar effect of comorbid panic disorder on the outcomes of treatment for depression.

These studies suggest that the life event of an illness (besides depression) may provide a useful focus as a role transition in IPT treatment (see also Koszycki et al. 2004). On the other hand, a large Canadian study recently showed no advantage for IPT plus clinical management versus clinical management alone in treating depressed patients with coronary artery disease (Lespérance et al. 2007).

The Prevention of Suicide in Primary Care Elderly: Collaborative Trial (the PROSPECT study) looked at IPT in an effectiveness setting, where IPT was offered as an alternative to or in combination with a serotonin reuptake inhibitor to enhance treatment of geriatric patients with major depression in primary care practices. Medical practices were randomized to provide usual care or to have a trained health care manager identify depressed patients. In those who received IPT, there was a larger decrease in depressive symptoms than in patients who received the usual care (Alexopoulos et al. 2005), and rates of suicidal ideation declined faster (Bruce et al. 2004). As primary care physicians became acquainted with IPT and its effects, their rate of prescribing IPT during the first study year rose from 11% to 27% (Schulberg et al. 2007).

Patients With Marital Disputes: Conjoint Interpersonal Therapy

Marital conflict can precipitate or complicate depressive episodes (Rounsaville et al. 1979); hence the IPT focus on role disputes. Some clinicians have believed that individual psychotherapy for patients in marital disputes may prematurely rupture marriages (Gurman and Kniskern 1978). A manual for conjoint therapy of depressed patients with marital disputes (IPT-CM) was developed (Klerman and Weissman 1993) that includes the spouse in all sessions and focuses on the current marital dispute. In a pilot study, 18 patients with major depression linked to the onset or exacerbation of marital disputes were randomly assigned to receive 16 weeks of either individual IPT or IPT-CM. Patients in the two treatment groups had similar reductions in depressive symptoms, but patients receiving IPT-CM reported significantly better marital adjustment, marital affection, and sexual relations (Foley et al. 1989). These pilot findings require replication in a larger trial using control groups.

Women With Peripartum and Postpartum Depression

Pregnancy and the postpartum period are times of heightened risk for depression, and times when women may wish to avoid antidepressant medication. Pregnancy and its aftermath also provide natural role transitions for an IPT focus. Spinelli (1997) used IPT first in an open trial to treat 13 women with antepartum depression. Exploring this role transition addresses the depressed pregnant woman's self-evaluation as a parent, physiological changes of pregnancy, and altered relationships with the spouse or significant other and with other children. Spinelli added *complicated pregnancy* as a fifth interpersonal problem area. Timing and duration of sessions are adjusted in response to bed rest, delivery, obstetrical complications, and child care. Postpartum mothers may bring children to sessions. As with depressed HIV-positive patients, pregnant women and postpartum mothers may require telephone sessions or hospital visits to receive IPT (Spinelli 1997). More recently, a controlled clinical trial compared acute treatment with IPT versus didactic parent education; this 16-week study involving 50 depressed pregnant women showed advantages of IPT (Spinelli and Endicott 2003).

O'Hara, Stuart, and their colleagues randomly assigned 120 women with postpartum depression to IPT or a waiting-list control group in a 12-week trial with an 18-month follow-up (O'Hara et al. 2000; Stuart and O'Hara 1995). The investigators assessed both the mothers' symptoms and their interactions with their infants. In the IPT group, 38% of subjects met Ham-D and 44% met Beck Depression Inventory (Beck 1978) remission criteria, compared with 14% (for each measure) in the waiting-list group. Sixty percent of IPT recipients, versus 16% of control subjects, reported more than a 50% reduction in BDI scores. Women receiving IPT also showed significant improvement in social adjustment compared with control subjects.

Other pregnancy-related trials of IPT have included group interventions for postpartum depression (Klier et al. 2001; Zlotnick et al. 2001) and a telephone intervention for women with subsyndromal depression postmiscarriage (Neugebauer et al. 2006, 2007).

Dysthymic Disorder

Medication benefits roughly half of dysthymic patients (Kocsis et al. 1988; Thase et al. 1996) but nonresponders may need psychotherapy, and even medication responders may benefit from combined treatment (Markowitz 1994). A modification of IPT for dysthymic disorder, IPT-D, encourages patients to reconceptualize what they have considered their lifelong character flaws as ego-dystonic, chronic mood-dependent symptoms: that is, as a chronic but treatable state rather than an immutable trait. Therapy itself is defined as an *iatrogenic role transition*, from believing oneself flawed in personality to recognizing and treating the lingering mood disorder. Markowitz (1994, 1998) openly treated 17 subjects with 16 sessions of IPT-D in a pilot study; none worsened, and in 11 subjects the disorder remitted.

Based on these results, a randomized trial at Weill Medical College of Cornell University compared 16 weeks of IPT-D alone, brief supportive psychotherapy, sertraline plus clinical management, and combined IPT plus sertraline. All groups improved, but IPT showed no greater acute benefits than brief supportive psychotherapy, and pharmacotherapy appeared more efficacious than either psychotherapy (Markowitz et al. 2005).

Browne, Steiner, and colleagues (2002) at McMaster University in Hamilton, Canada, treated 707 dysthymic patients in the community with either 12 sessions of standard IPT over a period of 4 months, sertraline (50–200 mg/day) for 2 years, or their combination. Patients were followed for 2 years. Using the criterion of a 40% reduction in score on the Montgomery-Åsberg Depression Rating Scale (MADRS) at 1-year follow-up, 51% of subjects treated with IPT alone improved, significantly fewer than the 63% of subjects treated with sertraline and 62% of those receiving combined treatment. On follow-up, however, IPT was associated with significant economic savings in use of family health care and social services. Thus combined treatment was as efficacious as but less expensive than treatment with sertraline alone.

de Mello and colleagues (2001) randomly assigned 35 dysthymic outpatients to receive moclobemide with or without 16 weekly sessions of IPT. Both groups improved, but there was a nonsignificant trend toward greater improvement in Ham-D and MADRS scores in the combined treatment group. Similarly, Hellerstein and colleagues (2001) found that fluoxetine plus a group psychotherapy combining interpersonal and cognitive elements improved outcomes more than fluoxetine alone among dysthymic patients responsive to fluoxetine.

Chronic depression is by and large more difficult to treat than acute depression, in part because of the ingrained despair that attends its very chronicity. IPT has not fared particularly well as a monotherapy for chronically depressed patients, but it may yet have benefit as an adjunct to medication, much as it may for patients with bipolar disorder.

Bipolar Disorder

Frank and colleagues at the University of Pittsburgh assessed the benefits of adjunctive IPT modified by *social zeitgeber theory*—behavioral scheduling of daily routines, and especially sleep patterns (Ehlers et al. 1988; Frank et al. 1999, 2000b; Malkoff-Schwartz et al. 2000)—as maintenance therapy. In this study of 175 bipolar patients treated with medication (Frank et al. 2005), IPSRT was compared with a medication clinic. The behavioral component of IPSRT helps to protect sleep patterns and limit the disruptions that may provoke mania; the psychotherapy's approach to treating depression remained largely the same as in IPT for unipolar depression.

Acutely ill bipolar patients were treated with medication and randomly assigned to receive IPSRT or clinical management with a medication clinic. After having achieved 4 weeks of stabilization, they were again randomly assigned to either IPSRT or clinical management for 3 years of maintenance treatment with continuing pharmacotherapy. Results of this complicated trial indicated that although the treatments did not differ in time to initial stabilization of symptoms, IPSRT with medication (before or after IPSRT) was superior to the comparison condition in delaying recurrence of depressive and manic episodes (Frank et al. 2005).

Other Psychiatric Disorders

Demonstration of the efficacy of IPT as an antidepressive treatment has led to its adaptation as a treatment for other psychiatric disorders.

Bulimia

Fairburn et al. (1993) altered IPT for patients with bulimia, eliminating the use of the sick role and of role-play in order to contrast distinct therapeutic strategies in comparing IPT and CBT. In an initial study, 75 patients with bulimia nervosa were randomly assigned to 19 sessions over 18 weeks of IPT, CBT, or a behavior therapy control. CBT worked faster to relieve bulimic symptoms, but on follow-up, IPT had benefits comparable to those of CBT and superior to those of the control condition. A subsequent multisite trial ($N=220$) found CBT superior to IPT (Agras et al. 2000). Nonetheless, IPT is one of the better-tested treatments for bulimia and is at least a second-line treatment after CBT. Wilfley and colleagues (1993, 2000, 2002) have also demonstrated the efficacy of a group adaptation of IPT for eating disorders.

A research group in Christchurch, New Zealand, applied IPT to anorexia nervosa. In their trial, 56 anorexic women were treated with 20 weekly sessions of IPT, CBT, or a supportive therapy control. Neither IPT nor CBT showed efficacy as an outpatient treatment, with both groups faring worse than the control group—a finding unfortunately consonant with anorexia outcome literature generally (Fairburn et al. 1995; McIntosh et al. 2005).

Social Phobia

IPT has not yet been tested in controlled studies for anxiety disorders. Two research groups have independently modified IPT for treating social phobia. Lipsitz and colleagues (1999) at Columbia University treated nine patients with social phobia in an IPT pilot study and reported promising results. They found that standard IPT ingredients such as the medical model, provision of the sick role, and the supportive therapeutic stance appear to benefit most patients. A small controlled trial has not yet been published.

Panic Disorder

Arzt and colleagues in Maastricht, the Netherlands, are comparing IPT with CBT as a treatment for panic disorder. Lipsitz and colleagues (2006) reported promising results of a small open trial of IPT for panic disorder, in which 9 of 12 subjects had reduced panic symptoms at the end of treatment.

Posttraumatic Stress Disorder

Posttraumatic stress disorder (PTSD) is an anxiety disorder defined by a stressful life event, suggesting the utility of IPT in its treatment. Krupnick and colleagues are assessing a group form of IPT for multiply victimized women in public sector gynecology clinics in Virginia. Markowitz and colleagues at Cornell University modified IPT as an alternative to exposure-based psychotherapies for PTSD and found excellent outcomes in a small ($N=14$) pilot trial (Bleiberg and Markowitz 2005). A controlled comparison is now planned.

Substance Abuse

IPT has failed to demonstrate efficacy in three clinical trials for patients with substance dependence. Rounsaville and colleagues (1983) studied 72 methadone-maintained opiate users and found that adding adjunctive IPT to standard substance abuse care (which already included a psychotherapy component) had no additional benefit in reducing psychopathology. Both treatment groups improved. The same research group treated 42 subjects with cocaine abuse who were attempting to achieve abstinence, and found 12 weeks of IPT ineffective and marginally worse than a behavioral control therapy (Carroll et al. 1991). They also treated 121 cocaine-dependent subjects in a 2 x 2–cell, 12-week trial with either IPT or CBT and disulfiram 250 mg or placebo (Carroll et al. 2004). CBT and disulfiram were superior to IPT and to placebo. These negative studies suggest limits to the range of utility of IPT but do not necessarily preclude its use for all substance abuse. IPT might be useful, for example, as a treatment for newly abstinent alcohol-dependent patients, who face psychosocial stressors that have been shown to precipitate relapse.

Applications and Adaptations to Other Disorders

Research groups are testing the applicability of IPT to body dysmorphic disorder, chronic somatization in primary care patients, depression in cancer patients, borderline personality disorder (Markowitz et al. 2006b), insomnia, and other disorders (Weissman et al. 2000). The IPT focus on life events suggests its potential applicability to patients with medical illness. Swartz and colleagues (2004) produced preliminary findings suggesting that IPT can be effective in a brief, eight-session form.

Interpersonal Counseling

Many patients present to primary care physicians reporting psychiatric symptoms that do not meet threshold criteria for a psychiatric disorder. These symptoms nonetheless can be debilitating and may result in high wasted utilization of medical procedures (Wells et al. 1989). Interpersonal counseling (IPC), based on IPT, was designed to treat distressed primary care patients who do not meet full syndromal criteria for psychiatric disorders. IPC is administered for a maximum of six sessions by health care professionals who lack formal psychiatric training, usually nurse practitioners. The first session can last up to 30 minutes; subsequent sessions are briefer.

IPC therapists assess the patient's current functioning, recent life events, occupational and familial stressors, and changes in interpersonal relationships. They assume that such events provide the context in which emotional and bodily symptoms occur. Klerman and colleagues (1987) studied 128 patients in a primary care clinic who scored 6 or higher on the Goldberg General Health Questionnaire, randomly assigning them to receive either IPC provided by medical nurses without prior psychotherapy training, or usual care without psychological treatment. Over an average of 3 months, IPC subjects—many of whom had had only one or two IPC sessions—showed significantly greater symptom relief and improvement in emotional symptoms on the General Health Questionnaire, especially mood improvement, than control subjects did. IPC subjects were more likely subsequently to make use of mental health services, suggesting a new awareness of the psychological aspect of their symptoms.

Mossey et al. (1996) noted that even depressive symptoms that do not reach the threshold for major depression impede recovery of hospitalized elderly patients. They conducted a 10-session trial of IPC for elderly hospitalized medical patients with minor depressive symptoms. Nonpsychiatric nurses delivered the treatment. Patients were seen for hour-long sessions on a flexible schedule to accommodate the patient's medical status. Hospitalized patients over age 60 ($N=76$) who had subsyndromal depressive symptoms on two consecutive assessments were randomly assigned to receive IPC or usual care. Researchers also followed an untreated control group of euthymic patients.

Patients found IPC feasible and tolerable. Assessment at 3 months showed nonsignificantly greater improvement in depressive symptoms and superiority in all outcome variables with IPC compared with usual care, whereas untreated control subjects showed a slight symptomatic worsening. Rehospitalization rates in the IPC and euthymic control groups were virtually identical (11% vs. 15%) and were significantly lower than in the subsyndromally depressed group of patients who received usual care (50%). Differences between the IPC and usual care groups reached statistical significance at 6 months in terms of depressive symptom reduction and self-rated health, but not physical or social functioning. The investigators felt that 10 sessions of counseling were insufficient for some patients and that a maintenance treatment phase might have been useful.

A dramatic study demonstrating the adaptability of IPT to a very different culture tested a group variant of IPC in randomly assigned villages in a poverty- and AIDS-stricken region of Uganda where depression rates are high. IPT was chosen as an intervention because antidepressant medication was unaffordable and other psychotherapies seemed incompatible with the local outlook. Researchers adjusted for cultural differences but applied the usual IPT paradigm. Local college graduates without mental health experience provided treatment. The group IPC intervention was impressively more effective than treatment as usual (Bolton et al. 2003), and gains persisted at 6-month follow-up (Bass et al. 2006).

Interpersonal Therapy by Telephone

Because many patients avoid or have difficulty reaching an office for face-to-face treatment, IPT and IPC are being tested as telephone treatments. Weissman and Miller at Columbia University conducted a successful pilot feasibility trial comparing IPT by telephone versus no treatment for 30 patients with recurrent major depression who had not received regular treatment (Miller and Weissman 2002). Neugebauer and colleagues (2006, 2007) found telephone IPC to be a helpful intervention for women with minor depression postmiscarriage.

Interpersonal Therapy Patient Guide

Weissman (2005) developed an IPT patient guide with worksheets for depressed individuals who want information about or are receiving IPT. Worksheets can be used to facilitate sessions or to monitor problem areas after treatment. The utility of the patient book in enhancing treatment has not been studied.

Differential Therapeutics

When two or more treatments have demonstrated comparable efficacy for a diagnosis such as major depressive disorder, when is one treatment more likely to provide a better outcome than another? Comparative trials are beginning to reveal moderating factors that may predict treatment outcome. Studies such as the NIMH TDCRP, which compared IPT and CBT (and included a comparison pharmacotherapy group), have suggested factors that might predict a better outcome with IPT versus CBT (see Table 12–2).

In the NIMH TDCRP study, Sotsky and colleagues (1991) found that depressed patients with a low baseline level of social dysfunction responded well to IPT, whereas those with severe social deficits (probably equivalent to the *interpersonal deficits* problem area) responded less well. Patients with greater symptom severity and difficulty concentrating responded poorly to CBT. Greater initial severity of major depression and of impaired functioning predicted a superior response to IPT and to imipramine than to CBT. Imipramine was the most efficacious treatment for patients with difficulty functioning at work, likely reflecting its faster onset of action compared with psychotherapy. Patients with atypical depression responded better to either IPT or CBT than to imipramine or placebo (Shea et al. 1999).

Barber and Muenz (1996), looking only at subjects who completed the NIMH TDCRP study, found IPT to be more efficacious than CBT for patients with obsessive personality traits, whereas patients with avoidant personality disorder fared better with CBT. Biological factors could also predict treatment response; for example, abnormal sleep profiles as shown on electroencephalograms predicted a significantly poorer response to IPT compared with normal sleep profiles (Thase et al. 1997). Frank and colleagues (1991; Frank 1991) found that psychotherapists' adherence to a focused IPT approach may enhance outcomes. For replication of initial study results and further elaboration, these predictive factors deserve ongoing study.

TABLE 12–2.   Indications for interpersonal psychotherapy (IPT) vs. cognitive-behavioral therapy (CBT)

Predictor	IPT	CBT
Life events	Present	Absent
Social dysfunction (baseline)	Low	Very high[a]
Symptom severity (baseline)	Higher	Lower
Personality disorder	Obsessive	Avoidant

[a]Interpersonal deficits.

Many psychiatrists recognize that medication and psychotherapy each have distinct benefits, making the combination of the two tempting. Yet monotherapy with either IPT or pharmacotherapy is likely to suffice for most patients with major depressive disorder. Hence combined treatment is probably best reserved for severely ill or chronically ill patients (Rush and Thase 1999). How best to combine time-limited psychotherapy with pharmacotherapy—for which patients, in what sequence, etc.—is an exciting area for future research.

Conclusion

IPT has demonstrated efficacy as acute and maintenance monotherapy, and as a component of combined treatment, for patients with major depressive disorder. It is a second-line treatment for bulimia, less tested and sometimes less efficacious than CBT. Encouraging research results suggest that IPT is applicable to anxiety disorders, although RCTs are necessary to confirm its initial promise in this area. IPT also seems adaptable to different lengths, formats, and cultures.

On the other hand, IPT has not shown benefit for treating substance use disorders or as a monotherapy for dysthymic disorder. Unlike some other therapies, IPT has been developed slowly: therapists have taken a modest approach in establishing the therapy's indications, relying on research to demonstrate its efficacy before applying the treatment clinically. It is unsurprising that this treatment, which was never intended for universal application, should have its limits.

The history of IPT has been a succession of outcome studies that have helped to define diagnostic indications for this treatment. Because psychotherapy is underfunded relative to pharmacotherapy, we have fewer studies and know far less about the dosage of and indications for IPT than we do about antidepressant medications. Future trials may continue to define the territory of IPT's utility. These should include trials of IPT for disorders other than mood disorders, such as the anxiety disorders, and at different dosages—to find the optimal frequency and duration of IPT sessions—and also studies of the sequencing of IPT with other treatments. For example, when, and for whom, is IPT best combined with pharmacotherapy? Is it best to start with pharmacotherapy and then add IPT? If so, at what interval, and with what frequency? When should IPT be used as augmentation for pharmacotherapy *and vice versa*? Other research may help to determine the cost-effectiveness of IPT, including its potential to offset health care costs, as a treatment that improves both symptoms and social functioning.

IPT has been anomalous among psychotherapies in its nearly pure research focus on outcome studies. Now that it is clear that IPT helps many patients, process research seems warranted to try to identify its active, mediating components. Little is known about the specific value of many IPT interventions. It is even unclear, for example, whether focusing on a role transition rather than a role dispute makes a difference for patients, or whether particular sorts of life events are helpful or unhelpful foci. It does appear that IPT therapists agree in choosing focal interpersonal problem areas (Markowitz et al. 2000), and that resolving an interpersonal problem correlates with treatment outcome, as IPT theory would predict (Markowitz et al. 2006a). Patient and therapist characteristics may also influence treatment outcome.

Clinical training in IPT is growing; how the use of IPT spreads will be a function of training programs. Training will eventually require formalized accreditation, both to ensure clinical competence and to satisfy managed care organizations. Research is needed on how best to teach and disseminate IPT, to ensure that IPT delivered by practitioners in clinical practice yields results comparable to those achieved by therapists in research trials (Markowitz 2001).

Key Points

- Interpersonal psychotherapy (IPT) is a time-limited, diagnosis-focused treatment adaptable to multiple diagnoses, formats, durations, and cultures.

- IPT has demonstrated efficacy as an acute treatment for patients with major depressive disorder or bulimia nervosa.

- IPT has demonstrated efficacy as a maintenance treatment for patients with major depressive disorder.

- IPT did not have demonstrated efficacy in three studies of substance abuse, and it appears to be less efficacious than pharmacotherapy as a monotherapy for dysthymic disorder.

References

Agency for Health Care Policy and Research, Depression Guideline Panel: Depression in Primary Care, Vol 1: Detection and Diagnosis. Clinical Practice Guideline Number 5 (AHCPR Publ No 93-0550). Rockville, MD, U.S. Department of Health and Human Services, April 1993

Agras WS, Walsh BT, Fairburn CG, et al: A multicenter comparison of cognitive-behavioral therapy and interpersonal psychotherapy for bulimia nervosa. Arch Gen Psychiatry 57:459–466, 2000

Alexopoulos GS, Katz IR, Bruce ML, et al; PROSPECT Group: Remission in depressed geriatric primary care patients: a report from the PROSPECT study. Am J Psychiatry 162:718–724, 2005

American Psychiatric Association: Diagnostic and Statistical Manual of Mental Disorders, 3rd Edition, Revised. Washington, DC, American Psychiatric Association, 1987

American Psychiatric Association: Practice Guidelines for the Treatment of Psychiatric Disorders: Compendium 2006. Arlington, VA, American Psychiatric Association, 2006

Barber JP, Muenz LR: The role of avoidance and obsessiveness in matching patients to cognitive and interpersonal psychotherapy: empirical findings from the Treatment for Depression Collaborative Research Program. J Consult Clin Psychol 64:951–958, 1996

Bass J, Neugebauer R, Clougherty KF, et al: Group interpersonal psychotherapy for depression in rural Uganda: 6-month outcomes: randomised controlled trial. Br J Psychiatry 188:567–573, 2006

Beck AT: Depression Inventory. Philadelphia, PA, Center for Cognitive Therapy, 1978

Beck AT, Rush AJ, Shaw BF, et al: Cognitive Therapy of Depression. New York, Guilford, 1979

Bleiberg KL, Markowitz JC: A pilot study of interpersonal psychotherapy for post-traumatic stress disorder. Am J Psychiatry 162:181–183, 2005

Bolton P, Bass J, Neugebauer R, et al: Group interpersonal psychotherapy for depression in rural Uganda: a randomized controlled trial. JAMA 289:3117–3124, 2003

Brown C, Schulberg HC, Madonia MJ, et al: Treatment outcomes for primary care patients with major depression and lifetime anxiety disorders. Am J Psychiatry 153:1293–1300, 1996

Browne G, Steiner M, Roberts J, et al: Sertraline and/or interpersonal psychotherapy for patients with dysthymic disorder in primary care: 6-month comparison with longitudinal 2-year follow-up of effectiveness and costs. J Affect Disord 68:317–330, 2002

Bruce ML, Ten Have TR, Reynolds CF 3rd, et al: Reducing suicidal ideation and depressive symptoms in depressed older primary care patients: a randomized controlled trial. JAMA 291:1081–1091, 2004

Carroll KM, Rounsaville BJ, Gawin FH: A comparative trial of psychotherapies for ambulatory cocaine abusers: relapse prevention and interpersonal psychotherapy. Am J Drug Alcohol Abuse 17:229–247, 1991

Carroll KM, Fenton LR, Ball SA, et al: Efficacy of disulfiram and cognitive behavior therapy in cocaine-dependent outpatients: a randomized placebo-controlled trial. Arch Gen Psychiatry 61:264–272, 2004

Cyranowski JM, Frank E, Winter E, et al: Personality pathology and outcome in recurrently depressed women over 2 years of maintenance interpersonal psychotherapy. Psychol Med 34:659–669, 2004

de Mello MF, Myczcowisk LM, Menezes PR: A randomized controlled trial comparing moclobemide and moclobemide plus interpersonal psychotherapy in the treatment of dysthymic disorder. J Psychother Pract Res 10:117–123, 2001

DiMascio A, Weissman MM, Prusoff BA, et al: Differential symptom reduction by drugs and psychotherapy in acute depression. Arch Gen Psychiatry 36:1450–1456, 1979

Donnelly JM, Kornblith AB, Fleishman S, et al: A pilot study of interpersonal psychotherapy by telephone with cancer patients and their partners. Psychooncology 9:44–56, 2000

Ehlers CL, Frank E, Kupfer DJ: Social zeitgebers and biological rhythms: a unified approach to understanding the etiology of depression. Arch Gen Psychiatry 45:948–952, 1988

Elkin I, Shea MT, Watkins JT, et al: National Institute of Mental Health Treatment of Depression Collaborative Research Program: general effectiveness of treatments. Arch Gen Psychiatry 46:971–982, 1989

Fairburn CG, Jones R, Peveler RC, et al: Psychotherapy and bulimia nervosa: longer-term effects of interpersonal psychotherapy, behavior therapy, and cognitive behavior therapy. Arch Gen Psychiatry 50:419–428, 1993

Fairburn C, Norman PA, Welch SL, et al: A prospective study of outcome in bulimia nervosa and the long-term effects of three psychological treatments. Arch Gen Psychiatry 52:304–312, 1995

Foley SH, Rounsaville BJ, Weissman MM, et al: Individual versus conjoint interpersonal psychotherapy for depressed patients with marital disputes. International Journal of Family Psychiatry 10:29–42, 1989

Frank E: Interpersonal psychotherapy as a maintenance treatment for patients with recurrent depression. Psychotherapy 28:259–266, 1991

Frank E: Treating Bipolar Disorder: A Clinician's Guide to Interpersonal and Social Rhythm Therapy. New York, Guilford, 2005

Frank E, Kupfer DJ, Perel JM, et al: Three-year outcomes for maintenance therapies in recurrent depression. Arch Gen Psychiatry 47:1093–1099, 1990

Frank E, Kupfer DJ, Wagner EF, et al: Efficacy of interpersonal therapy as a maintenance treatment of recurrent depression: contributing factors. Arch Gen Psychiatry 48:1053–1059, 1991

Frank E, Swartz HA, Mallinger AG, et al: Adjunctive psychotherapy for bipolar disorder: effects of changing treatment modality. J Abnorm Psychol 108:579–587, 1999

Frank E, Shear MK, Rucci P, et al: Influence of panic-agoraphobic spectrum symptoms on treatment response in patients with recurrent major depression. Am J Psychiatry 157:1101–1107, 2000a

Frank E, Swartz HA, Kupfer DJ: Interpersonal and social rhythm therapy: managing the chaos of bipolar disorder. Biol Psychiatry 48:593–604, 2000b

Frank E, Kupfer DJ, Thase ME, et al: Two-year outcomes for interpersonal and social rhythm therapy in individuals with bipolar I disorder. Arch Gen Psychiatry 62:996–1004, 2005

Frank E, Kupfer DJ, Buysse DJ, et al: Randomized trial of weekly, twice-monthly, and monthly interpersonal psychotherapy as maintenance treatment for women with recurrent depression. Am J Psychiatry 164:761–767, 2007

Gurman AS, Kniskern DP: Research on marital and family therapy: progress, perspective, and prospect, in Handbook of Psychotherapy and Behavior Change, 2nd Edition. Edited by Garfield SL, Bergin AE. New York, Wiley, 1978, pp 817–902

Hamilton M: A rating scale for depression. J Neurol Neurosurg Psychiatry 23:56–62, 1960

Hellerstein DJ, Little SA, Samstag LW, et al: Adding group psychotherapy to medication treatment in dysthymia: a randomized prospective pilot study. J Psychother Pract Res 10:93–103, 2001

Klein DF, Ross DC: Reanalysis of the National Institute of Mental Health Treatment of Depression Collaborative Research Program General Effectiveness Report. Neuropsychopharmacology 8:241–251, 1993

Klerman GL, Weissman MM: New Applications of Interpersonal Psychotherapy. Washington, DC, American Psychiatric Press, 1993

Klerman GL, Dimascio A, Weissman M, et al: Treatment of depression by drugs and psychotherapy. Am J Psychiatry 131:186–191, 1974

Klerman GL, Weissman MM, Rounsaville BJ, et al: Interpersonal Psychotherapy of Depression. New York, Basic Books, 1984

Klerman GL, Budman S, Berwick D, et al: Efficacy of a brief psychosocial intervention for symptoms of stress and distress among patients in primary care. Med Care 25:1078–1088, 1987

Klier CM, Muzik M, Rosenblum KL, et al: Interpersonal psychotherapy adapted for the group setting in the treatment of postpartum depression. J Psychother Pract Res 10:124–131, 2001

Kocsis JH, Frances AJ, Voss C, et al: Imipramine treatment for chronic depression. Arch Gen Psychiatry 45:253–257, 1988

Koszycki D, Lafontaine S, Frasure-Smith N, et al: An open-label trial of interpersonal psychotherapy in depressed patients with coronary disease. Psychosomatics 45:319–324, 2004

Lespérance F, Frasure-Smith N, Koszycki D, et al; CREATE Investigators: Effects of citalopram and interpersonal psychotherapy on depression in patients with coronary artery disease: the Canadian Cardiac Randomized Evaluation of Antidepressant and Psychotherapy Efficacy (CREATE) trial. JAMA 297:367–379, 2007

Lipsitz JD, Markowitz JC, Cherry S, et al: Open trial of interpersonal psychotherapy for the treatment of social phobia. Am J Psychiatry 156:1814–1816, 1999

Lipsitz JD, Gur M, Miller NL, et al: An open pilot study of interpersonal psychotherapy for panic disorder (IPT-PD). J Nerv Ment Dis 194:440–445, 2006

Malkoff-Schwartz S, Frank E, Anderson BP, et al: Social rhythm disruption and stressful life events in the onset of bipolar and unipolar episodes. Psychol Med 30:1005–1016, 2000

Markowitz JC: Psychotherapy of dysthymia. Am J Psychiatry 151:1114–1121, 1994

Markowitz JC: Interpersonal Psychotherapy for Dysthymic Disorder. Washington, DC, American Psychiatric Press, 1998

Markowitz JC: Learning the new psychotherapies, in Treatment of Depression: Bridging the 21st Century. Edited by Weissman MM. Washington, DC, American Psychiatric Press, 2001, pp 281–300

Markowitz JC, Klerman GL, Perry SW, et al: Interpersonal therapy of depressed HIV-seropositive patients. Hosp Community Psychiatry 43:885–890, 1992

Markowitz JC, Kocsis JH, Fishman B, et al: Treatment of depressive symptoms in human immunodeficiency virus-positive patients. Arch Gen Psychiatry 55:452–457, 1998

Markowitz JC, Leon AC, Miller NL, et al: Rater agreement on interpersonal psychotherapy problem areas. J Psychother Pract Res 9:131–135, 2000

Markowitz JC, Kocsis JH, Bleiberg KL, et al: A comparative trial of psychotherapy and pharmacotherapy for "pure" dysthymic patients. J Affect Disord 89:167–175, 2005

Markowitz JC, Bleiberg KL, Christos P, et al: Solving interpersonal problems correlates with symptom improvement in interpersonal psychotherapy: preliminary findings. J Nerv Ment Dis 194:15–20, 2006a

Markowitz JC, Skodol AE, Bleiberg K: Interpersonal psychotherapy for borderline personality disorder: possible mechanisms of change. J Clin Psychol 62:431–444, 2006b

McIntosh VV, Jordan J, Carter FA, et al: Three psychotherapies for anorexia nervosa: a randomized, controlled trial. Am J Psychiatry 162:741–747, 2005

Miller L, Weissman M: Interpersonal psychotherapy delivered over the telephone to recurrent depressives: a pilot study. Depress Anxiety 16:114–117, 2002

Mossey JM, Knott KA, Higgins M, et al: Effectiveness of a psychosocial intervention, interpersonal counseling, for subdysthymic depression in medically ill elderly. J Gerontol Biol Sci Med Sci 51:M172–M178, 1996

Mufson L, Weissman MM, Moreau D, et al: Efficacy of interpersonal psychotherapy for depressed adolescents. Arch Gen Psychiatry 56:573–579, 1999

Mufson L, Dorta KP, Moreau D, et al: Interpersonal Therapy for Depressed Adolescents, 2nd Edition. New York, Guilford, 2004a

Mufson L, Dorta KP, Wickramaratne P, et al: A randomized effectiveness trial of interpersonal psychotherapy for depressed adolescents. Arch Gen Psychiatry 61:577–584, 2004b

Mufson L, Gallagher T, Dorta KP, et al: A group adaptation of interpersonal psychotherapy for depressed adolescents. Am J Psychother 58:220–237, 2004c

Neugebauer R, Kline J, Markowitz JC, et al: Pilot randomized controlled trial of interpersonal counseling for subsyndromal depression following miscarriage. J Clin Psychiatry 67:1299–1304, 2006

Neugebauer R, Kline J, Bleiberg K, et al: Preliminary open trial of interpersonal counseling for subsyndromal depression following miscarriage. Depress Anxiety 24:219–222, 2007

O'Hara MW, Stuart S, Gorman LL, et al: Efficacy of interpersonal psychotherapy for postpartum depression. Arch Gen Psychiatry 57:1039–1045, 2000

Paykel ES, DiMascio A, Haskell D, et al: Effects of maintenance amitriptyline and psychotherapy on symptoms of depression. Psychol Med 5:67–77, 1975

Practice guideline for major depressive disorder in adults. American Psychiatric Association. 150 (4, suppl):1–26, 1993

Reynolds CF 3rd, Frank E, Perel JM, et al: Nortriptyline and interpersonal psychotherapy as maintenance therapies for recurrent major depression: a randomized controlled trial in patients older than 59 years. JAMA 281:39–45, 1999

Reynolds CF 3rd, Dew MA, Pollock BG, et al: Maintenance treatment of major depression in old age. N Engl J Med 354:1130–1138, 2006

Rosselló J, Bernal G: The efficacy of cognitive-behavioral and interpersonal treatments for depression in Puerto Rican adolescents. J Consult Clin Psychol 67:734–745, 1999

Rothblum ED, Sholomskas AJ, Berry C, et al: Issues in clinical trials with the depressed elderly. J Am Geriatr Soc 30:694–699, 1982

Rounsaville BJ, Weissman MM, Prusoff BA, et al: Marital disputes and treatment outcome in depressed women. Compr Psychiatry 20:483–490, 1979

Rounsaville BJ, Glazer W, Wilber CH, et al: Short-term interpersonal psychotherapy in methadone-maintained opiate addicts. Arch Gen Psychiatry 40:629–636, 1983

Rounsaville BJ, Chevron ES, Weissman MM, et al: Training therapists to perform interpersonal psychotherapy in clinical trials. Compr Psychiatry 27:364–371, 1986

Rush AJ, Thase ME: Psychotherapies for depressive disorders: a review, in Depressive Disorders. Edited by Maj M, Sartorius N (World Psychiatric Association Series: Evidence and Experience in Psychiatry, Vol 1). Chichester, UK, Wiley, 1999, pp 161–206

Schulberg HC, Scott CP: Depression in primary care: treating depression with interpersonal psychotherapy, in Psychotherapy in Managed Health Care: The Optimal Use of Time & Resources. Edited by Austad CS, Berman WH. Washington, DC, American Psychological Association, 1991, pp 153–170

Schulberg HC, Scott CP, Madonia MJ, et al: Applications of interpersonal psychotherapy to depression in primary care practice, in New Applications of Interpersonal Psychotherapy. Edited by Klerman GL, Weissman MM. Washington, DC, American Psychiatric Press, 1993, pp 265–291

Schulberg HC, Block MR, Madonia MJ, et al: Treating major depression in primary care practice. Arch Gen Psychiatry 53:913–919, 1996

Schulberg HC, Post EP, Raue PJ, et al: Treating late-life depression with interpersonal psychotherapy in the primary care sector. Int J Geriatr Psychiatry 22:106–114, 2007

Shea MT, Elkin I, Imber SD, et al: Course of depressive symptoms over follow-up: findings from the National Institute of Mental Health Treatment of Depression Collaborative Research Program. Arch Gen Psychiatry 49:782–787, 1992

Shea MT, Elkin I, Sotsky SM: Patient characteristics associated with successful treatment: outcome findings from the NIMH Treatment of Depression Collaborative Research Program, in Psychotherapy Indications and Outcomes. Edited by Janowsky DS. Washington, DC, American Psychiatric Press, 1999, pp 71–90

Sholomskas AJ, Chevron ES, Prusoff BA, et al: Short-term interpersonal therapy (IPT) with the depressed elderly: case reports and discussion. Am J Psychother 36:552–566, 1983

Sloane RB, Stapes FR, Schneider LS: Interpersonal therapy versus nortriptyline for depression in the elderly, in Clinical and Pharmacological Studies in Psychiatric Disorders. Edited by Burrows GD, Norman TR, Dennerstein L. London, John Libbey, 1985, pp 344–346

Sotsky SM, Glass DR, Shea MT, et al: Patient predictors of response to psychotherapy and pharmacotherapy: findings in the NIMH Treatment of Depression Collaborative Research Program. Am J Psychiatry 148:997–1008, 1991

Spinelli MG: Interpersonal psychotherapy for depressed antepartum women: a pilot study. Am J Psychiatry 154:1028–1030, 1997

Spinelli MG, Endicott J: Controlled clinical trial of interpersonal psychotherapy versus parenting education program for depressed pregnant women. Am J Psychiatry 160:555–562, 2003

Stuart S, O'Hara MW: Interpersonal psychotherapy for postpartum depression: a treatment program. J Psychother Pract Res 4:18–29, 1995

Swartz HA, Frank E, Shear MK, et al: A pilot study of brief interpersonal psychotherapy for depression in women. Psychiatr Serv 55:448–450, 2004

Thase ME, Fava M, Halbreich U, et al: A placebo-controlled, randomized clinical trial comparing sertraline and imipramine for the treatment of dysthymia. Arch Gen Psychiatry 53:777–784, 1996

Thase ME, Buysse DJ, Frank E, et al: Which depressed patients will respond to interpersonal psychotherapy? The role of abnormal EEG profiles. Am J Psychiatry 154:502–509, 1997

Weissman MM: Mastering Depression Through Interpersonal Psychotherapy: Patient Workbook. New York, Oxford University Press, 2005

Weissman MM: A brief history of interpersonal psychotherapy. Psychiatr Ann 36:553–557, 2006

Weissman MM, Klerman GL, Paykel ES, et al: Treatment effects on the social adjustment of depressed patients. Arch Gen Psychiatry 30:771–778, 1974

Weissman MM, Prusoff BA, Dimascio A, et al: The efficacy of drugs and psychotherapy in the treatment of acute depressive episodes. Am J Psychiatry 136:555–558, 1979

Weissman MM, Klerman GL, Prusoff BA, et al: Depressed outpatients: results one year after treatment with drugs and/or interpersonal psychotherapy. Arch Gen Psychiatry 38:51–55, 1981

Weissman MM, Markowitz JC, Klerman GL: Comprehensive Guide to Interpersonal Psychotherapy. New York, Basic Books, 2000

Weissman MM, Markowitz JC, Klerman GL: Clinician's Quick Guide to Interpersonal Psychotherapy. New York, Oxford University Press, 2007

Wells KB, Stewart A, Hays RD, et al: The functioning and well-being of depressed patients: results of the Medical Outcomes Study. JAMA 262:914–919, 1989

Wilfley DE, Agras WS, Telch CF, et al: Group cognitive-behavioral therapy and group interpersonal psychotherapy for the nonpurging bulimic individual: a controlled comparison. J Consult Clin Psychol 61:296–305, 1993

Wilfley DE, MacKenzie KR, Welch RR, et al: Interpersonal Psychotherapy for Group. New York, Basic Books, 2000

Wilfley DE, Welch RR, Stein RI, et al: A randomized comparison of group cognitive-behavioral therapy and group interpersonal psychotherapy for the treatment of overweight individuals with binge-eating disorder. Arch Gen Psychiatry 59:713–721, 2002

Zlotnick C, Johnson SL, Miller IW, et al: Postpartum depression in women receiving public assistance: pilot study of an interpersonal-therapy-oriented group intervention. Am J Psychiatry 158:638–640, 2001

Suggested Readings

Frank E: Treating Bipolar Disorder: A Clinician's Guide to Interpersonal and Social Rhythm Therapy. New York, Guilford, 2005

Frank E, Kupfer DJ, Wagner EF, et al: Efficacy of interpersonal therapy as a maintenance treatment of recurrent depression: contributing factors. Arch Gen Psychiatry 48:1053–1059, 1991

International Society for Interpersonal Psychotherapy (Web site: http://www.interpersonalpsychotherapy.org/)

Mufson L, Dorta KP, Moreau D, et al: Interpersonal Therapy for Depressed Adolescents, 2nd Edition. New York, Guilford, 2004

Weissman MM, Markowitz JC, Klerman GL: Comprehensive Guide to Interpersonal Psychotherapy. New York, Basic Books, 2000

Weissman MM, Markowitz JC, Klerman GL: Clinician's Quick Guide to Interpersonal Psychotherapy. New York, Oxford University Press, 2007

Chapter 13

Combining Interpersonal Psychotherapy With Medication

Oriana Vesga-López, M.D.
Carlos Blanco, M.D., Ph.D.

Both interpersonal psychotherapy (IPT) and antidepressants have come to be regarded as empirically supported treatments for major depressive disorder (MDD). Each treatment has its potential advantages and disadvantages. When discussing treatment selection with their patients, clinicians want to know which treatment modality is preferable for a particular patient, including when combined treatment should be recommended. Questions that often arise when discussing these topics include

---

Supported in part by National Institutes of Health grants DA-00482, DA-019606, and DA-020783 and by the New York State Psychiatric Institute (Dr. Blanco).

- Is there empirical evidence to prefer one course of action over another?
- What is the role of patients in treatment selection?
- Are there concerns about treatment cost, and if so, what are the relative costs of each course of treatment?
- Should all patients receive combined treatment?

In order to answer those questions, we review the empirical evidence of efficacy for IPT, medication, and their combination; propose a framework for treatment selection; and suggest some areas for future research.

Efficacy of Interpersonal Psychotherapy Versus Medication and Combined Treatment

Acute Studies of Major Depressive Disorder

Six studies of the acute treatment of MDD have examined the efficacy of IPT either following medication treatment, as a comparator to antidepressants, or as part of combined treatment (see Table 13–1). In the first study (Klerman et al. 1974; Paykel et al. 1975), patients ($N=150$) who had responded to amitriptyline (100–200 mg/day) were randomly assigned to receive 8 months of maintenance treatment with either IPT or a "nonscheduled treatment" in which patients could contact a psychiatrist whenever they felt a need for treatment. (This condition is referred to in other manuscripts as once-a-month supportive psychotherapy or low-intensity contact therapy group.) Within their therapy group assignment, patients were further randomly assigned to receive maintenance treatment with amitriptyline, placebo, or no pill, resulting in a six-cell design. Rates of relapse were similar for those receiving amitriptyline and IPT (12% vs. 16%). Patients who received both amitriptyline and IPT had better depression outcomes and better scores on a range of social adjustment measures, including overall adjustment, work performance, and communication, than those taking amitriptyline alone, suggesting an additive effect of IPT on medication treatment (Weissman et al. 1974).

In the second study (DiMascio et al. 1979; Weissman et al. 1979), 97 patients diagnosed with MDD according to the Schedule for Affective Disorders and Schizophrenia (SADS; Endicott and Spitzer 1978) were randomly assigned to receive 16 sessions of IPT delivered over 12 weeks, flexible-dose amitriptyline (maximum dosage=200 mg/day), combined treatment, or a nonscheduled treatment as described in the preceding paragraph. Patients in the nonscheduled treatment group who needed to see the psychiatrist more than once a month were considered to have experienced treatment

TABLE 13–1. Studies of interpersonal psychotherapy in major depressive disorder

Study	Study type	N	Groups	Outcome
Klerman et al. 1974 Paykel et al. 1975	Acute	150	IPT plus amitriptyline Placebo No pill SP plus amitriptyline Placebo No pill	Rates of relapse were 12% and 16% for those receiving amitriptyline and IPT, respectively; depression outcomes and social adjustment rating scores were better in patients who received both amitriptyline and IPT than in those who received amitriptyline alone.
Weissman et al. 1979 DiMascio et al. 1979	Acute	97	IPT Amitriptyline IPT plus amitriptyline Nonscheduled treatment	Combined group had higher retention rates, higher efficacy, and delayed onset of symptomatic failure than either treatment alone or nonscheduled treatment.

TABLE 13–1.   Studies of interpersonal psychotherapy in major depressive disorder (continued)

Study	Study type	N	Groups	Outcome
Elkin et al. 1989	Acute	250	IPT CBT Imipramine plus clinical management Placebo plus clinical management	In severely depressed and functionally impaired patients, IPT alone and imipramine plus clinical management were superior to placebo plus clinical management. CBT was intermediate in efficacy between IPT and imipramine and not significantly different from either. In less severely depressed patients, there were no significant differences among treatments.
Schulberg et al. 1996	Acute	276	Nortriptyline IPT Usual care	Remission rates were superior in the nortriptyline (48%) and IPT (46%) groups compared with the usual care group (18%).
Markowitz et al. 1998	Acute	101	IPT SP CBT SP plus imipramine	Patients randomly assigned to receive IPT or imipramine had significantly better improvement than those receiving SP or CBT.

TABLE 13–1. Studies of interpersonal psychotherapy in major depressive disorder *(continued)*

Study	Study type	N	Groups	Outcome
Frank et al. 1990	Maintenance	128	IPT-M IPT-M plus imipramine IPT plus placebo Imipramine Placebo	Both IPT and imipramine were significantly superior to placebo in delaying MDD relapse. Imipramine was superior to IPT-M in preventing relapse.
Reynolds et al. 1999	Maintenance	187	Nortriptyline IPT-M plus nortriptyline IPT-M plus placebo Placebo	Maintenance treatment with nortriptyline or IPT was superior to placebo in preventing or delaying recurrence. Combined treatment with IPT and nortriptyline was superior to IPT, placebo, and nortriptyline alone.
Reynolds et al. 2006	Maintenance	116	IPT-M plus paroxetine IPT-M plus placebo Paroxetine plus clinical management Placebo plus clinical management	Combined treatment with paroxetine plus IPT-M led to lower rates of recurrence than IPT-M plus placebo, paroxetine, or placebo alone. Monthly IPT-M did not prevent recurrence of depression.

Note. CBT=cognitive-behavioral therapy; IPT=interpersonal psychotherapy; IPT-M=monthly maintenance interpersonal psychotherapy; MDD=major depressive disorder. SP=supportive psychotherapy.

failure and were withdrawn from the study. An important finding of this study was that retention was much higher (67%) in the combined treatment group than in IPT alone (48%), pharmacotherapy alone (33%), and nonscheduled treatment (30%). All active treatments showed higher efficacy than nonscheduled treatment on depression measures. Furthermore, the combined treatment group was superior to both monotherapies. The effects of medication and IPT were additive.

The investigators suggested that the reason for this additive effect was the differential effect of the two treatments on symptoms: the effect of medication appeared to be more marked on sleep disturbances, somatic complaints, and appetite, whereas the effect of IPT appeared to be most marked on depressed mood, suicidal ideation, work and interests, and guilt. The onset of action was faster for amitriptyline than for IPT. A follow-up study (Weissman et al. 1981) found that social functioning did not differ across the groups at the 4-month posttreatment assessment, but at the 1-year posttreatment assessment social functioning was superior in patients receiving IPT, regardless of whether they had been taking medication. The authors interpreted this finding as indicating that the effects of psychotherapy take longer to develop on social functioning than on depressive symptoms.

Probably the most important comparison between medication and IPT to date has been the National Institute of Mental Health Treatment of Depression Collaborative Research Program (NIMH TDCRP). In that study (Elkin et al. 1989), 250 patients meeting SADS criteria for MDD were randomly assigned to receive imipramine plus clinical management, placebo plus clinical management, IPT, or cognitive-behavioral therapy (CBT). In the context of this trial, clinical management was also a manualized intervention, in which clinicians were instructed to empathically query patients regarding their symptoms and medication side effects but were discouraged from actively giving advice, using any CBT technique, directly addressing interpersonal issues, or making psychodynamic interpretations. An initial analysis of the results showed that regardless of the outcome measure under consideration, placebo plus clinical management always had the more symptomatic scores, imipramine plus clinical management had the least, and the two psychotherapies were generally in the middle (Elkin et al. 1989). There were no significant differences between imipramine plus clinical management and the two psychotherapies. However, post hoc analyses showed that although improvement was seen in the milder cases, in the more severe cases (i.e., Hamilton Rating Scale for Depression [Ham-D] score = 20) imipramine and IPT were superior to placebo, whereas CBT was in between and not statistically separable from placebo. In some analyses, IPT appeared to be slightly superior to CBT. However, a reanalysis of the same data set by other researchers using slightly different statistical assumptions found that although IPT was comparable to imipramine plus clinical management for cases in the less severe range of depression, imipramine was significantly superior to IPT in the more severe cases (Klein and Ross 1993). This frequently cited finding has never been replicated, and therefore caution is warranted in generalizing this important result to other samples.

As part of the NIMH TDCRP, researchers conducted an 18-month naturalistic follow-up study of patients who participated in the acute treatment phase (Shea et al. 1992). For the purposes of the study, recovery was defined as 8 weeks of minimal or no symptoms following the end of treatment. Of all patients entering treatment and having follow-up data for at least 6 months (N=200, 84%), the percentage who recovered and remained well during follow-up did not differ significantly across treatments: 30% for the CBT group, 26% for the IPT group, 19% for the imipramine group, and 20% for the placebo group. Thus, this study suggests that 16 weeks of treatment is insufficient for most patients to achieve full recovery and lasting remission, regardless of treatment modality. A secondary result of the NIMH TDCRP naturalistic follow-up study was that no significant differences were found among any of the treatment conditions in social functioning at 6 or 12 months. At 18 months, IPT was significantly superior to imipramine and approached significance over CBT on global social functioning. This result supports the finding of Weissman et al. (1981), although in that study significant differences in social functioning were evident at 12 months (and no follow-up was conducted at 18 months).

IPT has also been compared with pharmacotherapy in the treatment of depressed primary care patients. Schulberg et al. (1996) randomly assigned patients (N=276) with MDD to receive nortriptyline, IPT, or usual care. Although patients improved in all three groups, the investigators found that by 8 months, patients in the IPT and nortriptyline groups were significantly better and improved faster than those in the usual care group. Remission rates were also significantly higher in the nortriptyline (48%) and IPT (46%) groups compared with the usual care group (18%). In contrast with the early DiMascio et al. (1979) study, there were no significant differences between IPT and nortriptyline either in improvement on the Ham-D or in rates of response. In a secondary analysis of the Schulberg et al. data, Brown et al. (1996) found that depressed patients with a comorbid anxiety disorder presented with significantly more psychopathology and tended to terminate treatment prematurely more frequently than patients with MDD alone. Both IPT and nortriptyline were efficacious for depressed patients with and without comorbid generalized anxiety disorder, but time to recovery was longer for the former. Patients with a lifetime history of panic disorder showed poor recovery in response to either psychotherapy or pharmacotherapy. The authors concluded that both treatments were effective in primary care patients with MDD and a comorbid anxiety disorder, and there were no significant differences between the two treatments.

The comparative efficacy of IPT and medication has also been examined in the treatment of depressive symptoms in HIV-positive patients (Markowitz et al. 1998). A total of 101 patients (85 male, 16 female) with known HIV seropositivity for at least 6 months were randomly assigned to 16 weeks of treatment with IPT, supportive psychotherapy with imipramine, supportive psychotherapy alone, or CBT. Patients randomly assigned to IPT or imipramine had significantly better improvement than those receiving supportive psychotherapy or CBT, possibly because IPT addresses significant real changes in one's life rather than attempting to correct distorted cognitions, and these patients were experiencing dramatic life changes. The results of this study are important in documenting the efficacy of IPT in a special population. In conjunction with the results of the studies in primary care, they suggest the potential of IPT for the treatment of depressed patients with general medical conditions such as diabetes, asthma, or cancer, although a recent study found no benefit of IPT in depressed patients with cardiovascular disease (Lespérance et al. 2007). The results are also reminiscent of the results of the NIMH TDCRP in that both studies showed comparable efficacy of imipramine and IPT and potential superiority over CBT.

Overall, these studies seem to indicate that IPT and antidepressant medications have similar efficacy in the acute treatment of MDD. The combination of IPT and medication seems to be superior to either treatment alone, consistent with findings from the general psychotherapy and combined treatment literature (Keller et al. 2000; Thase et al. 1997b). Several not mutually exclusive mechanisms may explain the superiority of combined IPT plus medication over either treatment alone. First, combined treatment seems to improve retention. Because both IPT and antidepressants are efficacious treatments, increased retention should result in improved outcome. Second, IPT and medication may have differential efficacy for specific symptoms. Their combination should result in an overall more powerful treatment. Third, it is possible that some patients respond only to IPT, whereas others respond only to medication, the same way that some patients respond to some medications but not to others. Providing both treatments would then cover a broader range of potential responders, resulting in a larger overall response.

Maintenance Studies of Major Depressive Disorder

Because of the success of IPT as an acute treatment for MDD, the recurrent nature of mood disorders, and the efficacy of medication in preventing relapse and recurrence, IPT was adapted as a once-monthly maintenance treatment for MDD (monthly maintenance IPT [IPT-M]) (Frank et al. 1991). The results are summarized in Table 13–1.

The use of IPT as maintenance treatment was a novel development and allowed the first real testing of psychotherapy as a maintenance treatment for patients who had experienced remission of acute depression. Because IPT-M begins with patients who have remitted, its goal is to maintain the remitted state. Both patient and therapist are vigilant for early signs of interpersonal problems similar to those the patient and therapist previously identified as associated with the onset of the patient's most recent depressive episode. At the same time, the therapist works to enhance strengths that appear to have been present prior to the patient's illness or that began to emerge as the most recent depressive episode remitted. In contrast with the acute-phase application of IPT, which usually focuses on one or at most two interpersonal problem areas, ITP-M may shift problem areas over time. Three studies have compared medication and IPT as maintenance treatment for MDD.

In the first study, Frank et al. (1990, 1991) treated patients with acute IPT and imipramine at a dosage of up to 300 mg/day to remission from MDD, which was defined as a Ham-D score of ≤7 and a score on the Raskin Three-Area Severity of Depression Scale of ≤5 for at least 3 weeks. Patients whose symptoms remitted were stabilized for several months, during which time IPT was tapered to once monthly and imipramine maintained at full dosage. These patients were then randomly assigned to one of five groups: 1) IPT-M alone, 2) IPT-M with imipramine, 3) IPT with placebo, 4) imipramine alone, or 5) placebo alone. Patients received the maintenance treatment for 3 years. Both IPT and imipramine were significantly superior to placebo in delaying MDD relapse. Imipramine was superior to IPT-M in the ability to prevent relapse, possibly because of the relatively low-dose characteristic of IPT-M compared with the high dose of imipramine (mean dosage >200 mg/day) used in this study. In contrast to the findings in some of the acute treatment studies (Klerman et al. 1974), there were no additive or synergistic effects in delaying relapse between IPT-M and imipramine. The study may not have had sufficient power to examine that particular question: the group that received IPT with imipramine had a numerically lower rate of recurrence at 1 year (16%) than the group taking imipramine alone (40%). At 2 years, the mean survival time was 92 weeks for the IPT-with-imipramine group compared with 83 weeks for the imipramine-alone group. A later reanalysis of this study also showed that the quality of IPT-M (i.e., whether IPT-M was truly given as prescribed by the therapy manual) was an important predictor of its efficacy in delaying relapse (Frank et al. 1991).

The second maintenance study extended the findings of the first by focusing on individuals 60 years and older. Reynolds et al. (1999) randomly assigned 187 patients who had achieved remission on nortriptyline alone and had successfully maintained remission for 16 weeks on combined nortriptyline with IPT-M to receive one of four treatments: nortriptyline alone, placebo alone, IPT-M with nortriptyline, or IPT-M with placebo. The investigators found that time to recurrence of MDD for all three active treatments was significantly longer than for placebo. Combined nortriptyline with IPT was significantly superior to IPT and placebo alone in rates of recurrence. The comparison between combined nortriptyline with IPT versus nortriptyline alone approached, but failed to reach, statistical significance ($P=0.06$). This study showed a clinically (and almost statistically significant) advantage of combined treatment over medication alone in elderly depressed patients—an advantage that was less clearly evident in the Frank et al. (1990) study but that was in line with the early DiMascio et al. (1979) study.

Given the clinical context of MDD in later life, with its medical and psychosocial complexities, Reynolds et al. (1999) concluded that combined treatment was the treatment of choice in old-age depression. They pointed out that their study suggested that a primary care physician could competently prescribe and monitor antidepressant medication, which would facilitate the provision of combined treatment. A potential limitation of this study is that the antidepressant used was nortriptyline, rather than one of the selective serotonin reuptake inhibitors (SSRIs), which now have essentially replaced the tricyclic antidepressants. A recent study by the same group (Reynolds et al. 2006) found that patients 70 years of age or older with MDD who had responded to initial treatment with paroxetine and IPT-M were less likely to have recurrent depression if they received 2 years of maintenance therapy with paroxetine. Monthly maintenance psychotherapy did not prevent recurrence of depression, suggesting IPT-M may not be useful in the "old-old," possibly because of cognitive dysfunction that interferes with psychotherapy.

In summary, these maintenance studies found that IPT-M helps delay or prevent MDD relapse. Furthermore, although data are limited, there may be an additive effect of antidepressants and IPT in preventing relapse. In conjunction with the follow-up findings of the NIMH TDCRP demonstrating the risk of relapse after acute antidepressant treatment (Shea et al. 1992), these results strongly suggest the usefulness of IPT-M for a substantial number of patients with a history of MDD, regardless of whether they achieved remission with medication treatment or IPT. Important questions for future research are whether the efficacy of IPT-M is dose dependent (i.e., would higher frequencies lead to lower rates of relapse?) and whether IPT-M needs to be administered indefinitely, can be delivered with less frequency/intensity later on in the maintenance period, or can even eventually be stopped.

IPT and Medication in Other Disorders

The success of IPT in treating MDD has led researchers to investigate its efficacy in other disorders (see Chapter 12, "Applications of Individual Interpersonal Psychotherapy to Specific Disorders: Efficacy and Indications"). Modified forms of IPT have been compared or combined with medication in the treatment of two other mood disorders: bipolar disorder and dysthymic disorder. The studies are summarized in Table 13–2.

Bipolar Disorder

The modification of IPT used as an adjunct to medication in the treatment of bipolar disorder is called *interpersonal and social rhythm therapy* (IPSRT). Its use rests on the hypothesis that disruptions of social rhythms are destabilizing for bipolar patients and contribute to trigger relapse. By decreasing the number and intensity of those disruptions, IPSRT should improve the course of bipolar disorder.

To test this hypothesis, after stabilizing bipolar I patients with appropriate pharmacotherapy and either IPSRT or intensive clinical management, Frank et al. (1999) randomly assigned patients again to either IPSRT or clinical management for preventive treatment. In an early analysis of the data ($N=82$), Frank et al. found that patients remaining in the same treatment for both acute and preventive phases had lower rates of recurrence (<20% vs. >40%) and lower levels of symptomatology over the 52 weeks than those reassigned to the alternative modality. A surprising finding of that study was that continuity of treatment had more powerful effects than treatment specificity. That is, transfer from clinical management to IPSRT (supposedly a more powerful treatment) worsened the outcome of patients already receiving clinical management.

In a full report including 175 patients followed for 2 years, Frank et al. (2005) found that participants assigned to IPSRT acutely had longer survival times to a new affective episode, irrespective of maintenance treatment assignment. Participants in the IPSRT group had higher regularity of social rhythms at the end of the acute treatment, and this increased regularity of social rhythms during the acute treatment mediated the reduced likelihood of recurrence during the maintenance treatment. Further research appears necessary to more firmly establish the optimal timing and treatment duration of IPSRT.

Dysthymic Disorder

Three studies have examined the efficacy of IPT in treating patients with dysthymic disorder. de Mello et al. (2001) randomly assigned 35 patients with an ICD-10 diagnosis of dysthymia with or without comorbid MDD to

TABLE 13–2. Studies of interpersonal psychotherapy beyond major depressive disorder

Study	Disorder	N	Groups	Outcome
Frank et al. 2005	Bipolar I disorder	175	IPSRT Intensive clinical management	Participants assigned to IPSRT in the acute treatment phase had a longer period without a new affective episode, higher regularity of social rhythms, and reduced likelihood of recurrence during maintenance phase.
de Mello et al. 2001	Dysthymic disorder	35	Moclobemide plus IPT Moclobemide (300 mg/day)	Both moclobemide-plus-IPT and moclobemide-alone groups showed statistically significant improvement in all measures across time. Moclobemide-plus-IPT group had higher retention and statistically better scores than group receiving moclobemide alone on all outcome variables at weeks 24 and 48.

TABLE 13–2. Studies of interpersonal psychotherapy beyond major depressive disorder (continued)

Study	Disorder	N	Groups	Outcome
Browne et al. 2002	Dysthymic disorder with or without past or current MDD	707	Sertraline alone (50–200 mg/day) IPT IPT plus sertraline	Sertraline group and sertraline plus IPT group had higher response rates after 6 months and greater reduction in depressive symptoms at 2 years compared with IPT group.
Markowitz et al. 2005	Dysthymic disorder without MDD in prior 6 months	94	IPT BSP Sertraline Sertraline plus IPT	Sertraline group had superior response and remission rates compared with groups receiving psychotherapy alone. Groups receiving sertraline or sertraline plus IPT had higher response rates compared with groups receiving psychotherapy alone.

Note. BSP=brief supportive psychotherapy; IPSRT=interpersonal and social rhythm therapy; IPT=interpersonal therapy; MDD=major depressive disorder.

receive either moclobemide alone (n=19) or moclobemide plus IPT (n=16). Patients in both groups were treated with flexible-dose moclobemide up to 300 mg twice per day. Patients in the moclobemide-plus-IPT group also received 16 weekly sessions during the acute treatment phase and 6 monthly booster sessions during the maintenance phase. Patients were assessed with the 17-item Ham-D, the Global Assessment Scale, and the Quality of Life and Satisfaction Questionnaire at baseline, 12, 24, and 48 weeks. Both groups showed statistically significant improvement in all measures across time. Eleven patients (57.9%) in the moclobemide-alone group and six patients (37.5%) in the combined treatment group dropped out of the study. There were no differences between the two treatments at week 12. However, patients in the combined group had statistically better scores than the patients in the moclobemide group on all outcome variables at weeks 24 and 48. Both the higher retention and superior outcome of the combined group over medication alone are consistent with the findings in MDD (DiMascio et al. 1979; Reynolds et al. 1999). The percentage of patients with comorbid MDD ("double depression") was 91%.

In the second study, a clinical trial with blind outcome assessors, Browne et al. (2002) randomly assigned 707 adults in a primary care clinic with DSM-IV-TR dysthymic disorder, with or without past and/or current MDD (15% of the sample had current MDD), to treatment with sertraline alone (50–200 mg/day), IPT alone (10 sessions), or sertraline with IPT combined. Response was defined as ≥40% improvement from baseline. At the end of treatment, response rates were 60% for sertraline alone, 47% for IPT alone, and 58% for sertraline with IPT. After an additional 18-month naturalistic follow-up phase, there were no statistically significant differences in symptom reduction between sertraline alone and sertraline with IPT. However, both were more effective than IPT alone in reducing depressive symptoms. It is important to note, though, that IPT was given as a brief treatment, whereas sertraline was generally continued for the full 2 years of the study.

A third study (Markowitz et al. 2005) compared IPT adapted for the treatment of dysthymia (IPT-D), brief supportive psychotherapy, sertraline, and combined IPT-D and sertraline for patients with pure dysthymic disorder (i.e., without MDD in the 6 months prior to presentation; not double depression) in 94 subjects treated over 16 weeks. Attrition by cell was 17% for IPT-D, 19% for combined IPT-D and sertraline, 21% for sertraline alone, and 42% for brief supportive psychotherapy. Unlike studies in patients with MDD, this study did not find a substantially higher retention rate in the combined group than in the monotherapy groups. Patients improved in all conditions, with the cells including sertraline pharmacotherapy showing superiority over psychotherapy alone in response and remission.

The results of this study are consistent with an emerging literature suggesting that pharmacotherapy may acutely benefit patients more than psychotherapy. However, the study failed to examine the long-term effects of IPT-D alone or in combination with sertraline (e.g., does the addition of IPT-D extend in time the acute beneficial effects of sertraline?). Differences with the de Mello et al. (2001) study may have been due to differences in the efficacy of sertraline versus moclobemide in the treatment of dysthymic disorder or differences in the sample, because the de Mello et al. study allowed the inclusion of individuals with double depression, whereas the Markowitz et al. study excluded those individuals. However, in conjunction with the Browne et al. (2002) study, the Markowitz et al. study suggests that IPT may not be an efficacious treatment for all mood disorders.

Predictors of Response to Interpersonal Psychotherapy

In addition to the Brown et al. (1996) study described earlier (see subsection "Acute Studies of Major Depressive Disorder"), which examined anxiety as a predictor of response, four studies have examined predictors of response to IPT. Sotsky et al. (1991) and Krupnick et al. (1996) analyzed data from the NIMH TDCRP to identify general predictors of response to MDD treatment, as well as predictors for specific treatment modalities. Eight patient characteristics predicted outcome across treatments: social dysfunction (more severe dysfunction predicted worse response), cognitive dysfunction (more severe dysfunction predicted worse response, particularly to CBT), expectation of improvement (higher expectation predicted better response), therapeutic alliance (higher levels of alliance predicted better response), endogeneity of depression (endogenous depression predicted better response), double depression (its presence predicted poorer outcome), personality traits (presence of certain traits predicted worse response), and duration of current episode (longer duration predicted worse response). In addition, Sotsky et al. found that prior social adjustment, as measured by previous attainment of a marital relationship and higher satisfaction with social relationships in general, differentially predicted good response to IPT. This finding is consistent with reports in the general psychotherapy literature documenting that various indicators of social competence or achievement are associated with good psychotherapy response, whereas social impairment is not. Sotsky et al. noted that all predictors together explained less than 10% of the variance in response, suggesting that our understanding of treatment-specific predictors is still rather limited.

In another study, Thase et al. (1997a) classified depressed individuals into a group with normal sleep profiles ($n=50$) and a group with abnormal sleep profiles ($n=41$) on the basis of a validated index score derived from three electroencephalogram sleep variables monitored for 2 nights: sleep efficiency, rapid eye movement (REM) latency, and REM density. They found that patients with abnormal sleep profiles had significantly poorer clinical outcomes in symptom ratings, attrition rates, and remission rates than patients with more normal sleep profiles. Seventy-five percent of the patients who had not responded to IPT had remissions during subsequent pharmacotherapy. The authors interpreted this finding as indicating that more "biologically disturbed" depressed episodes are less responsive to psychotherapy. A limitation of this study is the use of sequential treatment without a control group in either part of the sequence, precluding an examination of whether failure to respond to IPT was due to a nonspecific delayed treatment response or to a lack of IPT for these types of patients.

The third study, as with the Brown et al. (1996) study, examined the effect of comorbidity on response to IPT. Frank et al. (2000b) compared the response to IPT in 61 depressed women participating in a larger randomized trial according to whether they scored high or low on the Panic-Agoraphobia Spectrum Self-Report. Women with high levels of panic-agoraphobia spectrum symptoms were less likely to respond to IPT alone than women with low scores on the Panic-Agoraphobia Spectrum Self-Report. A Kaplan-Meier survival analysis showed that high anxiety scores were also associated with a longer median time to remission with sequential treatment (addition of an SSRI when no remission in depression was seen with IPT alone). A limitation of this study is the lack of a control arm, which precluded examination of the specificity of IPT to these findings.

Overall, these findings suggest that comorbidity tends to worsen the prognosis of treatment with IPT alone. It is possible that patients with comorbidity may benefit from combined treatment.

Choosing Interpersonal Psychotherapy or Medication Treatment

Because treatment needs to be individualized for each patient, it is often useful to establish some rules to systematize treatment selection. We believe that, in general, five factors should be considered when choosing one treatment over other alternatives: 1) strength of the evidence for the efficacy of the treatment under consideration; 2) contraindications to the use of the treatments; 3) patient preference; 4) feasibility of treatment delivery, including economic factors that may influence treatment availability; and 5) clinician preference and competence.

Strength of the Evidence for the Efficacy of the Treatment Under Consideration

With the exception of the reanalyses of the NIMH TDCRP (Klein and Ross 1993), which suggested that medication may be superior to IPT in patients with more severe global impairment, there is no evidence that medication alone is superior to IPT alone in any domain in acute or as maintenance treatment. There is some evidence that IPT may actually improve long-term social functioning, possibly because of the new acquisition or restoration of interpersonal skills, which probably provides an enduring effect of IPT over medication. The situation is different regarding combined treatment, in which the weight of the evidence suggests that combined treatment is superior in both acute and maintenance treatment of MDD. It is important to note, however, that patients who achieved remission while taking medication can be maintained with IPT alone (Frank et al. 1990), suggesting that patients who achieved remission with combined treatment might also be maintained with IPT alone.

Contraindications to Use of the Treatments

We are not aware of any contraindications to IPT for mood disorders. In addition, there is substantial evidence that IPT is efficacious for a variety of populations, ages, and cultures, and in a diversity of formats and modes of delivery (see Chapter 12). It is also uncommon for all antidepressant medications (and by implication combined treatment) to be contraindicated for a patient. Pregnancy may be the only situation in which all antidepressants raise concern, and even this is still an active area of research. At present, pregnancy is at most a relative contraindication. Although each case deserves individual consideration, given its proven efficacy in the treatment of depressed pregnant women (Spinelli 1997; Spinelli and Endicott 2003), a course of IPT appears reasonable in most cases before prescribing an antidepressant.

Patient Preference

Patient preference should also be an important factor in treatment selection. As recently highlighted by the Institute of Medicine of the National Academies (2006), preference is a value in its own right. Furthermore, patient preference is likely to influence treatment adherence and thus its effectiveness (Roy-Byrne et al. 2002). The reasons for patient preferences are diverse and may include prior experience with the treatments, patients' knowledge and beliefs about treatment, and logistical reasons.

Some patients may prefer IPT alone for several reasons: IPT is devoid of medication side effects, it avoids potential interactions with any other medications (or with alcohol consumption), and it may not require ongoing treatment (although maintenance IPT may be advisable in cases of recurrent depression). It may also be perceived by the patient or others as less stigmatizing: the patient may see psychotherapy as indicating less severity than a disorder that requires medication, may value the psychological-mindedness that is necessary to engage in psychotherapy, may appreciate the IPT model of solving one's current life problems as a route to remission, or may consider that not taking medication avoids the possibility of others accidentally finding the patient's pills and labeling him or her as a psychiatric patient.

Other patients may prefer medication alone. Although the onset of action of IPT has not been systematically studied, clinical impression suggests that it may take 4–6 weeks before depressive symptoms start to improve. By contrast, it is generally accepted that the onset of action of antidepressants is generally 2–4 weeks, and two recent meta-analyses suggest that the onset of action of antidepressants might be even faster (Posternak and Zimmerman 2005; Taylor et al. 2006). Antidepressants may also require less time commitment (i.e., fewer and shorter treatment visits, particularly during the acute episode) than IPT treatment. This may be important for individuals with busy schedules or for those (e.g., low-income patients) who have changing job schedules or cannot afford child care. Some patients may also have limited interest in addressing psychological issues or shy away from affect, which could make medication a more appealing option.

Finally, some patients may prefer combined treatment. Some patients may be aware that combined treatment has shown superiority over monotherapy not only when IPT is used but also when other psychotherapies are involved. They may want to use the best available treatment and not risk using potentially inferior alternatives. Other patients may believe that medication treatment may provide relief for their symptoms but not solve the psychological conflicts that originate them or resolve life stressors that could trigger future episodes. Still others may believe that their depression has both biochemical and psychological roots and want to address both sources of symptoms.

Feasibility of Treatment Delivery

A fourth factor influencing treatment selection is the availability of different treatments. As an example, whereas many nonpsychiatric physicians can competently deliver antidepressant treatment, relatively few psychotherapists have received formal training in IPT. Thus, finding an IPT therapist might be difficult or might require traveling a long distance. Some patients may be willing to make that effort to obtain their preferred treatment, but others with less marked preferences may be willing to accept treatment with medication if it is more easily accessible. These issues are more dramatically evident in the treatment of special populations. Finding Spanish-speaking IPT therapists can be challenging. Finding a psychiatrist with expertise in the treatment of depressed pregnant women outside cities without major universities can also be difficult.

Economic considerations can also influence treatment availability and selection. Provision of IPT generally requires weekly 50-minute visits, whereas medication management can be accomplished in much shorter and less frequent visits. However, the cost of pharmacotherapy also involves the medication cost. This cost can be substantial if the patient requires maintenance treatment. IPT is often delivered by nonphysicians, and therefore the cost of visits may be lower. Most antidepressants are prescribed by psychiatrists or other physicians. The timing of the treatment costs may also influence treatment selection, because IPT costs occur up front, whereas medication costs are generally spread over a longer period of time. Reimbursement of the different aspects of the treatment may also powerfully influence treatment preference and selection.

Clinician Preference and Competence

Although often overlooked, clinician factors are also important determinants of treatment selection. Like patients, clinicians have information and beliefs about the efficacy and acceptability of different treatments. Although clinicians may not be influenced in their decision by the side effects of treatment, they may have different degrees of familiarity or competence with particular treatments. Given the same amount of empirical evidence, most clinicians are most likely to recommend treatments in which they feel well trained or which they feel confident they can provide. Economic factors, such as reimbursement policies, may also subliminally influence clinicians in their treatment recommendations. Clinicians' awareness of their own beliefs and potential biases, and systematic presentation of the available treatments to patients, may help decrease the influence of some of these on treatment selection.

In summary, the choice of treatment is a complex process in which several factors, not only the empirical support for each type of treatment, play an important role. Being aware of the tension between evidence and preference and availability of treatment should facilitate informed treatment selection.

Combining and Sequencing Interpersonal Psychotherapy With Medication

To date, there are no controlled studies that have investigated the addition of IPT to medication treatment in patients who have had partial or no response to the medication. The pharmacological literature (Quitkin et al. 1996, 2003, 2005) suggests that 4–8 weeks of medication treatment should be completed before declaring the treatment failed. If we consider IPT as equivalent to an antidepressant, 4–8 weeks appears a reasonable time frame to consider addition of IPT, unless patient preference or other factors suggest a different course. Similarly, there are no controlled studies of medication augmentation of IPT. However, two observational studies, both involving women (Frank et al. 2000a, 2000b), have suggested that addition of medication to patients who did not respond to a full trial of IPT can result in an increase in the number of treatment responders. Although both studies added the medication after a full course (12 weeks) of IPT, it appears reasonable to add medication earlier (6–8 weeks after the beginning of IPT) if no improvement in mood symptoms has been detected, unless there are reasons to delay this augmentation strategy.

Another issue to consider is medication adherence in the context of combined treatment. There are no systematic studies on how to improve medication adherence in combined treatment. From clinical experience, we believe that the framework presented earlier in the subsection "Feasibility of Treatment Delivery" can serve to explore potential reasons for poor adherence. Reasons may include new or previously nonverbalized concerns about medications; emergent side effects; cost of medication; and symptomatic improvement, which leads the patient to consider a less intensive treatment (i.e., only IPT, or possibly medication only). In our view, rather than the therapist focusing on persuading the patient to improve medication adherence, it is more productive to explore the potential reasons for nonadherence and attempt to negotiate an approach that balances scientific evidence and patient preference. This may include continuing with the combined treatment regimen after the patient is reassured that this course of action is superior to others; but temporary or permanent discontinuation of the medication might also ensue. Because IPT has proven to be a useful maintenance treatment for patients who have achieved remission while taking medication, it is likely to be useful also for those who have improved on combined treatment.

Finally, when combined treatment is provided, the issue is raised of how to structure the IPT session. Although there are no empirical studies or established protocols to guide this aspect of the treatment, we have found it useful to address medication issues generally early in the session. This approach allows for an initial exploration of the symptoms and frees up the rest of the session, preventing the need to cut short a potential discussion at the end of the session in order to be able to address pharmacological treatment. However, as with any clinical rule, exceptions may have to be made to accommodate the needs of patients or the urgency to discuss other aspects of the treatment.

Conclusion

As this review shows, there is substantial evidence that the combination of IPT with medication is at least as efficacious as either approach alone in adults. It is important to note that in almost all the MDD studies, the antidepressant medication used was a tricyclic. Given the current preeminent role of SSRIs in the treatment of MDD, an obvious direction for future studies would be to compare the efficacy of SSRIs versus IPT and their combination in the treatment of MDD. To date, only one study has addressed this issue (Reynolds et al. 2006), but it focused on the old-old and on maintenance treatment rather than on acute treatment. Given the scarcity of health care resources, studies in large samples that may allow for the identification of predictors of differential response to IPT versus combined treatment may also help in determining how to best allocate these resources.

There is also evidence that both antidepressant medication and IPT adapted for adolescents (IPT-A) are effective treatments for MDD in adolescents (Mufson et al. 1994, 1999, 2004). Given recent concerns about increased suicidal ideation in adolescents treated with antidepressants, a natural research step would be to compare the acceptability, efficacy, and safety of medication versus IPT in the treatment of MDD in adolescents. Another natural next research step would be to examine the relative efficacy, acceptability, and cost-effectiveness of combined IPT plus medication in the treatment of this population. Combined treatment might make more sense than sequential treatment for most adolescents. Depressed adolescents might get discouraged and not have the patience to try an augmentation strategy if the initial treatment does not lead to response or recovery.

A final area for future research is to compare medication to IPT and combined treatment for patients with non–mood disorders. IPT has shown efficacy in the treatment of bulimia and has had promising results in several trials of anxiety disorders, including social anxiety disorder, panic disorder, and posttraumatic stress disorder. Although a growing body of evidence has also established the efficacy of pharmacotherapy in the treatment of these disorders, many patients do not respond or have residual symptoms after treatment with medication or psychotherapy alone. Therefore, examining the efficacy of sequential or combined treatment in these disorders also appears an area of high research priority.

In conclusion, although the empirical basis of the efficacy of IPT, medication, and their combination is solidly established, there are still substantial opportunities for future research and potential patient benefit in this area.

Key Points

- Interpersonal psychotherapy (IPT) has demonstrated efficacy as an acute treatment for patients with major depressive disorder (MDD) or bipolar disorder.

- IPT and antidepressant medications have similar efficacy in the acute treatment of outpatients with MDD without psychotic features.

- The combination of IPT and medication seems to be superior to either treatment alone in the acute treatment of MDD.

- Monthly maintenance IPT helps delay or prevent relapse as maintenance treatment of MDD.

- Comorbidity tends to worsen the prognosis of treatment with IPT alone (as is also true for other treatments). It is possible that patients with comorbidity may benefit from combined treatment.

- When choosing IPT over other treatment alternatives, the therapist should take into account the strength of the evidence of the efficacy of the treatments under consideration, contraindications for the use of the treatments, patient preference, the feasibility of delivering the treatment, and the clinician's competence.

References

Brown C, Schulberg HC, Madonia MJ, et al: Treatment outcomes for primary care patients with major depression and lifetime anxiety disorders. Am J Psychiatry 153:1293–1300, 1996

Browne G, Steiner M, Roberts J, et al: Sertraline and/or interpersonal psychotherapy for patients with dysthymic disorder in primary care: 6-month comparison with longitudinal 2-year follow-up of effectiveness and costs. J Affect Disord 68:317–330, 2002

de Mello MF, Myczcowisk LM, Menezes PR: A randomized controlled trial comparing moclobemide and moclobemide plus interpersonal psychotherapy in the treatment of dysthymic disorder. J Psychother Pract Res 10:117–123, 2001

DiMascio A, Weissman MM, Prusoff BA, et al: Differential symptom reduction by drugs and psychotherapy in acute depression. Arch Gen Psychiatry 36:1450–1456, 1979

Elkin I, Shea MT, Watkins JT, et al: National Institute of Mental Health Treatment of Depression Collaborative Research Program: general effectiveness of treatments. Arch Gen Psychiatry 46:971–982, 1989

Endicott J, Spitzer RL: A diagnostic interview: the Schedule for Affective Disorders and schizophrenia. Arch Gen Psychiatry 35:837–844, 1978

Frank E, Kupfer DJ, Perel JM, et al: Three-year outcomes for maintenance therapies in recurrent depression. Arch Gen Psychiatry 47:1093–1099, 1990

Frank E, Kupfer DJ, Wagner EF, et al: Efficacy of interpersonal psychotherapy as a maintenance treatment for recurrent depression: contributing factors. Arch Gen Psychiatry 48:1053–1059, 1991

Frank E, Swartz HA, Mallinger AG, et al: Adjunctive psychotherapy for bipolar disorder: effects of changing treatment modality. J Abnorm Psychol 108:579–587, 1999

Frank E, Grochocinski VJ, Spanier CA, et al: Interpersonal psychotherapy and antidepressant medication: evaluation of a sequential treatment strategy in women with recurrent major depression. J Clin Psychiatry 61:51–57, 2000a

Frank E, Shear MK, Rucci P, et al: Influence of panic-agoraphobic spectrum symptoms on treatment response in patients with recurrent major depression. Am J Psychiatry 157:1101–1107, 2000b

Frank E, Kupfer DJ, Thase ME, et al: Two-year outcomes for interpersonal and social rhythm therapy in individuals with bipolar I disorder. Arch Gen Psychiatry 62:996–1004, 2005

Institute of Medicine: Improving the Quality of Health Care for Mental and Substance-Use Conditions. Washington, DC, National Academies Press, 2006

Keller MB, McCullough JP, Klein DN, et al: A comparison of nefazodone, the cognitive behavioral-analysis system of psychotherapy, and their combination for the treatment of chronic depression. N Engl J Med 342:1462–1470, 2000

Klein DF, Ross DC: Reanalysis of the National Institute of Mental Health Treatment of Depression Collaborative Research Program General Effectiveness Report. Neuropsychopharmacology 8:241–251, 1993

Klerman GL, Dimascio A, Weissman M, et al: Treatment of depression by drugs and psychotherapy. Am J Psychiatry 131:186–191, 1974

Krupnick JL, Sotsky SM, Simmens S, et al: The role of the therapeutic alliance in psychotherapy and pharmacotherapy outcome: findings in the National Institute of Mental Health Treatment of Depression Collaborative Research Program. J Consult Clin Psychol 64:532–539, 1996

Lespérance F, Frasure-Smith N, Koszycki D, et al; CREATE Investigators: Effects of citalopram and interpersonal psychotherapy on depression in patients with coronary artery disease: the Canadian Cardiac Randomized Evaluation of Antidepressant and Psychotherapy Efficacy (CREATE) trial. JAMA 297:367–379, 2007

Markowitz JC, Kocsis JH, Fishman B, et al: Treatment of HIV-positive patients with depressive symptoms. Arch Gen Psychiatry 55:452–457, 1998

Markowitz JC, Kocsis JH, Bleiberg KL, et al: A comparative trial of psychotherapy and pharmacotherapy for "pure" dysthymic patients. J Affect Disord 89:167–175, 2005

Mufson L, Moreau D, Weissman MM, et al: Modification of interpersonal psychotherapy with depressed adolescents (IPT-A): phase I and II studies. J Am Acad Child Adolesc Psychiatry 33:695–705, 1994

Mufson L, Weissman MM, Moreau D, et al: Efficacy of interpersonal psychotherapy for depressed adolescents. Arch Gen Psychiatry 56:573–579, 1999

Mufson L, Dorta KP, Wickramaratne P, et al: A randomized effectiveness trial of interpersonal psychotherapy for depressed adolescents. Arch Gen Psychiatry 61:577–584, 2004

Paykel ES, Dimascio A, Haskell D, et al: Effects of maintenance amitriptyline and psychotherapy on symptoms of depression. Psychol Med 5:67–77, 1975

Posternak MA, Zimmerman M: Is there a delay in the antidepressant effect? A meta-analysis. J Clin Psychiatry 66:148–158, 2005

Quitkin FM, McGrath PJ, Stewart JW, et al: Chronological milestones to guide drug change. When should clinicians switch antidepressants? Arch Gen Psychiatry 53:785–792, 1996

Quitkin FM, Petkova E, McGrath PJ, et al: When should a trial of fluoxetine for major depression be declared failed? Am J Psychiatry 160:734–740, 2003

Quitkin FM, McGrath PJ, Stewart JW, et al: Remission rates with 3 consecutive antidepressant trials: effectiveness for depressed outpatients. J Clin Psychiatry 66:670–676, 2005

Reynolds CF 3rd, Frank E, Perel JM, et al: Nortriptyline and interpersonal psychotherapy as maintenance therapies for recurrent major depression: a randomized controlled trial in patients older than 59 years. JAMA 281:39–45, 1999

Reynolds CF 3rd, Dew MA, Pollock BG, et al: Maintenance treatment of major depression in old age. N Engl J Med 354:1130–1138, 2006

Roy-Byrne P, Russo J, Dugdale DC, et al: Undertreatment of panic disorder in primary care: role of patient and physician characteristics. J Am Board Fam Pract 15:443–450, 2002

Schulberg HC, Block MR, Madonia MJ, et al: Treating major depression in primary care practice: eight-month clinical outcomes. Arch Gen Psychiatry 53:913–919, 1996

Shea MT, Elkin I, Imber SD, et al: Course of depressive symptoms over follow-up: findings from the National Institute of Mental Health Treatment of Depression Collaborative Research Program. Arch Gen Psychiatry 49:782–787, 1992

Sotsky SM, Glass DR, Shea MT, et al: Patient predictors of response to psychotherapy and pharmacotherapy: findings in the NIMH Treatment of Depression Collaborative Research Program. Am J Psychiatry 148:997–1008, 1991

Spinelli MG: Interpersonal psychotherapy for depressed antepartum women: a pilot study. Am J Psychiatry 154:1028–1030, 1997

Spinelli MG, Endicott J: Controlled clinical trial of interpersonal psychotherapy versus parenting education program for depressed pregnant women. Am J Psychiatry 160:555–562, 2003

Taylor MJ, Freemantle N, Geddes JR, et al: Early onset of selective serotonin reuptake inhibitor antidepressant action: systematic review and meta-analysis. Arch Gen Psychiatry 63:1217–1223, 2006

Thase ME, Buysse DJ, Frank E, et al: Which depressed patients will respond to interpersonal psychotherapy? The role of abnormal EEG sleep profiles. Am J Psychiatry 154:502–509, 1997a

Thase ME, Greenhouse JB, Frank E, et al: Treatment of major depression with psychotherapy or psychotherapy-pharmacotherapy combinations. Arch Gen Psychiatry 54:1009–1015, 1997b

Weissman MM, Klerman GL, Paykel ES, et al: Treatment effects on the social adjustment of depressed patients. Arch Gen Psychiatry 30:771–778, 1974

Weissman MM, Prusoff BA, Dimascio A, et al: The efficacy of drugs and psychotherapy in the treatment of acute depressive episodes. Am J Psychiatry 136:555–558, 1979

Weissman MM, Klerman GL, Prusoff BA, et al: Depressed outpatients: results one year after treatment with drugs and/or interpersonal psychotherapy. Arch Gen Psychiatry 38:51–55, 1981

Suggested Readings

Elkin I, Shea MT, Watkins JT, et al: National Institute of Mental Health Treatment of Depression Collaborative Research Program: general effectiveness of treatments. Arch Gen Psychiatry 46:971–982, 1989

Frank E, Kupfer DJ, Perel JM, et al: Three-year outcomes for maintenance therapies in recurrent depression. Arch Gen Psychiatry 47:1093–1099, 1990

Frank E, Kupfer DJ, Thase ME, et al: Two-year outcomes for interpersonal and social rhythm therapy in individuals with bipolar I disorder. Arch Gen Psychiatry 62:996–1004, 2005

PART 4

Individual Supportive Psychotherapy

Section Editor
Arnold Winston, M.D.

Chapter 14

Theory of Supportive Psychotherapy

Arnold Winston, M.D.
Michael Goldstein, M.D.

Supportive psychotherapy is a broadly defined approach with wide applicability that uses direct measures to ameliorate symptoms and maintain, restore, or improve self-esteem, ego function, and adaptive skills (Pinsker 1994; Pinsker et al. 1991; Winston et al. 2004). *Self-esteem* involves the patient's sense of efficacy, confidence, hope, and self-regard. *Ego functions* or *structural functions* include relation to reality, object relations, defenses, regulation of impulses and affects, thinking, and others (Bellak 1958; Beres 1956; Winston et al. 2004). *Adaptive skills* are actions associated with effective functioning. To accomplish these objectives, treatment involves examination of symptoms, relationships, everyday functioning, and patterns of emotional responses and behaviors.

The theory of supportive psychotherapy is based on a number of approaches, including psychoanalytic, cognitive-behavioral, and learning theories (see Table 14–1). These theoretical approaches help to guide the clinician in understanding the indications, strategies, goals, and types of

TABLE 14–1. Theoretical approaches

Psychoanalytic approaches

    Ego psychology and development

    Object relations and attachment

    Self psychology

    Interpersonal and relational approach

Cognitive-behavioral therapy

Learning theory technique

interventions used in supportive psychotherapy, as well as the nature and configuration of the patient–therapist relationship. Psychotherapists must be able to integrate the various theoretical approaches into a cohesive and well-organized psychotherapy that should be based on the needs of the patient.

The Psychopathology–Psychotherapy Continuum

An important concept in understanding the indications for supportive psychotherapy and its relationship to expressive or exploratory psychotherapy is the psychopathology–psychotherapy continuum, as shown in Figure 14–1 (Dewald 1971, 1994; Winston et al. 2004).

Individuals function along a psychopathology or health–sickness continuum according to their level of psychopathology, adaptive capacity, self concept, and ability to relate to others. The continuum is conceptualized as extending from the most impaired patients to the most intact individuals. Impairments consist of symptoms and behaviors that interfere with an individual's ability to think clearly and realistically, function in everyday life, form relationships, and behave in a relatively adaptive and mature manner. Those individuals on the healthy side of the continuum tend to function well, have good relationships, lead productive lives, and are able to enjoy a wide range of activities relatively free of conflict. At the center of the continuum are patients whose adaptation and behavior are uneven and who have significant problems in maintaining consistent functioning and stable relationships.

Placement of individuals on the continuum is associated with diagnosis. Patients with schizophrenia, bipolar disorder, or borderline personality disorder generally lie on the more disabled side of the continuum. Individuals with better adaptation, such as patients with Cluster C personality disor-

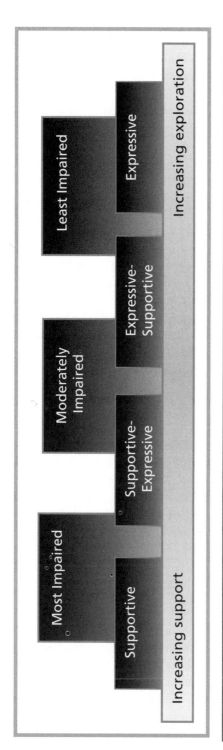

FIGURE 14–1. Psychopathology–psychotherapy continuum.

ders, dysthymia, and adjustment disorders, are generally on the healthier side of the continuum. Although diagnosis can provide a general idea of where a person might reside on the continuum, the actual placement depends on the individual's level of psychopathology and adaptation (Winston and Winston 2002).

Matching psychotherapy technique to patient locus on the health–sickness continuum is of crucial importance. On the left side of the continuum are supportive approaches directed toward building psychological structure, stability, self-esteem, a cohesive sense of self, and improved interpersonal relationships in sicker patients with significant psychopathology. At the healthier end of the continuum are expressive therapies, which generally use an interpersonal/conflict model (see Figure 14–1). *Expressive therapy* has been used as a collective term for a variety of approaches that seek personality change through analysis of the relationship between therapist and patient and through development of insight into previously unrecognized feelings, thoughts, needs, and conflicts, following which the patient attempts to consciously resolve and better integrate such conflicts. In reality many patients lie at neither end of the continuum and have both conflicts and structural problems and require a supportive–expressive treatment. In fact, even the most exploratory therapies include some supportive components, and supportive therapy may involve elements of exploratory therapy (Dewald 1994; de Jonghe et al. 1992).

Psychoanalytic Theory

Psychoanalytic theory extends from traditional drive-conflict theory, to ego psychology, object relations theory, self-experience, and interpersonal/relational models. Pine (1989) argues that all of the analytic approaches are connected and inform our understanding of adult functioning. Drive/conflict and ego psychology models can be considered to be the foundation for all psychoanalytic approaches. Models that focus less on conflicts and drives may have more explanatory power for patients with more serious psychopathology. In this chapter, we concentrate on these later models, which are more applicable to supportive psychotherapy.

Ego Psychology

Ego psychology, which encompasses developmental theory, offers insight into patients with serious impairment. Ego functions as outlined by Freud's (1923) structural approach of ego, id, and superego can serve as the basis for a theoretical review of ego psychology. The structural approach attempts to capture the relatively fixed characteristics of an individual's personality and symptoms, which are understood within a functional context. In general, the greater the disturbance in ego functions, the more likely the indication for a more supportive approach. The following description of psychological or ego functions is based on the work of Beres (1956) and Bellak (1958) (see Table 14–2).

Relation to Reality

Reality testing, sense of reality, and adaptation to reality are major components of relation to reality. *Reality testing* describes an individual's ability to assess reality. Reality testing is impaired in the presence of faulty judgment and is grossly disturbed in a patient with hallucinations or delusions. Disturbances in reality testing indicate significant structural problems and should point the clinician toward a more supportive psychotherapy approach designed to directly help the patient test reality. *Sense of reality* relates to a person's ability to distinguish self from other and is generally indicative of a stable and cohesive body image (Mahler et al. 1975). Again, problems in this area generally call for a more supportive approach. *Adaptation to reality* describes how an individual functions in the world and everyday life, including work, school, social situations, and relationships.

Patients with impaired relation to reality require a supportive approach that generally does not include the exploration of dreams and fantasies or extensive examination of past issues. Patients with more severe psychopathology will generally need a reality-based approach with an emphasis on their current functioning and everyday life.

Object Relations

The evaluation of object relations is based on an individual's capacity to relate in a meaningful and consistent way to significant individuals in his or her life. This capacity includes the ability to form intimate relationships, tolerate separation and loss, and maintain independence and autonomy. It also involves the sense of self, knowing what is within the self and outside the self, and the ability to form a cohesive and stable self-image (Mahler et al. 1975) without diminishing or over-idealizing self or others (Mitchell and Black 1995). Patients with significant impairment in interpersonal relationships, such as chaotic relationships, withdrawal from others, narcissistic or highly dependent needs, and/or impairment in sense of self, generally require a supportive approach, including a supportive/empathic relationship.

Affects, Impulse Control, and Defenses

Affects are complex psychophysiological states composed of subjective feelings and physiological expressions such as crying, sweating, facial expression, and tone of voice.

TABLE 14–2.   Components of the structural approach (ego and superego)

Relation to reality

Object relations

Affect

Impulse control

Defenses

Thought processes

Autonomous functions (perception, intention, intelligence, language, and motor development)

Synthetic functions (ability to form a cohesive whole or gestalt)

Conscience, morals, and ideals (superego)

Tomkins (1992) has described a number of affects, including excitement, joy, surprise, fear, anger, rage, irritation, anguish, shame, humiliation, sadness, and depression. An individual's inability to experience a wide range of affects at some depth and differentiate between affects (Jacobson 1964) generally indicates a need for a supportive approach to provide concrete help in this area.

The capacity to control impulses and modulate affect in an adaptive manner indicates a well-functioning defensive structure. This capacity involves the ability to delay gratification and tolerate frustration. When impulse control is impaired, the individual may engage in socially unacceptable behavior such as physically or verbally lashing out at others or making unreasonable demands.

Defenses mediate between a person's wishes, needs, feelings, and both internal prohibitions and prohibitions from the external world (A. Freud 1936). Individuals tend to use the same kinds of behavior as patterned responses in reaction to perceived danger, difficult situations, or painful affects. Primitive defenses, poor impulse control, severe affective instability, and shallow affect are indicators of structural deficits and suggest the need for a more supportive approach.

The process of exploration in expressive psychotherapy includes working with and exploring affects, impulses, and defenses with patients who are able to tolerate in-depth exploration of these issues. For patients with more severe psychopathology, exploration of affects, impulses, and defenses would be disruptive and anxiety provoking. In supportive psychotherapy, defenses, especially adaptive defenses, are strengthened to promote stability and adaptive functioning.

Thought Processes

The inability to think clearly, logically, and abstractly is a good indicator of significant psychopathology and again suggests that a supportive approach is indicated. Automatic thoughts and negative self-schemas as developed by cognitive-behavioral theorists are important elements to be considered when evaluating thought processes. Impaired adaptive skills and poor interpersonal functioning often result from automatic thoughts and negative self-schemas, which may need to be addressed in supportive psychotherapy (see section "Cognitive-Behavioral Theory" later in this chapter).

Autonomous Functions

Perception, intention, intelligence, language, and motor development are autonomous functions that are believed to develop in a relatively conflict-free manner (Hartmann 1939). These functions can be impaired in patients with significant psychopathology, indicating that a supportive approach may be more appropriate than an expressive or exploratory approach.

Synthetic Function

An individual's ability to organize himself or herself and the world in a productive fashion to form a cohesive whole or gestalt is indicative of synthetic functioning (Nunberg 1931). This function involves putting together the other ego functions and organizing them so that the individual can function in an integrated manner.

Conscience, Morals, and Ideals

Conscience, morals, and ideals derive from internalization of aspects of parental figures and societal mores and are considered superego functions. Severe impairments in these functions may interfere with the patient–therapist relationship. For instance, if a patient cannot be truthful with the therapist, achieving success in psychotherapy may be difficult.

The ego or psychological functions can be used as the basis of a case formulation summarizing a patient's strengths and impairments. The following clinical example provides the basis for a structural formulation.

> Sandra, a 28-year-old woman, is confused about herself and her identity as a woman. She has the belief that people in the street are saying derogatory things about her. She is unable to form relationships with others, tends to keep to herself, but is needy and demanding with her parents. She had great difficulty in college and dropped out when she was 20 years old. She has been unable to work for the past 6 or 7 years and blames others for her fail-

ure to find a job. At times she becomes enraged about minor issues and reacts with outbursts of anger toward her family.

This example illustrates a number of structural deficits. The patient has an impaired sense of reality, consisting of confusion about her self and her identity as a woman. Her reality testing is impaired, as she believes that others are talking about her, and object relations are on a need-satisfying and schizoid basis. Adaptation to reality is severely impaired, as indicated by her inability to work, finish school, and form relationships. She exhibits poor frustration tolerance and impaired impulse control. She uses immature defenses such as projection, acting out, and denial.

Object Relations Theory

The object relations approach developed in Great Britain and involved a number of psychoanalysts, including Fairbairn, Winnicott, and Bowlby. They viewed children as directed toward real people and seeking a satisfying relationship with their parents. Unfortunately, many individuals encounter inadequate or faulty parenting and, according to Fairbairn (1952, 1994), absorb certain pathological traits of their parents to remain connected to them. These prototypes of past relationships, which are present in internal object relations, come into play in the therapeutic relationship. For the patient, giving up old patterns connected to painful affects may lead to isolation and abandonment. The patient must be able to experience the therapist in a new and more positive manner. Winnicott (1965, 1971) described this as the therapist becoming the "good enough mother" by providing a "holding environment" in which content and interpretations are relatively unimportant. The patient is encouraged to experience the self in relation to the therapist, and the therapist becomes a new object for the patient. Fairbairn, like Winnicott, did not believe that insight produces change but rather that change develops from the capacity for relatedness based on connecting to the therapist in a different manner.

Bowlby's (1969, 1988) contributions added an important dimension to the patient–therapist relationship, namely, the concept of attachment. He proposed that the nature of an infant's attachment to a parent will become internalized as a working model of attachment and that children will develop secure or insecure attachment based on parents' sensitivity to the infant's signals. Parents can aid in reducing uncomfortable emotions in their children such as fear, anxiety, and sadness. In patients with insecure attachment, relationship ruptures generally are not followed by repair and connection to the person involved. The therapist's ability to repair ruptures in the therapeutic alliance contrasts with the abilities of parents of insecurely attached children. This process of repair is related to the concept of what

Alexander and French (1946) called the "corrective emotional experience." The corrective emotional experience takes place when the patient is exposed to emotional situations within the patient–therapist relationship that he or she previously could not handle or found traumatic. These authors explained that "because the therapist's attitude is different from that of the authoritative person of the past, he (or she) gives the patient an opportunity to face again and again, under more favorable circumstances, those emotional situations which were formerly unbearable and to deal with them in a manner different from the old" (p. 67). The following vignette illustrates how the therapist may provide the patient with an opportunity to experience a different kind of relationship in contrast to past experiences with significant people in the patient's life.

> **Patient:** You kept me waiting and I'm furious. Once I get angry and start to not trust someone…I write them off.
> **Therapist:** You got angry with me because I was late, and I'm sorry to have kept you waiting.
> **Patient:** I didn't think you were coming.
> **Therapist:** I disappointed you. I know that's hard.

In this example with a highly vulnerable patient, the therapist does not react to or address the patient's anger and lack of trust, but instead responds in an accepting and empathic manner, providing the patient with a corrective emotional experience. In Fairbairn's (1952) terms, maintaining a positive transference relationship is critical; "otherwise," he noted, "the patient will never acquire a sufficient sense of security to enable him to risk a release of his buried bad objects" (p. 74). In addition, the therapist focuses on the current situation and does not explore symbolic or transference issues.

Self Psychology

Kohut (1971, 1977), like Fairbairn and Winnicott, believed that early object relations are of crucial importance in the development of the self. When parents' empathic responsiveness to their children is repeatedly distorted or inappropriate, developmental problems of the self may occur. According to Kohut, the therapist offers this kind of patient a new kind of experience, namely, an empathic/introspective stance. The goal of Kohut's psychoanalytic approach is to promote patient development through accurately and empathically understanding the patient's needs and interpreting these needs to the patient. However, the therapist will inevitably fail to always meet these needs. In supportive psychotherapy the therapist does not interpret the patient's needs but instead acknowledges such failures in meeting the patient's needs and works to reestablish the patient–therapist alliance using supportive techniques. Repairs of alliance ruptures of this sort will generally lead to a strengthening of self-structures and an internalization by the patient of the therapist's good qualities. The following vignette illustrates this process.

> **Patient:** I was really upset with you since we last met. You really didn't understand me. You defended my boy friend, who was being horrible to me.
> **Therapist:** Yes, I see what you mean. I was suggesting not to get rid of him immediately rather than focusing on your hurt feelings.

In this example, the therapist acknowledges his mistake and immediately attempts to repair the misalliance. If a misalliance or rupture is not attended to in a timely fashion, the possibility of the patient leaving treatment is increased.

The Therapeutic Relationship

The therapeutic relationship or patient–therapist relationship may be the most important variable in producing a positive psychotherapy outcome (Gaston 1990; Horvath and Symonds 1991). The therapeutic relationship may be divided into three components: the transference/countertransference configuration, the real relationship, and the therapeutic alliance (Greenson 1967, 1971) (see Table 14–3). Transference and real relationship issues play a role in every transaction within the therapeutic relationship. At certain times transference may be more important, whereas at other times the real relationship may predominate. Expressive psychotherapy places more emphasis on transference, whereas supportive and cognitive-behavioral therapies focus more on the real relationship.

Transference has been described as a special type of object relationship consisting of behaviors, thoughts, feelings, wishes, and attitudes directed at the therapist that are related to important people in the patient's past (Greenson 1967). The real relationship exists in the here and now of the therapeutic interaction between patient and therapist, encompassing a genuine liking for each other without the distortions that are characteristic of transference (Greenson 1967, 1971). The real relationship includes the patient's hopes and aspirations for help, care, understanding, and love, as well as the everyday interactions that take place on a social level between individuals.

In supportive psychotherapy, the real relationship is paramount and transference issues are minimized. At the same time, the therapist is mindful of the transference but generally does not explore it unless the transference is negative. Negative transference must be discussed with the patient

TABLE 14–3. Components of the therapeutic relationship
Transference/countertransference configuration
Real relationship
Therapeutic alliance

because it can disrupt the psychotherapy and often results in the patient dropping out of treatment (Samstag et al. 1998).

The following examples illustrate how positive and negative transference reactions are managed in supportive psychotherapy.

> A 31-year-old man tells his therapist that things at work have greatly improved and that he is now getting along well with his boss. He no longer is afraid of losing his job. He attributes his gains in this area of his life to the therapist's helpfulness and understanding. The therapist accepts the patient's compliment by saying, "I'm pleased that you're doing better at work and that our work together has helped."

In this example the therapist does not explore the compliment but instead accepts what the patient has said. At the same time, the therapist indicates that this positive outcome was the result of a joint effort of both patient and therapist.

> A 43-year-old divorced woman was having great difficulty with her 19-year-old son, Ted, who was away at college. At the same time, Ted had a very good relationship with his father, her ex-husband. Ted refused to return his mother's phone calls or e-mails, complaining that she plagued him and had been abusive to him when he was a youngster. The therapist urged the patient to wait and not continue to phone and send so many critical e-mails. The patient became furious with the therapist for not understanding her pain and need to contact Ted. The therapist responded, "I think I understand how hard this is for you and how much anguish you feel. I was so eager to help your relationship with Ted that I neglected to respond to your needs."

In this example the patient becomes angry with the therapist, who immediately addresses the negative transference and attempts to repair it through an empathic intervention and by taking responsibility for her error.

Countertransference from a narrow or classical point of view is essentially the therapist's transference to the patient (Gabbard 2001; Greenson 1967). A broader definition of countertransference includes the real relationship, consisting of reactions most people would have to the patient determined by moment-to-moment interactions in the therapeutic relationship. In this sense, countertransference may be viewed as a transactional construct, affected by what the therapist brings to the situation as well as what the patient projects (Gabbard 2001; Kiesler 2001). The therapist's countertransference reactions can lead to a misunderstanding of the patient and can result in inappropriate behavior toward the patient. However, countertransference reactions that the therapist is aware of can be a powerful tool for understanding and empathizing with the patient. The use of empathy is important in facilitating countertransference awareness (Wolf 1983). The ability to empathize by accurately sensing and understanding what a patient is experiencing will enable the therapist to attend to countertransference reactions. The following is an example of the use of countertransference in supportive psychotherapy.

> A 28-year-old mother of two young children spoke about being angry with her 3-year-old daughter and smacking her across the face. The therapist began to get upset, anxious, and angry. She quickly recognized that she had strong feelings about what the patient had done to her daughter. The therapist realized that the patient had shared this behavior with her as a way of asking for help and testing the therapist to see if she would get angry and retaliate or reject her. The therapist was then able to respond in a helpful manner: "I'm glad you told me about what you did with your daughter. Let's try and understand what you were thinking and see if we can come up with a better way of dealing with your daughter when she acts up."

The therapeutic alliance is part of the real relationship and is necessary to support the work of psychotherapy (Zetzel 1956, 1966). In supportive psychotherapy, a positive therapeutic alliance early in therapy is predictive of outcome (Hellerstein et al. 1998; Luborsky 1984). Freud recognized the importance of a positive patient–therapist relationship, which he called the "friendly or affectionate feelings" that were "unobjectionable." These friendly, affectionate, and unobjectionable feelings the patient feels toward the therapist are called "the vehicle of success in psychoanalysis" (Freud 1912). Greenson (1967) emphasized the collaborative nature of the alliance, in which patient and therapist work together to promote therapeutic change. Bordin (1979) and Gaston (1990) further clarified and broadened the concept of the therapeutic alliance to include the following components: the affectionate bond between patient and therapist, their agreement on goals and tasks of therapy, the patient's capacity to perform the work of therapy, and the therapist's empathic relatedness and involvement. All of these components of the alliance are important elements of supportive psychotherapy.

In supportive psychotherapy, alliance ruptures occur less often than in expressive psychotherapy, possibly because the alliance in supportive psychotherapy is not threatened by challenging confrontations or interpretations, which may heighten patient anxiety (Hellerstein et al. 1998). When a misalliance does occur in supportive psychotherapy, the use of supportive measures should be considered as the initial approach to repair the misalliance (Bond et al. 1998). The therapist addresses the rupture in a practical manner, within the context of the current situation, before examining transference issues (Pinsker 1997). (For examples of rupture repair, see subsections "Object Relations Theory" and "Self Psychology" earlier in this chapter.)

Cognitive-Behavioral Theory

Cognitive-behavioral techniques are an indispensable part of supportive psychotherapy and can be applied to targeted problems such as panic, depression, obsessive-compulsive symptoms, and dysfunctional thinking. *Cognition* refers to the content of thought (what we think), the processes involved in thinking (how we think), and self-schemas (what structures our thinking). Cognitive-behavioral techniques focus on how individuals make use of information to understand the meaning of events in their lives. Behavior and feelings are viewed as deriving from the nature and characteristics of thinking. Maladaptive behavior is believed to be the result of idiosyncratic dysfunctional thinking.

Key concepts of cognitive-behavioral therapy include schemas (cognitive structures), dysfunctional attitudes, automatic thoughts, and cognitive distortions or errors. Schemas are relatively enduring beliefs and attitudes that reflect experientially derived abstractions about one's view of oneself or one's identity (Kovacs and Beck 1978). These beliefs and attitudes are based on early learning experiences and are thought to account for problems in screening and encoding information. Automatic thoughts and cognitive errors, which are reflections of self-schemas activated by events that are similar in content to the self-schemas, involve such things as arbitrary inference, overgeneralization, magnification, personalization, selective abstraction, and absolute thinking. Examples of automatic thoughts include "If I am not wealthy then I am a failure," "If my children are not successful, then I am a terrible parent," and "If I have an illness, then I did something wrong and deserve it."

In supportive psychotherapy the therapeutic process involves identifying and challenging automatic thoughts and subjecting them to empirical testing. Patients are taught to monitor automatic thoughts, test their validity, and develop alternative ways of thinking. Reframing is another cognitive technique often used to correct cognitive distortions.

A clinical example of this is a mother who exhibited absolute or dichotomous thinking regarding her 2-year-old. She complained to her therapist that her toddler kept running away from her and laughing when she came into his room. She said, "My child hates me." The therapist reframed this distortion by saying, "He doesn't hate you. He can run off and laugh because he has the strength, independence, and playfulness to be able to do it, based on what he has gotten from you."

Learning Theory

Basic Concepts

Many of the therapeutic interventions used in supportive psychotherapy can be viewed as a form of teaching, a process of imparting knowledge. The encoding of the information taught by the therapist constitutes the other half of the therapeutic process. In general, learning is the cognitive process of acquiring skill or knowledge. Memory is the retention of learned information. Psychotherapy can be considered a controlled form of learning (Etkin et al. 2005) through the acquisition of a combination of skills and knowledge. Incorporating the research on adult learning into supportive psychotherapy may enhance its effectiveness.

Learning theory has been applied primarily to adult education, and the studies in this area have tended to focus on how to enhance learning. The history of learning theory can be considered to have begun with Socrates and Plato, and evolved through the contributions of Piaget (1937), Skinner (1938), Thorndike (1932), and Bandura (1974). More recent contributors to this evolving field are Knowles' (Knowles et al. 1998) and Brookfield's (1995) adult learning theory and Geake and Cooper's (2003) brain-based learning. The work of Knowles, Brookfield, and Geakes and Cooper has been applied to the practice of adult education, corporate functioning, and marketing.

Researchers in the cognitive and affective neurosciences have made major contributions to the understanding of learning and learning impairments, and their findings have added to our knowledge of the molecular and neural basis of learning (Kandel et al. 2000), cognition (Gazzaniga 2004), and emotion (Panskeep 1998). These authors have provided the basis for understanding how impairments in neural functioning may impede psychotherapy and how neural growth may enhance psychotherapy. Patients with schizophrenia (Ongur et al. 2006), major depressive disorder (Burt et al. 1995), bipolar disorder (Thompson et al. 2005), borderline personality disorder (Judd 2005; Monarch et al. 2004), attention-deficit/hyperactivity disorder (Doyle et al. 2005; Fuggetta 2006), as well as individuals who have encountered significant psychological trauma (Bremner 2006; Navalta et al. 2006), have been shown to have learning impairments. Even transient mood shifts and transient stress can effect encoding and the ability to process information (Buchanan et al. 2006; Dreisbach 2006; Dreisbach and Goschke 2004; Lewis et al. 2005; Liston et al. 2006). Therefore, altered neural processing with cognitive deficits may be present in these patients. The use of learning theory techniques in these situations may be advantageous in helping the patient process information (see subsection "Techniques" later in this chapter). Little has been written about the consideration of learning impairments when applying supportive psychotherapy to these populations. Historically, learning deficits were viewed within the context of traumatic brain injury, pervasive developmental disorder, mental retardation, and other developmental disabilities. The recent research in neuroscience just described suggests that learning styles should be evaluated and the presence of learning deficits considered when evaluating patients with psychiatric disorders for psychotherapy. This type of evaluation involves monitoring a patient's ability to encode information from one session to the next or within a session.

Learning does not take place as a simple recording process. Learning requires active processing during the psychotherapy session through an interpretive process in which new information is stored by relating it to what is already known. New information is stored in relation to its meaning, associations, and relationships to existing knowledge. From this perspective, it is important for the therapist to facilitate effective processing during psychotherapy sessions using the techniques of interpretation, elaboration, and generation (see subsection "Techniques" later in this chapter) (deWinstanley and Bjork 2002; Richland et al. 2005). It is important to note that interpretation as a technique of learning theory is not the classical technique of interpretation in dynamic psychotherapy but more of a linkage to preexisting knowledge.

Strategies

Therapeutic Alliance

As in all forms of psychotherapy, the patient–therapist (student–teacher) relationship must be maintained on a positive level. In the event of a patient–therapist misalliance the rupture or misunderstanding must be repaired. A positive learning experience takes place in a supportive relationship in which the patient can be challenged and results in enhanced learning (Caine and Caine 1994). Patients need to understand that learning may involve taking risks by embracing uncertainty and change, which often requires that the therapist be reassuring and helpful. Patients should be involved in mutual planning with the therapist in setting relevant goals and objectives in a collaborative manner (Knowles et al. 1998). When patients participate in determining their goals and objectives, motivation will be enhanced, and they will have more control over their learning. On the other hand, a threatening environment may inhibit learning.

Standards and Expectations

In a learning theory–informed approach to supportive psychotherapy, patients are viewed as participating in an educational process. At times they may feel uncertain or puzzled and may make mistakes requiring support and reassurance from the therapist. Patients should understand that learning is an important part of supportive psychotherapy and that preparation and homework may be required to enhance the learning process.

Resource Identification

Patients should be encouraged to identify resources and devise strategies for using the resources to achieve their objectives. Resources include libraries, information from the Internet, books, journals, videos, and so on. At the same time, patients should be involved in evaluating their own learning, thereby promoting the skill of critical reflection (see subsection "Techniques" below) (Brookfield 1995). In addition, patients should be encouraged to utilize the process of self-assessment to help identify their strengths, weaknesses, and problems.

Techniques

A major approach to facilitate learning is *effective processing* (deWinstanley and Bjork 2002) (see Table 14–4). Processing involves interpretation that is focused and accurate, accompanied by thorough elaboration. Information that can be interpreted (linked) through associations with preexisting knowledge will be easier to learn than information that is not interpreted. *Elaborative processing* has to do with information being thought of in a number of different ways and connected with other previously known information. In addition to interpretation and elaboration, generation and interleaving are other important components of the learning process (Richland et al. 2005). *Generation* is defined as the producing of information during learning rather than being presented with that information by a teacher or therapist. *Interleaving* is the method of learning two or more sets of information such that instruction and focus alternate between the sets. This is in contrast to learning in which each set is focused on separately. In supportive psychotherapy these techniques can be utilized by asking questions designed to help patients think about their problems in a number of different ways and not supplying the answers. The patient is encouraged to engage in processing information in collaboration with the therapist.

TABLE 14–4. Learning theory technique

Processing

    Interpretation

    Elaboration

    Generation

    Interleaving

Critical reflection

Critical reflection (Mezirow 1998) is the process by which a patient questions and then replaces or reframes an assumption. Alternative perspectives are formed on previously taken for granted ideas, actions, and forms of reasoning. Supportive psychotherapy and other psychotherapy approaches use reframing and attempt to provide patients with alternative ways of thinking about the world, relating to others, and solving problems.

The following is a clinical example illustrating the use of processing in a patient with bipolar disorder with a history of medication noncompliance.

A 52-year-old single mother with bipolar disorder had been recently discharged from an inpatient hospital stay for an exacerbation of her illness. She came into her therapist's office saying that she was not sleeping well. The psychiatrist asked if she was taking her medication regularly. She replied that she was taking her medication some of the time, sort of on and off. The psychiatrist, feeling a mixture of concern and irritation, wondered if she was again becoming noncompliant with her medication. He stated that perhaps her sleeping problem had something to do with her not taking her medication regularly. Rather than admonishing her, he tried to find out about what she was thinking and experiencing when she did not take her medication. She said, "It's just cumbersome, and I don't like it, because it reminds me that something's wrong with me." The therapist continued to explore her difficulty taking medication, and the patient stated that "if I have to take medication it means I'm crazy." The therapist asked about her understanding of her illness and what helps this kind of illness (generation). He then asked the patient about her sister who has diabetes and what would happen if her sister stopped her diabetes medication. The patient was able to compare her illness with her sister's illness and began to question herself about not taking her medication (interleaving).

Exploration of this type promotes encoding and the processing of information (generation, elaboration, interleaving, and linkage to preexisting knowledge). Using these teaching techniques to deal with medication compliance can have a deeper impact than reviewing the risks and benefits of compliance in the usual manner.

Conclusion

Supportive psychotherapy is a broadly defined approach with wide applicability that uses direct measures to ameliorate symptoms and maintain, restore, or improve self-esteem, ego function, and adaptive skills. The theory of supportive psychotherapy is based on a number of approaches, including psychoanalytic, cognitive-behavioral, and learning theories. The concept of a psychopathology continuum ranging from sickness to health matched with a psychotherapy continuum ranging from supportive psychotherapy to expressive or exploratory psychotherapy is useful to determine the therapeutic approach based on the needs of the patient. The majority of patients most likely will fall in the middle of the continuum and benefit from a combined approach of supportive and expressive psychotherapy. A supportive approach is strengthened when the therapist is accepting and empathic and is attentive to maintaining a positive patient–therapist relationship or therapeutic alliance. In addition, combining and integrating approaches from cognitive-behavioral and learning theories can enhance the practice of supportive psychotherapy.

Key Points

- The theory of supportive psychotherapy is based on a number of approaches, including psychoanalytic, cognitive-behavioral, and learning theories.

- Matching psychotherapy technique to patient locus on the psychopathology continuum is of crucial importance.

- Psychoanalytic models that focus less on conflicts and drives (i.e., ego psychology, object relations theory, attachment theory, self psychology) have greater utility in patients with higher levels of psychopathology.

- Prototypes of past relationships, which are present in internal object relationships, appear within the patient–therapist relationship.

- In supportive psychotherapy the therapist offers the patient a new kind of experience, namely an empathic/introspective stance, so that the therapist is experienced in a new and positive manner.

- Generally, positive transference reactions are not addressed in supportive psychotherapy, whereas negative transference reactions are always examined to help prevent major alliance ruptures.

- Cognitive-behavioral concepts, including schemas, dysfunctional attitudes, automatic thoughts, and cognitive distortions, underlie many of the techniques of supportive psychotherapy.

- Psychotherapy can be considered as a controlled form of learning.

- Learning during psychotherapy requires active processing so that new information is stored by relating it to what is already known.

References

Alexander F, French TM: Psychoanalytic Psychotherapy. New York, Ronald Press, 1946

Bandura A: Behavior theory and the models of man. Am Psychol 29:849–869, 1974

Bellak L: The schizophrenic syndrome: a further elaboration of the unified theory of schizophrenia, in Schizophrenia: A Review of the Syndrome. Edited by Bellak L. New York, Logos, 1958, pp 3–63

Beres D: Ego deviation and the concept of schizophrenia. Psychoanal Study Child 11:164–235, 1956

Bond M, Banon E, Grenier M: Differential effects of interventions on the therapeutic alliance with patients with personality disorders. J Psychother Pract Res 7:301–318, 1998

Bordin E: The generalizability of the psycho-analytic concept of the working alliance. Psychotherapy: Theory, Research and Practice 16:252–260, 1979

Bowlby J: Attachment and Loss, Vol 1: Attachment. New York, Basic Books, 1969

Bowlby J: A Secure Base: Parent-Child Attachment and Healthy Human Development. New York, Basic Books, 1988

Bremner JD: The relationship between cognitive and brain changes in posttraumatic stress disorder. Ann N Y Acad Sci 1071:80–86, 2006

Brookfield S: Adult learning: an overview, in International Encyclopedia of Education. Edited by Tuinjman A. Oxford, UK, Pergamon Press, 1995, pp 375–380

Buchanan TW, Tranel D, Adolphs R: Impaired memory retrieval correlates with individual differences in cortisol response but not autonomic response. Learn Mem 13:382–387, 2006

Burt DB, Zembar MJ, Niederehe G: Depression and memory impairment: a meta-analysis of the association, its pattern, and specificity. Psychol Bull 117:285–305, 1995

Caine RN, Caine G: Making Connections: Teaching and the Human Brain. Lebanon, IN, Dale Segmore Publications, 1994

de Jonghe F, Rijnierse P, Janssen R: The role of support in psychoanalysis. J Am Psychoanal Assoc 40:475–499, 1992

Dewald PA: Psychotherapy: A Dynamic Approach, 2nd Edition. New York, Basic Books, 1971

Dewald PA: Principles of supportive psychotherapy. Am J Psychother 48:505–518, 1994

deWinstanley PA, Bjork RA: Successful lecturing: presenting information in ways that engage effective processing, in Applying the Science of Learning to University Teaching and Beyond (New Directions for Teaching and Learning No 89). Edited by Halpern DF, Hakel MD. San Francisco, CA, Jossey-Bass, 2002, pp 19–31

Doyle AE, Biederman J, Seidman LJ, et al: Neuropsychological functioning in relatives of girls with and without ADHD. Psychol Med 35:1121–1132, 2005

Dreisbach G: How positive affect modulates cognitive control: the costs and benefits of reduced maintenance capability. Brain Cogn 60:11–19, 2006

Dreisbach G, Goschke T: How positive affect modulates cognitive control: reduced perseveration at the cost of increased distractibility. J Exp Psychol Learn Mem Cogn 30:343–353, 2004

Etkin A, Phil M, Pittenger C, et al: Toward a neurobiology of psychotherapy: basic science and clinical applications. J Neuropsychiatry Clin Neurosci 17:145–158, 2005

Fairbairn WRD: An Object-Relations Theory of the Personality. New York, Basic Books, 1952

Fairbairn WRD: From Instinct to Self: Selected Papers of WRD Fairbairn, Vols 1–2. Edited by Birtles ED, Sharff DE. Northvale, NJ, Jason Aronson, 1994

Freud A: The ego and the mechanisms of defense (1936), in The Writings of Anna Freud, Vol 2. New York, International Universities Press, 1966

Freud S: The dynamics of transference (1912), in The Standard Edition of the Complete Psychological Works of Sigmund Freud, Vol 12. Edited by Strachey J. London, Hogarth Press, 1958, pp 99–108

Freud S: The ego and the id (1923), in The Standard Edition of the Complete Psychological Works of Sigmund Freud, Vol 19. Edited by Strachey J. London, Hogarth Press, 1961, pp 12–66

Fuggetta GP: Impairment of executive functions in boys with attention deficit/hyperactivity disorder. Child Neuropsychol 12:1–21, 2006

Gabbard GO: A contemporary psychoanalytic model of countertransference. J Clin Psychol 57:983–991, 2001

Gaston L: The concept of the alliance and its role in psychotherapy: theoretical and empirical considerations. Psychotherapy 27:143–153, 1990

Gazzaniga MS: The Cognitive Neurosciences, III. Cambridge, MA, MIT Press, 2004

Geake J, Cooper P: Cognitive neuroscience: implications for education? Westminster Studies in Education 26:7–20, 2003

Greenson RR: The Technique and Practice of Psychoanalysis. New York, International Universities Press, 1967

Greenson RR: The real relationship between the patient and the psychoanalyst, in The Unconscious Today. Edited by Kanzer M. New York, International Universities Press, 1971, pp 213–232

Hartmann H: Ego Psychology and the Problem of Adaptation (1939). Translated by Rapaport D. New York, International Universities Press, 1958

Hellerstein DJ, Rosenthal RN, Pinsker H, et al: A randomized prospective study comparing supportive and dynamic therapies: outcome and alliance. J Psychother Pract Res 7:261–271, 1998

Horvath AO, Symonds BD: Relation between working alliance and outcome in psychotherapy: a meta-analysis. J Couns Psychol 38:139–149, 1991

Jacobson E: The Self and the Object World. New York, International Universities Press, 1964

Judd PA: Neurocognitive impairment as a moderator in the development of borderline personality disorder. Dev Psychopathol 17:1173–1196, 2005

Kandel ER, Schwartz JH, Jessell TM: Principles of Neural Science. Maidenhead, UK, McGraw-Hill, 2000

Kiesler DJ: Therapist countertransference: in search of common themes and empirical referents. J Clin Psychol 57:1053–1063, 2001

Knowles MS, Holton EF, Swanson RA: The Adult Learner: The Definitive Classic in Adult Education and Human Resource Development. Burlington, MA, Gulf Professional Publishing, 1998

Kohut H: The Analysis of the Self. New York, International Universities Press, 1971

Kohut H: The Restoration of the Self. New York, International Universities Press, 1977

Kovacs M, Beck AT: Maladaptive cognitive structures in depression. Am J Psychiatry 135:525–533, 1978

Lewis PA, Critchley HD, Smith AP, et al: Brain mechanisms for mood congruent memory facilitation. Neuroimage 25:1214–1223, 2005

Liston C, Miller MM, Goldwater DS, et al: Stress-induced alterations in prefrontal cortical dendritic morphology predict selective impairments in perceptual attentional set-shifting. J Neurosci 26:7870–7874, 2006

Luborsky L: Principles of Psychoanalytic Psychotherapy: A Manual for Supportive-Expressive Treatment. New York, Basic Books, 1984

Mahler MS, Pine F, Bergman A: The Psychological Birth of the Human Infant. New York, Basic Books, 1975

Mezirow J: On critical reflection. Adult Education Quarterly 48:185–198, 1998

Mitchell SA, Black MJ: Freud and Beyond. New York, Basic Books, 1995

Monarch ES, Saykin AJ, Flashman LA: Neuropsychological impairment in borderline personality disorder. Psychiatr Clin North Am 27:67–82, 2004

Navalta CP, Polcari A, Webster DM, et al: Effects of childhood sexual abuse on neuropsychological and cognitive function in college women. Neuropsychiatry Clin Neurosci 18:45–53, 2006

Nunberg H: The synthetic function of the ego. Int J Psychoanal 12:123–140, 1931

Ongur D, Cullen TJ, Wolf DH, et al: The neural basis of relational memory deficits in schizophrenia. Arch Gen Psychiatry 63:356–365, 2006

Panskeep J: Affective Neuroscience: The Foundations of Human and Animal Emotion. New York, Oxford University Press, 1998

Piaget J: The Construction of Reality in the Child (1937). London, Routledge & Kegan Paul, 1999

Pine F: Motivation, personality organization and the four psychologies of psychoanalysis. J Am Psychoanal Assoc 37:31–64, 1989

Pinsker H: The role of teaching in supportive therapy. Am J Psychother 48:530–542, 1994

414   Textbook of Psychotherapeutic Treatments

Pinsker H: A Primer of Supportive Psychotherapy. Hillsdale, NJ, Analytic Press, 1997

Pinsker H, Rosenthal R, McCullough L: Dynamic supportive psychotherapy, in Handbook of Short-Term Dynamic Psychotherapy. Edited by Crits-Christoph P, Barber JP. New York, Basic Books, 1991, pp 220–247

Richland LE, Bjork RA, Finley JR, et al: Linking cognitive science to education: generation and interleaving effects, in Proceedings of the 27th Annual Conference of the Cognitive Science Society. Mahwah, NJ, Erlbaum, 2005, pp 1850–1855

Samstag LW, Batchelder ST, Muran JC, et al: Early identification of treatment failures in short-term psychotherapy: an assessment of therapeutic alliance and interpersonal behavior. J Psychother Pract Res 7:126–143, 1998

Skinner BF: The Behavior of Organisms: An Experimental Analysis. New York, Appleton-Century, 1938

Thompson JM, Gallagher P, Hughes JH, et al: Neurocognitive impairment in euthymic patients with bipolar affective disorder. Br J Psychiatry 186:32–40, 2005

Thorndike E: The Fundamentals of Learning. New York, Teachers College Press, 1932

Tomkins SS: Affect, Imagery, and Consciousness, Vol 4: Cognition. New York, Springer, 1992

Winnicott DW: The Maturational Process and the Facilitating Environment: Studies in the Theory of Emotional Development. London, Hogarth Press, 1965

Winnicott DW: Playing and Reality. New York, Basic Books, 1971

Winston A, Winston B: Handbook of Integrated Short-Term Psychotherapy. Washington, DC, American Psychiatric Publishing, 2002

Winston A, Rosenthal RN, Pinsker H: Introduction to Supportive Psychotherapy (Core Competencies in Psychotherapy). Washington, DC, American Psychiatric Publishing, 2004

Wolf ES: Empathy and countertransference, in The Future of Psychoanalysis. Edited by Goldberg A. New York, International Universities Press, 1983, pp 309–326

Zetzel E: Current concepts of transference. Int J Psychoanal 37:369–375, 1956

Zetzel E: The analytic situation, in Psychoanalysis in America. New York, International Universities Press, 1966, pp 86–106

Suggested Readings

Dewald PA: Principles of supportive psychotherapy. Am J Psychother 48:505–518, 1994

Knowles MS, Holton EF, Swanson RA: The Adult Learner: The Definitive Classic in Adult Education and Human Resource Development. Burlington, MA, Gulf Professional Publishing, 1998

Novalis PN, Rojcewicz SJ, Peele R: Clinical Manual of Supportive Psychotherapy. Washington, DC, American Psychiatric Press, 1993

Pinsker H: A Primer of Supportive Psychotherapy. Hillsdale, NJ, Analytic Press, 1997

Rockland LH: Supportive Therapy: A Psychodynamic Approach. New York, Basic Books, 1989

Winston A, Winston B: Handbook of Integrated Short-Term Psychotherapy. Washington, DC, American Psychiatric Publishing, 2002

Winston A, Rosenthal RN, Pinsker H: Introduction to Supportive Psychotherapy (Core Competencies in Psychotherapy). Washington, DC, American Psychiatric Publishing, 2004

Chapter 15

Techniques of Individual Supportive Psychotherapy

Richard N. Rosenthal, M.D.

Pinsker and Rosenthal (1988) define *supportive therapy* as

> a dyadic treatment characterized by use of direct measures to ameliorate
> symptoms and to maintain, restore, or improve self-esteem, adaptive skills,
> and psychological function. To the extent necessary to accomplish these
> objectives, treatment may utilize examination of relationships, real or trans-
> ferential, and both past and current patterns of emotional response or be-
> havior. (p. 1)

The therapist's use of direct measures means that the patient's response of
symptom reduction or adoption of more adaptive behavioral patterns is not
the result of insight into unconscious conflict and its working through, but
rather because the patient has greater self-esteem, ego functioning, and
adaptive skills as a result of therapist interventions. Self-esteem, deemed
the critical factor in this model, can be arranged as the top pole of a triangle
resting on the two foundations of ego functioning and adaptive skills. These
objectives are accomplished through specific supportive techniques deliv-

ered in a conversational style that are responsive to the patient's stated goals and are targeted to the specific developmental or reparative tasks that the clinician has identified.

As the patient's psychological development can be arrayed upon a continuum, so can the defensive operations be arrayed from the most primitive to the most individuated (Vaillant 1977, 1992). Primitive defenses such as projection, splitting, and denial recruit different supportive interventions than more mature defenses such as rationalization, displacement, suppression, or sublimation. Within the scope of supportive psychotherapy, defenses are respected and are usually not addressed directly unless they are grossly maladaptive or threaten the frame of therapy. Hence, the more primitive the defensive operations used, the more likely it is the therapist will need to intervene with awareness-expanding interventions, because the primitive defenses tend to be more globally maladaptive. This is one reason early psychotherapists viewed supportive therapy as keyed to severely mentally ill patients, whereas healthier people with more sophisticated defenses were able to make use of more expressive techniques. However, studies demonstrate that healthier patients are also helped by supportive psychotherapy (Hellerstein et al. 1998; Rosenthal et al. 1999). Generally, the typical interventions used with a healthier patient will be different from those used with a patient who has more severe psychopathology.

There are two levels of technique the therapist uses when conducting supportive psychotherapy: contextual and tactical. The contextual techniques are used in all supportive therapies with all patients and so form the groundwork of treatment. The tactical techniques are therapist responses based on the content of current communication, patient characteristics and goals, and therapist objectives. Table 15–1 presents a noncomprehensive list of basic supportive psychotherapy techniques.

Contextual Techniques

Adopt a Conversational Style

An active, conversational style is a basic supportive technique that is contextual rather than tactical (based on specific content of patients' utterances). The rationale for its use is that it emulates familiar social interaction and thus tends not to raise anxiety such as that seen with the therapist's more abstaining, exploratory stance when conducting an expressive treatment. The therapist tends to be more active than in traditional expressive therapies, in which, even if not abstinent in the classical sense, the therapist practices restraint as the default position (Gabbard 2004). Although supportive psychotherapy does not use abstinence as the primary therapeutic

TABLE 15–1.	Supportive psychotherapy techniques

Contextual techniques

Adopting a conversational style

Maintaining the frame of treatment

Being like a good parent

Focusing on real relationships

Tactical techniques

Alliance building

    Expression of interest

    Expression of empathy

    Expressing understanding

    Repairing a misalliance

    Self-disclosure

    Sustaining comments

Esteem building

    Praise

    Reassurance

    Encouragement

    Exhortation

    Inspiration

Enhancement of ego functioning

    Anxiety-reducing interventions

        Structuring the environment

        Maintaining a protected environment

        Setting limits

        Designating the topic explicitly

        Modulating affect

        Supporting defenses

        Universalizing

        Naming the problem

        Rationalizing

            Reframing

            Minimization

TABLE 15-1. Supportive psychotherapy techniques *(continued)*

Tactical techniques *(continued)*

Enhancement of ego functioning *(continued)*

    Awareness-expanding interventions

        Clarification

        Using humor

        Confrontation

        Interpretation

            Intellectualized

            Inexact

            Incomplete

Skills building

Giving advice

Teaching

Modeling adaptive behavior

Providing anticipatory guidance

Redirecting

Promoting autonomy

---

stance, because the intent is not to remain neutral so as to assist in the development of intense transferences, the therapist will still have a therapeutic rationale for his or her interventions. Sometimes the therapist will make bridging comments simply to keep the flow of the conversation going, because awkward silences can raise a patient's anxiety. At other times, the therapist waits with interest and concern for the patient to finish formulating his or her thoughts, or to get a handle on a difficult feeling, before he or she responds. Finishing patient's statements is supportive and empathic only if accurate and tempered to the characteristics of the patient. In addition, an interrogatory style consistent with medical student history taking peppers the patient with "why" questions that may be perceived as accusatory or attacking, so the supportive therapist uses a more conversational, nonchallenging approach to gather information (Pinsker 1997).

    The therapist is charged with the responsibility of keeping the conversation going in a balanced way. Free association, a fundamental process of psychoanalysis and related expressive therapies that uncovers defenses in the form of resistances, is not germane to the objectives of supportive psychotherapy and is thus neither expected nor promoted. Similarly, a patient may proceed to expand on a narrative with much affect, which reduces tension, provides relief, and may support self-esteem, but leaves no room for dialogue. Does one allow the patient to continue to ventilate? The therapist should determine what purpose it serves. Should one try to attempt to have conversation? To cut the ventilation off prematurely may be unsupportive. However, unless we see that the patient is benefiting from ventilation, it is best to redirect it after a time in order to move the treatment in the direction of improving ego functioning and adaptive skills. Clearly, a patient's strong pattern of ventilating over time precludes addressing these objectives. The therapist must instead figure out an empathic way to keep the conversation moving without sounding critical.

Maintain the Frame of Treatment

The frame of treatment entails common components and processes such as the office setting, the therapist's role, and expected interactions. The frame also includes explaining the rules of therapy: the patient's role, setting fees, scheduling, beginning and ending sessions, and how missed sessions are handled. The therapist conducts these discussions, in addition to history taking, setting of goals, and discussing the length of treatment, much in the same way as the rest of the supportive treatment. Sometime during the first session, the therapist covers the rules of treatment. With overly anxious patients, this discussion can take place at the beginning of the session as a way of structuring and reducing anxiety with relatively benign protocol.

The broad context in which therapy takes place should be structured, predictable, and reliable. The "holding environment" as described by Winnicott (1960, 1971) and others is the optimized interpersonal space that offers nurture, relatedness, organizing feedback, and mirroring to the developing ego.

By creating a holding environment, the frame of treatment in supportive psychotherapy lowers anxiety through providing consistency and structure, and offering and augmenting this environment is a central facet of supportive psychotherapy (Pine 1984). However, the frame does not include contextual techniques from the frame of expressive therapies such as technical neutrality and abstinence, which are artifacts in supportive therapy. The technically neutral therapist holds himself or herself equidistant from the patient's ego, id, and superego. In contrast, in conducting supportive psychotherapy, the therapist is not technically neutral because he or she is an active proponent of the patient's ego functioning and self-esteem. Because the therapist does not rely upon technical neutrality, he or she must remain aware of the risk of acting out on countertransference feelings or supporting regressive behavior (Kernberg 1999). The therapist conducting supportive therapy must also balance the need to maintain the integrity of the therapy frame with clinical judgment, whereas at times it may be judicious to be more flexible (Gold and Cherry 1997). Obviously, the patient abruptly terminating therapy destroys the frame of treatment. Therefore, the frame of treatment also includes therapist interventions that address a potential rift in the therapeutic alliance or frank evidence that the patient may terminate prematurely because of psychopathology and/or a rupture in the therapeutic alliance.

The traditional expressive response has been to state something akin to "Our time is up for today" to signal the end of the session. In the least, it is not conversational. This carryover of classical psychoanalytic technique might be experienced as abrupt and unsupportive to a patient in supportive therapy, especially one who is in a crisis, or for whom anticipation of the soon-to-come ending of the session would be helpful in organizing whatever time remains. The clinician conducting supportive therapy will anticipate the end of a session and clue in the patient by remarking about the time left as well as making concluding or summarizing statements at the end.

Be Like a Good Parent

The clinician conducting supportive psychotherapy needs to continually reevaluate the developmental strengths and deficits of the patient (Misch 2000). Using expectations about what responsibilities are age appropriate, and empathic and experiential feedback about a child's current functioning, a good parent balances the wish to protect the child from harm against the child's need to develop autonomy. That balance moves toward autonomy as the child matures and his or her procedural knowledge and capacity to exercise judgment improve. However, it may swing back toward needing adult intervention in times of crisis, novelty associated with risk, or other situations requiring the parent to comfort, protect, or set limits. In a manner analogous to good parenting, the supportive therapist's goal is to increase the individuation and autonomous functioning of the patient. At times, this means dealing with developmental immaturity in a mentoring and reassuring manner (e.g., giving expert advice or leading anticipatory guidance so that the patient has a clearer understanding of the potential positive and negative consequences of his or her choices). At others, it means backing off (in spite of a wish to "fix it") and witnessing as the patient makes his or her own choices and deals with the consequences. Regardless of the parenting-like roles of the therapist, we do not substitute our own wishes or values for the patient's, and although we may have strong reactions, we never punish the patient for negative attitude, thoughts, or behavior. In regard to the parenting-like role of the therapist conducting supportive psychotherapy, part of the art of working with patients is to support without fostering regression and to confront without punishing the patient (Rosenthal 2002).

Focus on Real Relationships

Whereas the focus of expressive therapies is the elucidation of the transference relationship as a means of revealing core neurotic conflicts, the actual relationship between therapist and patient is also a context within which supportive treatment unfolds but is not necessarily a focus of treatment. The patient and therapist collaborate to understand interpersonal and other patterns in order to discover what can be changed, not to discover reasons for the existence of the behavior or feelings that should be changed (Rosenthal et al. 1999). Self-understanding, or emotional insight, is not a core indicator of treatment success, and it is pursued only to the extent that it supports the accomplishment of patient goals and therapist objectives. The therapist keeps the focus on relationships that are in the here and now, including the therapist relationship when appropriate, and only makes connections to genetic figures when the therapist can do so in order to describe a current maladaptive pattern in a rationalized and practical way, or if the patient is demonstrating real insight and driving a more expressive process. Although supportive psychotherapy is not a transference-focused treatment, the therapist must still be mindful of transference material and object relationship patterning (Westen and Gabbard 2002). Generally, positive transference is allowed to build without interpretation or confrontation because it tends to strengthen and deepen the therapeutic alliance. Similarly, negative transference is not interpreted unless the continuity of the treatment is threatened. However, distinct from positive transference, negative transference is typically confronted and distortions corrected because a buildup of negative transference threatens the therapeutic alliance and, thus, the frame of treatment.

Tactical Techniques

The tactical techniques of supportive psychotherapy can be organized into four general categories that correspond to the establishment and maintenance of a working relationship in order to effectively conduct treatment: alliance building, and the three core objectives of supportive psychotherapy: esteem building, enhancing ego functioning, and skills building. Alliance building could also be thought of as a set of contextual techniques, the goal of which is to support the development of a strong working alliance within which to conduct the treatment. However, because the techniques that fall under the rubric of alliance building also have tactical utility in that they are responsive to patients' statements, they are included in this section. Esteem building might otherwise be included under ego functioning, but because it is a primary objective of supportive psychotherapy and has many core techniques specifically associated with it, it is given its own category. In addition, many of the interventions could be placed in more than one category because effects are often multimodal. For example, expression of empathy is often reassuring depending on the context and thus could support self-esteem, but the primary intent is to strengthen the therapeutic alliance. Similarly, encouragement is esteem building but also allays anxiety. For simplicity, each technique is organized in relation to its main effect.

Alliance Building

Barber et al. (2001) argue that a positive therapeutic alliance, although clearly an indicator of positive outcome in psychotherapy, is not in itself a technique. That stated, supportive psychotherapy focuses on the development of a strong therapeutic alliance as a purposive, core strategy and thus offers several proactive techniques that can be used to support that goal.

Expression of Interest

Deliberately reiterating material from past sessions is a way to deliver the message that the patient is important to the therapist (self-esteem). Whenever the therapist forgets specifics of a patient's experience or recalls them incorrectly and casually reveals this to the patient, it is nonsupportive. Although interest can be expressed in the therapist's questions, the therapist should endeavor to not ask questions that put the patient on the spot (so as to reduce anxiety). In addition, for some patients, being asked too many questions, particularly "why" questions, can be experienced as an intrusion or an attack.

Expression of Empathy

Empathic relatedness underscores a core relational aspect of positive regard and so forms part of the patient's experience of the therapist that the therapist cares in a meaningful way. Empathic relating goes beyond simple caring and concern. Being known by the therapist in this way is intrinsically supportive and provides the patient a sense of recognition and connection, strengthening the self and influencing the unconscious affective bonds often described as "implicit relational knowing" (Lyons-Ruth et al. 1998). When the opportunity presents itself in treatment, the therapist gives feedback in the form of relating his or her own internal emotional experience to corroborate that of the patient (e.g., "You must have felt humiliated when he treated you that way"). This empathic validation demonstrates the "therapist's empathic attunement with the patient's internal state" (Gabbard 2005) and serves to deepen the patient's experience of being understood in an essential way.

Expression of Understanding

In parallel to the emotional sense of regarding the patient, the clinician also communicates his or her alignment with the patient in a cognitive way. Letting the patient know that one understands what he or she is communicating supports the patient's experience that he or she is "in synch" with the therapist. This function of witnessing and feeding back clinician understanding tends to support the development of a strong working alliance, even when what the patient communicates is painful or problematic. The risk that the therapist may miss the point of a patient's statements and may say something incorrect necessitates that the therapist solicit the patient's feedback that he or she is on target. At other times, the statements by the patient may be vague or otherwise unclear. As a basic therapeutic strategy, the therapist always wants to know more about unclear communications and asks for clarification. Authenticity is an intersubjective experience that supports the therapeutic alliance. If a patient experiences that the therapist does not actually understand but is "coasting" by acting as if he or she does, it damages the therapist's credibility and thus the alliance.

Repairing of a Misalliance

General principles of supportive psychotherapy related to the patient–therapist relationship are described in Winston et al. (2004), building upon the work of Pinsker (1997), Misch (2000), and Novalis et al. (1993). Some of the principles related to addressing a misalliance are as follows (Winston et al. 2004, p. 83):

1. When a patient–therapist problem is not resolved through practical discussion, the therapist moves to discussion of the therapeutic relationship.
2. The therapist can modify the patient's distorted perceptions using clarification and confrontation and not interpretation.
3. If indirect means to address negative transference or therapeutic impasses fail, then more explicit discussion about the relationship may be warranted.
4. The therapist uses only the amount of expressive technique necessary to address negative transference.
5. The therapeutic alliance may allow the patient to listen to the therapist present material he or she would not accept from anyone else.

6. Sometimes the therapist will have to frame what the patient will experience as criticism in a palatable or supportive manner, or first offer anticipatory guidance.

The therapist typically uses standard supportive techniques to address a misalliance because supportive measures are the first line of repair for ruptures in the alliance (Bond et al. 1998). This approach means the problem should first be addressed in a practical way, related to the current situation, before symbolic or transference issues are addressed. With lower-functioning patients, the therapist may need to alter his or her stance, as one does in normal social discourse when the person is becoming distant or more obviously angry (Pinsker et al. 1991).

Self-Disclosure

Although it is not inappropriate for the patient to know something about the therapist as a person in the real world, in general the information should be that which might be available in the public record, such as the Internet or other media. When the therapist chooses to reveal less obvious personal information, it should be for a clearly therapeutic purpose. In expressive therapies one buys out of the direct question about what the therapist's experience is by asking why the patient is interested or by interpreting. In supportive psychotherapy, if it seems reasonable, one may self-disclose, being careful not to be seductive, competitive, or unnecessarily gratifying, or otherwise exploit the patient. As a contrast, it may be useful to state here that some of the best self-disclosure occurs through a process wherein the therapist reveals himself or herself by modeling appropriate behavior—thinking through a problem collaboratively, being steadfast and compassionate in a crisis, manifesting patience and emotional strength, demonstrating flexibility when necessary, exercising both wisdom and humility, and teaching the patient how to emulate these qualities when possible.

> **Patient:** I don't think you like me.
> **Therapist 1:** It's important for you to know how I feel. (Traditional clarification doesn't reveal the therapist's feelings but is responsive.)
> **Therapist 2:** I hear a question in your statement and I will answer it, but first I'd like to know what it means to you. (One can answer with a question as long as it is not avoiding answering or off-putting and it is combined with anticipatory guidance.)
> **Therapist 3:** Sure I like you. What makes you think differently? (This response is used with a fragile, lower-functioning patient.)

Sometimes a patient will ask for an opinion that draws on the therapist's subjective experience and that may have direct impact on the patient's self-esteem. The therapist is best off responding with a teaching moment based on principle.

> **Patient:** I brought in some of my drawings. What do you think of them?
> **Therapist:** It's important that you've been putting your creative impulses into action, and I'd like to see your work. However, it's generally unwise for psychotherapists to make comments on things that he or she is not expert in, so I'm not going to comment as if I were. It's one of those unwritten rules of psychotherapy. (Sets limits in a nonpunitive way, softens potential rejection through praise and generalization, frames expected patient behavior through declaration of a principle.)

Sustaining Comments

As discussed previously (see subsection "Adopt a Conversational Style"), it is not always possible to continue with statements about adaptive skills and self-esteem, so one must make bridging statements or return to important issues by refocusing the patient in a supportive way.

> **Patient:** Hi [*then several minutes of silence*].
> **Therapist:** Hello.
> **Patient:** [*After more minutes of silence*] Mmmm...
> **Therapist:** Well, I've been doing a lot of thinking about what you said last week about your situation at home. (Validating, alliance-building, anxiety-reducing; lets the patient know that he has been on the therapist's mind and that the therapist remembers the patient's concerns and, thus, that the patient is important.)

Esteem Building

Self-esteem is the collection of beliefs and experiences that a person has of his or her inherent value and includes the individual's actual competence or self-efficacy. Interventions that augment psychological functioning or adaptive skills raise the patient's capacity to function appropriately in the world and support increased self-esteem. There are, however, supportive interventions that are intended to directly restore or improve self-esteem.

Praise

Praise, along with the other esteem-building interventions, is used proactively and liberally in supportive treatment. In one sense, praise is a clarification that raises self-esteem by raising the patient's awareness about his or her accomplishments. However, in order for praise to be effective, it must be data based, that is, grounded in the therapist's understanding of the patient's values and experience. Thus, the therapist must be careful not to impose his or her values on the patient. If the patient does not experience the therapist's statements as praise, because what has been identified is not felt by the patient to be praiseworthy, then the therapist has not been supportive. Praise that is empty or undeserved is likely to be experienced negatively. One is better off not saying anything in that situation, because praise for something the patient does not feel is praiseworthy belittles the patient. Similarly, it is important that the therapist choose words that do not deliver a subtly denigrating, dismissive, or patronizing message or tone (Pinsker 1997).

Honest praise can be given for positive movement in the usual objectives of supportive therapy—an accomplishment of a stated task, use of a more adaptive skill, or demonstration of a more mature emotional strategy.

> **Patient:** So I walked into his office and decided I had to put my cards on the table. Like usual, he started to put up a fuss, but I said he needed to hear me out because I'd had other offers, which wasn't true [*grins*]! Inside, I was sort of watching myself deal with him. Some part of me couldn't believe I was doing that. But he listened to me and then he gave me the raise!
>
> **Therapist:** That's great! [*smiles, mirroring*] You knew the right way to deal with your boss. In contrast to your statements that you're a pushover, here you demonstrated real initiative and got what you wanted. Are there other times when you act so self-assured? (Praises the patient's successful bargaining; attempts to broaden the role in the patient's self-concept.)

The therapist can praise the patient's ability to negotiate (i.e., his or her adaptive skills), an intervention firmly in the realm of the supportive approach, and here we are the experts. Patients are often unaware of the gains they have made, so the therapist can build self-esteem by making strengths explicit.

A patient is able to talk about his or her experiences of failure, but in a balance, as he or she has other things of value in his or her life:

> **Patient:** I've screwed up plenty of relationships over the years—we've talked about that. Also, my attempt at law school was a bust. I kept trying and trying but just couldn't cut it. I've also blown through a bunch of jobs since then, especially 2 years ago when I had that billing supervisor job at the medical clinic. Boy, was I in way over my head! I tried to ride it out, figuring I'd get the hang of it, but it didn't work out. I like the numbers, but I don't like the pressure. But now I'm doing pretty well at this new place. I track their inventory on a computer, and I've been there 8 months with no major upheaval. It suits me better. And of course, now I have Lisa in my life....
>
> **Therapist:** So now, your confidence is much more realistic! (Clarifies.)
>
> **Patient:** I just get myself into these situations and then find out I'm not prepared or it's too stressful.

Therapist: But I'm struck by your ability to go round after round and see things through. You always land on your feet. (Self-esteem building by making strengths explicit.)

Reassurance

Reassurance is used as a supportive intervention within supportive psychotherapy as well as in other situations in which one person allays the fears of another by delivering truthful information in a caring way. In general medical practice, reassurance is used frequently to dispel patients' negative expectations about the course of an illness, or sequelae of a treatment or surgery, and thus to alleviate their anxieties. When supportive psychotherapy is being conducted, reassurance is best when it is data based or based on principle. It usually is not good to reassure without knowledge of patient's life and expectations. Similarly, one should first let the patient voice his or her concerns before attempting to be reassuring, lest such reassurance be perceived as hollow or nonspecific to the patient's needs.

Normalizing is a particular form of reassurance that relies on comparisons with others whom the patient is likely to deem normal or "regular." The therapist's message that "other people do it too" normalizes by recategorizing the patient's beliefs about his or her or others' experience or behavior.

Patient: It's really difficult. I know I have to move forward with my plan, but I'm really scared about what could happen. There must be something wrong with me. I should be able to "just do it" [*anxious smile*]. I feel guilty, too, 'cause I see Dad in my head saying, "Feeling scared is just so ridiculous. Look at your opportunity!"
Therapist: Anyone would be afraid and proceed with caution in your situation. (Depathologizes, empathizes.)

The therapist's comments when normalizing must be targeted, specific, and helpful. Empty comments are not supportive, even if accurate:

Patient: I'm the weirdest person there is. I'm all alone—isolated and no friends, no interests, and no prospects [*frowns, stares into space*].
Therapist: Many people feel this way. (Fatuous.)

Encouragement

When patients are discouraged in the face of difficult external obstacles, or their own incapacities, they may be provided encouragement. Frequently, patients present in therapy in a demoralized state—they experience distress at an inability to rectify a problem against what is experienced as great odds, combined with subjective incompetence and decreased self-esteem (de Figueiredo 1993; Frank 1974). When patients are demoralized, they do not try new things to improve their quality of life, because they presume that they have no power to effect change (Pinsker et al. 1991). Patients can be demoralized because of moral beliefs they have about their own behavior, externalizing defenses that promote the experience of powerlessness, disempowering responses of others to their maladaptive behavior, or their experience of treatment systems that communicate their low expectation of real change (Rosenthal 2002). With the patient faced with problems that appear to loom large, the therapist can provide encouragement by assisting the patient in taking one step at a time. This means that the therapist acts to spur on or to instill hope, an elemental factor that may contribute to therapeutic change (Yalom 1995). There are many common adages ("Rome wasn't built in a day"; "Every cloud has a silver lining") that present an encouraging or hopeful message.

Exhortation

Exhortation is a more insistent form of encouragement in which the clinician urges or eggs on the patient to pursue a goal. Typically, this is done with a more impaired patient, who, though reluctant, must have a high likelihood of accomplishing the task (Pinsker 1997). Because of the risk of overwhelming or disempowering the patient, caution must be used in tempering the manner and the message so that the patient feels the strong alliance with and conviction of the therapist that what the therapist is suggesting is the right course of action.

> **Patient:** I'm not sure I have what it takes to get through this....I have to tell them whether I'll take their offer in the next week.
> **Therapist 1:** I've seen what you are capable of. You can do this! (Frank cheerleading.)
> **Therapist 2:** You've spent many weeks convincing me that this is the goal you want to pursue, and you were quite eloquent in laying out the arguments as to why it was appropriate for you. It's not unusual to have some doubts along the way, especially before you commit yourself, but I think you have a great rationale for making this choice. (Reiterates the patient's own arguments to counter the patient's ambivalence, normalizes doubts, adds the weight of the therapist's reasoning to the decisional process.)

Inspiration

The aim of inspiration is to support the patient's experience of self-esteem and self-efficacy through self-transcendence, a powerfully validating experience. Inspiration is seen more commonly in the context of religious or spiritual guidance or participation or when spontaneously experiencing a noble or heroic action by another. However, as a purposive technique in supportive psychotherapy, it is difficult and infrequently used because it requires a situation in which the therapist experiences an opportunity both to self-transcend and to communicate his or her authentic experiences or beliefs or those of another in a manner that the patient experiences as elevating. Inspiration goes beyond reassurance and encouragement, because in this highly motivated state the patient's fear and the experienced need for small steps are supervened. When one is inspired, there is an increase in motivation for self-actualizing behavior.

Enhancement of Ego Functioning

The domain of ego functioning includes the various functions of the mental operations of the self, including reality testing, sense of reality, affect regulation, defensive functions, synthetic function, object relations, thought processes, and superego (conscience, morals, ideals) (Bellak 1958; Beres 1956). Because anxiety tends to exacerbate impairments in ego functioning, as well as amplifying symptoms of major mental disorders, supportive psychotherapy offers several interventions that directly address it.

Anxiety-Reducing Interventions

Interventions that reduce anxiety are fundamental to the repertoire of supportive psychotherapy. The rationale of many of the contextual techniques is that they reduce anxiety or prevent its exacerbation. Anxiety in supportive psychotherapy generally is framed as psychopathological or at least as contributing to the patient's sense of dysphoria and maladaptation. When anxiety or fear is experienced as overwhelming, people have difficulty trying new things and as a result may not master important adaptive skills, such as asking someone out for a date, driving a car, or learning to swim. Thus, in supportive treatment, anxiety is usually reduced through direct means except when the therapist is purposefully titrating it (e.g., through exposure) or working with skills to help the patient cope more adaptively. In contrast, in expressive therapies, unless anxiety is at the disorder level, it is seen as a motivator of the psychotherapeutic work or as a signal to the participants that conflictual unconscious content is emergent (A. Freud 1936).

Structuring the environment. When patients have more severe psychopathology and are relatively low functioning, the therapist acts to increase the amount of structure available to the patient through therapeutic interventions and interactions with the patient's environment. These mechanisms may include interaction with case managers, family members, employers, and so on (Rockland 1989). With higher-functioning patients, the clinical necessity to intervene directly in the patient's life or environment is greatly reduced and, in respect to the patient's actual functional autonomy, becomes intrusive or otherwise inappropriate.

Maintaining a protected environment.   Although maintaining a protected environment is not supportive psychotherapy proper, at times the most supportive activity is to provide a holding environment that literally contains the patient. Clearly for safety reasons, as when a patient cannot be relied on to contain self-destructive or other destructive impulses, and there is insufficient community support, hospitalization can provide respite and containment.

Setting limits.   At times, the therapist will choose to exercise professional and relational power to set limits when the patient is behaving in a way that is maladaptive in that the patient is not following the rules of therapy. A patient's transgression can take the form of behaviors that are unresponsive to therapists' cueing and feedback, such as being threatening or seductive, arriving intoxicated, not leaving the session when the time is up, or acting in an otherwise inappropriate manner. The intoxicated patient, assuming that he or she can leave the session safely, must do so with the clear message to come back in a nonintoxicated state. Otherwise, if the patient is able to pull back on the behavior and discuss it in session after being made aware, many of these behaviors are amenable to discussion in the context of supporting ego function and adaptive skills.

The therapist decides when to alter the structure of the session. For example, with a patient in crisis and also under other circumstances, it may be therapeutically appropriate to extend the time of a session. The therapist pays proper attention to not gratuitously satisfying patients' infantile wishes but tempers this with reasonableness, which is the therapist modeling reasonable behavior and judgment (Winston et al. 2004). At other times, for example, with a patient who has a pattern of continuing to engage and speak after the end of a session, the therapist can choose not to extend the session because it would enable maladaptive, regressive behavior without reasonable clinical or environmental justification. In this case, the therapist gets up and shows the patient the door.

Designating the topic explicitly.   Because of the inherent power imbalance in the therapeutic relationship, the therapist attempts to empower the patient by involving him or her as a decision-making participant in what is discussed. Compared with free association, which is anxiety provoking, agenda setting gives the patient a structured topic on which to focus and reduces anxiety by putting the patient into the position of acceding or refusing to discuss the topic.

Modulating affect.   *Modulating affect* pertains to how people manage emotions: their own and their responses to the feelings of others or to an emotionally charged situation. When patients have impairments in this area of ego functioning, they may respond disproportionately to the situation with an overly intense, overly constricted, dysphoric, or otherwise maladaptive manner. The patient's loss of control of affect is typically maladaptive. For patients with an inability to contain their expression of affect, continuing to focus on what is making the person angry only escalates the problem, so often it is best to change the subject (Pinsker 1997). Gaining emotional competence improves self-esteem, so in the context of a good therapeutic alliance the therapist focuses the patient on how to better contain affects and intervenes in ways that help the patient develop his or her capacity for affective regulation. Reducing the patient's reactions to environmental or intrapsychic stress or altering the inclination toward negative emotional states and misinterpretations of his or her physical states can improve self-efficacy (Bandura 1994).

Supporting defenses. Defenses are usually not confronted unless they are clearly maladaptive (e.g., primitive denial, regression, projection, splitting) or threaten the frame of treatment. Adaptive defenses such as repression, rationalization, intellectualization, and reaction formation are generally and specifically supported:

> **Patient:** I spend too much time thinking about everything. (Bemoans obsessional style.)
> **Therapist:** Standing in front of the closet deciding what to wear helps you stall some and put off what would be very anxiety provoking [i.e., having to make a decision]. (Supports obsessional defenses.)

Universalizing. Rather than personalizing a comment to the patient, an approach that may be received as an attack or a criticism, the supportive therapist can cloak the comment in an impersonal remark.

> **Therapist 1:** You heard what you wanted to hear. (Confronts directly.)
> **Therapist 2:** The mind has a tendency to hear what it wants to hear. (Declares a general principle.)

Naming the problem. Identifying and naming a problem helps a patient to conceptualize it and thus to better understand and cope with it. For example, with a patient who is overly digressive, making the pattern of communication with the therapist the exemplar for a more general pattern can focus the patient on working to be better understood, if it is his or her desire to do so.

> **Therapist:** I notice that when you are explaining something, you tend to use a lot of extra words and refer to subjects that are not necessary to get the point across. I'm finding it hard to understand. Has anyone ever brought that up as an issue?

Patient: People always seem to get huffy and impatient with me when I talk about things.

Therapist: So, that I'm having some difficulty following your train of thought is not something unusual for you?

Patient: I don't think so.

Therapist: Maybe your experience of people's negative responses is related to their having trouble with easily understanding you, too. Should we put this pattern of speaking to others on the problem list? (Connects people's responses to his style; offers it as something that can be worked on.)

The patient could answer that and have his autonomy supported.

Rationalizing. Rationalization allows a patient to explain unacceptable attitudes, beliefs, or behaviors so as to make them bearable (Gabbard 2004). When the therapist offers a rationalizing comment, he or she is shoring up healthier defensive mode for the patient that is adaptive in that it aids the patient in coping with realities that tend to reduce a patient's self-esteem.

Reframing. Reframing is a rationalization strategy in which the therapist offers a different point of view given the same information, with the intended effect of interfering with the patient's maladaptive beliefs about his or her thoughts or behavior.

Patient: I really want to talk to him but then I get tongue-tied and I walk away. Then I try again and end up somewhere else, like at the front desk, or one time right out the door. Last time, I actually walked right by him, but all I could manage was a weak smile. I'm sure it looked goofy because I was so anxious. I'm so inept; I'll never connect with him this way.

Therapist: Being shy around someone you are really attracted to is pretty common, so in this you are definitely not alone. (Normalizes.) Sometimes it takes a bunch of tries in order to be successful. It's like testing the shallow part before you go out to the deep end of the water. (Relabels approach-avoidance behavior as "getting used to.")

Reframing can soften the impact of an unpleasant reality on the patient's self-esteem:

Patient: Ugh, sometimes I'd get through the voir dire, but by the end of it they'd rejected me from five juries. Five juries! I couldn't believe it [*scowls*].

Therapist: You can be rejected for being too well educated. (Esteem building by reframing and rationalizing.)

At times, reframing can be used in a more traditional way within the context of supportive psychotherapy. Pointing out maladaptive behavior as part of an illness is reframing it to make it ego-dystonic, a standard psychotherapeutic technique to increase motivation for change. Given the rationale of supportive psychotherapy, the delivery must be couched in a reassuring and hopeful manner that minimizes anxiety, reduces potential blows to self-esteem, and outlines an achievable pathway for change.

Here, a patient recognizes the pattern that his life is unstable and blames himself for its damaging his interpersonal relationships.

> **Patient:** I've been really down since Tuesday, when Beth broke up with me. I screwed it up because my life isn't together. But I know it's my fault…it happens with every relationship. When I was going out with Sandi, the same thing happened. Same with Leslie. I should have acted like I was more in charge. I'm such a loser.
>
> **Therapist:** Is there a utility in your rehashing old relationships? Let's make a distinction between the use of analyzing interpersonal patterns and self-punishing. It seems that each time you bring it up, rather than looking objectively for ways to be more successful in going forward, you use it to underscore your failures and beat yourself up. This has a direct negative effect on your self-esteem, so it's not adaptive for you. Maybe we can use the patterns you recognize to be more successful? (Reframing, which proposes that the patient change his perspective on the same information.)

Minimization. Another form of rationalization is one in which the therapist substitutes minimization for the patient's denial of affect in order to make the affect more palatable for the patient to accept it: "So, there was *some* resentment?"

Awareness-Expanding Interventions

The aim of expanding awareness is contrasted with development of insight, which in psychodynamic terms is emotional awareness based on genetic material, usually via the transference. Clarification, confrontation, and, more rarely, interpretation are useful techniques in supportive psychotherapy, but there is no requirement that the unconscious be made conscious or that full linkage of impulses, wishes, or affects be made with early important figures. In supportive psychotherapy, the therapist clarifies frequently, confronts periodically, but interprets infrequently.

Clarification. Without elaboration, the therapist using clarification reduces cognitive distortion or points out patterns by restating, acknowledging, summarizing, paraphrasing, or organizing a patient's statements.

> **Patient:** I'm so mad Beth dumped me. Maybe if she told me earlier that she was getting unhappy and frustrated, I could've changed things [*frowns*]. I was really trying to be a good partner. It's so painful—I

> don't understand why she did this. Things were going pretty well. I
> miss her and want her back.
>
> **Therapist:** Can we look at what happened?
>
> **Patient:** I took her out for dinners and always had to fit everything to her
> schedule. I even went to plenty of events with her and did lots of other
> stuff that I didn't really want to do. And then, nothing. When's it my
> turn? It's just not fair! [*reddens*]
>
> **Therapist:** Did you tell her about what you were dissatisfied about?
>
> **Patient:** Not so much.
>
> **Therapist:** So, your experience is that you made a lot of adjustments to
> sustain the relationship with her, but it makes you angry that she
> didn't reciprocate the effort before she broke up with you. (Clarifies.)

Using humor.   Sometimes framing a clarification in a humorous wrapper softens the potential esteem-lowering impact of finding out that what one is doing is getting in one's own way.

> **Patient:** I'm still so lonely. I think a lot about how it would be to meet
> someone and have a relationship, but it doesn't happen.
>
> **Therapist** [*sees issue of procrastinating*]: It's difficult for you to meet men.
> (Clarification.)
>
> **Patient:** I've been getting things done, but I have so much to do: I'm busy
> at work, then there's dating, answering personals, going online, and
> so on…
>
> **Therapist:** If you can use your creativity to find ways of doing what you say
> is your intention instead of making creative excuses, you'll probably
> be successful. (Avuncular.)

The content in this case might be the same as what a friend or family member would tell her, but a therapist saying it might give it more power.

Confrontation.   Confrontation is an intervention that brings to the patient's awareness something he or she is avoiding or suppressing, or an unrecognized maladaptive pattern of behavior. If the therapist in the previous interaction went further and elaborated on the information in a way that brought into awareness the maladaptive pattern of behavior the patient is avoiding looking at, it would be a confrontation:

> **Therapist:** I notice that you tend to say "I don't understand" about things
> you actually do understand. (Confronts without giving rationale.)
>
> **Therapist:** I'm going to point out something I think will help you to better
> get your needs met in relationships. It seems that you expect that people
> should know what you need. Then when you don't get it, you get
> angry. (Gives rationale for confronting, confronts.)

When the therapist chooses to confront in supportive psychotherapy, he or she puts the confronting into a specific context and gives a clear rationale for it (e.g., to increase adaptive skills), making sure there is ample feedback that the patient understands the therapist's intent. "I'm bringing this to your awareness so that the next time you get into a dispute with your father that makes you angry, you can respond in a way that makes you feel more competent." This is especially useful in working with a patient's more primitive defenses:

Patient: It made me so angry and jealous when I caught him looking at another woman. Then he has the nerve to claim that he wasn't looking at her.

Therapist: Is that not possible? Did you actually see him looking at her? (Continues to reality test the basis of her assessment.)

Patient: I could sense that he was looking, but, well, no, I didn't actually see him looking. You think he might be doing it on purpose?

Therapist: I'm thinking maybe that question is a little far-fetched. Is it offensive to you that I point this out? (In dealing with a paranoid style, the therapist encourages the patient to "consider the alternatives.")

Patient: No, it's okay. I just get angry when he's checking out another woman. I've told him about that.

Therapist: I understand, but since you didn't actually see him, is it possible that he really didn't look at her? It seems that you assume that if a woman you think he thinks is attractive walks by, he will look at her, even though you've made it clear that it upsets you.

Patient: Don't know. Maybe I do that. There have been times I've accused people of stuff and they denied it, they even had what looked like proof, so I backed off. But I get the feeling anyway that somehow they got away with it.

Therapist: So, you've described a pattern where people disagree with your take on things, and even with some evidence they are speaking honestly, you have this vexing sense they are not. Is it a possibility that somehow things may be at times a little different from how you experience them? (Clarifies, then points out that this is not an isolated experience for her, but part of a pattern [confrontation]; softens and minimizes the observation that she is distorting.)

Patient: I guess it's possible. It just doesn't seem that way, but I see your point about the pattern—I do that a lot, and not just with him. (Responds to the confrontation with increased awareness.)

Denial is a common defense that can be adaptive or maladaptive. The supportive task here is how to improve a patient's reality testing, in this case about the end of a relationship, without damaging his or her self-esteem.

Therapist: I see that it is difficult or maybe painful for you to look at, but this may help you to think about moving forward. You are acting toward these women as if you still had a relationship so you don't have to let go. (Confronts pattern of denial that relationships are in the past.)

Patient: I still think about Beth. She should call me so we could discuss things.

Therapist: However, you are no longer in a relationship with her. (Reiterates confrontation more specifically.)

Patient: But I still care for her. [*Long silence*] She's out having a wonderful time. I think it's bad for me to think she didn't have any genuine feelings for me.

Therapist: That's an assumption. Why would she have feelings for you now since the relationship is over? That's probably why she hasn't called. But that doesn't mean that she was not genuine when you were together. (Confronts distortion.)

Patients will at times talk in a vague manner. This manner can be due to a vague style, which may be the result of cognitive, interpersonal, or cultural factors, or a situational vagueness caused by obsessional defenses that are aroused in response to a conflictual feeling, wish, or impulse.

Therapist: How did you feel when again, she didn't give you what you had clearly asked for?

Patient: Oh, this happens all the time [*shrugs*]. We ended up going out to the movies instead. (Uninformative.)

Therapist 1: You are being vague. (Confronts the defense without contextual support, potentially raising anxiety.)

Therapist 2: Could you be more specific? I'm not sure what you are getting at, but I hear you aren't getting what you want from her. (Confronts in a more diluted and empathic fashion, lowering the risk of raising anxiety.)

Therapist 3: People often talk around a topic when they are uncomfortable about how they feel or how they may be perceived. I hope you understand that I've pretty much heard it all and am comfortable with the issues people are most uncomfortable with. (Confronts in a softened and normalized fashion, balancing with alliance building and reassurance, thus lowering anxiety.)

Patient: Well, I get upset when she does this. She does this all the time. [*Reddens, clenches hands together.*]

Therapist 3: How upset?

Patient: I was disappointed. It makes me feel wimpy and hopeless.

Therapist 3: Did you communicate your feelings to her so that she might address your concerns?

Patient: We went to the movies like nothing happened.

Therapist 3: So, we can see that though you are able to initially ask her for what you want, she frequently dismisses this and you get dejected and feel a loss of self-esteem because you feel ineffective in getting your needs met. Maybe we can work on a way for you to more effectively address getting your needs met. (Confronts, encourages by offering a path toward increased self-efficacy.)

Similarly, patients may have a digressive style or only become digressive as a defensive posture. Do you intervene when the patient digresses, or do you let him or her move toward the point? Focusing too early with confrontation may cut off the final point, but letting him or her digress too much may avoid the adaptive context. One must make a data-based intervention based on the patient's goals and the objectives of supportive psychotherapy.

Indirect or impersonal suggestion is a confrontive technique that does not engage defenses directly in order to raise awareness. Rather than asking something that the patient must answer such as, "Are you angry?" one can embed it in the conversation:

> **Patient:** And then he said he was sorry I was mad he didn't pick me up and I wasn't even mad. He's just a jerk sometimes! [*loudly and emphatically*]
> **Therapist:** When people raise their voices, sometimes they're angry. (Sidesteps defenses and doesn't arouse anxiety.)

Interpretation. Interpretation focuses awareness on a thought, behavior, affect, defense, or symptom by connecting it to its unconscious origin or meaning. Transference interpretation is used infrequently in supportive psychotherapy, although it may be used provided it is aimed toward adaptive functioning or to maintain the frame of treatment. Interpretive ideas can be offered in a variety of more supportive configurations (Winston et al. 1986). Linkages can be made at times even to genetic figures, but waiting to make the interpretation until the patient is not in the grip of the affect or impulse ("striking while the iron is cold") decreases the likelihood of anxiety generation (Pine 1984). One can also structure an interpretation by removing or reducing key elements in order to reduce its potential to arouse anxiety or dysphoria.

Intellectualized interpretation. Intellectualized interpretation ignores specific dynamic referents, transferential aspects, and nonverbal communication, and gives a rationale connecting phenomena about which the patient is already conscious. There is no connection made to a purported unconscious fantasy or mechanism (Rockland 1989, p. 96).

Inexact interpretation. Inexact interpretation (Glover 1931) protects the fragile patient by offering an explanation about impulses or behavior that is plausible but not the whole truth about infantile fears. This is related to what Langs (1973) would call "interpretation upward," in which, as a means of reducing anxiety and supporting ego function, there is a tying together of the conflictual affect or impulse to a more mature (and ego-syntonic) or triadic conflict rather than the actual pre-oedipal, dyadic construct.

> **Patient:** I'm so mad I want to make a fat hamburger out of him.
> **Therapist:** It makes you angry that he asked her out when you wanted to see her—so you want your rival out of the way, so you can get the girl.

(Focuses the affect on rivalry, sidesteps exploring or interpreting primitive incorporative aspects of fantasy.)

Incomplete interpretation.   Incomplete interpretation (Pinsker et al. 1991), an intervention formulated within the supportive psychotherapy frame, leaves out the genetic references in an interpretation and generalizes the subject in order to decrease the generation of anxiety while increasing the patient's awareness of avoided material.

> **Patient:** They hold the meetings at inconvenient times, so I'm usually a few minutes late. My boss gets a little annoyed at waiting, but nothing comes of it.
> **Therapist:** So, habitually coming a few minutes late to the meeting is a way for you to show people that you resent conforming to expected behavior that doesn't take your needs into account, and that you can do things your way and exert some control. (Makes a connection to the angry feeling, supports self-esteem, contrasts the patient's behavior with a real-world expectation.)

Skills Building

The intention of skills building is to impart factual or procedural knowledge the patient can use to increase adaptive functioning.

Giving Advice

Giving advice is a mainstay of supportive psychotherapy. Within the context of "being like a good parent," advice is given when needed but tempered against the patient's developmental needs. The therapist judges whether a patient needs to be told what to do (with an eye toward it being learned), will benefit from being pointed in the direction of information, or can simply be reassured that he or she already has what is needed to make a decision. Advice needs to be specific and individualized and should come from the therapist's expertise in areas such as mental illness, adjustment, and reasonable living in society (Winston et al. 2004). Advice is usually not helpful when not asked for—as with most supportive interventions, advice that is perceived as not relevant to the patient's issues is not helpful, even if it is reasonable advice.

Teaching

Teaching is the imparting of information as an expert or as a wise, adaptive person. Moreover, teaching is the realm in which a patient can be given principles that he or she may internalize so as to be able to make more adaptive judgments and decisions. Teaching principles tends to be a more powerful tactic than giving advice about a particular issue, because principles are more easily generalized and used adaptively over time in different situations.

> **Therapist:** The mind tends to lump unconnected problems together to make sense of chaos. The result is we fear a scary monster outside the house, when the truth is that it is the wind that is howling, it is the window shutter banging in the wind, and the lights are flickering because a tree fell on the power lines a few blocks away.

Modeling Adaptive Behavior

Because one of the hypothesized mechanisms of change in supportive psychotherapy is through identification with a well-compensated and effective therapist, he or she must consistently demonstrate adaptive, reasonable, and organized thinking and behavior to the patient (Pinsker et al. 1991). However, at times in therapy, as in any human relationship, the therapist is going to get it wrong—as manifested in incorrect understanding, assumption, statement, or action. How the therapist is able to address these blunders with honesty, grace, humility, and resilience can impart an important message to the patient and offer a more interpersonally flexible and adaptive model of character with which the patient can identify.

Providing Anticipatory Guidance

Rehearsing before the actual need to perform a task or decision allows the patient to consider what problems might arise and to come up with coping strategies in advance. In addition to building up the patient's behavioral repertoire, working through a task in advance can reduce performance-related or decisional anxiety.

> **Patient:** When I'm in school, I get flustered about things I know don't really matter. I know it's about dealing with her. I end up clamming up or focusing on minutiae and not getting my ideas across.
> **Therapist:** Who?
> **Patient:** The school principal.
> **Therapist:** So, talking to her is anxiety provoking for you and you find yourself getting upset over stuff you think is trivial. (Clarifies.)
> **Patient:** Yeah, I've never been good around powerful people, but I used what we talked about before—I go over what the play of the hand is going to be before I go into the meeting. I know better now what she's going to ask and I rehearse my responses. Last meeting, I was okay and I noticed that I didn't get all twisted up. I was still nervous, but not so much [*smiles*].
> **Therapist:** So, because you rehearsed it, you were able to interact with the principal in a way that was more effective. The old adage "practice makes perfect" comes to mind. (Clarifies, adds a confirmatory slogan.)

In sessions focused on an upcoming termination of treatment, anticipatory guidance can play a major role. The therapist, in addition to reviewing the accomplishments achieved, can use anticipatory guidance to outline issues to explore in the future. Further, because it is typical for patients to have a range of feelings about the end of treatment, and about the therapist after treatment, it is useful to help the patient anticipate how he or she will deal with them.

> **Therapist:** Later when you wish to talk about something, you might be angry at feeling cut off. What might you do?
> **Patient:** Well, I wouldn't be able to talk it out with you.
> **Therapist:** Not exactly, but when things come up, you can remember similar things that would come up in treatment and how we would deal with it then. (Helps the patient model his own holding environment.)

Redirecting

Steering the patient away from painful affects through distraction is a strategy that the patient can learn to do. The therapist works with the patient to identify alternatives that are more adaptive when anxious. The patient's attention can be diverted to either increased activity (cleaning, distraction) or decreased activity (relaxation tape, good old memories). Remembering good things when things are bad adds perspective and may temper dysphoria or hopelessness.

> **Patient:** Often when it's getting late I feel sad and afraid, like I need to eat something to calm myself down. So I chow down comfort food from the pantry or the freezer. Now I'm gaining weight because of it!
> **Therapist:** Maybe there are other things you can do that can help you cope with those feelings in a healthier way. You've spoken about how you are so busy with work and your other responsibilities you can't seem to get the time to get things put away and clean up.
> **Patient:** What does that have to do with feeling bad and then eating too much?
> **Therapist:** Perhaps rather than overeating, which you also feel bad about, you can distract yourself from the uncomfortable feelings by using that time to focus on putting things away and cleaning up.

Promoting Autonomy

The patient is only allowed to depend on the therapist to the extent that he or she actually needs it, as he or she would depend on a good parent or mentor. The therapist sets limits when appropriate, and when appropriate, imparts the message that the patient is capable of working a task through on his or her own.

Key Points

- Supportive psychotherapy objectives of maintaining or increasing self-esteem, ego functioning, and adaptive skills are promoted through the use of contextual and tactical interventions.

- The main contextual techniques applicable in all treatments are the use of a conversational style, the maintenance of the frame of treatment including the purposive establishment of a strong therapeutic alliance, relating to the developmental needs of the patient as would a good parent, and focusing generally on here-and-now relationships.

- Tactical techniques based on the content of current communication, patient characteristics and goals, and therapist objectives are therapist responses that address the therapeutic alliance or aim to bolster self-esteem, ego functioning, or adaptive skills.

- As with other psychotherapy interventions, supportive techniques have an intrinsic logic but must have an appropriate rationale for being implemented. These techniques can be mastered over time with proper attention, supervision, and practice.

References

Bandura A: Self-efficacy, in Encyclopedia of Human Behavior, Vol 4. Edited by Ramachaudran VS. New York, Academic Press, 1994, pp 71–81

Barber JP, Stratt R, Halperin G, et al: Supportive techniques: are they found in different therapies? J Psychother Practic Res 10:165–172, 2001

Bellak L: The schizophrenic syndrome: a further elaboration of the unified theory of schizophrenia, in Schizophrenia: A Review of the Syndrome. New York, Logos, 1958, pp 3–63

Beres D: Ego deviation and the concept of schizophrenia. Psychoanal Study Child 11:164–235, 1956

Bond M, Banon E, Grenier M: Differential effects of interventions on the therapeutic alliance with patients with personality disorders. J Psychother Pract Res 7:301–318, 1998

de Figueiredo JM: Depression and demoralization: phenomenologic differences and research perspectives. Compr Psychiatry 34:308–311, 1993

Frank J: Psychotherapy: the restoration of morale. Am J Psychiatry 131:271–274, 1974

Freud A: The ego and the mechanisms of defense (1936), in The Writings of Anna Freud, Vol 2. New York, International Universities Press, 1966

Gabbard GO: Long-Term Psychodynamic Psychotherapy: A Basic Text. Washington, DC, American Psychiatric Publishing, 2004

Gabbard GO: Psychodynamic Psychiatry in Clinical Practice, 4th Edition. Washington, DC, American Psychiatric Publishing, 2005, pp 100–104

Glover E: The therapeutic effect of inexact interpretation: a contribution to the theory of suggestion. Int J Psychoanal 12:397–411, 1931

Gold SN, Cherry EF: The therapeutic frame: on the need for flexibility. Journal of Contemporary Psychotherapy 27:147–155, 1997

Hellerstein DJ, Rosenthal RN, Pinsker H, et al: A randomized prospective study comparing supportive and dynamic therapies: outcome and alliance. J Psychother Pract Res 7:261–271, 1998

Kernberg OF: Psychoanalysis, psychoanalytic psychotherapy and supportive psychotherapy: contemporary controversies. Int J Psychoanal 80:1075–1091, 1999

Langs R: The Technique of Psychoanalytic Psychotherapy, Vol 1. New York, Jason Aronson, 1973

Lyons-Ruth K; Members of the Change Process Study Group: Implicit relational knowing: its role in development and psychoanalytic treatment. Infant Ment Health J 19:282–289, 1998

Misch DA: Basic strategies of dynamic supportive therapy. J Psychother Pract Res 9:173–189, 2000

Novalis PN, Rojcewicz SJ, Peele R: Clinical Manual of Supportive Psychotherapy. Washington, DC, American Psychiatric Press, 1993

Pine F: The interpretive moment: variations on classical themes. Bull Menninger Clin 48:54–71, 1984

Pinsker H: A Primer of Supportive Psychotherapy. Hillsdale, NJ, Analytic Press, 1997

Pinsker H, Rosenthal RN: Beth Israel Medical Center Supportive Psychotherapy Manual. Social and Behavioral Sciences Documents 18, #2886. Washington, DC, American Psychological Association, 1988

Pinsker H, Rosenthal R, McCullough L: Dynamic supportive psychotherapy, in Handbook of Short-Term Dynamic Psychotherapy. Edited by Crits-Christoph P, Barber JP. New York, Basic Books, 1991, pp 220–247

Rockland LH: Supportive Therapy: A Psychodynamic Approach. New York, Basic Books, 1989

Rosenthal RN: Group treatments for schizophrenic substance abusers, in The Group Psychotherapy of Substance Abuse. Edited by Brook DW, Spitz HI. New York, Haworth Press, 2002, pp 327–349

Rosenthal RN, Muran JC, Pinsker H, et al: Interpersonal change in brief supportive psychotherapy. J Psychother Pract Res 8:55–63, 1999

Vaillant GE: Adaptation to Life. Boston, MA, Little, Brown, 1977

Vaillant GE (ed): Ego Mechanisms of Defense: A Guide for Clinicians and Researchers. Washington, DC, American Psychiatric Press, 1992

Westen D, Gabbard GO: Developments in cognitive neuroscience, II: implications for the theory of transference. J Am Psychoanal Assoc 50:99–134, 2002

Winnicott DW: The theory of the parent-child relationship. Int J Psychoanal 41:585–595, 1960

Winnicott DW: Playing and Reality. New York, Basic Books, 1971

Winston A, Pinsker H, McCullough L: A review of supportive psychotherapy. Hosp Community Psychiatry 37:1105–1114, 1986

Winston A, Rosenthal RN, Pinsker H: Introduction to Supportive Psychotherapy (Core Competencies in Psychotherapy). Washington, DC, American Psychiatric Publishing, 2004

Yalom ID: The Theory and Practice of Group Psychotherapy, 4th Edition. New York, Basic Books, 1995

Suggested Readings

AADPRT Supportive Therapy Competencies. Available at: http://www.aadprt.org/training/competency.aspx. Accessed January, 8, 2008.

Barber JP, Stratt R, Halperin G, et al: Supportive techniques: are they found in different therapies? J Psychother Pract Res 10:165–172, 2001

de Jonghe F, Rijnierse P, Janssen R: Psychoanalytic supportive psychotherapy. J Am Psychoanal Assoc 42:421–446, 1994

Hellerstein DJ, Pinsker H, Rosenthal RN, et al: Supportive psychotherapy as the treatment model of choice. J Psychother Pract Res 3:300–306, 1994

Novalis PN, Rojcewicz SJ, Peele R: Clinical Manual of Supportive Psychotherapy. Washington, DC, American Psychiatric Press, 1993

Pinsker H: A Primer of Supportive Psychotherapy. Hillsdale, NJ, Analytic Press, 1997

Rosenthal RN: Group treatments for schizophrenic substance abusers, in The Group Psychotherapy of Substance Abuse. Edited by Brook DW, Spitz HI. New York, Haworth Press, 2002, pp 327–349

Winston A, Rosenthal RN, Muran JC: Supportive psychotherapy, in Handbook of Personality Disorders. Edited by Livesley WJ. New York, Guilford, 2001, pp 344–358

Winston A, Rosenthal RN, Pinsker H: Introduction to Supportive Psychotherapy (Core Competencies in Psychotherapy). Washington, DC, American Psychiatric Publishing, 2004

Chapter 16

Applications of Individual Supportive Psychotherapy to Psychiatric Disorders

Efficacy and Indications

Peter J. Buckley, M.D.

All effective psychotherapies are, ipso facto, "supportive." This adage extends even to classical psychoanalysis. As de Jonghe, Rijnierse, and Janssen (1992) concluded in an examination of psychoanalytic treatment:

> [A]dequate support given by the analyst and the resulting specific experience occurring in the analysand contribute significantly to the power of psychoanalysis—[which] applies not only to the treatment of severely disturbed patients by "modified psychoanalysis" or psycho-analytically oriented psychotherapy but is valid even for "ordinary analysis" in the treatment of "ordinary neurosis." Without minimizing the importance of the interpretation–insight factor, we contend that the support–experience factor is the

mute and underestimated power of psychoanalysis; it is its "silent force." (p. 476)

This insightful observation highlights the increasing awareness of the importance of the therapeutic relationship and its "supportive" components as a central agent of change in any psychotherapy relationship, extending along the continuum from "pure" supportive psychotherapy to "classical" expressive psychoanalysis. Crucial to a clinical theory of effective supportive psychotherapy, therefore, is an understanding of the two-person relational aspect of the clinical situation. Maintaining the positive transference and thus enhancing the therapeutic alliance together with a high degree of therapist empathy for the patient is a key element in what makes supportive psychotherapy work (Buckley 1986).

Efficacy Studies

Relatively few controlled empirical studies of the efficacy of supportive psychotherapy have been conducted. Those that exist, however, suggest, but are far from concluding, that it is an effective ancillary or primary treatment for a number of psychiatric disorders.

The Menninger Psychotherapy Research Project

Wallerstein and his coworkers (Wallerstein 1986, 1989) conducted a naturalistic, comprehensive outcome study comparing supportive and expressive psychotherapy with psychoanalysis in the treatment of 42 psychiatric inpatients. Supportive psychotherapy achieved far more positive change than had been predicted. Wallerstein (1986) summarized this finding as follows:

> [W]ith the patients treated via primarily supportive modes (of all the varieties specified), changes have been substantially in excess of concomitant achieved insights; furthermore, they have seemed over the course of the follow-up observation to be just as stable, as enduring, as proof against subsequent environmental vicissitudes and as free (or not free) from the requirement for supplemental post treatment contact, support, or further therapeutic help as the changes in those patients treated in a centrally expressive mode (psychoanalysis). (p. 719)

Although this study was a naturalistic one conducted without control subjects or random assignment of patients, it highlights the efficacy of supportive psychotherapy in the treatment of quite seriously disturbed psychiatric patients, many of whom suffered from the spectrum of severe narcissistic and borderline conditions. The effectiveness of supportive psychotherapy in this patient group was an unexpected finding for the investigators. This study also had the merit of rigorously defining the supportive psychotherapy used in treatment.

Anxiety Disorders

Zitrin et al. (1978) randomly assigned 111 subjects with agoraphobia (and panic attacks), mixed phobias (and panic attacks), or simple phobias to treatment with behavior therapy plus imipramine, behavior therapy and placebo, or supportive psychotherapy and imipramine. No differences in effectiveness were found between behavior therapy and supportive psychotherapy, with both producing moderate to marked beneficial effects. Klein et al. (1983) attributed the lack of differential success to the fact that for patients with phobias "both treatments operate through nonspecific expectancy effects that incite the specific remedial action, i.e., maintained exposure in vivo" (p. 143). This study defined the supportive psychotherapy utilized (i.e., "non-judgmental, non-directive with patients encouraged to ventilate feelings and discuss problems and interpersonal relationships").

Shear et al. (1994) compared "nonprescriptive" psychotherapy with cognitive-behavioral therapy (CBT) in the treatment of patients with panic disorder with or without agoraphobia. Both psychotherapies were equally efficacious. In a follow-up study (Shear et al. 2001), patients with more "pure" panic disorder (i.e., with no more than mild agoraphobia) were studied for their response to emotion-focused psychotherapy versus CBT. In this study, the investigators found lower efficacy for the emotion-focused therapy than for CBT. Emotion-focused psychotherapy, as defined by these investigators, consisted of "a reflective listening approach with systematic exploration of the circumstances and details of emotional reactions. The treatment is based on the premise that unrecognized emotions trigger panic attacks and contribute to the maintenance of the disorder" (p. 195). Although these investigators posited that emotion-focused psychotherapy is a form of supportive therapy, it is not the usual type of supportive therapy. Even so, patients receiving this therapy had the highest completion rate in this study.

Schizophrenia

A National Institute of Mental Health (NIMH) study investigated the relative benefit of exploratory insight-oriented psychotherapy versus reality-adaptive supportive psychotherapy in the treatment of schizophrenia patients (Gunderson et al. 1984; Stanton et al. 1984). These therapies were provided by experienced clinicians, with insight-oriented therapy occurring three times a week and the supportive therapy once a week. Both were given over 2 years, with standard psychopharmacological treatment provided simultaneously. The results demonstrated a better outcome for supportive psychotherapy, particularly in significant positive gains in patients' coping styles. This is a striking finding given that the supportive psychotherapy was only once per week. It suggests that supportive psychotherapy, in combination with psychopharmacological management, is the treatment of choice in chronic schizophrenia and that more intensive and psychically intrusive, exploratory psychotherapeutic treatments may in fact be contraindicated.

Rosenbaum et al. (2005) examined the effects of early, rapid, and year-long sustained psychosocial intervention after a first psychotic episode of a schizophrenic spectrum disorder. Patients were assigned to receive supportive psychodynamic psychotherapy as a supplement to treatment as usual, an integrated assertive psychosocial and educational treatment program, or treatment as usual. They found that integrated treatment and supportive therapy in addition to treatment as usual improved outcome, particularly in social functioning, after 1 year for patients with first-episode psychosis compared with treatment as usual alone.

In a methodologically rigorous study of individual psychotherapeutic approaches to the treatment of schizophrenia, Hogarty et al. (1997) examined the effectiveness of personal therapy over a period of 3 years after hospital discharge among 151 patients. Personal therapy was defined by the investigators as a therapy that

> sought to enhance personal and social adjustment through the identification and effective management of affect dysregulation that was believed to either precede a psychotic relapse or provoke inappropriate behavior that was possibly generated by underlying neuropsychological deficits.... Through a process called "internal coping," personal therapy encouraged the patient to identify the affective, cognitive, and physiological experience of stress....Personal therapy focused on the patient's characteristic response to stress in general rather than on the idiosyncratic response to a specific stressor. It avoided symbolic interpretation and clarification of unconscious motives and drives. (p. 1506)

The patients, all of whom were taking antipsychotic medication, were randomly assigned to receive personal therapy or contrasting therapies that included supportive therapy in one of two concurrent trials. One trial studied patients who were living with family; the other studied patients who were living independent of family. The personal therapy was supplemented by techniques of supportive therapy, defined by the investigators as "active listening, correct empathy, appropriate reassurance, reinforcement of patient health–promoting initiatives, and reliance on the therapist for advocacy and problem solving in times of crisis" (p. 1507). Among patients living with family, personal therapy was more effective than family or pure supportive therapy in preventing psychotic and affective relapse. Among patients living independent of family, those who received personal therapy had significantly more psychotic episodes than those who received supportive therapy. These investigators noted that

> the supportive therapy condition in the current study was the most comprehensive of any previously tested by us. It included not only an explicit treatment contract but also the principles of supportive therapy, minimum effective dosing, patient psychoeducation, and case management addressed to needed services. This change in supportive therapy was made to enhance treatment compliance, and it apparently maintained the clinical remission of most patients who remained in treatment. (p. 1511)

Depressive Disorders

Few controlled studies of supportive psychotherapy in the treatment of depressive disorders have been reported. Thompson and Gallagher (1985) randomly assigned 30 elderly depressed patients to receive behavior therapy, cognitive therapy, or supportive therapy. Improvement was comparable in all three modalities from pre- to postevaluation, but in follow-up, patients in the cognitive and behavioral treatments maintained greater gains than those who received supportive psychotherapy. Conte (1994) criticized this study because of the small number of patients in each treatment group as well as the limited nature of the supportive psychotherapy, which did not emphasize the development of skills for living and dealing with stressful events, all hallmarks of effective supportive psychotherapy.

In the NIMH Treatment of Depression Collaborative Research Program, CBT and interpersonal therapy (both rigorously defined) were compared with an antidepressant–clinical management condition and a control condition consisting of drug placebo and clinical management (Elkin 1994; Elkin et al. 1989; Imber et al. 1990). The clinical management condition was a somewhat diffuse supportive psychotherapy approach. The two psychotherapies were found to be efficacious but not greatly different from the placebo–clinical management condition on measures of improvement in depressive symptoms and overall functioning.

Renaud et al. (1998) examined the differential course and treatment outcome of 100 adolescent patients with major depressive disorder who were randomly assigned to receive cognitive, family, or supportive psychotherapy. Their findings suggested that supportive psychotherapy was efficacious for milder forms of depression but less so for more severe depressions. Maina et al. (2005) compared brief dynamic psychotherapy with brief supportive psychotherapy in the treatment of minor depressive disorders (DSM-IV-TR dysthymic disorder). Patients treated with either psychotherapy showed a significant improvement after treatment in comparison to nontreated control subjects, but brief dynamic psychotherapy was shown to be more effective at follow-up evaluation.

Personality Disorders

Hellerstein et al. (1998) compared brief supportive therapy with short-term dynamic psychotherapy in the treatment of personality disorder patients. Similar efficacy posttreatment was found on measures of symptomatology, presenting complaints, and interpersonal functioning. However, these investigators demonstrated lasting positive change in interpersonal functioning in subjects treated with supportive psychotherapy.

Piper et al. (1998) conducted a randomized clinical trial investigating the efficacy of interpretive versus supportive therapy in the treatment of personality disorders. The drop-out rate was higher for interpretive therapy than supportive therapy. Patients in both types of therapy improved, but the therapies did not differ in outcome from each other. These investigators concluded that "when treatment is carried out by experienced therapists who follow a treatment manual, time-limited supportive therapy can be as efficacious as time-limited interpretive therapy" (p. 564).

Anecdotal evidence for the efficacy of supportive psychotherapy in the treatment of severe personality disorders can be found in the published case reports of Waldinger and Gunderson (1989). They examined the successful psychotherapeutic treatment of five patients with severe borderline personality disorder. Successful treatment occurred when a supportive and nonexpressive approach was used in the first half of treatment. A more expressive interpretive approach was utilized in the second half of these roughly 5-year treatments, but only after the supportive psychotherapy had, in these clinicians' opinion, provided a framework for the intrapsychic internalization of a positive patient–therapist interaction that then enabled these patients to tolerate and use a more insight-oriented therapy.

Perry et al. (1999) found positive outcome at termination and follow-up for patients with personality disorders who received psychotherapy. The psychotherapies in the studies these authors examined included psychodynamic psychotherapy, CBT, supportive therapy, and interpersonal group therapy. They recommended that future studies examine the differential responses of specific types of personality disorders to specific psychotherapies. Bateman and Fonagy (2000) conducted a systematic literature review of outcome studies on psychotherapeutic treatment of personality disorders. They noted that "our knowledge of effective psychological treatments is rudimentary" (p. 141). Although acknowledging that the majority of the studies they reviewed were uncontrolled, these authors concluded that they consistently demonstrated "modest gains associated with relatively high doses of treatment" (p. 141). They also noted that these effective treatments had the common factor of the therapist being active in the context of a well-established therapeutic relationship—both central aspects of supportive psychotherapy.

Clarkin et al. (2007) examined the differential effectiveness of three 1-year-long outpatient psychotherapy treatments for borderline personality disorder. Ninety patients with rigorously diagnosed borderline personality disorder were randomly assigned to receive one of three treatments: dialectical behavioral therapy (which focused directly on skills to help the patient regulate emotion), transference-focused psychotherapy (which employed transference interpretation as a possible mechanism of change), and dynamic supportive psychotherapy. The therapists in the supportive psychotherapy modality provided emotional support, gave advice on daily problems, and followed and managed the transference, but they explicitly did not use interpretation. The dialectical behavioral therapy consisted of weekly individual and group sessions and telephone consultation as requested. Transference-focused psychotherapy consisted of two individual sessions weekly, and supportive psychotherapy consisted of one weekly session that could be supplemented with additional sessions as needed. These investigators found that patients in all three treatment modalities demonstrated significant positive change in many areas, including depression, anxiety, global functioning, and social adjustment. Both transference-focused psychotherapy and dialectical behavioral therapy were significantly associated with improvement in suicidality. Transference-focused psychotherapy and supportive psychotherapy were associated with improvement in anger and impulsivity. Only transference-focused psychotherapy was significantly predictive of change in irritability and verbal and direct assault. The authors concluded that all three structured treatments for borderline patients were generally equivalent with regard to broad positive change in borderline personality disorder symptoms; they noted, however, that the specific differential findings suggest that there may be different routes to symptom change in patients with borderline personality disorder.

Substance Abuse

In the National Institute on Drug Abuse Collaborative Cocaine Treatment Study, Crits-Christoph et al. (1997) compared four treatments delivered in an ambulatory setting: 1) cognitive therapy plus group drug counseling, 2) supportive-expressive psychotherapy plus group drug counseling, 3) individual drug counseling plus group drug counseling, and 4) group drug counseling alone. This large, rigorously controlled study involved more than 400 patients who were heavy users of crack cocaine. All groups showed substantial reductions in cocaine use, but patients receiving individual and group drug counseling had the best results. Luborsky et al. (1985) demonstrated that the clinician who established a positive therapeutic alliance with the substance abuse patient right from the start of treatment (a sine qua non of supportive psychotherapy) was much more likely to achieve an effective outcome as measured by the patient's staying in treatment and stopping drug use.

Medical Disorders

Few controlled studies of the efficacy of supportive psychotherapy in the ancillary treatment of medical conditions have been conducted. Sjodin et al. (1986) randomly assigned 103 outpatients with chronic peptic ulcer disease to receive either medical treatment only or the same medical treatment plus supportive psychotherapy. Follow-up indicated significant positive differences in favor of those assigned to medical treatment plus supportive psychotherapy. Mumford et al. (1982) found increased compliance and speed of recovery, as well as fewer complications and days in the hospital, in patients recovering from myocardial infarctions and surgery when they received supportive psychotherapy as an ancillary treatment.

Indications

Although there is an urgent need for rigorous, controlled, randomized outcome studies that compare supportive psychotherapy with other treatments, the research data that currently exists suggest some clinical indications.

Psychotic illnesses appear to be a specific indication for the use of supportive psychotherapy alongside psychopharmacological management. Studies by Stanton et al. (1984) demonstrated that supportive psychotherapy, compared with insight psychotherapy, resulted in better outcome in terms of patients' coping styles for those suffering from chronic schizophrenia. Supportive psychotherapy enhanced treatment compliance and reduced the number of psychotic episodes in patients living independent of family in the Hogarty et al. (1997) study.

Personality disorder patients were found by Hellerstein et al. (1998) to have lasting improvement in interpersonal functioning when treated with supportive psychotherapy. In current clinical practice many personality disorder patients, including those with more severe forms such as the borderline patient, are treated with expressive psychotherapy, and only future controlled outcome studies contrasting psychotherapies such as dialectical behavioral therapy, transference-focused therapy, and supportive psychotherapy will determine specific indications. It is possible that both supportive and expressive psychotherapy have a differential role to play in the treatment of patients with personality disorders contingent on the degree of the patient's pathology and interpersonal functioning, but this remains to be demonstrated empirically.

Supportive psychotherapy can be useful in depressive and anxiety disorders, as the Elkin (1994) and Zitrin et al. (1978) studies have suggested. Supportive psychotherapy is also indicated alongside counseling and group treatment in substance abuse patients, for whom the maintenance of a positive therapeutic alliance is crucial (Luborsky et al. 1985).

Applications

Gill (1954) has provided a clear outline of how supportive psychotherapy should be applied:

> The therapist engages in various kinds of activity. He is not neutral, but is willing to take a definite hand in decisions and values, though he usually tries to avoid being too active in these areas if he can. He does not foster a regressive transference neurosis, since he does not employ the devices which would lead to this, but on the contrary actively discourages the development of such a transference by conducting the interview more like a social interchange of equals, by avoiding free association, by emphasizing reality rather than fantasy, by creating an atmosphere of temporariness, and similar measures. He observes various elements of transference developing anyhow—which he correctly calls transferences rather than a transference neurosis—and he may or may not interpret these. If they become obtrusive and seem to be hindering the treatment, or if he sees an opportunity to make a valuable point by interpreting a piece of transference, he will do so. But if reasonably positive and desirable behavioral changes are occurring, or if the hostile transference seems too hot to handle, he will remain silent about it and permit the transference to persist unresolved. (pp. 783–784)

Although Gill's emphasis was on the real relationship, he also astutely observed that in supportive psychotherapy the transference cannot always be ignored, because the spontaneous development of strong and regressive transference manifestations may be inevitable—for instance, in borderline patients. He noted that such transferences may be "florid, wild, and fluctuating," requiring considerable therapist activity designed to promote the development of a more stable object relationship within the therapeutic situation itself.

Personality Disorders

Patients with borderline personality disorder are often the most difficult to treat, reflecting the fluid and volatile state of many aspects of their psychological structure and functioning. Affective instability, unstable interpersonal relationships, identity disturbances, rejection sensitivity, impulsivity, self-destructive behavior, suicidality, and so on—all present a daunting therapeutic task for the clinician. Supportive psychotherapy, with its emphasis on the therapist as a real person and not an anonymous figure who promotes transference, has a crucial role to play in effective treatment. Providing an external ego, promoting reality testing, and not angrily responding in the countertransference to these patients often provocative and aggressive behavior both within and outside the clinical situation can be therapeutic. Given the stable instability of the borderline patient, the countertransference demands on the clinician can be enormous, but the sober, reality-based, and empathic connection to the patient that supportive psychotherapy provides can lead to positive change and growth. Appropriate therapist activity in the context of an established therapeutic alliance as opposed to passivity is an important clinical posture with these patients and has a positive impact on outcome. Empathically confronting self-destructive behavior such as drug abuse, promiscuity, and endangering the self through suicidal gestures and acts is an aspect of this supportive activity.

Kohut's (1971, 1977) work on the treatment of narcissistic patients catalyzed a revolution in American psychoanalysis. He highlighted psychological deficits, emphasized the power of the therapeutic relationship, and advocated a highly "empathic introspective" stance by the therapist toward the patient. This clinical posture was successful in the treatment of patients who had previously been quite refractory to psychotherapeutic intervention, and he postulated that therapeutic change occurred through the internalization by the patient of positive aspects of the clinical interaction alongside interpretive work. Many of these concepts have been incorporated into supportive psychotherapy, particularly Kohut's emphasis on the critical importance of the clinician's empathic-introspective immersion in the treatment of the patient with significant self-deficits.

Anxiety Disorders

Anxiety disorders, phenomenologically united by the subjective experience of overwhelming and disabling anxiety that has little basis in reality, have been classified into various discrete entities in DSM-IV-TR (American Psychiatric Association 2000). However, with the exception of obsessive-compulsive disorder, this taxonomy may be more illusory than real because "pure" forms of these disorders are not common, and comorbidity studies (Brown and Barlow 1992) have shown that one type frequently overlaps with another.

CBT has been well established in the effective treatment of anxiety disorders. Supportive psychotherapy, by incorporating CBT principles, also has a role to play, allowing, for example, the phobic patient to slowly address his or her avoidance behavior in the context of the safety of the empathic supportive psychotherapy situation. The patient with posttraumatic stress disorder (PTSD) may also benefit greatly from supportive psychotherapy. PTSD can be thought of as a disorder of memory. Most experiences, pleasurable or painful, fade over time. The patient with PTSD remains bound to the past traumatic experience, which has not diminished in memory. The traumatized patient often fears reexperiencing the trauma if he or she talks about it in the clinical situation. Supportive psychotherapy can reassure the patient that he or she can explore the past trauma and its impact at the patient's own pace, thus preventing retraumatization. An empathic supportive interest in the patient as a *person*, not a *victim*, shifting the treatment into an examination of the patient's life, history, social supports, and so on, can be highly therapeutic.

Depressive Disorders

Pharmacotherapy and psychotherapy are of roughly equal efficacy in the treatment of mild to moderate depression, and most patients respond best to a combination of medication and psychotherapy. CBT, with its focus on the content of the patient's negative thoughts about the self and core beliefs, has been shown to be highly effective in the treatment of patients with depression. Supportive psychotherapy with the depressed patient incorporates CBT techniques within the overarching context of a positive empathic therapeutic relationship. The supportive psychotherapy of the depressed patient requires considerable activity by the clinician, exploring, in particular, dependent relations with others because the disruption of such a relationship is a common precipitant of depressive symptoms. Presence of suicidal thoughts also must be actively explored. The active discussion of suicidal thoughts aimed at increasing supportive understanding of the patient is often the most effective therapeutic measure against suicidal impulses.

Chronic Psychotic Illnesses

Supportive psychotherapy has an important role to play as an ancillary treatment in chronic psychotic illnesses. Gunderson et al. (1984) demonstrated that patients with schizophrenia had a better outcome when provided with weekly supportive treatment as compared with more intensive expressive psychotherapy. Supportive psychotherapy for patients with schizophrenia should incorporate psychoeducation about the nature of the illness and its treatment. Addressing issues of medication side effects and thus enhancing compliance is an important element of supportive psychotherapy with these patients. An empathic supportive approach to the impact of the illness on the patient's self-esteem and adaptive skills, and addressing deficits in social skills, can be highly therapeutic and lead to improvements in self-esteem (Glynn et al. 2002).

Patients with bipolar disorder can also benefit greatly from supportive psychotherapy. The clinician can provide an observing ego, helping the patient self-monitor his or her affective state and recognize when the appearance of increased irritability, euphoria, sleep disturbance, increased energy, and so on may presage a hypomanic episode and require somatic intervention. The supportive psychotherapist can use psychoeducation concerning the nature of the illness, its biological origins, its fluctuating course, and specific psychopharmacological treatment to help the patient understand his or her disease. Placing the illness empathically in the larger context of the patient's psychological strengths, creativity, personal life history, and personality can enhance his or her self-esteem. Being aware of the danger of suicide with the bipolar patient and monitoring for the presence of suicidal thoughts are important aspects of the supportive psychotherapy with these patients.

Substance Abuse

A combination of counseling and psychotherapy is central to the effective treatment of addiction disorders. Counseling focuses on the immediate external problems of the substance abuser and provides support, monitors behavior, encourages abstinence, and addresses concrete real-life issues such as job placement, housing, and so on. A positive therapeutic alliance is at the core of effective psychotherapeutic treatment of substance abuse. Mercer et al. (2004) have perceptively noted that

> to promote a positive therapeutic alliance, therapists should refrain from being judgmental and may occasionally need to extend themselves more with addicted patients than with persons who have other types of psychiatric disorders. The dependence needs of addicted patients often express themselves in the therapist–patient relationship, and occasional appropriate concrete, supportive responses can be useful especially in the early phases of treatment. (p. 381)

Hence, supportive psychotherapy, with its more activist approach than expressive psychotherapy and its focus on bolstering a positive therapeutic alliance, has a major role to play in the treatment of the substance abuse patient.

Motivational interviewing (Rollnick and Miller 1995) as a directive intervention that aids the substance abuse patient in addressing his or her ambivalence about giving up drugs has also been shown to be useful in treatment.

Motivational interviewing should be incorporated as a central element of the supportive psychotherapy of the substance abuse patient. In motivational interviewing, the therapist is highly empathic, closely examines the patient's ambivalence, and places the onus on the patient to initiate change. Miller et al. (1993) demonstrated that high levels of therapist confrontations were associated with poorer outcomes. Carroll et al. (2004) note that

> confrontation is regarded as counterproductive because it leads to a defensive movement away from change on the part of the patient. Although the therapist may not always agree with the patient, the therapist accepts the patient's position and perspective. The therapist is not globally neutral, given that education is sometimes provided and advice is given if specifically requested, but he or she is neutral about what the patient does with this education or advice. The core principles of motivational interviewing include expression of empathy, development of discrepancy, avoidance of argument, patience in the face of resistance, and support of self-efficacy—the important assumption is made that ambivalence and fluctuating motivations define substance abuse recovery and need to be explored rather than harshly confronted. (pp. 371–372)

The incidence of comorbidity of substance abuse and severe psychiatric illness is considerable. Supportive psychotherapy is highly indicated for patients' with co-occurring substance abuse and severe mental illness. The supportive psychotherapy for these dual-diagnosis patients synthesizes the techniques that are used for each disorder. Maintaining a positive therapeutic alliance, aiding medication compliance, improving adaptive skills, and closely monitoring for the onset of relapse are all central to their supportive psychotherapy with these patients.

Conclusion

Both the empirical studies that exist and a welter of anecdotal clinical reports suggest that supportive psychotherapy can be applied usefully to a wide variety of psychiatric and medical conditions. The central technical components of effective supportive psychotherapy have been adumbrated by Winston et al. (2004). I would add to their list the importance in the supportive psychotherapeutic situation of the therapist's empathic-introspective stance advocated by Kohut (1971, 1977). The effective use of empathy immeasurably aids the maintenance of the therapeutic alliance and facilitates the internalization by the patient of positive transference aspects of the interactive process of therapy, thus facilitating change and growth (Loewald 1980).

Two and a half millennia ago, Plato recognized the healing power of what we would come to call supportive psychotherapy when he wrote:

If the head and body are to be well you must begin by curing the soul—that is the first essential thing. And the cure of the soul, my dear youth, has to be effected by the use of certain charms, and these charms are fair words, and by them temperance is implanted in the soul, and where temperance comes and stays, then health is speedily imparted, not only to the head but to the whole body. (Plato 1987, p. 181)

Key Points

- Extant studies of the efficacy of supportive psychotherapy indicate that it is a potent and effective treatment in a variety of psychiatric disorders. More systematic empirical studies need to be conducted.

- Supportive psychotherapy can be usefully applied in the treatment of severe personality disorders, chronic psychotic illnesses, anxiety and depressive disorders, and substance abuse.

- Maintaining the positive transference, and thus enhancing the therapeutic alliance, combined with a high degree of therapist empathy for the patient is a key element in what makes supportive psychotherapy work.

References

American Psychiatric Association: Diagnostic and Statistical Manual of Mental Disorders, 4th Edition, Text Revision. Washington, DC, American Psychiatric Association, 2000

Bateman AW, Fonagy P: Effectiveness of psychotherapy treatment of personality disorder. Br J Psychiatry 177:138–143, 2000

Brown TA, Barlow DH: Comorbidity among anxiety disorders: implications for treatment and DSM-IV. J Consult Clin Psychol 60:835–844, 1992

Buckley PJ: Supportive psychotherapy: a neglected treatment. Psychiatr Ann 16:515–521, 1986

Carroll KM, Ball SA, Martino S: Cognitive, behavioral and motivational therapies, in The American Psychiatric Publishing Textbook of Substance Abuse Treatment, 3rd Edition. Edited by Galanter M, Kleber HD. Washington, DC, American Psychiatric Publishing, 2004, pp 365–376

Clarkin JF, Levy KN, Lenzenweger MF, et al: Evaluating three treatments for borderline personality disorder: a multiwave study. Am J Psychiatry 164:922–928, 2007

Conte HR: Review of research in supportive psychotherapy: an update. Am J Psychother 48:494–504, 1994

Crits-Christoph P, Siqueland L, Blaine J, et al: The National Institute on Drug Abuse Collaborative Cocaine Treatment Study: rationale and methods. Arch Gen Psychiatry 54:721–726, 1997

de Jonghe F, Rijnierse P, Janssen R: The role of support in psychoanalysis. J Am Psychoanal Assoc 40:475–499, 1992

Elkin I: The NIMH Treatment of Depression Collaborative Research Program: where we began and where we are, in Handbook of Psychotherapy and Behavioral Change. Edited by Bergin AE, Garfield SL. New York, Wiley, 1994, pp 114–139

Elkin I, Shea MT, Watkins JT, et al: National Institute of Mental Health Treatment of Depression Collaborative Research Program: general effectiveness of treatments. Arch Gen Psychiatry 46:971–982, 1989

Gill MM: Psychoanalysis and exploratory psychotherapy. J Am Psychoanal Assoc 2:771–797, 1954

Glynn SM, Marder SR, Liberman RP, et al: Supplementing clinic-based skills training with manual-based community support sessions: effects on social adjustment of patients with schizophrenia. Am J Psychiatry 159:829–837, 2002

Gunderson JG, Frank AF, Katz HM, et al: Effects of psychotherapy in schizophrenia, 11: comparative outcome of two forms of treatment. Schizophr Bull 10: 564–598, 1984

Hellerstein DJ, Rosenthal RN, Pinsker H, et al: A randomized prospective study comparing supportive and dynamic therapies: outcome and alliance. J Psychother Pract Res 7:261–271, 1998

Hogarty GE, Kornblith SJ, Greenwald D, et al: Three-year trials of personal therapy among schizophrenic patients living with or independent of family, I: description of study and effects on relapse rates. Am J Psychiatry 154:1504–1513, 1997

Imber SD, Pilkonis PA, Sotsky SM, et al: Mode-specific effects among three treatments for depression. J Consult Clin Psychol 58:352–359, 1990

Klein DF, Zitrin CM, Woerner MG, et al: Treatment of phobias, II: behavior therapy and supportive psychotherapy: are there any specific ingredients? Arch Gen Psychiatry 40:139–145, 1983

Kohut H: The Analysis of the Self. New York, International Universities Press, 1971

Kohut H: The Restoration of the Self. New York, International Universities Press, 1977

Loewald HW: On the therapeutic action of psychoanalysis, in Papers on Psychoanalysis. New Haven, CT, Yale University Press, 1980

Luborsky L, McLellan AT, Woody GE, et al: Therapist success and its determinants. Arch Gen Psychiatry 82:602–611, 1985

Maina G, Forner F, Bogetto F: Randomized controlled trial comparing brief dynamic and supportive therapy with waiting list conditions in minor depressive disorders. Psychother Psychosom 74:43–50, 2005

Mercer D, Woody GE, Luborsky L: Individual psychotherapy, in The American Psychiatric Publishing Textbook of Substance Abuse Treatment, 3rd Edition. Edited by Galanter M, Kleber HD. Washington, DC, American Psychiatric Publishing, 2004, pp 377–389

Miller WR, Benefield RG, Jenigan JS: Enhancing motivation for change in problem drinking: a controlled comparison of two therapist styles. J Consult Clin Psychol 61:455–461, 1993

Mumford E, Schlesinger HJ, Glass CV: The effects of psychological intervention on recovery from surgery and heart attacks: an analysis of the literature. Am J Public Health 72:141–151, 1982

Perry JC, Banon E, Ianni F: Effectiveness of psychotherapy for personality disorders. Am J Psychiatry 156:1312–1321, 1999

Piper WE, Joyce AS, McCallum M, et al: Interpretive and supportive forms of psychotherapy and patient personality variables. J Consult Clin Psychol 66:558–567, 1998

Plato: Charmides, in Early Socratic Dialogues. Translated by Watt D. New York, Penguin Books, 1987, p 181

Renaud J, Brent DA, Baugher MMA, et al: Rapid response to psychosocial treatment for adolescent depression: a two-year follow up. J Am Acad Child Adolesc Psychiatry 37:1184–1190, 1998

Rollnick S, Miller WR: What is motivational interviewing? Behavioral and Cognitive Psychotherapy 23:325–334, 1995

Rosenbaum B, Valbak K, Harder S, et al: The Danish National Schizophrenia Project: prospective, comparative longitudinal treatment study of first-episode psychosis. Br J Psychiatry 186:394–399, 2005

Shear MK, Pilkonis PA, Cloitre M, et al: Cognitive behavioral treatment compared with nonprescriptive treatment of panic disorder. Arch Gen Psychiatry 51:395–401, 1994

Shear MK, Houck P, Greeno C, et al: Emotion-focused psychotherapy for patients with panic disorder. Am J Psychiatry 158:1993–1998, 2001

Sjodin L, Svedland J, Otlosson JO, et al: Controlled study of psychotherapy in chronic peptic ulcer disease. Psychosomatics 27:187–197, 1986

Stanton AH, Gunderson JG, Knapp PH, et al: Effects of psychotherapy in schizophrenia, I: design and implementation of a controlled study. Schizophr Bull 10:520–563, 1984

Thompson LW, Gallagher D: Depression and its treatment. Aging 348:14–18, 1985

Waldinger RJ, Gunderson JG: Effective Psychotherapy With Borderline Patients. Washington, DC, American Psychiatric Press, 1989

Wallerstein RS: Forty-Two Lives in Treatment: A Study of Psychoanalysis and Psychotherapy. New York, Guilford, 1986

Wallerstein RS: The psychotherapy research project of the Menninger Foundation: an overview. J Consult Clin Psychol 57:195–205, 1989

Winston A, Rosenthal RN, Pinsker H: Introduction to Supportive Psychotherapy (Core Competencies in Psychotherapy). Washington, DC, American Psychiatric Publishing, 2004

Zitrin CM, Klein DF, Woerner MG, et al: Behavior therapy, supportive psychotherapy, imipramine, and phobias. Arch Gen Psychiatry 35:307–316, 1978

Suggested Readings

Gabbard GO: Psychodynamic Psychiatry in Clinical Practice, 4th Edition. Washington, DC, American Psychiatric Publishing, 2005

MacKinnon RA, Michels R, Buckley PJ: The Psychiatric Interview in Clinical Practice, 2nd Edition. Washington, DC, American Psychiatric Publishing, 2006

Perry S, Cooper AM, Michels R: The psychodynamic formulation: its purpose, structure and clinical application. Am J Psychiatry 144:543–550, 1987

Wallerstein RS: Forty-Two Lives in Treatment: A Study of Psychoanalysis and Psychotherapy. New York, Guilford, 1986

Winston A, Rosenthal RN, Pinsker H: Introduction to Supportive Psychotherapy (Core Competencies in Psychotherapy). Washington, DC, American Psychiatric Publishing, 2004

Chapter 17

Combining Supportive Psychotherapy With Medication

David J. Hellerstein, M.D.

It is commonly believed that optimal outcome of treatment for many psychiatric disorders can be achieved by combining pharmacotherapy and psychotherapy. Supportive psychotherapy (SPT) is most likely the most frequently used modality of psychotherapy in current clinical practice (Tanielian et al. 2001). In the 1998 National Survey of Psychiatric Practice, 36% of patients treated by psychiatrists received supportive psychotherapy versus 19% receiving insight-oriented therapy, 6% receiving cognitive-behavioral therapy (CBT), and 1% receiving psychoanalysis (Tanielian et al. 2001). Recently, the development of competency in SPT has become a requirement of residency training in the United States, and a number of texts about SPT have been published in recent years. Since the introduction of selective serotonin reuptake inhibitors (SSRIs) in the late 1980s, an increasing proportion of psychiatric patients have been treated with pharmacotherapy. From 82% to 90% of patients in psychiatrists' caseloads receive medications (Pincus et al. 1999; Tanielian et al. 2001).

Paradoxically, however, there is a relative lack of research about the effectiveness of combining SPT with pharmacotherapy and an almost entire absence of data on particular supportive therapy approaches or techniques that are the most (or least) effective when combined with pharmacotherapy. This paucity of empirical data no doubt results from a number of factors, including overall low levels of funding for psychotherapy research and the relatively low standing of SPT (as a broad-spectrum, nonspecific treatment approach) when compared with other more targeted psychotherapies such as dialectical behavioral therapy (DBT) (Linehan 1993), CBT (Beck et al. 1979), or interpersonal psychotherapy (IPT) (Weissman and Klerman 1991).

Furthermore, there are relatively few studies of the combination of psychotherapy and pharmacotherapy using any psychotherapy approach—and the few existing studies generally provide data on narrowly focused treatments such as CBT or IPT. In addition, when SPT has been studied in psychotherapy research, it has often been studied as a control or comparison treatment against other, more specific and presumably more active approaches, which may have more rigorous therapist training, greater therapeutic zeal, and even a larger number of therapy hours. Thus, the quality of the few existing data about SPT is often suspect. Nevertheless, there has been a growing literature suggesting that SPT is an active and efficacious treatment approach that often achieves lasting and significant results (Buckley 1986; Hellerstein et al. 1995, 1998; Maina et al. 2005; Novalis et al. 1993; Pinsker 1997; Rosenthal et al. 1999; Wallerstein 1989). However, as mentioned, the paucity of research on the combination of SPT and pharmacotherapy does not permit definitive conclusions.

The clinical literature on SPT also has relatively few discussions on how it can be combined with pharmacotherapy. Despite the growing number of SPT texts and manuals, they relatively rarely provide extensive discussions on the best ways of combining SPT and pharmacotherapy. Such discussions are absent from many SPT texts: both older ones, including those by Luborsky (1984) and Rockland (1989), and newer ones, including those by Pinsker (1997) and Winston et al. (2004), provide only limited guidance, although Novalis et al. (1993) do devote a chapter to this topic. Texts and reviews of the combination of psychopharmacology and psychotherapy (Beck et al. 1979; Chiles et al. 1991; Gabbard and Kay 2001; Gitlin 1996; Hersen 1986; Hyland 1991; Kahn 1990; Klerman 1991; Krupnick et al. 1996; Lader and Bond 1998; Ostow 1962; Preskorn 2006; Winston and Winston 2002) describe numerous issues related to combining these modalities that are applicable to many different psychotherapeutic approaches, including SPT.

The goal of this chapter is to describe major issues in the combination of SPT and pharmacotherapy. I briefly review the literature for SPT, both broadly and narrowly defined; define these two modalities; and differentiate SPT from the supportive relationship required for good clinical psychopharmacological management. I then summarize the possible advantages (and disadvantages) of combined SPT and pharmacotherapy treatment. Finally, I discuss particular SPT approaches and provide examples of the ways in which they may be combined with pharmacotherapy over the course of treatment. Because of the limited quantitative data on combined SPT and pharmacotherapy, the scientific literature will be cited where relevant, but it cannot currently be used as a reliable guide to therapeutic approaches. We are a long way from being able to provide detailed evidence-based practice guidelines for combining SPT with pharmacotherapy.

Theoretical Rationale

There are a number of reasons, both implicit and explicit, why SPT may have particular benefit in combination with psychopharmacology. Particularly since the introduction of the SSRIs in the late 1980s, a growing percentage of psychiatric patients have received medications in a wide range of settings, often for many years. However, medication treatment may often reach a stage of diminishing returns. After the major symptoms of Axis I disorders have responded to treatment, patients may continue to have significant impairment, resulting from a number of causes. Some residual symptoms of Axis I disorders may not respond well to pharmacotherapy yet may increase the risk of relapse. Also, many patients have significant comorbidities (including Axis I substance abuse problems, Axis II personality disorder diagnoses, and Axis III medical problems) for which psychotropic medication does not provide significant relief. Adverse life circumstances (e.g., traumas, losses) or long-standing coping styles may lead to continued impairment despite significant relief of depression, anxiety, or other Axis I symptoms. Alternatively, a robust response to psychotropic medication may enable patients who were previously preoccupied by severe and/or chronic symptoms to begin to address significant interpersonal and psychological issues: patients with prolonged remission (see Markowitz's [1993] discussion of "postdysthymic" patients) uniquely may be ready to benefit from psychotherapy.

These rationales (e.g., of the benefits of adjunctive psychotherapy in pharmacologically treated patients) could justify the use of a variety of psychotherapy approaches, including psychodynamic therapy, CBT, IPT, and others, not only SPT. However, there are particular reasons why SPT may be frequently the psychotherapy of choice (Hellerstein et al. 1994) for combining with medication. SPT is a broad-spectrum treatment approach that may be used for an extremely wide range of patient populations and in many settings. Numerous meta-analyses of the efficacy of psychotherapy have demonstrated the overall benefit of psychotherapy, the importance of development of a good therapeutic alliance, and the lack of superiority of one particular form of psychotherapy over another in many disorders (Smith and Glass 1977). (Exceptions are the anxiety disorders panic disorder, phobias, and posttraumatic stress disorder, in which evidence favors CBT, and obsessive-compulsive disorder, in which evidence favors exposure and response prevention.) Also, unlike some forms of psychodynamic psychotherapy, SPT does not require patients to have a high level of motivation or psychological-mindedness. SPT also does not require homework exercises or other types of out-of-session patient-initiated activities that are often an essential component of CBT. These findings and characteristics of SPT have been used to justify the use of SPT as the "default" psychotherapy model (Hellerstein et al. 1994).

On a practical level, SPT approaches are consistent with the methods of case management and crisis management, and SPT therapists often "switch gears" between psychotherapy and case management depending on a patient's condition. SPT is also philosophically compatible with the use of psychotropic medication. In addition, the SPT relationship is more of a socially "real" relationship than traditional psychoanalytic relationships and thus may be less vulnerable to possible role confusion between psychotherapist and psychopharmacologist than some schools of psychodynamic psychotherapy. SPT has been described by some authors (Novalis et al. 1993; Pinsker 1997) as an atheoretical treatment model, which may make it relatively appealing for psychiatrists from a wide range of theoretical backgrounds, including interpersonal, cognitive-behavioral, learning theory, and psychodynamic backgrounds. (It is worth noting however that other authors [Kernberg 1982; Rockland 1989; Winston et al. 2004] have written of psychodynamic supportive therapy as a treatment falling within psychodynamic models.) Finally, the addition of a required competency in SPT during psychiatry residency training is likely to ensure a growing cadre of psychiatrists comfortable with its use.

Research on the Combination of Supportive Psychotherapy and Pharmacotherapy

What exactly is (or is not) SPT? A narrow definition of SPT would include only treatments specifically defined as SPT. A broader definition would include psychotherapies that primarily use techniques and approaches within the SPT umbrella (Novalis et al. 1993; Pinsker 1997; Winston et al. 2004). These treatments could include motivational enhancement therapy (Miller et al. 1994), IPT (Markowitz and Weissman 2004; Weissman and Klerman 1991), positive psychology treatments (Seligman 2002), and possibly other approaches such as problem-solving treatment (Mynors-Wallis et al. 2000), an approach that uses a combination of supportive and behavioral approaches. Such broadly defined SPTs primarily may use techniques that are subsets of the broader SPT armamentarium as defined by Pinsker, Novalis, and others, or they may include primarily SPT techniques but also incorporate some approaches outside the customary range of SPT approaches. Such a broad definition of SPT generally would exclude studies of behavior therapy, DBT, or classical psychoanalysis (although these all contain some "supportive" elements), but might include variants of CBT such as the Cognitive-Behavioral Analysis System of Psychotherapy (CBASP; Keller et al. 2000), which combines aspects of CBT and IPT and variants of expressive therapy such as Luborsky's (1984) supportive-expressive therapy. It is beyond the scope of this chapter to review the efficacy of such broadly defined supportive therapies; however, it is worth stating that each of these approaches has been shown to be effective for treatment of many disorders, including depression, anxiety disorders, and substance use disorders. Winston and Winston (2002) have reviewed the efficacy of combined psychotherapy and pharmacotherapy and conclude that there is evidence for their benefit in schizophrenia, bipolar disorder, anxiety disorders, some types of depression, and other conditions. Many of the therapies used in such studies would fit within the broader rubric of SPT.

Thus, there are, strictly speaking, few studies of SPT and pharmacotherapy. Viewed more broadly, the literature on SPT and pharmacotherapy would include a wider range of studies, as noted. The literature review for combined treatments in major depression in the following subsection illustrates many of the issues that are relevant to combined treatment using SPT.

Combined Treatment for Major Depression

In a review of antidepressants and psychotherapy, Frank et al. (2005) evaluated the use of combination treatments, both from the initiation of treatment and in various combinations, including psychotherapy added to incompletely effective pharmacotherapy, and pharmacotherapy added to an incompletely effective psychotherapy. They concluded that "the number of research reports available to address these questions is small relative to their importance for clinical practice" (p. 263).

Thase (1999) argues that the combination of psychotherapy and pharmacology in treatment of major depression may be of advantage in "treatment of patients with more complex depressive disorders, including characteristics such as comorbidity, chronicity, treatment resistance, episodicity, and severity" (p. 333). In contrast, milder acute depressions may not warrant the routine use of combined treatment. Jindal and Thase (2003) reviewed the efficacy of integrated psychotherapy and pharmacotherapy for patients with mood disorders in light of new understandings about clinical trial design and concluded that there is a "systematic underestimation of the benefits of combined treatments for certain subgroups of patients" (p. 1484). Thase and Jindal (2004; as discussed in Piper 2004) expanded this review to other Axis I disorders and have suggested that evidence supports the superiority of combined pharmacotherapy and psychotherapy, not only for recurrent and severe major depression but also for schizophrenia, obsessive-compulsive disorder, and bipolar affective disorder.

In a meta-analysis, Friedman et al. (2004) reviewed combined psychotherapy and pharmacotherapy for the treatment of major depressive disorder. They concluded that "combined treatment is associated with a small improvement in efficacy" across studies and that benefit was most notable for patients with chronic or severe depression.

Pampallona et al. (2004) reviewed 16 studies of combined versus pharmacological treatment of depression. Psychotherapy approaches included social skills training, CBT, cognitive therapy, group cognitive therapy, IPT, problem-solving treatment, psychodynamic psychotherapy, psychodynamic SPT, and group cognitive-interpersonal psychotherapy. They found that combined treatment had an overall odds ratio of 1.86 for treatment response, although counter to expectation combined treatment did not lead to lower drop-out rates. In addition, studies greater than 12 weeks in length showed a significant benefit for combined treatment over medication treatment alone.

Combined Treatment With Other Forms of Supportive Psychotherapy

As noted previously, there are very few studies specifically studying the effect of combined treatment with a narrowly defined SPT and pharmacotherapy versus single treatments. de Jonghe et al. (2001, 2004) have published two studies on combining medication and "short psychodynamic supportive psychotherapy"—a treatment consistent with Werman's (1984) SPT and Rockland's (1989) psychodynamically oriented supportive therapy—for treatment of major depression. The first study compared medication alone ($n = 84$ subjects) versus medication combined with psychotherapy ($n = 83$ subjects) and found a significantly better response rate for combined treatment over a 6-month period, with a 59.2% response rate in combined treatment versus 40.7% in medication treatment alone.

Interestingly, in a secondary analysis of de Jonghe et al.'s 2001 study, Kool et al. (2003) reported that combined psychodynamic SPT and medication was more efficacious than medication alone for depressed patients with comorbid personality disorders but not for those without personality disorders. This finding is notable in view of the extensive literature that suggests that depressed patients with comorbid personality disorders have worse outcome with pharmacotherapy than those without personality disorders (Newton-Howes et al. 2006).

In their second study, de Jonghe et al. (2004) studied the effectiveness of psychotherapy alone and in combination with pharmacotherapy for the treatment of depression in ambulatory patients with mild or moderate DSM-IV diagnosed major depression. They reported on 208 participants, of whom 107 were assigned to psychotherapy and 101 to combined treatment, and found that clinicians and independent observers were not able to discern additive benefits for combined treatment, although patients experienced combined treatment as more efficacious. Efficacy on various measures ranged from 32% to 69% for psychotherapy alone versus 42%–79% with combined treatment.

Of note, neither of de Jonghe's studies contains randomization to placebo versus medication, and neither compares SPT with another psychotherapy approach. Thus, it is not possible to determine the potential role of placebo response or nonspecific treatment effects. (It is also worth noting that there have been no studies comparing psychodynamically oriented SPT with atheoretical SPT, with or without medication.) The much-cited CBASP study (Keller et al. 2000) of chronic major depression treated with nefazodone, CBASP, or combined nefazodone and CBASP, which found a higher rate of response to combined treatment, also lacked such comparison groups. (As mentioned previously, CBASP, as a treatment combining CBT and IPT treatment approaches, may conceivably be considered to be within the broader construct of SPTs, although it clearly falls within the construct of CPT as well.)

Stanley (2006) conducted a medication versus psychotherapy efficacy study among 75 patients with borderline personality disorder who had a history of recent self-injurious or suicidal behavior. Her four-cell study compared 1-year outpatient treatments with DBT versus SPT (based on models of Novalis [Novalis et al. 1993] and Pinsker [1997] and adapted for borderline personality disorder) and fluoxetine versus placebo. Results have not been published to date, although descriptions of the SPT approach have been published (Aviram et al. 2004; Hellerstein et al. 2004).

Key Definitions

Supportive Psychotherapy

Supportive psychotherapy has been defined in various ways by different authors, including Kernberg (1982), Luborsky (1984), Rockland (1989),

Novalis (Novalis et al. 1993), Pinsker (1997), and others. Some authors have consistently defined SPT as a treatment with minimal goals and only suitable for very impaired patients. Karasu (2005), for instance, defines SPT as "the creation of a therapeutic relationship as a temporary buttress or bridge for the deficient patient." However, our view is that this definition more closely approximates what we would call the supportive relationship. Earlier authors such as Rockland and Kernberg often defined SPT within a psychoanalytic framework, but more recently authors (Novalis et al. 1993; Pinsker 1997) often define SPT without specific reference to psychodynamic psychotherapy, in a way that may be characterized as atheoretical.

In Pinsker's (1997) model, SPT is defined as an active verbal treatment involving a conversational style that has the goals of maintaining or improving self-esteem, adaptive skills, and psychological functioning. It commonly uses techniques, including clarification, suggestions, praise, reassurance, cognitive restructuring, normalization, and rehearsal and anticipation. In Novalis et al.'s (1993) model, SPT is defined as a form of psychotherapy that uses empirically based techniques to achieve several aims: promoting a supportive patient–therapist relationship; enhancing the patient's strengths, coping skills, and ability to use environmental supports; reducing distress and behavioral dysfunction; achieving independence from psychiatric illness; and maximizing autonomy for the patient's treatment decisions. Novalis and Pinsker use a similar range of techniques (see Table 17–1). In both models, relationships and patients' emotional responses and/or behavior are examined, with the goal of improving psychosocial functioning. These new models of SPT as a change- and improvement-oriented treatment are in marked contrast to those writers (e.g., Karasu 2005) who have viewed SPT as a treatment that is best suited to low-functioning patients and that should have the limited goal of stabilization or prevention of decompensation.

In both Pinsker and Novalis's models, SPT therapists respect adaptive defenses or coping mechanisms. The "real" relationship rather than the transference is emphasized, although the therapist monitors the status of the therapeutic alliance and may make interpretations or otherwise address the therapeutic relationship if the treatment is threatened. There is no effort to enhance the development of what a psychodynamic therapist might call a *transference* (or what other schools might call an intense emotional relationship and dependency on the therapist)—in fact, transference is avoided by trying to decrease the patient's in-session anxiety and to minimize regression. The SPT therapeutic relationship is one in which the therapist maintains a conversational style, rather than allowing prolonged silences, and demonstrates involvement, empathy, nonjudgmental acceptance, and an appropriate level of interest in the patient and his or her life. The SPT therapist is not as concerned about anonymity as a psychodynamic therapist might be. He or she might respond briefly to direct questions by the patient and may otherwise use judicious self-disclosure.

The goals of SPT commonly are set in a process of discussion between therapist and patient and may vary over the course of treatment. Goal setting in SPT is a collaborative process based on both the patient's and the clinician's assessment of significant life issues. SPT is primarily present- and future-focused, although it does not ignore past issues. Past experiences are explored in the context of present life issues rather than the present being used as a means of entry to exploring past issues.

Pharmacotherapy

Pharmacotherapy can be defined as the use of medications to treat illness, disorders, or symptoms. For the purposes of this chapter, we restrict discussions to psychopharmacotherapy, or the use of psychotropic somatic treatments to treat mental illnesses, disorders, or symptoms. Therapeutic interventions in pharmacotherapy include not only medication but also other somatic treatments such as electroconvulsive treatment, magnetic stimulation treatment, and phototherapy, as well as nonprescription additives such as St. John's wort or omega-3 fatty acids. Education about illness, or psychoeducation in psychiatric illnesses, is also a key component of pharmacotherapy. Pharmacotherapy is provided within a context of competent clinical management, which generally follows a medical model and which assumes the development and maintenance of what I describe later in this chapter as a supportive relationship. A good doctor–patient relationship is obviously key to the success of pharmacotherapy.

The goals of pharmacotherapy generally are framed by the definition of the illness, disorder, or condition being treated, but the primary goal is to alleviate symptoms. Pharmacotherapy cannot begin until there is clarification of the particular type or types of disorder that a patient has, the primary symptoms of that disorder, and the severity and impact of the symptoms on a patient's life. The prior course of illnesses, including duration of symptoms and prior episodes, must be defined, and family history and prior treatment response are obtained as well. Initial goals for treatment of Axis I disorders often include achieving a therapeutic response, which is defined differently for various disorders (commonly, a 50% or more decrease in severity of symptoms of depression or panic disorder, or a 20% or more decrease in symptoms in more refractory conditions such as obsessive-compulsive disorder or schizophrenia). Symptoms are commonly defined on the basis of DSM-IV-TR diagnoses, and their severity is assessed by use of diagnostic criteria or rating scales such as the Hamilton Rating Scale for

TABLE 17-1. Basic features of supportive psychotherapy for patients with depression

Conceptual basis and goals

> Ameliorate symptoms and maintain, restore, or improve self-esteem, adaptive skills, and psychological functioning.
>
> Examine relationships and patients' emotional responses and/or behavior.
>
> Respect adaptive defenses.
>
> Emphasize real relationship.
>
> Maximize treatment autonomy and independence from psychiatric disorder.

Therapeutic relationship

> Be conversationally responsive.
>
> Demonstrate involvement, empathy, nonjudgmental acceptance, interest, and liking.
>
> Collaborate with patient in goal setting.
>
> Regulate distance.
>
> Use judicious self-disclosure.
>
> Be aware of transference, but only make interpretations when treatment is threatened.

Interventions

> Clarification
>
> Suggestion
>
> Advice, guidance, and education
>
> Limit setting
>
> Reframing
>
> Rationalization
>
> Encouragement
>
> Modeling
>
> Rehearsal and anticipation
>
> Cognitive restructuring

TABLE 17–1.　Basic features of supportive psychotherapy for patients with depression *(continued)*

Application to depression

　Discuss in clear terms the expectations for supportive psychotherapy, and clarify the goals of therapy.

　Make early (and ongoing) efforts to develop therapeutic alliance.

　Provide psychoeducation about depression and likely outcomes of treatment, starting from initiation of treatment and continuing throughout course of treatment.

　Make an ongoing effort to limit self-destructive behavior and to assess risk of suicide.

　Support patient's efforts to deal with symptoms of depression, to reregulate circadian rhythms, and to maximize daily functioning.

　Address situations (interpersonal, behavioral, intrapsychic) that predispose to or maintain depression.

　Ensure that treatment progresses from an early focus on acute depressive state (including risk of self-injury); to attaining and maintaining remission from depression; to working toward recovery from depression, including enhancing interpersonal and social skills and problem-solving abilities.

　Work to prevent recurrence of depression and development of chronicity.

Source.　Adapted from Aviram et al. 2004; Hellerstein 2008; Novalis et al. 1993; Pinsker 1997.

Depression or the Brief Psychiatric Rating Scale. Later in treatment, treatment goals may be more ambitious and often include remission (symptoms of the disorder are absent) and even recovery (the patient has returned to a normal level of psychosocial functioning).

　The therapeutic interactional style in pharmacotherapy follows the venerable rituals of the physician visit, in which patients commonly report symptoms and side effects in detail and also describe significant life events and concurrent illnesses. In pharmacotherapy, the physician has traditionally been viewed as the expert on treatment of particular illnesses, and the patient as a subject to be treated, although in recent decades the patient has increasingly become a partner in care who may obtain information about disorders from a variety of sources, including the Internet, and who may be engaged to monitor and manage his or her disorder, with a variety of behavioral changes, including diet and exercise. Nevertheless, the roles of pharmacologist and patient follow a traditional medical model, in which the patient's involvement in treatment may be measured by "compliance" or "adherence" to medication versus "noncompliance." Visits are brief, as little as 5–10 minutes, compared with 45- or 50-minute psychotherapy sessions, and are often highly structured, with little time to discuss anything other than symptoms, side effects, and the need for prescription refills or dosage adjustments. In pharmacotherapy, medication may be seen as the primary treatment of the disorder and even as the only active treatment.

Supportive Relationship

The supportive relationship is a type of relationship that underlies physician–patient interactions in all medical specialties, although it is often implicit rather than explicit. It is hardly limited to medical settings but is seen in all helping professions, in educational processes, and throughout society. Good outcome in medical care commonly is believed to require a good doctor–patient relationship, if nothing else to ensure adherence to prescribed treatment and a willingness to keep scheduled appointments. Pharmacotherapy cannot proceed in a reliable fashion without the development of an adequate supportive relationship. For that matter, neither can SPT. The supportive relationship of pharmacotherapy (SR-PMT) shares many key components with SPT (see Table 17–2), but there are also some key differences.

Both SR-PMT and SPT use techniques such as normalization, appropriate rationalization, education, anticipatory guidance, and reframing. However, discussions of psychological responses to life stressors are an essential part of SPT but may only infrequently occur in an SR-PMT. The therapeutic alliance is continually monitored and managed in SPT and is a key component of SPT treatment but is only addressed to a limited degree in the SR-PMT. SPT obviously requires that the patient and clinician believe that they are in an ongoing process of psychotherapy, whereas they do not believe such a process is ongoing in an SR-PMT, although there may be occasional psychotherapeutic moments. Clinical visits in SPT will generally be more regular and longer than those for medication management. Overall, SPT contains numerous components and approaches that are not regularly present in an SR-PMT. In clinical practice, it is possible that boundaries between an SR-PMT and SPT may at times be blurred, especially because they share many common components. However, because the goals of SPT are significantly different from the goals of an SR-PMT, it appears to be sensible for clinicians to decide whether they are providing SPT to a patient and for the patient to know whether he or she is making a commitment to a formal course of SPT.

Another shared characteristic for SPT and an SR-PMT is the traditional assumption that anyone can do it. Whereas psychiatric training has traditionally provided extensive training in psychodynamic psychotherapy and the technical aspects of psychopharmacology, until recently there was minimal training in SPT. Similarly, it is only recently that medical schools in the United States have devoted attention to the development of competency in the doctor–patient relationship. Furthermore, because SPT and pharmacotherapy are often provided by contemporary psychiatrists, either concurrently or in split treatment, it makes sense for psychiatrists in training to be assessed for their competency in combining SPT with medication treatment.

Benefits and Risks of Combining Supportive Psychotherapy and Pharmacotherapy

Possible Efficacy

To summarize findings from the previous literature review: combined treatments may be particularly effective in more severe, chronic, and highly comorbid disorders. Whereas specific benefits may be obtained by combining focused treatments like CBT or DBT with pharmacotherapy in many disorders, the therapeutic superiority of such focused psychotherapy approaches has been demonstrated only in limited cases, generally in efficacy studies with diagnostically purified treatment samples in academic settings. There is a paucity of effectiveness studies of such treatment approaches with broadly based community samples, which may include more varied populations with higher rates of comorbidities, more socioeconomic and cultural variability, and more active psychosocial and health issues. Thus, in view of the limited research findings, there is a strong rationale for using SPT as the psychotherapy for combined treatments in many cases, if only because of its socially comfortable conversational style, broad applicability, relative simplicity, and flexibility.

Combined SPT and pharmacotherapy could possibly lead to better outcome in a variety of ways—for Axis I disorders and for Axis II, Axis III, and other comorbidities—and to improved psychosocial functioning and/or interpersonal relationships. It is possible, although not certain, that combining SPT with pharmacotherapy might lead to better therapeutic alliance/relationships, especially for patients with comorbid personality disorders. It is also possible that retention in treatment might be improved with better medication compliance or adherence as a result of concurrent psychotherapy, although currently there are no definitive data to support this. It has been reported that patients have growing dissatisfaction with 5- to 10-minute psychiatric medication check visits (Morgan 1999).

TABLE 17-2. **Characteristics of the supportive relationship in pharmacotherapy (SR-PMT) compared with supportive psychotherapy**

Item	SR-PMT	Supportive psychotherapy
Empathy	++	++
Reassurance	+	++
Clarification	+	++
Anticipatory guidance	+	++
Normalization	+	++
Reframing	+	++
Limit setting	+	+
Discussion of symptoms and side effects	+++	+
Psychoeducation about disorder	+++	+
Psychoeducation about interpersonal and psychological issues	+	+++
Extensive assessment of psychiatric disorder and related medical conditions	+++	+
Extensive assessment of psychological issues		++
Ongoing detailed discussion of psychological issues		++
Patient and clinician believe they are engaged in ongoing psychotherapy		++
Patient and clinician believe they are engaged in ongoing pharmacotherapy	++	
Clinician is aware of transference/ therapeutic alliance on ongoing basis	+/−	++
Rehearsal and anticipation		++

TABLE 17-2. Characteristics of the supportive relationship in pharmacotherapy (SR-PMT) compared with supportive psychotherapy *(continued)*

Item	SR-PMT	Supportive psychotherapy
Cognitive restructuring	+	++
Appropriate rationalization		++
Examination of relationships and patient's emotional responses and/or behaviors		++
Efforts to limit self-destructive behavior, assessment of suicide risk	++	++
Support patient's efforts to deal with symptoms of disorder	++	++
Systematic attempts to enhance self-esteem, psychological functions, adaptive skills		++
Average duration of sessions	5–25 minutes	30–50 minutes
Average frequency of sessions	Monthly[a]	Weekly[b]
Model of interaction	Physician–patient	Therapist–patient

[a]Range: 1 per week to 1 per 3 months.
[b]Range: 2 per week to 1 per month.

Practical Rationales

In addition to the theoretical reasons why it may be beneficial to combine SPT with pharmacotherapy, there are a number of other practical rationales that may apply over the course of treatment. Many pharmacotherapy patients may need psychotherapy; many if not most psychotherapy patients are treated with SPT—and possibly SPT may be the treatment of choice for many patients. Also, many patients treated with SPT can benefit from pharmacotherapy. From a practical goal of achieving optimal therapeutic outcome, it may be useful, in many cases, to provide patients with both SPT and pharmacotherapy if resources are sufficient. SPT is designed to be an open, flexible treatment approach, with a goal of improvement that allows for and encourages appropriate medication use, in contrast to some traditional psychodynamic approaches, which are concerned with the patients' loss of motivation if their symptoms are relieved too quickly.

Pharmacotherapy may enhance SPT in a number of ways. Symptom control through medication treatment may enable a patient to work productively in psychotherapy. In particular, improving sleep, normalizing mood, and decreasing anxiety may allow the patient to feel calm and more stable. Particular effects of specific medications such as SSRIs and various mood stabilizers may allow for increased resiliency, decreased rejection sensitivity, and decreased mood lability. On a biological level, medications may decrease hyperarousal of hypothalamic-pituitary-adrenal stress response systems as well as decreasing amygdala activation, enhancing adaptive brain plasticity, and even enhancing hippocampal neurogenesis, which has been hypothesized to allow for less black-and-white thinking and more modulated behavioral responses (Viamontes and Beitman 2006a, 2006b). All of these factors may allow patients to work more productively in psychotherapy.

SPT may also enhance pharmacotherapy, particularly in dealing with individuals with comorbid Axis II diagnoses. Behaviors such as avoidance and social isolation, impulsivity, affective instability, dependency in relationships, black-and-white thinking, and unpracticed social skills may make it difficult for them to keep appointments, take medication regularly, and otherwise become engaged in the patient role. Whereas the limited scope of the supportive relationship may make it difficult to address these issues, the conversational dialogues of SPT may engage such patients in a therapeutic process to enable them to benefit from pharmacotherapy.

Possible Risks or Negative Effects

There are possible negative effects of combining SPT and pharmacotherapy. Many of these effects have been described (Marcus 1990) as present for any combined psychotherapy and pharmacotherapy, and others have been described specifically in the context of SPT (Novalis et al. 1993).

Combined treatment may lead to worse compliance among some patients, who may only want one treatment approach (e.g., wanting only medication within a medical model of treatment) and who may resist being in psychotherapy. Engagement in SPT may lead to an increased intensity of the therapeutic relationship and possibly may destabilize some patients. For patients currently engaged in SPT, the recommendation for initiation of pharmacotherapy may be experienced as a rejection or an admission of failure and might theoretically interfere with the therapist–patient relationship (Marcus 1990; Novalis et al. 1993, pp. 295–309). Combined treatment may be too costly for some patients or mental health care systems, especially in situations with limited resources. Also, as mentioned previously, more specific psychotherapy approaches may be more effectively combined with pharmacotherapy than SPT—for instance, CBT or CBASP plus pharmacotherapy might be more effective for treatment of chronic depression than well-performed SPT plus pharmacotherapy.

It is possible that some medication choices might interfere with the gains of SPT: for instance, benzodiazepine use may interfere with incorporation of new memories as patients expand their interpersonal or behavioral repertoires.

Split Versus Unified Treatment

Finally, there is the issue of whether therapy and medication should be provided by the same individual. Either combined or split pharmacotherapy and SPT may be advantageous for some patients and disadvantageous for others (Chiles et al. 1991; Gitlin 1996, pp. 436–442). Gitlin (1996) suggests that split treatment has the advantages of keeping psychotherapy focused on psychotherapy, allowing for different interviewing styles to be used most effectively, permitting better management of overwhelming transferences, and having lower cost. Gitlin also cites disadvantages, including the possibility of fostering resistance, increased difficulty in integrating biological and psychological experiences, and possible communication difficulties, especially around suicide risk. Novalis has suggested that paranoid patients, patients easily overwhelmed by authority, "angry medical patients," and most patients with borderline personality disorder may benefit from split treatment, whereas patients with schizophrenia, patients with a high degree of dependency, and those who need frequent medication changes may benefit from a single therapist/medicator (Novalis et al. 1993, p. 308).

Frame of Treatment

It is important when combining SPT and pharmacotherapy to set a frame for treatment to decide whether a patient in pharmacotherapy is receiving SPT and then to determine frequency and duration of visits. Neither SPT nor pharmacotherapy requires inflexible commitments to frequent ongoing visits, but treatment planning should be within the frame of treatment goals—generally, initial visits will be more frequent and regular for both pharmacotherapy and SPT treatments. Unlike psychodynamic treatments, SPT also allows patients time to work on issues between sessions; the intensity of frequent visits is not a requirement of treatment. Pharmacotherapy also permits flexibility of scheduling but depends on pharmacological stability, symptoms, and side effects. With combined treatment, one issue for each visit becomes whether it is a pharmacotherapy visit, SPT visit, or both. Priority issues may range from practical issues such as refilling prescriptions to therapy-related issues such as current life crises.

Phases of Treatment

Pharmacotherapy and SPT approaches may vary over the course of treatment, as outlined later in this section and illustrated with examples. In early treatment, the phase of initiation of medication treatment and psychotherapy, there is a focus on developing therapeutic relationships and the collaborative development of treatment goals. In the middle phase of treatment, the goals tend to be achieving relief of the major symptoms of a disorder and addressing psychosocial issues. During continuation of treatment, the goals include remission of the disorder and improvement in life functioning.

Early Treatment

Major goals of early treatment include the following:

- Assessment, diagnosis, and formulation
- Crisis management
- Prevention of self-injury and suicide
- Toleration and alleviation of symptoms
- Management of side effects
- Setting of goals for further treatment

Examples of the use of combined pharmacotherapy and SPT in early treatment are presented below.

Ms. A

Ms. A, a 28-year-old woman with a diagnosis of borderline personality disorder and recurrent major depression, had a history of multiple severe suicide attempts. She was treated with an SSRI antidepressant, with a significant response: she reporting feeling euthymic for the first time in her adult life. However, she continued to self-injure, particularly after fights with her boyfriend. Her psychotherapist used SPT techniques to develop a therapeutic alliance with Ms. A, a difficult task given her long history of mistrust of clinicians and an extensive history of physical and sexual abuse. Supportive interventions included many empathic statements, clarifications, and normalizations ("Your rage is totally understandable given your life experiences") but also allowed Ms. A to maintain sufficient distance to avoid feeling overwhelmed. Ms. A's emotional outbursts were consistently put in the context of her being a "person of strong passions" and "a complicated person," and by the use of the techniques of reframing and normalization. The therapist addressed her self-cutting within the context of multiple choices Ms. A had for dealing with her anger: "You can cut yourself and you can go for a walk and you can talk to a friend and you can call me—there are a lot of things you can choose from." Anticipatory guidance was also used when Ms. A was calm and not upset—an approach consistent with Pine's (1984) advice to "strike while the iron is cold": "How might you deal with things the next time you and your boyfriend have a fight?"

Mr. B

Mr. B, an unemployed man in his early 20s with a history of many depressive episodes, had begun drinking alcohol heavily, initially to control his moods but eventually to the extent that his symptoms met the criteria for alcohol dependence as well as major depression. He had never received a therapeutic trial of medication, having prematurely dropped out of treatment. Diagnosis was made of bipolar II disorder, and Mr. B responded well to mood stabilizers. The psychiatrist worked hard to develop a therapeutic alliance with Mr. B in weekly SPT sessions, using empathic responses. The psychiatrist clarified how angry and humiliated Mr. B felt because of his financial dependence on family members, and gradually worked with Mr. B to assess the impact of alcohol on his life. Mr. B agreed to try to discontinue alcohol use, enrolling in a rehabilitation program, and maintained sobriety for a number of months, then abruptly stopped antidepressant medication and relapsed into both depression and alcohol use.

Mr. B's psychiatrist worked to manage the crisis engendered by recurrent depression and alcohol use, reengaging him in weekly supportive therapy sessions, in which it became clear that Mr. B felt "like a total failure" because of his inability to remain sober. His psychiatrist reframed Mr. B's feelings of "being a failure" as "a normal feeling except one that doesn't recognize that you are really succeeding in starting to address these problems." His recurrent alcohol use was normalized in the context of being an understandable "slip" on the road to recovery, and the goals for further treatment were to return to medication treatment and Alcoholics Anonymous meetings, and to try to figure how he could consolidate his gains and then to gradually work on other issues such as financial independence from his family. Discussion focused on anticipatory guidance of how to deal with interactions with family members, which often left him feeling angry and depressed.

Midtreatment

Once patients have responded to treatment, SPT may also enable patients who have benefited from pharmacotherapy to make additional psychological and behavioral changes. Patients who have achieved "response" of major depression or other Axis I disorders, particularly chronic disorders, often have residual impairment. Friedman et al. (1999), in studying chronically depressed patients who had achieved remission following antidepressant treatment, found that only one-quarter had functioning within the normal range on the Social Adjustment Scale. SPT may help medication-responsive patients to decrease avoidance and social isolation and to enhance the development of new skills.

Such psychological and behavioral changes could include

- Adopting healthy behaviors: exercise, diet, medication compliance, decreasing substance abuse.
- Developing interpersonal skills: increasing appropriate risk-taking, increasing assertiveness, practicing new behavioral interactions, working

on modulating interactions with others ("getting what you want and need").

* Addressing residual cognitive and intrapsychic issues, such as low self-esteem, risk averseness, all-or-nothing thinking, and catastrophization.

Anxiety and avoidance can be addressed by means of SPT techniques such as normalization and reframing, given the overall context of medication-induced treatment response: "It's good that you're feeling better. And it's understandable that you spend most of your time in your apartment—that makes sense because during the time you were so depressed it was the only place you felt comfortable. Now it makes sense for you to try to get out more, to take more chances." Residual depressive symptoms and mood instability, especially when they result from interpersonal interactions, can be addressed as well: "Your mood is really a lot more stable now, and you're feeling pretty good. You don't even have as many ups and downs, but you do tend to crash when you encounter setbacks at work, especially after your weekly sales meeting. Let's talk about how you can deal better with your co-workers and boss at these meetings: what might you do next time?"

The following are examples of combined pharmacotherapy and SPT in midtreatment:

Ms. C

Ms. C, a young married woman, presented with depression, temper outbursts, and intrusive obsessive thoughts that verged on paranoia. Her symptoms met the criteria for bipolar II disorder, with a history of recurrent depressive episodes interspersed with clear hypomanic episodes. She responded well to a combination of SSRI medication and lithium, with a notable stabilization of her mood, a significant decrease in intrusive thoughts, and improved work functioning. Concurrent with medication treatment, Ms. C participated in SPT, which focused on helping her to improve adaptive skills (especially at work, where she tended to withdraw rather than address issues with coworkers, or become explosive and angry), psychological functions or defenses (she tended to project her feelings onto others, to deny the existence of problems until they were overwhelming, and to regress into childlike helplessness), and self-esteem (which was worsened by each explosive outburst, and her dependence on her husband). During the many years of Ms. C's illness, her husband had taken over most decision making, because she had felt helpless to participate. As her depression improved, she began to become more assertive about her opinions and preferences, which led to conflicts with her husband. Supportive therapy helped to clarify that many of these issues were important to her and that she should work on trying to find solutions that made sense to both of them. Concurrently, she needed to decide when not to respond reflexively to her feelings of rage, to figure out how she wanted to respond, and then to find a useful way to address the issues that bothered her, whether at home or work. Over the course of many months, she developed new skills in relationships and at work and was able to find a rewarding new job and to move to a new home with her husband.

Ms. D

Ms. D, a clerical worker in her early 60s, had a long history of depressive symptoms, marginal social adjustment, and social isolation. She had been severely abused and neglected as a child and had had few relationships as an adult. She engaged in concurrent weekly SPT and pharmacotherapy. Antidepressant medication successfully put her mood disorder into remission, enabling her to improve her work performance. Over time, it became clear that Ms. D had numerous interests that she had never felt well enough to pursue. She described severe fears around pursuing these interests, fearing that she would become depressed again after doing artwork or if she pursued the development of a small business she had dreamed of for years.

Using SPT techniques, the psychiatrist helped Ms. D to clarify her fears, reframed them as normal in the context of her prior history of abuse, and encouraged her to gradually pursue these interests, first in a limited and tentative way, then taking more risks. Normalization, cognitive restructuring, rehearsal and anticipation, and encouragement were commonly used, and over time Ms. D began to pursue both interests with a significant degree of success, being able to show artwork and to complete a number of business deals. After successes in these areas Ms. D initially had severe depressive reactions, lasting several days, sometimes leading to suicidally depressed mood. Ms. D and her psychiatrist worked on finding ways to ameliorate these reactions, including rationalization, suppression, reaching out to others, and doing things that she enjoyed. Over time, Ms. D's postsuccess depressive reactions appeared to become less severe.

Continuation Treatment

The major goals of the continuation phase (this phase often begins after a year or more of treatment) include

- Enhancing medication response: moving from remission toward recovery
- Preventing relapse, recurrence, and chronicity
- Developing skills and modulating developmental issues
- Helping the patient to "extend himself or herself" (in cases in which extended remission of a disorder has been achieved)
- Helping the patient to tolerate chronic symptoms of chronic, severe, or progressive disorders; realistically optimize adaptation to the disorder; and engage in care issues, including competency and guardianship

Ms. D *(continued)*

Ms. D's major depression remained in remission over several years. Over time, her long-standing social withdrawal emerged as a psychotherapy issue, with Ms. D describing feelings of extreme loneliness and isolation, especially around weekends and holidays. Her supportive psychotherapist encouraged her to reach out to others, and helped Ms. D to address difficult feelings (of rejection, anger, disappointment) that emerged at times. She began working actively to develop an ability to sort out "which relationships are good for you and which ones aren't" (e.g., to avoid dependency on unreliable people and to allow herself to experience the pleasure of mutual, reciprocal friendships). Over time Ms. D became able to develop closer friendships, and she established the first social support system she had had in many years. Several years into combined pharmacotherapy and SPT treatment, Ms. D commented that she felt she had "extended [her]self" over the course of treatment; her therapist complimented her on the aptness of her description, in that she had indeed gone from a life of withdrawal, depression, fearfulness, and avoidance to one of engagement and thoughtful risk taking.

Mr. E

Mr. E was a man in his late 30s who had received a diagnosis of chronic paranoid schizophrenia and was unable to work. He gained nearly 100 pounds after treatment with an atypical antipsychotic medication, which had successfully stabilized his psychotic disorder. He was largely housebound and often fought with his elderly father. Mr. E's psychiatrist worked with Mr. E in intermittent SPT to find activities that he enjoyed and to help him become more adaptive within the limits imposed by his disorder. Mr. E liked to walk around his neighborhood, so his doctor supported this adaptive functioning, as well as the benefits of taking medications, and praised him when he helped his elderly father with household chores. SPT techniques were used to encourage Mr. E to ignore auditory hallucinations and intrusive thoughts, and to focus on being a good son. Overall the treatment was primarily within the supportive relationship of pharmacotherapy, with some SPT techniques, including realistic planning and normalization ("We all have to watch our weight; we have to find ways to exercise more"). Over time, Mr. E lost over 50 pounds and remained psychiatrically stable, with fewer conflicts with his father.

Supportive Psychotherapy Techniques in the Context of Pharmacotherapy

Specific SPT techniques may be particularly useful throughout the course of pharmacotherapy. Some of the most useful of these techniques are presented below in the form of therapist statements (see Table 17–1 for a more extensive listing of SPT techniques).

Reframing

You describe feeling like a "total failure" because it is difficult for you to travel in the city. But it's clear that you are really improving, because a few months ago you had difficulty leaving your apartment, and now the medication has blocked your panic attacks, it's much easier for you to get out. And you are really succeeding in pushing the envelope of where you feel comfortable.

Normalizing

Your feelings are very intense, since you are a very passionate person. Medicine has helped you to bounce back when these feelings overwhelm you, but it still takes you a while to figure out the best way to respond to those feelings. Your gut sense of what to do is sometimes right, and sometimes it gets you in trouble if you don't take a moment to think things through first.

Anticipatory Guidance

It sounds like that was a rough time seeing your family, so that your depressive symptoms even started coming back. It sounds like you might have some thoughts of how you might prepare yourself for the next visit so it won't be so hard on you. We can talk about adjusting medication dosage, but what other options are there?

Confrontation

One question is, Does it make sense pharmacologically to start and stop the antidepressant medication? You feel good one day so you don't take it because that makes you feel healthier and the next day you crash. We've talked about how the blood levels of the medication have to stay stable in order for you to feel good. So we really need to decide if you need medicine or not and then come to a consensus of what is the best way for you to take it. Or if you want to come off medication, we can discuss the best way to do that so you don't get worse.

The Therapeutic Relationship in Concurrent Supportive Psychotherapy and Pharmacotherapy

Clinicians treating patients concurrently in SPT and pharmacotherapy need to be aware of a range of transference and countertransference issues resulting from the complex and at times contradictory relationships between SPT and SR-PMT. Principles of SPT suggest that these issues must be addressed when the frame of the treatment is threatened (e.g., if the patient's medication adherence is affected by feelings toward the doctor). A patient in concurrent treatment who is working on intimacy issues and appears to be developing romantic feelings toward the psychiatrist may raise numerous boundary issues, which need to be addressed. At the other extreme, patients may avoid significant psychotherapy issues by diverting the discussion into technical aspects of pharmacotherapy, rather than discussing interpersonal problems or troubling emotions. Whereas psychodynamic therapists address both positive and negative transference, SPT therapists usually address only the negative transference.

Combining and Phasing Treatments

SPT and medications may be combined in numerous different ways. A full discussion of these is beyond the scope of this chapter, but it is useful for clinicians to actively decide how they are phasing treatments.

Concurrent Treatment

Both SPT and pharmacotherapy can be used concurrently from the start of treatment, which may be especially beneficial for patients with chronic, severe, and/or comorbid disorders.

Augmentation (or Sequencing) of Treatment

Single treatments, whether pharmacotherapy or SPT, can be augmented. Treatment may start with pharmacotherapy, with the goal of symptom response, and SPT may be added at a later date if the patient continues to have significant impairment or life stresses. Also, with severe symptoms, patients may not be able to participate in psychotherapy until symptoms abate. Alternatively, many patients may start treatment with a course of SPT, and pharmacotherapy may be added later.

Switching Treatments

Occasionally, patients may try a course of SPT and then decide to switch to pharmacotherapy, or patients treated with medications may decide to change treatments to psychotherapy. This approach is probably less common with SPT than with more targeted treatments such as CBT, which may focus narrowly on treatment of disorders such as panic disorder or phobias.

Intermittent Use of One or the Other Modality

It is likely that the most common way in which SPT and pharmacotherapy are combined is through intermittent use of one or the other modality. A patient who is in ongoing psychotherapy may require intermittent medication use, or a patient who is receiving pharmacotherapy may require a brief course of SPT.

Mr. F

Mr. F was a 55-year-old lawyer who had had recurrent depression since his early 20s. He was being treated with maintenance pharmacotherapy, which had helped him to remain in a euthymic state over many years. Periodically Mr. F would enter several-month courses of weekly psychotherapy: during a time of job transition, several years later when he was having marital and family problems, and a decade later when his mother was undergoing serious medical procedures. Each time he worked productively on these psychotherapy issues and then returned to monthly or bimonthly brief medication visits.

In each phase in which the patient enters SPT, there is a similar process of setting goals, deciding on the frame of treatment, evaluating the patient's progress over time, and then reviewing the treatment once major goals have been achieved.

Incorporating Other Treatment Approaches

On both a theoretical and practical basis, SPT is a flexible psychotherapy approach that enables clinicians to incorporate techniques and interventions derived from other psychotherapies. As noted by Novalis et al. (1993, p. 20), SPT can be seen as an overarching therapeutic "matrix in which more specific techniques of therapy can be embedded" (see also Misch 2000). Commonly, clinicians incorporate techniques from CBT, psychodynamic therapy, and IPT, which can be flexibly combined with pharmacotherapy treatments as well.

Ms. G

Ms. G, a 32-year-old woman with major depression, generalized anxiety disorder, and personality disorder not otherwise specified had a good work history but had problems in her personal life. She had difficulty achieving intimacy with others, and she experienced anger attacks and frequent superficial arm scratching. After receiving combined pharmacotherapy and SPT, Ms. G was able to become engaged in treatment, to work on keeping her mood euthymic, and to decrease her marijuana use. Her psychotherapist focused on Ms. G's tendency to collapse either positive or negative experiences into strong feelings of anxiety or depression, often leading to arm scratching. SPT techniques such as clarifications, normalization, and reframing were used with some benefit. However, it became clear that Ms. G often became extremely anxious in day-to-day life and had difficulty calming herself, even if sitting in traffic or standing in line at a store, and even more if she was at a party or on a date. Her psychiatrist decided to incorporate some techniques from CBT, including asking Ms. G to keep a diary of her feelings and responses, and practicing mindfulness exercises, including "closing your eyes and listening carefully to what is around you." Ms. G found listening exercises a more effective way to calm herself than breathing or muscle relaxation exercises. Although incorporating these two CBT elements in an ongoing way into treatment, Ms. G's psychotherapy remained primarily SPT in orientation.

Clearly, because of the proliferation of psychotherapy approaches, and the ever-growing variety of somatic and pharmacological interventions, clinicians must be thoughtful and consistent in applying these approaches in order to avoid confusing the patient and unnecessarily changing treatment directions or approaches. The case of Ms. G therefore describes a way in which CBT approaches such as exposure, relaxation exercises, or mindfulness exercises can be incorporated in the treatment of a patient with mood and anxiety disorders without losing the overall frame of SPT.

Limits of Supportive Psychotherapy When Added to Pharmacotherapy

There may be patients for whom adding SPT to pharmacotherapy may be insufficient. These may include patients who need a different treatment setting or level of care or who are unwilling or unable to participate in a verbal therapy. Patients urgently requiring inpatient care, medical hospitalization, detoxification, and so on are likely to be unsuitable for SPT. Other patients may benefit from structured programs such as vocational rehabilitation programs instead of individual SPT. It is worth noting that SPT can be a model for psychotherapy treatments provided in many settings, however, including day treatment programs and acute psychiatric hospital settings, and among patients with high levels of symptom severity, comorbidity, and impairment. For instance, we have published studies of group SPT with severely ill patients diagnosed with chronic schizophrenia and substance abuse (Hellerstein et al. 1995; Miner et al. 1997) in which a high level of engagement and retention in treatment and significant improvement in psychiatric and substance abuse severity were demonstrated.

Other patients may need and benefit more from other (more specific) treatment approaches, including CBT, DBT, and psychodynamic therapies. It is possible that DBT may be a more specific antisuicide treatment than other psychotherapies, including SPT. Therefore, DBT may be the psychotherapy of choice for some bipolar disorder patients—especially those with severe suicidality (Stanley 2006). For other patients with bipolar disorder diagnoses, it is possible that equally good outcome may be achieved with SPT or other psychotherapy approaches. Patient preference for a therapeutic modality may play a role for many such choices.

Psychoanalytic/psychodynamic therapy may be preferable to SPT for some patients as well. Some patients may experience SPT as "superficial" or "inadequately intense or powerful," and may benefit from more classic exploratory treatment that allows them to explore fantasies, dreams, and in-session affective states. Such approaches may be essential for therapeutic progress for some patients, although there is little empirical evidence to determine who such patients may be. Clearly, however, patients who have previously failed to improve with competently performed SPT should be candidates for other treatment approaches.

Conclusion

The present review of relevant research, theoretical writings, and clinical practice suggests that pharmacotherapy and SPT are logically combined in clinical practice with a wide range of psychiatric patients. There is a growing cohort of trained psychiatric clinicians who are competent in performing combined pharmacotherapy and SPT—and also in managing split treatments where other therapists provide SPT. The limited research on narrowly defined SPT alone and in combination with pharmacotherapy is clearly insufficient to guide treatment in a detailed fashion. There is a need for more research on SPT because often it may be the default treatment in clinical practice as well as being a treatment of choice, given the large population of patients with chronic, comorbid, and severe disorders, and given the general high level of acceptability of SPT both to practitioners and patients.

It would be useful to have more research on the overall efficacy of combining SPT with pharmacotherapy as well as more research on the specific processes of treatment: we currently have little idea which SPT interventions are or are not particularly efficacious, especially when combined with pharmacotherapy.

It is also clear that psychotherapy researchers should use a robust, active model of SPT (as in Novalis's, Pinsker's, and Rockland's models) when studying putatively more active or specific treatments such as DBT or CBT, rather than using hobbled SPT treatments that are closer to what is defined here as a supportive relationship.

Finally, it would be helpful to train psychiatrists and other mental health professionals to think more rigorously about the best ways to combine pharmacotherapy and SPT, and about issues raised by these combined modalities in their work with patients.

Key Points

- Supportive psychotherapy (SPT) is the most commonly practiced form of psychotherapy and is often combined with pharmacotherapy.

- SPT is a broad-spectrum treatment with well-defined techniques and is applicable to a wide range of patients in various treatment settings.

- Research findings, although limited, suggest the benefit of combined psychotherapy and pharmacotherapy in many cases, particularly for patients with chronic, recurrent, severe, comorbid, or treatment-resistant disorders.

- SPT may be the psychotherapy of choice in many cases of combined treatment.

- Possible benefits of combined treatment include better management of Axis I, II, and III disorders as well as improved psychosocial functioning.

- There are numerous ways to combine SPT and pharmacotherapy, including concurrent, sequential, and augmenting treatment strategies, and treatment can also include components of other treatments such as cognitive-behavioral therapy.

- There is a need for more research on rigorously performed SPT, both with and without pharmacotherapy.

References

Aviram RB, Hellerstein DJ, Gerson J, et al: Adapting supportive psychotherapy for individuals with borderline personality disorder who self-injure or attempt suicide. J Psychiatr Pract 10:145–155, 2004

Beck AT, Rush AJ, Shaw BF, et al: Cognitive therapy and antidepressant medications, in Cognitive Therapy of Depression. New York, Guilford, 1979, pp 354–396

Buckley PJ: Supportive psychotherapy: a neglected treatment. Psychiatr Ann 16:515–521, 1986

Chiles JA, Carlin AS, Benjamin GAH, et al: A physician, a nonmedical psychotherapist and a patient: the pharmacotherapy-psychotherapy triangle, in Integrating Pharmacotherapy and Psychotherapy. Edited by Beitman BD, Klerman GL. Washington, DC, American Psychiatric Press, 1991, pp 105–120

de Jonghe F, Kool S, van Aalst G, et al: Combining psychotherapy and antidepressants in the treatment of depression. J Affect Disord 64:217–229, 2001

de Jonghe F, Hendricksen M, van Aalst G, et al: Psychotherapy alone and combined with pharmacotherapy in the treatment of depression. Br J Psychiatry 185:37–45, 2004

Frank E, Novick D, Kupfer DJ: Antidepressants and psychotherapy: a clinical research review. Dialogues Clin Neurosci 7:263–272, 2005

Friedman MA, Detweiler-Bedell JB, Leventhal HE, et al: Combined psychotherapy and pharmacotherapy for the treatment of major depressive disorder. Clinical Psychology: Science and Practice 11:47–68, 2004

Friedman RA, Markowitz JC, Parides M, et al: Six months of desipramine for dysthymia: can dysthymic patients achieve normal social functioning? J Affect Disord 54:283–286, 1999

Gabbard GO, Kay J: The fate of integrated treatment: whatever happened to the biopsychosocial psychiatrist? Am J Psychiatry 158:1956–1963, 2001

Gitlin MJ: The split treatment model: interactions between psychotherapy and pharmacotherapy, in The Psychotherapist's Guide to Psychopharmacology, 2nd Edition. New York, Free Press, 1996, pp 431–466

Hellerstein DJ: Supportive psychotherapy (Chapter 1: Double Depression and James Avery), in Approach to the Psychiatric Patient: Case-Based Essays. Edited by Barnhill JW. Washington, DC, American Psychiatric Publishing, 2008, pp 45–49

Hellerstein DJ, Pinsker H, Rosenthal RN, et al: Supportive psychotherapy as the treatment model of choice. J Psychother Pract Res 3:300–306, 1994

Hellerstein DJ, Rosenthal RN, Miner CR: A prospective study of integrated outpatient treatment for substance-abusing schizophrenic patients. Am J Addict 4:33–42, 1995

Hellerstein DJ, Rosenthal RN, Pinsker H, et al: A randomized prospective study comparing supportive and dynamic therapies: outcome and alliance. J Psychother Pract Res 7:261–271, 1998

Hellerstein DJ, Aviram R, Kotov K: Beyond "handholding": supportive therapy for patients with borderline personality disorder and self-injurious behavior. Psychiatric Times 21:58–61, 2004

Hersen M (ed): Pharmacological and Behavioral Treatment: An Integrative Approach. New York, Wiley, 1986

Hyland JM: Integrating psychotherapy and pharmacotherapy. Bull Menninger Clin 55:205–215, 1991

Jindal RD, Thase ME: Integrating psychotherapy and pharmacotherapy to improve outcomes among patients with mood disorders. Psychiatr Serv 54:1484–1490, 2003

Kahn D: The dichotomy of drugs and psychotherapy. Psychiatr Clin North Am 13:197–208, 1990

Karasu TB: Psychoanalysis and psychoanalytic psychotherapy, in Kaplan and Sadock's Comprehensive Textbook of Psychiatry, Eighth Edition. Edited by Sadock BJ, Sadock VA. Philadelphia, PA, Lippincott Williams & Wilkins, 2005, pp 2472–2498

Keller MB, McCullough JP, Klein DN, et al: A comparison of nefazodone, the cognitive behavioral-analysis system of psychotherapy, and their combination for the treatment of chronic depression. N Engl J Med 342:1462–1470, 2000

Kernberg OF: The psychotherapeutic treatment of borderline personalities (Part V: Borderline and Narcissistic Personality Disorders), in Psychiatry 1982: The American Psychiatric Association Annual Review, Vol 5. Edited by Grinspoon L. Washington, DC, American Psychiatric Press, 1982, pp 470–487

Klerman GL: Ideological conflicts in integrating pharmacotherapy and psychotherapy, in Integrating Pharmacotherapy and Psychotherapy. Edited by Beitman BD, Klerman GL. Washington DC, American Psychiatric Press, 1991, pp 3–21

Kool S, Dekker J, Duijsens IJ, et al: Efficacy of combined therapy and pharmacotherapy for depressed patients with or without personality disorders. Harv Rev Psychiatry 11:133–141, 2003

Krupnick JL, Sotsky SM, Simmens S, et al: The role of the therapeutic alliance in psychotherapy and pharmacotherapy outcome: findings in the National Institute of Mental Health Treatment of Depression Collaborative Research Program. J Consult Clin Psychol 64:532–539, 1996

Lader MH, Bond AJ: Interaction of pharmacological and psychological treatments of anxiety. Br J Psychiatry 34(suppl):42–48, 1998

Linehan M: Cognitive-Behavioral Treatment of Borderline Personality Disorder. New York, Guilford, 1993

Luborsky L: Principles of Psychoanalytic Psychotherapy: A Manual for Supportive-Expressive Methods. New York, Basic Books, 1984

Maina G, Forner F, Bogetto F: Randomized controlled trial comparing brief dynamic and supportive therapy with waiting list condition in minor depressive disorders. Psychother Psychosom 74:43–50, 2005

Marcus ER: Integrating psychopharmacotherapy, psychotherapy, and mental structure in the treatment of patients with personality disorders and depression. Psychiatr Clin North Am 13:255–264, 1990

Markowitz JC: Psychotherapy of the postdysthymic patient. J Psychother Pract Res 2:157–163, 1993

Markowitz JC, Weissman MM: Interpersonal psychotherapy: principles and applications. World Psychiatry 3:136–139, 2004

Miller WR, Zweben A, DiClemente CC, et al: Motivational Enhancement Therapy Manual (Project MATCH Monogr Ser, Vol 2; NIH Publ No 94-3723). Rockville, MD, National Institute on Alcohol Abuse and Alcoholism, 1994

Miner CR, Rosenthal RN, Hellerstein DJ, et al: Prediction of compliance with outpatient referral in patients with schizophrenia and psychoactive substance use disorders. Arch Gen Psychiatry 54:706–712, 1997

Misch DA: Basic strategies of dynamic supportive therapy. J Psychother Pract Res 9:173–189, 2000

Morgan DG: "Please see and advise": a qualitative study of patient experiences of outpatient care. Soc Psychiatry Psychiatr Epidemiol 34:442–450, 1999

Mynors-Wallis LM, Gath DH, Day A, et al: Randomised controlled trial of problem solving treatment, antidepressant medication, and combined treatment for depression in primary care. BMJ 320:26–30, 2000

Newton-Howes G, Tyrer P, Johnson T: Personality disorder and the outcome of depression: meta-analysis of published studies. Br J Psychiatry 188:13–20, 2006

Novalis PN, Rojcewicz SJ, Peele R: Clinical Manual of Supportive Psychotherapy. Washington, DC, American Psychiatric Press, 1993

Ostow M: Drugs in Psychoanalysis and Psychotherapy. New York, Basic Books, 1962

Pampallona S, Bollini P, Tibaldi G, et al: Combined pharmacotherapy and psychological treatment for depression. Arch Gen Psychiatry 61:714–719, 2004

Pincus HA, Zarin DA, Tanielian TL, et al: Psychiatric patients and treatments in 1997: findings from the American Psychiatric Practice Research Network. Arch Gen Psychiatry 56:441–449, 1999

Pine F: The interpretive moment: variations on classical themes. Bull Menninger Clin 48:54–71, 1984

Pinsker H: A Primer of Supportive Therapy. Hillside, NJ, Analytic Press, 1997

Piper WE: Implications of psychotherapy research for psychotherapy training. Can J Psychiatry 49:221–229, 2004

Piper WE, Joyce AS, McCallum M, et al: Interpretive and supportive forms of psychotherapy and patient personality variables. J Consult Clin Psychol 66:558–567, 1998

Preskorn SH: Psychopharmacology and psychotherapy: what's the connection? J Psychiatr Pract 12:41–45, 2006

Rockland LH: Supportive Therapy: A Psychodynamic Approach. New York, Basic Books, 1989

Rosenthal RN, Muran JC, Pinsker H, et al: Interpersonal change in brief supportive psychotherapy. J Psychother Pract Res 8:55–63, 1999

Seligman M: Authentic Happiness: Using the New Positive Psychology to Realize Your Potential for Lasting Fulfillment. New York, Simon & Schuster, 2002

Smith ML, Glass GV: Meta-analysis of psychotherapy outcome studies. Am Psychol 32:752–760, 1977

Stanley BH: Treatment of suicidal behavior and self-injury in borderline personality disorder: fluoxetine and dialectical behavior therapy. Paper presented at the 46th Annual Meeting of the New Clinical Drug Evaluation Unit, Boca Raton, FL, June 12–14, 2006

Tanielian TL, Marcus SC, Suarez AP, et al: Datapoints: trends in psychiatric practice, 1988–1998, II: caseload and treatment characteristics. Psychiatr Serv 52:880, 2001

Thase ME: When are psychotherapy and pharmacotherapy combinations the treatment of choice for major depressive disorder? Psychiatr Q 70:333–346, 1999

Thase ME, Jindal RD: Combining psychotherapy and psychopharmacology for treatment of mental disorders, in Bergin and Garfield's Handbook of Psychotherapy and Behavior Change, 5th Edition. Edited by Lambert MJ. New York, Wiley, 2004, pp 743–766

Viamontes GI, Beitman BD: Neural substrates of psychotherapeutic change, I: the default brain. Psychiatr Ann 36:225–236, 2006a

Viamontes GI, Beitman BD: Neural substrates of psychotherapeutic change, II: beyond default mode. Psychiatr Ann 36:238–245, 2006b

Wallerstein RS: The psychotherapy research project of the Menninger Foundation: an overview. J Consult Clin Psychol 57:195–205, 1989

Weissman MM, Klerman GL: Interpersonal psychotherapy for depression, in Integrating Pharmacotherapy and Psychotherapy. Edited by Beitman BD, Klerman GL. Washington DC, American Psychiatric Press, 1991, pp 379–394

Werman D: The practice of supportive psychotherapy. New York, Brunner/Mazel, 1984

Winston A, Winston B: The partnership: medication and psychotherapy, in Handbook of Integrated Short-Term Psychotherapy. Washington, DC, American Psychiatric Publishing, 2002, pp 95–106

Winston A, Rosenthal RN, Pinsker H: Introduction to Supportive Psychotherapy (Core Competencies in Psychotherapy). Washington, DC, American Psychiatric Publishing, 2004

Suggested Readings

Chiles JA, Carlin AS, Benjamin GAH, et al: A physician, a nonmedical psychotherapist and a patient: the pharmacotherapy-psychotherapy triangle, in Integrating Pharmacotherapy and Psychotherapy. Edited by Beitman BD, Klerman GL. Washington, DC, American Psychiatric Press, 1991, pp 105–120

Novalis PN, Rojcewicz SJ, Peele R: Medication and compliance, in Clinical Manual of Supportive Psychotherapy. Washington, DC, American Psychiatric Press, 1993, pp 295–310

Novalis PN, Rojcewicz SJ, Peele R: Principles (Section I), in Clinical Manual of Supportive Psychotherapy. Washington, DC, American Psychiatric Press, 1993, pp 3–125

Pampallona S, Bollini P, Tibaldi G, et al: Combined pharmacotherapy and psychological treatment for depression. Arch Gen Psychiatry 61:714–719, 2004

Pinsker H: A Primer of Supportive Therapy. Hillside, NJ, Analytic Press, 1997

Thase ME, Jindal RD: Combining psychotherapy and psychopharmacology for treatment of mental disorders, in Bergin and Garfield's Handbook of Psychotherapy and Behavior Change, 5th Edition. Edited by Lambert MJ. New York, Wiley, 2004, pp 743–766

Winston A, Winston B: The partnership: medication and psychotherapy, in Handbook of Integrated Short-Term Psychotherapy. Washington, DC, American Psychiatric Publishing, 2002, pp 95–106

PART 5

Group, Family, and Couples Therapy

Section Editor
James Griffith, M.D.

Chapter 18

Family Systems Theory and Practice

John S. Rolland, M.D.
Froma Walsh, Ph.D.

Over the past three decades, family systems approaches to practice have become essential to the understanding and treatment of individual and relational disorders. These approaches are guided by a developmental, multisystemic conceptual orientation to human problems and processes of change, attending to the family and social context of functioning and well-being. Current research evidence supports involving families in assessment and treatment (Heru 2006).

In this chapter we provide an overview of family systems assessment and intervention in psychiatry. We begin with a description of basic principles of a systemic orientation to practice and a framework for assessment of family functioning. We offer a brief outline of foundational models and more recent advances in family therapy theory and practice. Next, we describe the utility of an array of systems approaches in psychiatry, including family or couple assessment, consultation, brief interventions, multisystemic approaches, multifamily groups, and more intensive therapy. We then consider how to combine family systems with other therapeutic modalities and how to use systemic thinking more generally in a variety of psychiatric treatment settings and specific psychiatric diagnoses.

Family Systems Orientation

A family systems orientation is distinguished by its view of the family as a transactional system. Stressful events and problems of an individual member affect the whole family as a functional unit, with ripple effects for all members and their relationships. In turn, the family response—how the family handles problems—contributes significantly to positive adaptation or to individual and relational dysfunction. Thus, individual problems are assessed and treated in the context of the family system. Relational problems are addressed directly in couple and family sessions with those involved.

Biopsychosocial Orientation

The practice of family therapy is grounded in a biopsychosocial orientation, recognizing the complex interplay of individual, family, and social processes (Engel 1980; von Bertalanffy 1969). The family is viewed as an open system that functions in relation to its broader sociocultural context and evolves over the life cycle (Minuchin 1974). Family systems theory advanced conceptualization of human functioning and dysfunction from a linear, dyadic, deterministic view of causality in traditional psychoanalytic theory to the recognition of multiple, recursive influences within and beyond the family that shape both individual and family functioning over the life course. This approach considers the family's interface with larger systems, such as school, the workplace, and health care systems. It attends to cultural and socioeconomic influences, including the impact of racism and other forms of discrimination for poor minority families and other marginalized groups (Boyd-Franklin 2003; McGoldrick and Hardy 2008). From an ecological perspective, individual dysfunction cannot be adequately understood and treated apart from its psychosocial context. Regardless of the origin of problems, or genetic predisposition, the family is regarded as an essential partner in treatment, with the potential for fostering optimal adaptation.

Multigenerational Family Life Cycle Perspective

In a systemic model of human development, individual and family development are seen to coevolve over the life course and across the generations (Carter and McGoldrick 1999). Relationships grow and change, boundaries shift, roles are redefined, and new members and losses require adaptation. Each developmental phase presents salient challenges; distress often occurs around major transitions such as the birth of the first child, entry into adolescence, launching young adults, or needs for elder care. All families must cope with stressful events, including both the predictable, normative stresses, as with child-rearing, and unexpected, disruptive circumstances, such as raising a child with disabilities (Walsh, in press). Divorce, single parenting, and stepfamily integration pose additional challenges for many families (Hetherington and Kelly 2002). Over an expanded life course, family members may transition in and out of single status, couple bonds, and varied family configurations, adding complexity to all relationships.

The increasing diversity of family forms, lifestyle options, and timing of nodal events makes it imperative that no single model or life trajectory be deemed as essential for healthy child development (Walsh 2003b).

Systemic Lens: Patterns That Connect

Family therapy is not simply a therapeutic modality in which all members are treated conjointly. In fact, individuals may be seen separately or brought together for some sessions in different combinations. A family systems approach is distinguished less by who is in the room and more by the clinician's attention to relationship systems in assessment and treatment planning. We consider how family members may contribute to—and are affected by—problem situations. Most importantly, regardless of the source of problems, we involve key family members who can contribute to needed changes. Therapy may focus on strengthening a couple's relationship; it might combine individual sessions with an adolescent and sessions with the whole family or with parents, siblings, or extended kin. Interventions are aimed at modifying dysfunctional patterns, tapping family resources, and strengthening both individual and family functioning.

Mutual Influences

Family members are interrelated such that each individual affects all others and the group as a whole in turn affects the first member in a circular chain of influence. Even for psychiatric conditions, such as depression, that are largely biologically based, it is important to understand how depression affects family interaction, how those transactions contribute to or reinforce symptoms, and how interactional changes can improve individual—and family—functioning and well-being. A circular tracking process is a key element in a systems-oriented assessment, providing an interactive view of the biological and relational influences to guide interventions.

In a chain of influence, every action is also a reaction: a mother's overly harsh response to a child's tantrum may exacerbate the child's out-of-control behavior. In tracking the *sequence of interactions* around a presenting problem, we often find repetitive patterns involving other family members. For example, if the father then criticizes the mother and sides with the child, it is likely to make matters worse. Regardless of how a sequence began, parents can be helped to pull together as a team to handle challenges more effectively. Skilled intervention involves interrupting vicious cycles to promote "virtuous cycles" and problem resolution.

Although processes may be circular, not all participants have equal power or influence. Clinicians are cautioned not to take a neutral stance or a "no fault" position in cases in which an abusive spouse or parent must be held accountable for any harmful behavior. Moreover, therapist neutrality tends to support the status quo and can perpetuate destructive patterns.

Clinicians should not reflexively type a family by the diagnosis of a member, such as an "alcoholic family." Such labels carry faulty attributions of blame. Individual disturbance may have social influences or a strong genetic predisposition. Family distress should not be presumed to have played a causal role in individual symptoms; it may result from unsuccessful attempts to cope with an overwhelming situation that has a significant genetic or other biological etiological component. For instance, marital conflict between parents of an adolescent with bipolar disorder may have been fueled by repeated unsuccessful attempts to deal with their child's emotional outbursts. With multiple influences, the impact of external stressors and socioeconomic conditions should be taken into account. For instance, a child's plummeting school grades must be seen in the context of his father's recent job loss and related family tensions. Sensitive family therapy intervention acknowledges family stress and frustrations and helps members find more effective ways to approach challenges and prevent problem behavior.

Assessment of Family Functioning

Mapping the Family System

In clinical practice, a broad conception of family is needed to encompass the wide range of family structures, relationship options, and cultural diversity in contemporary society (Coontz 1997).Clinicians need to be mindful of cultural, personal, and professional assumptions and biases when assessing families. Myths of the ideal family can compound a sense of deficiency and failure for struggling families that do not fit the intact nuclear family model. Decades of research clearly confirm that children can grow up healthy in a variety of family arrangements (Walsh 2003b). What matters most is the quality of relationships and the effectiveness of family processes.

At the outset, it is essential to learn who is in the family system. This includes all household members and the extended kin network as well as other significant relationships (e.g., intimate partner, informal kin, caregivers). It is crucial to assess relationships with nonresidential parents and stepfamily members.

The *genogram* and *time line* (McGoldrick et al. 2008) are essential tools for mapping the family system, noting relationship information, and tracking system patterns to guide intervention planning. A resilience-oriented assessment searches for positive influences and potential resources, such as models and mentors, alongside problematic patterns and troubled relationships. Clinicians need to inquire about a family's organizational shifts and coping strategies in response to past stressors such as major losses. Such inquiry helps to understand the family's current meaning making, coping, and adaptation to current or threatened loss. It is important to identify strengths, such as courage and perseverance, in the midst of past struggles and to draw out positive stories and experiences in overcoming past adversity (Walsh 2006).

Family functioning is assessed in the context of the multigenerational system moving forward over time (Carter and McGoldrick 1999). A time line can be sketched to note the timing and sequence of critical events or a pileup of stressors in the family. Frequently symptoms and dysfunction coincide with developmental transitions (e.g., starting a family) or relationship changes or in the context of stressful events such as unemployment. Because family members may not initially mention such connections, the genogram and time line can guide inquiry and reveal patterns to explore.

Although all change is stressful, strain increases exponentially when current stressors intersect with vulnerable multigenerational issues. Nodal events are likely to reactivate past unresolved conflicts and losses, particularly when similar developmental challenges are confronted. An impending separation may reactivate past losses. Families may conflate current situations with past adverse experience, generating catastrophic fears. One mother became anxiously preoccupied that her 16-year-old daughter would become pregnant, the same age that the mother, herself, became pregnant. In another case, a husband's avoidance of intimacy and conflict over his wife's desire to have a second child became more understandable in learning that his mother had died in childbirth with his younger sibling. Family intervention explores such covert linkages, helping families to heal and learn from their past to make a difference in their current relationships.

Clinicians routinely should note family histories of traumatic loss that often contribute to depression, substance abuse, and self-destructive behavior (Walsh 2007; Walsh and McGoldrick 2004). It is particularly important to note critical events that occurred at the same age as the patient or current nodal point in the family system, as in the following case:

In a family session after the suicide attempt of 13-year-old Daniel, he remained silent and his parents were unable to comprehend his actions. They made no mention of an older deceased brother. In doing a family genogram, it was learned that Daniel had been named for his brother, who had died — at age 13 shortly before Daniel's birth. When the family response and ripple effects were explored, it emerged that the family, to avoid their sorrow, never talked about him. With communication opened, Daniel related that he had worn his brother's handed-down clothes and had tried to take his place to ease his parents' grief. Now, as he was turning 14, he didn't know how to be, so he had decided to join his brother in heaven.

Components of Family Functioning

Family process research over the past three decades has provided considerable empirical grounding for assessment of family functioning (Walsh 2003b). The family resilience framework in Table 18–1 was developed as a conceptual map for clinicians to assess family functioning and to target and strengthen key processes that foster positive adaptation (Walsh 2003a, 2006). This framework, informed by social science and clinical research, can be useful to identify key processes for effective family functioning in three domains: family belief systems, organizational patterns, and communication processes.

Family Belief Systems

Shared belief systems are at the core of all family functioning (Reiss 1981). Relationship rules, both explicit and unspoken, provide a set of expectations about roles, actions, and consequences that guide family life and members' behaviors. Shared values and assumptions evolve through transactions with significant others and the larger social world (Hoffman 1990) and are influenced by cultural, ethnic, and religious beliefs (Falicov 1995; McGoldrick et al. 2005; Walsh 1999). Psychiatrists should routinely explore a family's beliefs concerning their problem situation: the meaning it holds for them, how it came about, and how it might be improved. For instance, beliefs about spirit possession or traditional faith healing practices, common in many immigrant families, may not be mentioned unless a therapist inquires respectfully about them (Falicov 1998).

Family history and patterns of relating and functioning are transmitted across the generations, influencing future expectations, hopes, and dreams. Multigenerational stories, secrets, and taboos become encoded into family scripts that can rally efforts or fuel catastrophic fears when a family is faced with a threatening situation (Byng-Hall 1995). Some families become stuck in the past; others cut off emotionally from painful memories and contacts. Well-functioning families are better able to balance intergenerational con-

TABLE 18–1.　Key processes in family resilience

BELIEF SYSTEMS

Making meaning of adversity

Resilience as relationally based

Normalization and contextualization of distress

A sense of coherence: crisis as meaningful, comprehensible, and manageable challenge

Appraisal of adverse situation, options, and future expectations

Positive outlook

Hope, optimistic bias; confidence in overcoming barriers

Courage/encouragement; affirmation of strengths and potential

Active initiative and perseverance

Mastering the possible; acceptance of what cannot be changed

Transcendence and spirituality

Larger values, purpose

Spirituality: faith, rituals and practices, congregational support

Inspiration: new possibilities, dreams; creative expression; social action

Transformation: learning, change, and growth from adversity

ORGANIZATIONAL PATTERNS

Flexibility

Adapting to meet new challenges; rebounding, reorganizing

Regaining of stability: continuity, dependability through disruption

Strong authoritative leadership: nurture, guide, protect

　　Varied family forms: cooperative parenting/caregiving teams

　　Couple/coparent relationship: equal partners

Connectedness

Mutual support, collaboration, commitment

Respect for individual needs, differences, and boundaries

Seeking of reconnection, reconciliation of troubled relationships

Social and economic resources

Mobilization of kin, social and community networks; recruit mentors

Financial security, work/family balance, institutional supports

TABLE 18–1. Key processes in family resilience *(continued)*

COMMUNICATION/PROBLEM SOLVING

Clarity

Clear, consistent messages (words and actions)

Clarification of ambiguous information; truth seeking/truth speaking

Open emotional expression

Sharing of range of feelings (joy and pain; hopes and fears)

Mutual empathy; tolerance for differences

Responsibility for own feelings, behavior; avoid blaming

Pleasurable interactions, respite; humor

Collaborative problem solving

Creative brainstorming; resourcefulness

Shared decision making; negotiation; resolve/repair conflicts

Focus on goals, concrete steps: build on success; learn from failure

Proactive stance: prevent crises; prepare for future challenges

tinuity and change, and to maintain links between their past, present, and future direction (Beavers and Hampson 2003).

Family identity and beliefs are conveyed through family rituals, including celebrations of holidays, rites of passage (e.g., bar/bat mitzvah), traditions, and routine interactions (e.g., family dinner). Rituals provide stabilization and continuity over time and also facilitate transitions such as the inclusion of children in a remarriage ceremony. Family therapists often use rituals in therapeutic intervention to foster change or healing (Imber-Black et al. 2003), as in cases such as suicide or stillbirth in which a loss has not been adequately marked.

Therapists aim to understand constraining beliefs and narratives and to expand those that facilitate positive change (Wright et al. 1996). Research suggests that clinicians can foster resilience by helping distressed families 1) make meaning of their crisis situation and their options; 2) regain a positive outlook, with hope for the future and conviction in success through shared efforts, perseverance, and focus on mastering what is possible; and 3) forge larger transcendent/spiritual values, purpose, and bonds in their lives (e.g., through connection to cultural roots, spiritual beliefs, practices, and a faith community) (Griffith and Griffith 2002).

Family Organizational Patterns

Family functioning requires effective organization to maintain integration as a family unit, foster healthy development of members, and master life challenges. Varying family structures, such as an intact two-parent family, a single-parent family, a binuclear divorced family, a stepfamily, and a three-generational household, have varied configurations, resources, and constraints.

Adaptability—a counterbalance of flexibility and stability—is a core requisite for effective family functioning (Beavers and Hampson 2003; Olson and Gorell 2003). To function well, a family needs strong leadership with predictable, consistent rules, roles, and patterns of interaction. The family must also adapt to changing circumstances or developmental priorities. Lacking this flexible structure, families at dysfunctional extremes tend to be either overly rigid and autocratic, or chaotically disorganized and leaderless. In times of crisis or disruptive transitions such as divorce or diagnosis of a serious illness (Rolland 1994), flexibility for change must be counterbalanced by efforts to restabilize, reorganize, and reestablish patterns in daily life. Significant losses may require major adaptational shifts in order to ensure the continuity of family life. For instance, when a husband becomes disabled, family roles change as the wife becomes the primary breadwinner and he assumes the bulk of homemaking/child-rearing responsibilities.

Connectedness, or cohesion, is another central dimension of family organization. Well-functioning families balance needs for closeness and mutual support with respect for separateness and individual differences. The functional balance of connectedness shifts as families move through the life cycle. Extremes of enmeshment or disengagement tend to be highly dysfunctional. However, with varying cultural norms, personal preferences, and situational demands, clinicians must be cautious not to reflexively label a highly cohesive family style as enmeshed or presume it is necessarily dysfunctional. For instance, research on families coping with a serious physical illness found that although they often scored at the high extreme on cohesion, the relationships were generally not pathologically fused, but were adaptive in meeting the illness challenges over time.

Equal power in the couple/parental unit, with an equitable sharing of authority, responsibility, and privilege, fosters healthy relationships (Goldner 1988; Gottman 1999). The complexity of divorced and stepfamily configurations poses a challenge to sustain workable parenting coalitions across households and to knit together biological and step-relations, including stepsiblings and extended kin.

Family boundaries are crucial structural requisites that need to be clear and firm yet permeable (Minuchin 1974). *Interpersonal boundaries* define and separate individual members, promoting differentiation and autonomous functioning. *Generational boundaries* maintain hierarchical organization in families. Leadership and authority need to be clear and firm, distinguishing grandparent, parent, and child roles, rights, and obligations. Generational boundaries are blurred when a parent abdicates leadership, assumes a child-like position, or uses a child as a parental surrogate. It may be functional, and even necessary, for older children to assist parents with responsibilities, particularly in single-parent or large families, and in cases of parental illness or disability (Rolland 1999). However, rigid role expectations can sacrifice a child's own development needs. Boundaries are breached most destructively in cases of violence and sexual abuse (Sheinberg and Fraenkel 2001).

The concept of the *triangle* and the dysfunctional process of *triangulation* (Bowen 1978) refer to the pattern when two members (e.g., spouses/parents) draw in or scapegoat a third person to deflect rising tension. A couple may avoid conflict to rally together in mutual concern about a symptomatic child. A triangulated child may assume the role of go-between for parents, thereby balancing loyalties and regulating tension and intimacy. In high-conflict marriage and divorce, one parent may draw a child into a coalition against the other parent. A grandparent–child coalition may be formed against a single parent. In more troubled families, these patterns are more rigid and likely to be replicated in multiple interlocking triangles throughout the family system. Efforts to help clients to detriangle from their own involvement are central to Bowen coaching methods (Carter and McGoldrick 2001).

Kin and community networks can be vital lifelines for family functioning (Bengston 2001) and for support in times of crisis. Family isolation contributes to dysfunction and blocks socialization and emancipation of growing children. Where families are not supportive, friendship networks can become valued "families of choice," as in gay and lesbian communities.

Communication Processes

Communication processes facilitate all family functioning. Family therapists attend to both the content and relationship aspects of communication. The statement "Eat your vegetables" conveys an order with expectation of compliance, implying a hierarchical differentiation of status or authority, as between parent and child. All verbal and nonverbal behavior, including silence (or spitting out the vegetables), conveys interpersonal messages (e.g., "I won't obey you!").

Clarity is essential. In family evaluation, psychiatrists assess family members' ability to communicate openly about both pragmatic and emotional issues (Ryan et al. 2005). Cultural norms vary considerably regarding directness and degree of expression of opinions and feelings (McGoldrick et al. 2005). Clear and congruent messages conveyed in words and actions are important. In ambiguous situations, such as unclear diagnosis or prognosis of an illness, anxiety and risk of depression are heightened, as in the following case:

> A mother brought her 5-year-old son for an evaluation, fearing he had been sexually abused in his preschool because she often found him fondling himself. Carefully ruling out sexual abuse, the therapist explored recent stressful events in the family. The mother reported that several months earlier her husband had had exploratory surgery for "stomach pains." A cancerous tumor and most of his stomach were removed. At hospital discharge, he told his wife, "Okay, they said they got it all; I just want to go back to life as normal and not talk about it." To respect her husband's wishes, she told the children, "Daddy's fine," and no more was said. A recent checkup found something suspicious, and the future prognosis was now unclear. The parents assumed the son wasn't worrying because he hadn't asked any questions. Then she recalled that when the family had said grace before dinner recently, he added, "And please, God, take care of Daddy's tummy." The parents were seen together to open their communication about the life-threatening situation and then were helped to discuss it sensitively with their children.

A climate of mutual trust encourages *open expression of a range of feelings and empathic responses,* with respect for differences. Troubled families, in contrast, tend to perpetuate mistrust, with repeated blaming and scapegoating. Highly reactive emotional expression can fuel destructive cycles of conflict escalating to violence. Cascading effects of criticism, stonewalling, contempt, and mutual withdrawal contribute to despair and divorce (Gottman 1999). It is important to note areas of conflict, as well as toxic or sensitive subjects, when communication is blocked (e.g., a fatal drug overdose). Also, clinicians should be aware of constraints of gender-based socialization—for instance, in expectations that men should be tough, instrumental problem-solvers and guarded in sharing emotions or revealing vulnerability.

Collaborative problem solving is crucial for family functioning and is facilitated in all approaches to family therapy. Families can have difficulties solving instrumental problems, such as juggling job and child care demands, and more affective aspects of problems, such as comforting of children in a time of crisis. Families can falter at various steps in the problem-solving process (Ryan et al. 2005): identifying the problem; communicating with appropriate people about it; brainstorming possible solutions; deciding on an approach, taking initiative, and following through; and evaluating the effectiveness of the approach. Resilient families build on small successes and view mistakes as learning experiences. Families become more resourceful as therapy focuses proactively to anticipate, prepare for, and avert future problems. A systemic assessment attends to the process of collaborative problem solving; how decisions are made can be as crucial as the decision itself, with negotiation, compromise, and reciprocity.

Table 18–1 summarizes key processes that support family resilience. Any assessment must consider functioning in context: relative to each family's structure, cultural values, resources, and life challenges. Whether patterns are functional or dysfunctional depends on the fit between patient/family and the psychosocial demands of their problematic situation (Rolland 1994, 2003). For example, when a serious health crisis, requiring close teamwork, strikes a family with low cohesion, in which members fend for themselves, family sessions would be useful to build more functional collaboration and mutual support to meet the overwhelming challenges.

Evolution in the Field of Family Therapy: From Deficits to Strengths

The family systems paradigm expanded the view of the family beyond the narrow focus on early childhood mother–child relationships to ongoing interactions in the broad family network. Reflecting psychiatry's focus on psychopathology, early family therapy tended to be skewed toward identifying dysfunctional family patterns in the maintenance of individual symptoms, if not their origin. It was thought that symptoms served a function for families, a view no longer held.

Over the past two decades, the field of family therapy has refocused attention from family deficits to family strengths (Nichols and Schwartz 2005; Walsh 2006). The therapeutic relationship has become more collaborative and empowering, with recognition that successful interventions depend more on tapping family resources than on therapist techniques. The language and discourse are respectful and avoid pathologizing labels and constructions. Assessment and intervention are redirected from how problems were caused to how solutions can be found, identifying and amplifying existing and potential strengths. The therapist and family work together to find new possibilities in problem-saturated situations and take steps to overcome impasses to change. This positive, future-oriented stance refocuses from how families have failed to how they can succeed.

A family resilience framework builds on these developments to draw out strengths in dealing with adversity (Walsh 2003a). It links symptoms of distress with stressful events and conditions. Families most often come for help in crisis, but frequently they do not initially connect presenting problems with relevant stressors. This family resilience framework can serve as a valuable conceptual map to guide intervention efforts to target and strengthen key processes as presenting problems are addressed. This approach alters the deficit-based lens, from regarding parents and families as *damaged* and beyond repair to seeing them as *challenged* by life's adversities, with potential to foster healing and growth in all members. As families become more resourceful, risk and vulnerability are reduced, and they are better able to meet future challenges. Thus, building resilience is also a preventive measure.

Postmodern perspectives (Anderson 1997; Freedman and Combs 1996; Hoffman 1990; White and Epston 1990) have heightened awareness that clinical views of normality, health, and pathology are socially constructed. Clinicians and researchers bring their own values and biases and thus co-construct the patterns they "discover" in families. Moreover, therapeutic objectives are influenced by both family and therapist beliefs about healthy functioning (Walsh 2003b). Clinicians and researchers need to be aware of their own implicit assumptions, values, and biases embedded in cultural norms, professional orientations, and personal experience.

Many varied family therapy models have been advanced over the past three decades. For a description and comparison of foundational family therapy models (Boscolo et al. 1987; Boszormenyi-Nagy 1987; Bowen 1978; Byng-Hall 1995; Framo 1980; Haley 1976; Minuchin 1974; Patterson et al. 1975; Weakland et al. 1974) and more recent approaches (e.g., Dattilio 2005; de Shazer 1988; White and Epston 1990), readers are referred to the family therapy textbooks of Nichols and Schwartz (2005) and Goldenberg and Goldenberg (2004). Despite many differences, all approaches are grounded in a systemic orientation and attend to ongoing transactional processes, relational connections, and their wider context. They differ in focus on particular aspects of functioning: meaning systems, structural patterns, communication, problem solving, relational dynamics, and multigenerational patterns. Table 18–2 presents an outline of major approaches to family therapy and their views of functioning/dysfunction, change processes, and therapeutic goals.

Most clinicians with a family systems orientation increasingly integrate elements of various approaches (Lebow 1997), as in multidimensional, multisystemic approaches with troubled adolescents (Liddle et al. 2002) and in emotionally focused therapy with couples (Johnson 1996), combining attachment theory and behavioral approaches to foster secure relationships.

Value of Systems Approaches in Psychiatry

It is important for clinicians to appreciate the value of a systemic approach in general practice, regardless of whether they are using individual, family, couples, or multifamily group treatment approaches. As a basic worldview, a systems perspective includes attention to

- Individuals, problems, and resources in family and sociocultural contexts

TABLE 18–2. Major approaches to family therapy

Family therapy model	View of problems	Therapeutic goals	Process of change
		Intergenerational/growth-oriented approaches	
Psychodynamic/ transgenerational Boszormenyi-Nagy 1987 Framo 1980 Byng-Hall 1995	Symptoms caused by shared family projection process; unresolved past conflicts, losses, loyalty, and trust issues in family of origin	• Resolve family-of-origin issues • ↓ Family projection processes • Individual and relational growth	• Insight-oriented, link covert past and present dynamics • Facilitate resolution of issues in current direct interaction • Encourage mutual empathy in couple relationships

Bowen approach Bowen 1978 Carter and McGoldrick 2001	Functioning impaired by unresolved family-of-origin issues, losses:
	• Poor differentiation
	• Anxiety (reactivity)
	• Triangulation
	• Cutoffs
		• Differentiation in relationships
		• ↑ Cognitive functioning
		• ↓ Emotional reactivity
		• Modify relationship patterns:
		  • Detriangulation
		  • Repair cutoffs
			• Survey multigenerational system (use of genogram, time line)
			• Plan-focused interventions to change self directly with family
			• Therapist coaches action outside session
			• Detoxify, use humor, reversals

TABLE 18–2. Major approaches to family therapy *(continued)*

Family therapy model	View of problems	Therapeutic goals	Process of change
Experiential Satir 1988 Whitaker 1992	Symptoms are nonverbal messages expressing current communication dysfunction in system	Direct, clear communication • Genuine expression of feelings • Individual and relational growth	Change here-and-now interaction • Share feelings about relationships • Facilitate direct communication • Experiential techniques to reveal hidden conflicts, needs • Therapist uses experience with family to catalyze change process
Structural Minuchin 1974	Symptoms result from current family structural imbalance: • Malfunctioning hierarchy, boundaries • Maladaptive reaction to developmental or environmental changes	Reorganize family structure: • Parental leadership, authority • Clear, flexible subsystems and boundaries • Promote adaptive coping	Therapist shifts interaction patterns • Join family • Enactment of problem • Map structure, plan stages of restructuring • Tasks and directives

TABLE 18–2. Major approaches to family therapy (continued)

Family therapy model	View of problems	Therapeutic goals	Process of change
Strategic/systemic Jackson 1965 Haley 1976 Boscolo et al. 1987	Symptoms maintained by family's unsuccessful problem-solving attempts	Solve presenting problem; specific behaviorally defined objectives	Pragmatic, focused, action-oriented: • Change symptom-maintaining sequence to new outcome • Interrupt feedback cycles • Relabeling, reframing, paradox • Circular questions; curiosity
Postmodern Solution-focused; de Shazer 1988 Narrative; White and Epson 1990 Conversational; H. Anderson 1997	• Normality is socially constructed • Problem-saturated narratives • Constrained, marginalized by dominant discourse	• Envision new possibilities; take positive steps to attain facilitative meaning-making • Reauthor, thicken life stories	• Future-oriented potential • Search for problem exceptions • Collaborative, respectful • Externalize problems to overcome

TABLE 18–2. Major approaches to family therapy *(continued)*

Family therapy model	View of problems	Therapeutic goals	Process of change
Cognitive-behavioral Patterson et al. 1975 Sexton and Alexander 2003 Dattilio 2005	Maladaptive, symptomatic behavior reinforced by • Family reward • Negative interaction cycles • Core beliefs (schemas)	Concrete behavioral goals Improved communication and problem solving Cognitive restructuring of distortions, misperceptions	• Therapist guides, shapes • Change interpersonal assumptions • Reward desired behavior • Negotiation and problem-solving skills
Psychoeducational C.M. Anderson et al. 1986 McFarlane 2002	• Biologically based disorders; stress/diathesis • Adaptational challenges (e.g., chronic illness)	• Optimal functioning • Reduce stress, stigma, isolation • Master adaptational changes	• Multifamily groups, social support, provide useful information • Offer management guidelines • Respectful collaboration
Multisystemic Santisteban et al. 2003 Liddle et al. 2002 Henggeler et al. 1998	Family, social, larger systems influence adolescent conduct disorders, substance abuse	Reduce risks, problem behaviors Promote positive youth adaptation	Collaborative involvement of families, peers, mentors, schools, community programs

- Transactional processes in the couple relationship, family unit, and kin network
- Multiple, ongoing mutual biopsychosocial influences
- Patterns, critical events, phases, and transitions across multigenerational family life cycles

Despite differences in particular strategies and techniques employed in various systemic therapy models, all approaches focus on direct assessment and change to improve functioning, adaptation, and relationships, rather than a narrow, deficit-focus on reducing pathology of the individual symptom bearer. This is perhaps the major distinction of a family systems orientation from traditional individual psychotherapy models.

A systemic lens enriches all forms of psychiatric intervention, from a biomedical model to psychodynamic and cognitive-behavioral approaches. From this clinical stance, inquiry includes the social and temporal context of a problem, relevant multigenerational patterns, interactional processes that contribute to problems, and relational resources that can be tapped for problem resolution and well-being. A systems viewpoint can be utilized to understand family processes regardless of how many people are in the room. However, a broader view is gained by multiple perspectives, and the tracking process is enhanced by observation of interactions. Moreover, engagement, collaboration, and building of family resources are all facilitated through direct contact with key members in the kin network.

In systemic intervention models, the therapist aims to promote change directly with significant family members. Also, the focus is broadened from dyadic to triangular and larger systemic patterns and their influence in problems and change. It is sometimes erroneously assumed that work with families is more superficial or diluted compared to individual therapy. In fact, family therapy is very powerful and sessions can be intense. When transference reactions occur, they are redirected for change back into the natural relationships. Countertransference issues can be easily stimulated because of the emotional power of a family system and the likelihood that some member or relationship may elicit therapist reactions. Thus, clinicians must be aware of interface issues between their own personal relationships and the families with whom they work.

Systemic Approaches in Clinical Practice

Family Consultation and Assessment

The often asked question "When is family or couples consultation/therapy indicated?" requires reframing from a systems perspective. When problems are conceptualized at the relationship level, an individual's problems cannot be understood or changed apart from the context in which they occur. An individual cannot be expected to change without reactions from others; positive changes in stressful transactions will facilitate individual change and growth. Thus, the question of "indications" raises the further question "What is the symptom-maintaining context of a problem, and how can it most effectively be altered?"

The assessment of most problems should therefore include a careful evaluation of the couple or family system, preferably in most cases by convening both spouses and/or significant family members for a conjoint session. Typically, this session is best framed as a consultation (Wynne et al. 1986). It is important to consider all key relationships in the evaluation, to clarify treatment objectives, and to decide whom to include in subsequent sessions. This approach will clarify diagnostic questions, treatment objectives, and the choice of therapeutic intervention. With conditions such as schizophrenia, acute mania, organic brain syndromes, and substance abuse, family members can provide more accurate information regarding symptoms and behavior. When it is feasible to do so, patients on medication or who are in danger of crises should routinely be seen early in treatment with their partner or family to develop a treatment plan. This plan should include education about the course of the illness and the role and side effects of medication; an agreement on what constitutes a relapse or crisis; clarification of situations in which the physician or hospital should be contacted; and the role of the family in medication monitoring.

The clinical advantages of meeting with family members far outweigh any drawbacks. Family members are less likely to interfere with any subsequent individual treatment, as with an adolescent, when they feel the therapist understands and respects their positions. Multiple perspectives more fully inform the clinician to make sound intervention decisions. Because a clinician's request for a family session may arouse concerns by parents or a spouse that they will be blamed or shamed for their loved one's problem, it is essential to explicitly convey the conviction that families are essential partners in all treatment, that they can make valuable contributions to patient gains, and that their stresses and concerns will be addressed. The invitation should convey respect for the family and interest in their experience. An initial family or couples assessment can lay the groundwork for timely conjoint sessions even if the therapy remains primarily individual. Systems-oriented therapists can use such sessions to share information, facilitate communication and change, consolidate new behaviors, or set the stage for the next phase of an individual treatment. An initial conjoint meeting tends to balance the alliance with an individual patient, permitting the therapist more latitude to bring other members in comfortably later, if needed.

Myths about the impossibility of a family meeting often are dispelled when other family members readily agree to convene. The initial act of sitting down together as a couple or family begins the therapeutic process. Even when a patient refuses to bring in a partner or other family members, or when they do not agree to a consultation, the process offers the clinician with useful diagnostic information.

At times, some therapists may be reluctant to convene a large family or include small children because of a fear of being overwhelmed or simply outnumbered, or because of concern about the impact on a child or vulnerable member. Actually, seeing all members conjointly can be easier when they are viewed as a system and when the therapist attends to stressful events, issues, or relationship patterns connecting members rather than addressing them as a collection of individuals. In an assessment session, it can be instructive to observe how a child climbs on a parent's lap when a sensitive or threatening issue arises or parents disagree. When a child misbehaves, a therapist can observe how parents handle the behavior.

For *child- and adolescent-focused problems,* an initial family assessment places the identified patient's behavior in context (Combrinck-Graham 2006). This is particularly true for a variety of conduct, eating, and anxiety-separation disorders. Problematic behavior often is connected to family dynamics, such as when a child is triangled into conflict between warring parents. A boy's angry, oppositional behavior toward his mother, a single parent, may be in part a deflection of anger and sense of abandonment with a nonresidential father's lack of contact, interest, or support. An individual intervention with the child or the mother would miss the crucial systemic context of the problem. For problems that have biological and/or social influences, it is especially important to reduce parental guilt and blame, often stoked by prior contacts with school or other authorities.

A therapist should join with parents to empower their authority and competence to handle child-focused problems. If a therapist takes an expert position in fixing or rescuing a child, it can communicate, "I am a better parent and can do what you couldn't." Adopting such a position can leave parents with a profound sense of deficiency and shame.

Many *inpatient programs* include a family orientation and assessment as part of their standard intake or initial evaluation process (Heru 2004). Family consultation/brief treatment often is seen as integral to inpatient evaluation and treatment and serves a number of functions. It promotes a joining process with the family system and helps in the identification and reduction of family resistances to treatment. It facilitates mutual familiarization about structure and functioning between the family and a treatment unit. It ensures opportunities for family psychoeducation related to the illness of the patient, pharmacological and psychosocial treatment options, and expected treatment and prognosis. It facilitates family members learning about the need for social support, respite, and self-care, and about family support organizations such as the National Alliance on Mental Illness (NAMI) and online resources. It also alerts the treatment team to dysfunctional transactional patterns that may be replicated within the treatment system, such as triangular conflicts involving the patient and two clinicians. Also, in situations in which the need for hospitalization versus less restrictive care is not clear-cut, assessment of the family as a support system is critical.

A prevention-oriented family consultation is extremely useful with the diagnosis or progression of a *serious illness or disability*. Most families lack a psychosocial map for the experience. In the *consultation-liaison or outpatient context*, families benefit enormously from information and support to cope and adapt to a family member's major illness. Family dynamics can influence compliance, disease course, and the well-being of the patient and key family caregivers (Campbell 2003; Weihs et al. 2002). Therefore, brief consultation with key family members near the time of initial diagnosis and at major nodal points over the course of the illness (e.g., rehospitalization, recurrence or progression of the illness, transfer to rehabilitation or hospice) can both facilitate the treatment process and support the family unit in a time of crisis (Rolland 1994, 2003). With the new era of genomics, family consultation will be increasingly needed in the context of genetic testing and living with risk information for a broad spectrum of medical and psychiatric conditions (Miller et al. 2006; Rolland and Williams 2005).

Research has demonstrated that a family-centered collaborative team approach that includes health and mental health care providers, patients, and their families fosters optimal biopsychosocial care (Blount 1998; McDaniel et al. 2007; Seaburn et al. 1997). Convening the family early on in an illness promotes this collaborative model of care. The rationale is more than crisis management: it is prevention oriented and psychoeducational, counteracting marginalization of family members. It encourages an ongoing relationship with a mental health care provider as the family proceeds with living with a serious illness. The Family Systems Illness Model developed by Rolland (1994, 2003) provides a useful framework for consultation with families facing chronic illness, disability, and loss. Convening families in the consultation-liaison context is not difficult, as family members typically visit their hospitalized member.

The therapist in a family-centered psychiatric consultation:

- Emphasizes that all family members are impacted by the strains and challenges of living with a major illness and addresses the immediate emotional and practical needs of the patient and family members, such as guilt, shame, helplessness, and the reactivation of old family conflicts around illness decision making.

- Provides information about the illness and treatment and ways in which family members can be helpful.
- Provides family psychoeducation regarding a psychosocial understanding of the particular illness over time in relation to family expectations, offering practical management guidelines. Such psychoeducation includes helping the family understand the illness in longitudinal and developmental terms: how different phases of the illness might affect plans and dreams for the patient, family members, and the family unit.
- Elicits history and information that may be vital to diagnosis and treatment decisions. Such information includes a family's multigenerational experience with illness and loss that may hinder or facilitate current coping and adaptation.
- Facilitates communication around illness, treatment-related, and caregiving issues and decisions.
- Understands the cultural and spiritual beliefs that guide the family. Such an understanding is essential to fostering culturally sensitive collaborative care and helping the family make meaning of the illness experience.
- Identifies high-risk, multistressed, or dysfunctional patients/families needing more intensive follow-up care.
- Educates the family about the usefulness of periodic family-centered consultations ("psychosocial checkups") and brief interventions at nodal points and transitions in the illness course, in the patient's or other family members' development, and in the family life cycle.

Brief Family Therapy

Brief family or couples therapy has been particularly useful when the chief complaint is a focal problem. Sometimes the complaint involves a problematic behavior, conflict, situation, life transition, or major life challenge, such as a serious chronic illness. A preventive, early intervention consultation-oriented approach with a family can avert a major crisis or spiraling of distress. Problematic behaviors can be helped by attention to the web of surrounding interactions. In the case of a child's sudden drop in school performance, intervention with the parents around their escalating conflict and threat of divorce would be imperative. Frequently, with focal problems, the therapist and family contract for a certain number of sessions, in which the goals are clearly delineated and progress can be objectively monitored. This approach is similar to individual brief treatment models. Depending on the kind of problem, structural, systemic/strategic, behavioral, and intergenerational models of family therapy are all well suited to brief, focal treatment. At completion of the contract, the therapist and family can re-negotiate a new contract or in complicated cases shift to more intensive long-term therapy. Some families learn to use family consultations and treatment in a periodic, time- and cost-effective way when family strains emerge over the life course. This approach is particularly useful for families coping with recurrence or exacerbation of psychiatric or physical disorders, who simply want to go on with their lives during periods of remission.

Intensive Family Therapy

More intensive family therapy may be needed in cases of multiple and chronic or entrenched difficulties. There is a myth that working with family members together is inherently more superficial than in one-to-one treatment. In fact, the experience is quite powerful, and lasting change can occur more rapidly than in individual therapy. First, in focusing only on the individual in pain, one is frequently trying to treat symptoms of a relationship problem involving others. In attending to the system, the therapist can anticipate reactivity to change and has more power to alter symptom-maintaining patterns. Second, intrapsychic issues are also interpersonal; the systems therapist working at the interactional level finds that behavioral change in the system is easier to bring about and facilitates intrapersonal change, regardless of the origin or chronicity of the problem. Third, direct intervention and change with significant family members, whether planned to occur in sessions or between sessions, has potential therapeutic benefit for all members, not only the current symptom-bearer.

Therapy may selectively focus on specific problems and those members most critically involved for problem solving. Different members may be brought in at different phases of intervention. Situations when involvement of additional members is indicated include 1) when they are part of the problem-maintaining system and 2) when they can be helpful in attaining treatment goals.

A family presenting with a child- or adolescent-focused problem is generally treated conjointly, including parents, siblings, and any other significant members of the household or extended family. In these situations, any marital problems identified during the assessment are best approached by strengthening the coparental alliance around solution of the presenting problem in the child's or adolescent's behavior or functioning. After the presenting child-focused issues are improved, the couple has established a working therapeutic alliance with the clinician, and there is a greater likelihood they will be willing to face their marital difficulties. With child or adolescent-focused issues, it is often preferable to have a single therapist meet individually with the identified patient and conjointly with the family.

Family therapy is useful for a range of other clinical situations. Separation, divorce, and remarriage involve myriad issues for a family that are often best addressed by conjoint sessions. Other clinical situations include chronic psychiatric and medical conditions, major stressful life events such as loss through death and work difficulties, and situations involving substance, sexual, or physical abuse. Problems identified as strongly connected to unresolved issues from the family of origin and in which key family members can participate are typically best treated conjointly.

Evidence-Based Multisystemic Intervention Models

The development of several evidence-based, multisystemic, multidimensional intervention models offers highly effective approaches with high-risk and seriously troubled youth through involvement of families and larger community systems (Henggeler et al. 1998, 2002; Liddle et al. 2002; Sexton and Alexander 2003; Szapocznik and Williams 2000). These family-centered approaches with adolescent conduct disorders and drug abuse also yield improvements in family functioning, including increased cohesion, communication, and parenting practices, which are significantly linked to more positive youth behavioral outcomes than in standard youth services. Multisystemic interventions may take a variety of forms and involve school counselors, teachers, coaches, and peer groups; these individuals may work with police officials, probation officers, and judges to address adolescent and family legal issues. They might help a youth and family access vocational services, youth development organizations, social support networks, and religious group resources.

With families that are often seen as unready, unwilling, or unmotivated for therapy, these approaches engage family members in a strengths-oriented, collaborative alliance. They develop a shared atmosphere of hope, expectation for change, a sense of responsibility (active agency), and empowerment (Sexton and Alexander 2003). Rather than troubled youths and their families being viewed as "resistant" to change, attempts are made to identify and overcome barriers to success in the therapeutic, family, and social contexts. Therapeutic contacts emphasize the positive and draw out systemic strengths and competencies for change. Clinicians maintain and clearly communicate an optimistic perspective throughout the assessment and intervention processes.

Couples Therapy

When couples problems are presented, the focus of therapy is on that relationship, with children being excluded, just as one would close the bedroom door. When individuals present with problems of intimacy and they are currently in a primary relationship, a couple evaluation and at least some couple

sessions are generally indicated. Interventions for couples with sexual difficulties have been highly successful with a range of presenting problems. Also,
when sexual problems are intertwined with relational difficulties, behavioral
techniques need to be applied within a systemic framework to address underlying issues. Couples therapy is also useful in situations in which one member
is affected by serious illness or disability and in which a relationship skew and
ongoing support or caregiving are likely (Rolland 1994, 2003).

An exclusive individual treatment lacking a systemic lens may achieve
certain individual goals for growth but at the cost of a marriage. Without
engaging the partner and directly assessing the relationship, the therapist
may gain a one-sided view of problems and an overly negative impression of
the partner. The empathic therapeutic bond may make the real-life relationship seem even less satisfactory by comparison. The therapist also risks
being triangled on the side of the client in scapegoating the spouse or in
futile attempts to change him or her ("My therapist agrees with me that it's
all your fault"). In couples therapy, the therapist takes a bipartial stance, reduces defensiveness and blame in vulnerability cycles, and facilitates mutual
understanding, communication, and support for positive relationship change
(Scheinkman and Fishbane 2004).

Couples therapy can facilitate individual therapy. The process of couples therapy typically leaves each partner with a clearer sense of issues that
he or she brought to the relationship, those of his or her partner, and those
that were co-constructed or caused by external factors. Usually, the pace of
individual treatment is faster, and relational issues that were initially fused
with personal ones have been ferreted out.

Individual Systemic Therapy

Individual systemic therapy involves a conceptual stance, incorporating sys-
tems-based thinking into individual treatment. This method is particularly
useful for young adults and older adults to better understand and repair
wounded, conflictual, or estranged family relationships; to gain perspective
and compassion for a parent's limitations; or to work on unresolved issues
with a parent who is deceased. Coaching methods are used for individuals to
become less anxious and reactive and more differentiated in order to change
their own part in "stuck" relational patterns (Carter and McGoldrick 2001).
First the individual is encouraged to gather more information and broader
perspectives from other key persons to enlarge his or her own subjective
view. With the aid of a genogram to note systemic patterns and their context, the clinician and client carefully plan meetings for change with key
family members outside sessions and later process those transactions. In this
approach, the focus is on changing oneself in transactions (rather than at-

tacking, blaming, or trying to change others), which interrupts old patterns and is more likely to generate positive response and client empowerment.

Family Psychoeducation

Family psychoeducation, empirically demonstrated to be an essential component of effective treatment with schizophrenia (Anderson et al. 1986), is widely used with a range of chronic mental and physical conditions and stressful life challenges (McFarlane et al. 2003). This approach counters the stigma, blame, and shame families too often experienced in traditional treatment settings. The clinicians respect families as valued partners in collaboration with health care providers. Family psychoeducation is based on the premise that families need vital information and support in the care of their loved one with challenging mental or physical conditions. The approach provides practical information about the condition, prognosis, medications, and treatment options, as well as support and guidelines for management and problem solving through predictable stressful periods and crises over the course of the disorder, and provides overall stress reduction for all family members.

Psychoeducational family interventions have been adapted to a variety of formats, including one-time or periodic family consultations, brief time-limited groups, and ongoing multifamily groups. Intervention "modules" can be timed with critical phases or transitions in a condition. This encourages families to accept and digest manageable portions of a long-term coping process. Examples include postdiagnosis or hospital discharge/community reentry and the initial crisis, chronic, terminal, or bereavement phases of a chronic or life-threatening illness (Rolland 1994). Psychoeducation is also valuable around such challenges as teen pregnancy, family separation and divorce, single parenting, and planned remarriage and stepfamily integration. It provides a cost-effective, preventive approach and can identify families at high risk of maladaptation or relapse for more intensive services.

Multifamily and Couples Groups

Multifamily group interventions, most often with a psychoeducational component, have been expanded to a wide range of psychiatric and medical populations (Fristad et al. 2003; Gonzalez and Steinglass 2002; McFarlane 2002). They have been utilized in inpatient, outpatient, and day treatment settings. Groups are typically composed of four or more patients with their spouses or with families, including parents, siblings, and significant kin or friends. Objectives may include the improvement of communication and structural patterns to reduce interactional stress and to facilitate optimal functioning, coping, and problem solving.

The group context provides opportunities for families to learn from one another and to try new adaptive patterns of relating and handling problems. Family members can relate to the experience of their counterparts in other families, gain perspective on their own stressful situation, reduce guilt and blame, and feel less stigma and isolation. Family relationship change is less threatening with the mutual supportive network the group provides.

Multifamily interventions tend to have a short-term structure, varying from a single daylong workshop (McFarlane 2002) to 6–8 weekly meetings, and may include monthly or occasional follow-up sessions. Psychoeducational groups, first developed by Anderson and colleagues (1986), have a strong informational component—for instance, teaching families about schizophrenia as a chronic biologically based illness and addressing related management and medication issues. Guidelines are offered for what to expect, common stressors, and ways to reduce tensions and support optimal functioning. This modular, time-limited format is particularly useful for a wide range of chronic psychiatric and physical disorders (Gonzalez and Steinglass 2002) and for life cycle challenges such as divorce and remarriage, single parenthood, and bereavement.

Ongoing multifamily or couples therapy groups, often meeting monthly, are useful and cost-effective alternatives or adjuncts to other modalities, particularly for situations of persistent biopsychosocial strain, as with chronic disorders. They establish support networks that extend well beyond the group sessions with families facing similar kinds of challenges.

Combined Interventions

With the expanding range of therapeutic approaches and the recognition that complex biopsychosocial problems are often not resolved by a single approach, combined modalities are increasingly common. For chronic disorders such as schizophrenia or serious physical conditions, research has documented the combined effectiveness of psychotropic interventions with individual, family, and group approaches (Anderson et al. 1986; Dixon et al. 2001; Goldstein et al. 1978). Treatment models for substance, physical, or sexual abuse also typically require a multimodality approach. It is essential for addiction and abusive behavior to be under control before couple or family intervention, for the safety of other family members.

A more complicated question is the advisability of a family therapist to conduct individual therapy with a family member or one or both members of a couple. Many family therapists include individual sessions in their therapeutic approach. Frequently, during an evaluation, meeting with individual members allows the clinician to gain a fuller picture, particularly when communication is guarded or volatile. Sometimes, in the course of treatment, individual sessions can help overcome reluctance to dialogue with other family members as a stepping-stone to the next phase of treatment. Likewise, systems-oriented therapists may include conjoint sessions in the course of an individual therapy. Careful planning, timing, and focus are important. Inpatient or partial hospitalization programs with built-in time limits of treatment may make it advantageous for the same therapist to conduct a number of treatment modalities. Family treatments that are intended for supportive or psychoeducational purposes can more easily be carried out by the individual therapist.

A family consultation or treatment component enhances collaboration with complex treatment plans. For example, compliance with pharmacotherapy is facilitated by discussing the treatment plan with the patient and family together. This approach encourages support for multimodality treatments, thereby reducing treatment resistance.

Conclusion

In this chapter we provided an overview of family systems concepts and approaches to clinical assessment and intervention. Applications of systems approaches in psychiatry were described, with guidelines for effective use of various family systems approaches and combination with other therapeutic modalities. More broadly, a developmental, systemic orientation has been shown to be valuable as an integrative framework for practicing a biopsychosocial model. It fosters an understanding of each person in family and sociocultural contexts, and facilitates respectful collaboration with families in any treatment plan for optimal functioning and well-being.

Key Points

Current family systems approaches to practice, despite some differences, are characterized by the following:

- A family-centered, collaborative model of care
- A biopsychosocial orientation: multiple, ongoing mutual influences
- A multigenerational, developmental, family life cycle perspective

Systemic approaches to practice attend to and address the following:

- Individual problems and functioning in family and sociocultural contexts
- The symptom-maintaining context of a problem and how it can effectively be altered
- Strengths, resources, and resilience alongside vulnerabilities, dysfunction, and risk

- Transactional processes in the couple relationship, family unit, and broad kin network

- Patterns, critical events, and transitions across the family life cycle and the generations, using a genogram and time line to track information

- Belief systems, organizational patterns, and communication/problem-solving processes

- Positive strivings, potential, and goals of every individual and family

- Relational resources that can be tapped for problem resolution and well-being

References

Anderson CM, Reiss D, Hogarty G: Schizophrenia and the Family. New York, Guilford, 1986

Anderson H: Conversation, Language, and Possibility: A Postmodern Approach to Therapy. New York, Basic Books, 1997

Beavers WR, Hampson R: Measuring family competence: the Beavers systems model, in Normal Family Processes: Growing Diversity and Complexity, 3rd Edition. Edited by Walsh F. New York, Guilford, 2003

Bengston VG: Beyond the nuclear family: the increasing importance of multigenerational bonds. J Marriage Fam 63:1–16, 2001

Blount S: Integrated Primary Care: The Future of Medical and Mental Health Collaboration. New York, WW Norton, 1998

Boscolo L, Cecchin G, Hoffman L, et al: Milan Systemic Family Therapy: Conversations in Theory and Practice. New York, Basic Books, 1987

Boszormenyi-Nagy I: Foundations of Contextual Family Therapy. New York, Brunner/Mazel, 1987

Bowen M: Family Therapy in Clinical Practice. New York, Jason Aronson, 1978

Boyd-Franklin N: Black Families in Therapy: Understanding the African American Experience, 2nd Edition. New York, Guilford, 2003

Byng-Hall J: Rewriting Family Scripts: Improvisation and Systems Change. New York, Guilford, 1995

Campbell T: The effectiveness of family interventions for physical disorders. J Marital Fam Ther 29:263–281, 2003

Carter B, McGoldrick M: The Expanded Family Life Cycle: Individual, Family, and Social Perspectives, 3rd Edition. New York, Allyn & Bacon, 1999

Carter B, McGoldrick M: Advances in coaching: family therapy with one person. J Marital Fam Ther 27:281–300, 2001

Combrinck-Graham L: Children in Family Contexts: Perspectives on Treatment, 2nd Edition. New York, Guilford, 2006

Coontz S: The Way We Really Are: Coming to Terms With America's Changing Families. New York, Basic Books, 1997

Dattilio FM: The restructuring of family schemas: a cognitive-behavioral perspective. J Marital Fam Ther 31:15–30, 2005 de Shazer S: Clues: Investigating Solutions in Brief Therapy. New York, WW Norton, 1988

Dixon L, McFarlane WR, Lefley H, et al: Evidence-based practices for services to families of people with psychiatric disabilities. Psychiatr Serv 52:903–910, 2001

Engel GH: The clinical application of the biopsychosocial model. Am J Psychiatry 137:535–544, 1980

Falicov CJ: Training to think culturally: a multidimensional comparative framework. Fam Process 34:373–388, 1995

Falicov CJ: Latino Families in Therapy: A Guide to Multicultural Practice. New York, Guilford, 1998

Framo J: Family of origin as a therapeutic resource for adults in marital and family therapy: you can and should go home again. Fam Process 15:193–210, 1980

Freedman J, Combs G: Narrative Therapy: The Social Construction of Preferred Realities. New York, WW Norton, 1996

Fristad MA, Goldberg-Arnold JS, Gavazzi SM: Multi-family psychoeducation groups in the treatment of children with mood disorders. J Marital Fam Ther 29:491–504, 2003

Goldenberg I, Goldenberg H: Family Therapy: An Overview, 6th Edition. Pacific Grove, CA, Thomson (Brooks/Cole), 2004

Goldner V: Generation and gender: normative and covert hierarchies. Fam Process 27:17–21, 1988

Goldstein M, Rodnick E, Evans J, et al: Drug and family therapy in the aftercare treatment of acute schizophrenics. Arch Gen Psychiatry 35:1169–1177, 1978

Gonzalez S, Steinglass P: Application of multifamily groups in chronic medical disorders, in Multifamily Groups in the Treatment of Severe Psychiatric Disorders. Edited by McFarlane WF. New York, Guilford, 2002, pp 315–341

Gottman J: The Marriage Clinic: A Scientifically Based Marital Therapy. New York, WW Norton, 1999

Griffith J, Griffith ME: Encountering the Sacred in Psychotherapy: How to Talk With People About Their Spiritual Lives. New York, Guilford, 2002

Haley J: Problem-Solving Therapy. San Francisco, CA, Jossey-Bass, 1976

Henggeler SW, Schoenwald SK, Borduin CM, et al: Multi-Systemic Treatment of Antisocial Behavior in Children and Adolescents. New York, Guilford, 1998

Henggeler SW, Clingempeel W, Brondino MJ, et al: Four-year follow-up of multisystemic therapy with substance-abusing and substance-dependent juvenile offenders. J Am Acad Child Adolesc Psychiatry 41:868–874, 2002

Heru A: Basic family skills for an inpatient psychiatrist: meeting ACGME core competency requirements. Fam Syst Health 22:216–227, 2004

Heru A: Family psychiatry: from research to practice. Am J Psychiatry 163:962–968, 2006

Hetherington M, Kelly J: For Better or Worse: Divorce Reconsidered. New York, WW Norton, 2002

Hoffman L: Constructing realities: an art of lenses. Fam Process 29:1–13, 1990

Imber-Black E, Roberts J, Whiting R (eds): Rituals in Families and Family Therapy, 2nd Edition. New York, WW Norton, 2003

Jackson D: Family rules: marital quid pro quo. Arch Gen Psychiatry 12:589–594, 1965

Johnson S: The Practice of Emotionally Focused Couple Therapy: Creating Connection. New York, Brunner/Mazel, 1996

Lebow J: The integrative revolution in couple and family therapy. Fam Process 36:1–17, 1997

Liddle HA, Santisteban DA, Levant RF, et al (eds): Family Psychology: Science-Based Interventions. Washington, DC, American Psychological Association, 2002

McDaniel S, Hepworth J, Doherty H: Medical Family Therapy: Psychosocial Treatment of Families With Health Problems, 2nd Edition. New York, Basic Books, 2007

McFarlane WF (ed): Multifamily Groups in the Treatment of Severe Psychiatric Disorders. New York, Guilford, 2002

McFarlane WR, Dixon L, Lukens E, et al: Family psychoeducation and schizophrenia: a review of the literature. J Marital Fam Ther 29:223–245, 2003

McGoldrick M, Hardy K (ed): Re-Visioning Family Therapy: Race, Culture, and Gender in Clinical Practice, 2nd Edition. New York, Guilford, 2008

McGoldrick M, Giordano J, Garcia-Preto N: Ethnicity and Family Therapy, 3rd Edition. New York, Guilford, 2005

McGoldrick M, Gerson R, Petry S: Genograms: Assessment and Intervention, 3rd Edition. New York, WW Norton, 2008

Miller S, McDaniel S, Rolland J, et al (eds): Individuals, Families, and the New Era of Genetics: Biopsychosocial Perspectives. New York, WW Norton, 2006

Minuchin S: Families and Family Therapy. Cambridge, MA, Harvard University Press, 1974

Nichols M, Schwartz R: Family Therapy: Concepts and Methods, 7th Edition. Needham Heights, MA, Allyn & Bacon, 2005

Olson DH, Gorell D: Circumplex model of marital and family systems, in Normal Family Processes, 3rd Edition. Edited by Walsh F. New York, Guilford, 2003, pp 514–544

Patterson GR, Reid JB, Jones RR, et al: A Social Learning Approach to Family Intervention. Eugene, OR, Castalia, 1975

Reiss D: The Family's Construction of Reality. Cambridge, MA, Harvard University Press, 1981

Rolland JS: Families, Illness, and Disability: An Integrative Model. New York, Basic Books, 1994

Rolland JS: Families and parental illness: a conceptual framework. J Fam Ther 21:242–267, 1999

Rolland JS: Mastering family challenges: coping with serious illness and disability, in Normal Family Processes, 3rd Edition. Edited by Walsh F. New York, Guilford, 2003, pp 460–489

Rolland JS, Williams JK: Toward a biopsychosocial model for 21st century genetics. Fam Process 44:1:3–24, 2005

Ryan C, Epstein N, Keitner G, et al: The McMaster Approach. New York, Routledge & Kegan Paul, 2005

Santisteban DA, Coatsworth J, Perez-Vidal A, et al: Efficacy of brief strategic family therapy in modifying Hispanic adolescent behavior problems and substance use. J Fam Psychol 17:121–133, 2003

Satir V: The New Peoplemaking. Palo Alto, CA, Science & Behavior Books, 1988

Scheinkman M, Fishbane M: The vulnerability cycle: working with impasses in couple therapy. Fam Process 43:279–299, 2004

Seaburn D, Gunn W, Mauksch L, et al: Models of Collaboration: A Guide for Mental Health Professionals Working With Health Care Practitioners. New York, Basic Books, 1997

Sexton T, Alexander J: Functional family therapy: a mature clinical model for working with at-risk adolescents and their families, in Handbook of Family Therapy. Edited by Sexton T, Weeks G, Robbins M. New York, Brunner-Routledge, 2003, pp 323–363

Sheinberg M, Fraenkel P: The Relational Trauma of Incest: A Family Based Approach to Treatment. New York, Guilford, 2001

Szapocznik J, Williams RA: Brief strategic family therapy: twenty-five years of interplay among theory, research and practice in adolescent behavior problems and drug abuse. Clin Child Fam Psychol Rev 3:117–134, 2000

von Bertalanffy L: General systems theory and psychiatry—an overview, in General Systems Theory and Psychiatry. Edited by Gray W, Duhl FJ, Rizzo D. Boston, MA, Little, Brown, 1969, pp 33–46

Walsh F (ed): Spiritual Resources in Family Therapy. New York, Guilford, 1999

Walsh F: Family resilience: a framework for clinical practice. Fam Process 42:1–18, 2003a

Walsh F (ed): Normal Family Processes, 3rd Edition. New York, Guilford, 2003b

Walsh F: Strengthening Family Resilience, 2nd Edition. New York, Guilford, 2006

Walsh F: Traumatic loss and major disasters: strengthening family and community resilience. Fam Process 46:207–227, 2007

Walsh F: Family transitions: risk and resilience, in The American Psychiatric Publishing Textbook of Child and Adolescent Psychiatry, 4th Edition. Edited by Dulcan M. Washington, DC, American Psychiatric Publishing (in press)

Walsh F, McGoldrick M (eds): Living Beyond Loss: Death in the Family, 2nd Edition. New York, WW Norton, 2004

Weakland J, Fisch R, Watzlawick P, et al: Brief therapy: focused problem resolution. Fam Process 13:141–168, 1974

Weihs K, Fisher L, Baird M: Families, Health, and Behavior—a section of the commissioned report by the Committee on Health and Behavior: Research, Practice and Policy, Division of Neuroscience and Behavioral Health and Division of Health Promotion and Disease Prevention, Institute of Medicine, National Academy of Sciences. Fam Syst Health 20:7–57, 2002

Whitaker C: Symbolic experiential family therapy: model and methodology, in The Evolution of Psychotherapy. Edited by Zeig JK. Philadelphia, PA, Brunner/Mazel, 1992, pp 13–23

White M, Epston D: Narrative Means to Therapeutic Ends. New York, WW Norton, 1990

Wright L, Watson WL, Bell JM: Beliefs: The Heart of Healing in Families and Illness. New York, Basic Books, 1996

Wynne LC, McDaniel S, Weber T (eds): System Consultation: A New Perspective for Family Therapy. New York, Guilford, 1986

Suggested Readings

Boyd-Franklin N: Black Families in Therapy: Understanding the African American Experience, 2nd Edition. New York, Guilford, 2003

Campbell T: The effectiveness of family interventions for physical disorders. J Marital Fam Ther 29:263–281, 2003

Carter B, McGoldrick M: The Expanded Family Life Cycle: Individual, Family, and Social Perspectives, 3nd Edition. New York, Allyn & Bacon, 1999

Combrinck-Graham L: Children in Family Contexts: Perspectives on Treatment, 2nd Edition. New York, Guilford, 2006

Falicov CJ: Latino Families in Therapy: A Guide to Multicultural Practice. New York, Guilford, 1998

Heru A: Family psychiatry: from research to practice. Am J Psychiatry 163:962–968, 2006

Liddle HA, Santisteban DA, Levant RF, et al (eds): Family Psychology: Science-Based Interventions. Washington, DC, American Psychological Association, 2002

McGoldrick M, Gerson R, Shellenberger S: Genograms: Assessment and Intervention, 3rd Edition. New York, WW Norton, 2007

Minuchin S: Families and Family Therapy. Cambridge, MA, Harvard University Press, 1974

Rolland JS: Families, Illness, and Disability: An Integrative Model. New York, Basic Books, 1994

Rolland JS, Williams JK: Toward a biopsychosocial model for 21st century genetics. Fam Process 44:1:3–24, 2005

Walsh F: Family resilience: a framework for clinical practice. Fam Process 42:1–18, 2003

Walsh F: Strengthening Family Resilience, 2nd Edition. New York, Guilford, 2006

Chapter 19

Couples Therapy

Jay L. Lebow, Ph.D.
Molly F. Gasbarrini

Couples therapy[1] has emerged in recent years as a crucial intervention modality in mental health treatment. This growing attention to couples therapy stems from a number of sources.

Perhaps the foremost of these sources is the epidemic of marital difficulties in the Western world. Epidemiological studies typically find 20% of the population to be experiencing marital distress at any particular moment in time (Gurman and Fraenkel 2002). Moreover, the divorce rate has stabilized, with approximately half of all marriages ending in divorce. A total of 10%–15% of couples separate in the first 4 years of marriage, and 70% of marriages last a decade (Emery 1999).

---

[1]The words *couple* and *marital* in this chapter are both employed to describe the full range of committed couple relationships, and thus the terms *marital therapy* and *couples therapy* are interchangeable in what follows.

Correspondingly, there is a high level of demand in society today for couples therapy, given the natural ecological fit between couples therapy and marital distress and the fact that couples therapy is the only evidence-based treatment available for this indication. By far the most frequent reason for seeking mental health treatment identified in surveys of those beginning treatment is relationship difficulties (typically so identified in 40% of clients) (Gurman and Fraenkel 2002). There has been an overwhelming change in public attitude about couples therapy over the last few decades. Whereas couples therapy was once stigmatized, increasingly it has become accepted as the most viable treatment for people experiencing problems in their relationships. Paradoxically, in many circles of Western society, the stigma has been reassigned to people who choose to end their marriages *without* seeking couples therapy. A survey of psychotherapists conducted by Orlinsky and colleagues found that 70% of therapists treat at least some couples (Orlinsky and Ronnestad 2005; Ronnestad and Orlinsky 2005). Much of this therapy is aimed at marital difficulties, but couples therapy also includes preventive and "enrichment" work (Gurman and Fraenkel 2002).

Another source for the increased attention to couples therapy is the individual and family comorbidities associated with couple distress. Persons with marital distress tend to have a higher level of work difficulty, more health problems, and more problems in their children, particularly in the wake of high conflict (Snyder and Whisman 2003; Whisman and Uebelacker 2006). Research has established that the causal pathways are circular: psychopathology leads to higher rates of marital difficulty, and marital distress leads to higher rates of psychopathology (Snyder et al. 2006; Whisman and McClelland 2005). The rates of various DSM-IV-TR (American Psychiatric Association 2000) disorders typically double in those who experience martial distress compared with those who do not (Whisman 1999). Whisman (1999) found a strong association between marital distress and the prevalence rates of psychiatric disorder, including each of the 15 major groups of psychiatric disorders. Among individuals with significant levels of marital distress, 15% had concurrent mood disorders, 28% had anxiety disorders, and 15% had alcohol or substance use disorders. Much research has also demonstrated the negative impact of marital distress on physical health and work productivity, as well as on the frequency and severity of problems in children (effects on children are especially pronounced when there are high levels of conflict) (Emery 1999; Wood and Miller 2002). Couples therapy has been demonstrated to be an effective treatment or component in the treatment of several individual disorders, including depression, anxiety, and substance abuse.

As the need for interventions for couples has grown and become more salient, couples researchers and clinicians have responded. Over the last 20 years, couples therapy has moved from a backwater in the field of psychotherapy to a field in which there are numerous well-articulated approaches and a strong evidence base for its efficacy (Gurman and Fraenkel 2002; Johnson and Lebow 2000).

In this chapter, we provide an overview of the field of couples therapy today. First, we review briefly the history of couples therapy. Second, we explore current research on couple processes that serve as the underpinning for today's couples therapy. After a brief discussion of couple assessment, we summarize today's most widely circulated couples therapies. We then briefly review the evidence for the impact of couples therapy.

History of Couples Therapy

Gurman and Fraenkel (2002) describe the theoretical and clinical history of couples therapy as having emerged in four phases. Phase I, which they call *atheoretical marriage counseling formation*, began in 1929 with the emergence of several pioneers who eventually established the American Association of Marriage Counselors. Phase I was also marked by the first legal recognition of marriage counseling as a profession in 1963 and the first publication of professional literature broaching the subject (Gurman and Fraenkel 2002). During that time, most clinicians were professionals who did not primarily identify themselves as psychotherapists, such as clergy and social workers (Broderick and Schrader 1991). Typically, they did not see the spouses conjointly, as is the common practice today. Michaelson (1963) estimated that in the 1940s, only 5% of couples experienced counseling conjointly; by the mid-1960s, this number had increased only to about 15%.

Phase II, which Gurman and Fraenkel call *psychoanalytic experimentation*, saw the development of couples therapy primarily as a conjoint approach, beginning with both spouses participating in therapy individually but being treated by the same therapist (Greene 1965), and gradually moving toward the currently espoused approach, wherein both spouses participate in conjoint sessions with a therapist (Gurman and Fraenkel 2002). As the title suggests, the approaches used most by therapists during this phase were psychoanalytic and included the use of free association and dream analysis, the interpretation of defenses, and examination of the unconscious. In Phase III, there was then an expansion of the theoretical breadth of couples therapies. The most recent era (Phase IV) has included the development of empirically supported treatments, the extension of therapies to include feminism and multiculturalism, a movement to integration, and a focus on utilizing couples therapy as part of multiformat therapies for treating Axis I and Axis II disorders.

Couple Processes

Couple treatment builds on the emerging science of couple relationships, a field in which John Gottman is arguably the world's most influential contributor. In his work he has explicated the differences between satisfied and unsatisfied couples and how couples move toward dissatisfaction and divorce (Asher and Gottman 1973; Gottman 1990, 1993, 1994, 1999; Gottman and Carrere 1994; Gottman and Krokoff 1989; Gottman and Notarius 2000, 2002; Gottman et al. 1998). If we are to know how to prevent and treat dissatisfaction, we must understand the characteristics of unsatisfied couples.

Gottman has identified several differences between satisfied and dissatisfied couples. First, satisfied couples manifest high rates of positive to negative behaviors in their exchanges, maintaining a ratio of 5 positive behaviors to 1 negative behavior, whereas dissatisfied couples manifest a ratio of about 0.8 to 1. Second, distressed and divorcing couples manifest high levels of what Gottman has called "The Four Horsemen": defensiveness, criticism, contempt, and stonewalling. Gottman has shown that these four characteristics, which manifest early in marriage and often display nonverbally, are the best predictors of later divorce and intractable marital distress (Gottman and Levenson 1992).

Gottman has also conducted research that indicates that most problems in marriages tend to be irreconcilable and stable over time, even in happy couples. Successful couples learn to problem-solve and navigate their differences through direct communication, whereas unsuccessful couples get stuck in a pattern of conflict. Similarly, Gottman has shown that, contrary to the general public's beliefs, satisfied couples do argue but that they resolve their differences successfully and avoid common traps such as too-rapid startup by the partner stating the issue (who often is the female spouse) and flooding on the part of the listener (who often tends to be the male spouse) (Gottman 1998).

Gottman (and numerous others) has also shown that not only our behaviors but also our cognitions contribute to the levels of satisfaction in marriage. *Positive sentiment override*, the sense of feeling positively about one's partner and viewing events and processes within the relationship in the context of that positive view, is crucial to couple satisfaction.

Other researchers have shown that many unhappy couples are engaged in sequences of demand/withdrawal (Bradbury et al. 2000; Roberts and Krokoff 1990). This type of interaction pattern is present when one partner tries to engage the other in communication, problem solving, or affection, and the other partner distances. More often than not, it is the male who withdraws and the female who pursues (Kluwer et al. 1997).

Yet another important line of research has shown that distressed couples are more likely to engage in violent behavior with each other than is typically thought (Fritz and O'Leary 2004).

This growing body of research about couple processes has informed newer treatments addressing marital distress. There is no universally accepted treatment for marital distress, but there *is* a set of universally shared process goals. These goals include providing a calm environment in which relationship difficulties can be communicated and negotiated, increasing mutual acceptance, ameliorating crisis, improving communication, improving problem solving, building attachment, improving marital friendship, and improving sexuality (Lebow 1999, 2003). Varying approaches differ in the extent to which they accentuate these goals.

Assessment of Marital Distress

There are numerous foci for assessment in couples. The most common concerns stated in couples therapy are communication, problem solving, affective connection, sexuality, conflict resolution, violence, parenting, finances, and relationships with extended family. Looking beyond such surface manifestations, couples can be assessed along a number of systemic levels, including behavior, cognition, affect, and the internal dynamics.

A number of assessment tools are available for couples therapists to use in tracking the degree of marital distress. Many of these tools are self-report questionnaires that the couple may fill out prior to their initial session. These questionnaires include the Marital Satisfaction Inventory—Revised (Snyder and Aikman 1999), which is used to assess marital satisfaction; the Weiss-Cerreto Marital Status Inventory (Weiss and Cerreto 1980), which is used to assess partners' thoughts about ending the relationship; the Dyadic Adjustment Scale (Spanier 1976), which is used to assess relationship satisfaction; the Area of Change Questionnaire (Weiss and Heyman 1990), which is used to assess areas of concern; and the Conflict Tactics Scale (Straus et al. 1996), which is used to assess violent and controlling behaviors. More complex measures utilized in the laboratory focus on the observation of behavior. These include Gottman's Rapid Couples Interaction Scoring System (Krokoff et al. 1989) and the Marital Interaction Coding System (Sperry 2004; Weiss and Heyman 1990).

Treatment Approaches

Numerous couples therapies have been developed. In the following sections, we summarize today's most prominent treatments, emphasizing those with the strongest evidence base.

Behavioral Couples Therapy

Behavioral couples therapy (BCT) is a treatment developed in various forms by Jacobson and Margolin, Stuart, and Weiss (Jacobson and Gurman 1995). Based in social exchange theory (Thibaut and Kelley 1959), BCT attempts, as its primary process goal, to increase the frequency of reciprocal positive behaviors demonstrated by each partner, with the understanding that each partner's behavior influences the other, creating a circular and reciprocal sequence of positive reinforcers. There are two main components to BCT (Jacobson and Christensen 1996): behavior exchange and communication/problem-solving training. The goal of behavioral exchange techniques is to increase positive behaviors and/or decrease negative behaviors in the couple's daily life. The therapist assigns behavioral exchange techniques as homework that the couple is asked to complete between therapy sessions. For example, the therapist may assign a couple to have a "love day," wherein each partner decides to enact specific behaviors, such as putting away the clean dishes or giving the other a neck rub, that will make the other person feel good. Communication or problem-solving training is administered in addition to behavioral exchange techniques to teach the couple skills that will enable them to solve future problems on their own. Therapists often teach a skill called *reflective listening*, whereby one partner expresses a feeling, thought, or emotion, and the other partner summarizes and restates what the other has just conveyed before responding. BCT has served as the foundation for the creation of the Prevention and Enhancement Rehabilitation Program, an evidence-based marital enrichment and divorce prevention program developed by University of Denver researchers Howard Markman and Scott Stanley that has gained considerable popularity and been evaluated in several longitudinal studies (e.g., Markman et al. 1993; Stanley et al. 1995). BCT has been widely investigated, and its efficacy has been demonstrated in more than 20 studies (Dimidjian et al. 2002).

Cognitive-Behavioral Couples Therapy

Cognitive-behavioral couples therapy (CBCT) was developed in accordance with the belief that relationship dysfunction occurs in part because people process information inappropriately or because they evaluate their relationship and their partners according to unreasonable standards. CBCT adds a cognitive emphasis to BCT. The assumption is that once people's distorted appraisals of events are altered, positive changes in behavior and emotion will ensue. CBCT therapists refer to two different types of stress in a relationship: primary distress and secondary distress. Primary distress results from the unmet fundamental needs of one partner (e.g., needs for intimacy, affiliation, achievement, autonomy). Secondary distress is the result of people using maladaptive strategies to address the conflict over primary distress (e.g., ignoring each other, verbally or physically attacking each other) (Epstein and Baucom 2002).

Typically CBCT is delivered within 8–25 sessions of weekly therapy (Baucom et al. 2002). The first 2–3 sessions are devoted to assessment and are followed by a feedback session, during which the couple and therapist work together to define treatment goals. Behavioral interventions may include behavioral exchange techniques and communication/problem-solving skills. Cognitive interventions may include *Socratic questioning* and *guided discovery*. Socratic questioning involves asking the client a series of questions that help him or her to reevaluate the logic or line of thinking that led the client to establish certain beliefs. This technique is often helpful in illuminating underlying issues affecting cognitive functioning that would not otherwise surface (Baucom et al. 2002). Guided discovery can include various techniques (such as role-playing or exploring the pros and cons of conducting the relationship according to each partner's standards) that will create experiences that lead one or both partners to develop a different perspective on the relationship.

CBCT has been demonstrated to be as effective as BCT in improving couple adjustment and communication and has demonstrated efficacy relative to wait-list control groups (Baucom and Lester 1986; Baucom et al. 1990).

Integrative Behavioral Couples Therapy

Recognizing the limits of BCT and CBCT in achieving lasting change, Jacobson and Christensen (1996) developed integrative behavioral couples therapy (IBCT), a treatment that adds the concept of emotional acceptance to the framework of BCT. IBCT integrates behavioral interventions to effect change along with strategies to promote mutual acceptance and increase positive sentiment. Jacobson and Christensen theorize that in the early stages of a relationship, couples appreciate the differences in personality and functioning between them as the source of their attraction to each other. However, as time goes on, these differences can become sources of concern, even of discontent, and distressed couples may respond with mutual coercion, vilification, and polarization (Dimidjian et al. 2002). Designed to help couples effectively navigate their differences and conflicts, IBCT focuses not only on the agent of behavior but also on the recipient of behavior, with the understanding that increased acceptance both reduces conflict and, paradoxically, serves as a catalyst for change. Change techniques are directed toward the perpetrator to alter some behavior or lack of behavior. Acceptance techniques are aimed at the recipient of the behavior to help soften the adversarial stance that partners often take toward each other (Doss et al. 2002). This acceptance work is based on Gottman's findings that some problems simply cannot be solved (Gottman 1998, 1999). Instead of aiming to resolve the conflict, IBCT "attempts to turn areas of conflict into sources of intimacy and closeness" (Jacobson 1992, p. 497).

IBCT therapists identify one central theme for each couple they treat. The theme is a summary of the central issue the couple is facing. From the IBCT viewpoint, as couples make efforts to change each other, a polarization process occurs that serves to exacerbate the conflict between partners. IBCT therapists call the result the *mutual trap*, the hopelessness and frustration the couples experience as a result of the defeat they face upon trying to change one another. In IBCT, the theme, polarization process, and mutual trap are collectively termed *the formulation*. Unlike BCT therapists, IBCT therapists are interested in the history of the relationship, the individuals' family-of-origin history, and an individual's previous romantic relationships. This information is gathered through the assessment portion of the treatment.

Doss et al. (2002) describe four broad methods for increasing emotional acceptance: 1) empathic joining around a problem (creating intimacy by examining the problem together), 2) unified detachment in examining a problem ("taking a step back" to examine the problem as objectively as possible), 3) increasing tolerance of an aversive problem (for example, by presenting the positive aspects of a negative behavior), and 4) increasing self-care until the problem is ameliorated or alleviated (this can include encouraging the distressed partner to call a friend, get a professional massage, engage in physical exercise, express negative emotions through journaling, etc.). Outcomes achieved with IBCT were at least comparable, and in some ways superior, to BCT in the largest randomized controlled trial of marital therapy thus far conducted (B. Baucom et al. 2005; Christensen et al. 1995, 2004, 2006).

Emotionally Focused Couples Therapy

Emotionally focused couples therapy (EFT), an experiential approach developed by Susan Johnson, focuses on couple emotion and attachment (Johnson 2004; Johnson and Denton 2002). The treatment focuses not on understanding and excavating the past but on recreating bonds in couples by "restructuring and expanding their emotional responses to each other" (Johnson and Denton 2002). The new secure bond enables couples to better cope with crises and life transitions and to experience a more satisfying cycle of interaction. Couples are also encouraged to explore their vulnerabilities together in order to increase attachment to one another and provide opportunities for mutual soothing.

Johnson and Denton (2002) outline three main tasks to be accomplished by the EFT therapist: "first, to create a safe, collaborative alliance; second, to access and expand the emotional responses that guide the couple's interactions; and third, to restructure those interactions in the direction of accessibility and responsiveness" (p. 222). The therapist uses techniques based on humanistic/experiential therapies (Greenberg et al. 1998; Rogers 1951) that focus on acceptance, empathy, and authenticity. The therapist creates a secure base for the therapy by refocusing the couple to see the negative interaction cycle as the common enemy—instead of seeing each other as the enemy. A variety of intervention techniques are used to achieve the goal of exploring and reformulating emotions within the couple. The therapist may use heightening techniques, such as repetition, images, or metaphors, to help the couple engage in a constructive emotional experience. Johnson and Denton (2002, p. 235) offer the following examples of heightening techniques: "So could you say that again, directly to her, that you do shut her out?" "It seems like this is so difficult for you, like climbing a cliff, so scary." Couples are also encouraged to engage in the process of softening, in which "hard" emotions like anger are explored deeper and transformed into "softer" emotions like fear, sadness, and shame. In these ways, partners are encouraged to be open and vulnerable, and helped to experience secure attachment with one another.

Research on EFT outcomes indicates that after concluding EFT (delivered in 10–12 sessions), 70%–75% of couples no longer view their relationship as distressed (Johnson et al. 1999).

Object Relations Couples Therapy

Object relations couples therapy (Scharff and de Varela 2005) is an offshoot of individual object relations–based treatments. Object relations theory views the infant as primarily driven by the desire to have a relationship with a nurturing figure (Scharff and Bagnini 2002). As the infant bonds, attachment develops. However, the attachment experience is inherently unsatisfying because the infant's needs cannot be met before they cause discomfort. In turn, the infant self is split into three distinct parts: 1) the central self, whose needs are satisfied and met by the mother; 2) the craving self, who is attached longingly and unsatisfyingly to an unavailable figure; and 3) the rejecting self, who is angrily attached to the rejecting figure. Object relations theory holds that couples seek lost parts of themselves in their spouses, and "that through marriage unacceptable parts of the self can be expressed vicariously" (Scharff and Bagnini 2002, p. 60). The success of the marriage depends on the spouses' ability to receive and return these projections to each other as well as contain and modify each other's views of the self and the other (the object). Object relations couples therapy provides a safe holding environment in which the couple is enabled to better understand their own defenses and anxieties, and ultimately free themselves from the confining pattern of projection and identification. Interpretation of the mutual transferences that emerge between the couple is a major agent of change. Object relations couples therapy is typically delivered as long as necessary, with an ideal average duration of 2 years. Sessions are longer, up to 90 minutes in length, and may occur once or twice weekly (Scharff and Bagnini 2002).

Affective Reconstruction

Affective reconstruction is a pluralistic, developmental approach whose theory is derived from the main assertion that couple difficulties often stem from injuries sustained in previous relationships that cause partners to develop defensive strategies that interfere with intimacy (Snyder and Schneider 2002). As defined by Snyder and Schneider (2002), affective reconstruction is "the interpretation of persistent maladaptive relationship patterns as having their source in previous developmental experiences" (p. 151). This process is a hierarchical, pluralistic model that incorporates structural, behavioral, and cognitive interventions to address six fundamental tasks: 1) developing a collaborative alliance, 2) containing disabling relationship crises, 3) strengthening the marital dyad, 4) promoting relevant relationship skills, 5) challenging the cognitive components of relationship distress, and 6) examining developmental sources of relationship distress. Affective reconstruction affords the therapist flexibility to move in a nonlinear fashion among these six tasks according to the couple's needs and level of functioning. Treatment length is 25 sessions, each 50 minutes in duration, although many couples require fewer sessions and some require more (Snyder and Schneider 2002). An earlier form of this treatment (then called *insight-oriented couples therapy*) proved not only effective but also highly durable in its effects, with most couples maintaining change at a 5-year follow-up (Snyder and Wills 1989).

Brief Integrative Marital Therapy

Brief integrative marital therapy (BIMT), developed by Alan Gurman at the University of Wisconsin, generally is focused on the present. It tends to be pragmatic, brief (as the name suggests) in duration, and problem focused in nature. Strongly influenced by both behavior therapy and object relations therapy, much of its theory rests on the foundation created by attachment theory and general family systems theory (Gurman 2002). BIMT operates according to the belief that both our interpersonal and intrapersonal worlds need attending to, that neither can exist meaningfully without the other, and that problems cannot be solved without addressing both factors.

The three central therapist goals in BIMT are to teach relationship skills, to challenge dysfunctional relationship rules, and to inculcate systemic thinking. This final goal involves helping clients become "more sensitive to the recurrent circular processes in their relationship that maintain their primary problems, including intrapsychic events and cues" (Gurman 2002, p. 200). This can often be achieved by asking pertinent questions that require the couple to observe and reflect on their own functioning. The BIMT therapist is equipped to intervene in a variety of ways to achieve these goals.

BIMT therapists believe that it is essential to modify the overt behaviors about which couples complain, as do behavior therapists. But BIMT therapists, much like object relations therapists, also believe it is essential to modify the patterns of *collusion*, or *mutual projective identification*, in a relationship. Collusion, as already described, is the process by which each partner projects the undesired parts of his or her own self onto the other partner, who thereby accepts the projection and behaves in accordance with it. Gurman (2002) has described the "implicit agreement, or 'collusion,' not to talk about or challenge the agreement": "The collusion is a joint, shared avoidance that involves both intrapsychic and interpersonal defenses against various fears (e.g., merger, attack, abandonment, etc.). Collusion is a bilateral process in which partners seek to maintain a consistent, if maladaptive, sense of self" (p. 186).

Blocking interventions are designed to interrupt collusive processes as they transpire during a session. *Cognitive restructuring* is one such blocking intervention that is derived from CBCT whose goal is to target the automatic thoughts generated about a partner, especially negative overgeneralizations about the partner's character or behavior. Alternatively, the therapist may choose to "shift affective gears," much like in EFT, in which the therapist refocuses one partner's "hard" feelings (e.g., anger) about the other partner's behavior to his or her "soft" feelings (e.g., sadness). The therapist may also use self-control coaching as a blocking strategy, in which the therapist trains the partner to alter his or her response to the other partner's undesired behavior using behavioral techniques. Another technique utilized is *anticollusive questioning*. During this process, the therapist asks specific but often rhetorical questions that illuminate the collusive processes taking place within the session and encourage the couple to reflect on them and address the roles they play in the relationship. BIMT sessions are typically 50–60 minutes long, with the average treatment lasting 12–15 sessions (Gurman 2002).

Narrative Couples Therapy

Narrative couples therapy, like BIMT, is grounded in the belief that change happens when couples modify their views of themselves and others, but the approach is dramatically different from these other approaches. Based on the postmodern view that we define ourselves and each other through the stories we tell ourselves concerning our lives, narrative couples therapy seeks to help couples create stories that better reflect the lives they want to live and the relationship they want to experience (Freedman and Combs 2002). Narrative couples therapists are not typically interested in the assessment of problems in a relationship, nor do they see people as having stable characteristics (Freedman and Combs 2002). Instead, they are interested in helping people generate new stories about themselves and their relationships, with the hope that these new stories invite the possibility for change and growth. Problems in a relationship are thought of as plots, and the problems are tackled by developing what narrative therapists call *projects*, which serve as counterplots. Couples may identify joint projects involving both partners, individual projects to be addressed by one person, or both. Treatment length in narrative couples therapy is not specified; some couples find that a story may be reworked and redefined in only a few sessions; other couples may take years to flesh out and reauthor the stories that define themselves. The time, duration, and date of the therapy session are not fixed. Rather, they are decided on by the couple in treatment on the basis of their perceived needs at the end of each session (Freedman and Combs 2002).

Integrative Problem-Centered Therapy

Integrative problem-centered therapy (IPCT), as conceptualized and formulated by Pinsof (1983, 1995), is a psychotherapeutic framework that approaches problem solving in therapy by integrating individual, family, and biological therapies. Developed with the belief that each psychotherapeutic approach has its domain of expertise, and that no single psychotherapeutic approach is sufficient to treat all presenting problems, IPCT is a hierarchical approach to therapy in which specific psychotherapeutic techniques are employed sequentially so that one picks up where the previous one failed. Therapy begins with the simplest, most direct, and least expensive form of treatment and progresses to more complex, indirect, and extensive strategies only if the previous methods have failed (Pinsof 2002).

One of the key concepts of IPCT is the *problem maintenance structure*. All of the people who are involved in maintaining or resolving a patient's presenting problem are collectively known as the *patient system*. All of the factors within the patient system that prevent a problem from being solved are known as the *problem maintenance structure*. Each of the factors that make up the problem maintenance structure can be assigned to one of six categories: social organization constraints, biological constraints, meaning constraints, family-of-origin constraints, object relations constraints, and self psychological constraints. Social organization constraints are addressed in therapy first, primarily through behavioral interventions. For example, if marital dissatisfaction is a result of a social constraint, such as not enough time spent together without the children present, the therapist intervenes behaviorally, helping the couple to modify their schedule to make it more conducive to the needs of the relationship. If this method of treatment fails, the therapist progresses to the other levels of intervention in turn, as needed.

IPCT is a process in which therapy progresses from the simplest to the complex, from outside in, and from the present (behavioral modification) to the past (analysis of childhood events and attachments). Movement from one orientation to the next is a result of the failure of the previous intervention to solve the problem. The progression is not always strictly linear; instead, the therapist may move back and forth as the problem maintenance structure reveals itself during therapy.

Feminist Couples Therapy

Feminist couples therapy has brought into focus issues of gender in marital therapy. As Rampage (2002) notes, "Although there is no monolithic feminist method of couples therapy, all feminist-informed approaches carefully attend to the ways in which power differences are manifested in the couple relationship" (p. 535). Feminist couples therapists believe that intimacy cannot be achieved without equality. Therefore, in the feminist approach, the therapist must evaluate the distribution of power in a relationship and work with the couple to balance it.

Special Problems

Special strategies of intervention are employed when couples present with certain specific problems. For distressed couples facing issues of sexuality, sex therapy is the treatment of choice (Leiblum 2007). Couples who suffer from the trauma and mistrust resulting from infidelity also require special intervention strategies, particularly to address issues surrounding trust and forgiveness (D.H. Baucom et al. 2005, 2006). Special strategies are also crucial in treating couples experiencing significant marital violence (Stith et al. 2002). The presence of violence in a relationship requires careful planning around safety as well as an ongoing evaluation of whether marital therapy might place women at greater risk. Still other specific strategies are indicated to address couples struggling with individual psychopathology or personality disorder. Evidence-based treatments are beginning to emerge for these specific populations (see section "Research Assessing Effectiveness of Couples Therapy" below).

Ethical Issues

Ethical considerations are essential aspects of couples therapy (Margolin 1982). The issues of confidentiality and of record keeping should be discussed and made clear at the onset of treatment. An issue of particular note is the sharing of secrets between a partner and the therapist. It is generally suggested that couples therapists refrain from harboring major individual secrets affecting a marriage.

The couples therapist must endlessly deal with interface issues in marital therapy and vexing issues of personal values (Doherty and Boss 1991). Sometimes, outlining the goal of couples therapy itself can present an ethical dilemma, such as when partners have very different goals for their relationship. Most marital therapists agree that it is a goal of therapy to try to preserve and build better relationships, not to save them at all costs. However, there are therapists whose unyielding purpose is to save a marriage, and in contrast there are those who place a greater value on personal rather than relational happiness.

Research Assessing Effectiveness of Couples Therapy

Meta-analyses have demonstrated that couples therapy has matched individual therapies in effectiveness (Lebow and Gurman 1995; Sprenkle 2002). In particular, traditional BCT, CBCT, IBCT, and EFT have a strong evidence base for effectiveness. Additionally, both an adapted version of BCT used to treat distressed couples that include a depressed individual (Beach et al. 1990), and an integrative therapy (including psychoeducation, promoting insight and forgiveness, and techniques from behavioral marital therapy) for treating couples who have experienced infidelity (D.H. Baucom et al. 2005), have produced promising results in single studies. Numerous other couples therapies have yet to undergo testing to determine their effectiveness.

One of the greatest challenges couples researchers developing treatments face is the high rate of return of problems in couples who have participated in couples therapy, which typically approaches 50% (Jacobson and Addis 1993). Nonetheless, Snyder and Wills (1989) demonstrated a very low rate of recidivism at 5-year follow-up of their insight-oriented approach, suggesting that such a return of problems can be avoided. The vicissitudes of life and the many transitions couples face throughout their life span often create conditions ripe for problems. Therefore, one frequently encountered notion is for clients to approach their couples therapy in an open-ended fashion and return to therapy if their problems resurface (Lebow 1995). Clearly, couples therapies must address the maintenance of change. Even when therapy is effective, many clients still experience some distress in their relationships; for example, Jacobson and Addis (1993) found in their quite successful BCT that only 35% were without any distress at the end of treatment.

Conclusion

Recent decades have seen tremendous growth in the field of couples therapy. Researchers and clinicians continue to strive for greater understanding of the complexities found in human relationships, with the goal of providing treatment to improve marital functioning and provide relief to those experiencing relationship distress. It is a propitious time in the field of couples therapy, as research on couple processes relevant to practice is blossoming, and evidence-based treatments that point to effective pathways for change have begun to emerge.

Key Points

- As the need for intervention in couples has developed and become more salient, couples therapy researchers and clinicians have responded.

- Recently, there has been a movement toward integration of various treatment modalities for couples and a focus on utilizing couples therapy as part of multiformat therapies for treating Axis I and Axis II disorders.

- Numerous couples interventions have been developed, many of which are strongly supported by empirical evidence.

- Couples therapy clinicians have a unique set of ethical considerations to address as they strive to create a therapeutic alliance with both partners.

References

American Psychiatric Association: Diagnostic and Statistical Manual of Mental Disorders, 4th Edition. Washington, DC, American Psychiatric Association, 2000

Asher SR, Gottman JM: Sex of teacher and student reading achievement. J Educ Psychol 65:168–171, 1973

Baucom B, Christensen A, Yi JC: Integrative behavioral couple therapy, in Handbook of Clinical Family Therapy. Edited by Lebow JL. Hoboken, NJ, Wiley, 2005, pp 329–352

Baucom DH, Lester GW: The usefulness of cognitive restructuring as an adjunct to behavioral marital therapy. Behav Ther 17:385–403, 1986

Baucom DH, Sayers SL, Sher TG: Supplementing behavioral marital therapy with cognitive restructuring and emotional expressiveness training: an outcome investigation. J Consult Clin Psychol 58:636–645, 1990

Baucom DH, Epstein N, LaTaillade JJ: Cognitive-behavioral couple therapy, in Clinical Handbook of Couple Therapy, 3rd Edition. Edited by Gurman AS, Jacobson NS. New York, Guilford, 2002, pp 26–59

Baucom DH, Gordon KC, Snyder DK: Treating affair couples: an integrative approach, in Handbook of Clinical Family Therapy. Edited by Lebow JL. Hoboken, NJ, Wiley, 2005, pp 431–463

Baucom DH, Gordon KC, Snyder DK, et al: Treating affair couples: clinical considerations and initial findings. Journal of Cognitive Psychotherapy 20:375–392, 2006

Beach SRH, Sandeen EE, O'Leary DK: Depression inMarriage: A Model for Etiology and Treatment. New York, Guilford, 1990

Bradbury TN, Fincham FD, Beach SRH: Research on the nature and determinants of marital satisfaction: a decade in review. J Marriage Fam 62:964–980, 2000

Broderick CB, Schrader SS: The history of professional marriage and family therapy, in Handbook of Family Therapy, Vol 2. Edited by Gurman AS, Kniskern DP. New York, Brunner/Mazel, 1991, pp 3–40

Christensen A, Jacobson NS, Babcock JC: Integrative behavioral couple therapy, in Clinical Handbook of Couple Therapy, 2nd Edition. Edited by Jacobson NS, Gurman AS. New York, Guilford, 1995, pp 31–64

Christensen A, Atkins DC, Berns S, et al: Traditional versus integrative behavioral couple therapy for significantly and chronically distressed married couples. J Consult Clin Psychol 72:176–191, 2004

Christensen A, Atkins DC, Yi J, et al: Couple and individual adjustment for two years following a randomized clinical trial comparing traditional versus integrative behavioral couple therapy. J Consult Clin Psychol 74:1180–1191, 2006

Dimidjian S, Martell C, Christensen A: Integrative behavioral couple therapy, in Clinical Handbook of Couple Therapy, 3rd Edition. Edited by Gurman AS, Jacobson NS. New York, Guilford, 2002, pp 251–277

Doherty WJ, Boss PG: Values and ethics in family therapy, in Handbook of Family Therapy, Vol 2. Edited by Gurman AS, Kniskern DP. New York, Brunner/Mazel, 1991, pp 606–637

Doss BD, Jones JT, Christensen A: Integrative behavioral couples therapy, in Comprehensive Handbook of Psychotherapy, Vol 4: Integrative/Eclectic. Edited by Lebow JL (Kaslow FW, series ed). Hoboken, NJ, Wiley, 2002, pp 387–410

Emery RE: Marriage, Divorce, and Children's Adjustment, 2nd Edition. Thousand Oaks, CA, Sage, 1999

Epstein N, Baucom DH: Enhanced Cognitive-Behavioral Therapy for Couples: A Contextual Approach. Washington, DC, American Psychological Association, 2002

Freedman JH, Combs G: Narrative couple therapy, in Clinical Handbook of Couple Therapy, 3rd Edition. Edited by Gurman AS, Jacobson NS. New York, Guilford, 2002, pp 308–334

Fritz PA, O'Leary K: Physical and psychological partner aggression across a decade: a growth curve analysis. Violence Vict 19:3–16, 2004

Gottman JM: How marriages change, in Depression and Aggression in Family Interaction (Advances in Family Research). Edited by Patterson GR. Hillsdale, NJ, Erlbaum, 1990, pp 75–101

Gottman JM: A theory of marital dissolution and stability. J Fam Psychol 7:57–75, 1993

Gottman JM: What Predicts Divorce? The Relationship Between Marital Processes and Marital Outcomes. Hillsdale, NJ, Erlbaum, 1994

Gottman JM: Psychology and the study of the marital processes. Annu Rev Psychol 49:169–197, 1998

Gottman JM: The Marriage Clinic: A Scientifically Based Marital Therapy. New York, WW Norton, 1999

Gottman JM, Carrere S: Why can't men and women get along? Developmental roots and marital inequities, in Communication and Relational Maintenance. Edited by Canary DJ, Stafford L. San Diego, CA, Academic Press, 1994, pp 203–229

Gottman JM, Krokoff LJ: Marital interaction and satisfaction: a longitudinal view. J Consult Clin Psychol 57:47–52, 1989

Gottman JM, Levenson RW: Marital processes predictive of later dissolution: behavior, physiology, and health. J Pers Soc Psychol 63:221–233, 1992

Gottman JM, Notarius CI: Decade review: observing marital interaction. J Marriage Fam 62:927–947, 2000

Gottman JM, Notarius CI: Marital research in the 20th century and a research agenda for the 21st century. Fam Process 41:159–197, 2002

Gottman JM, Coan J, Carrere S, et al: Predicting marital happiness and stability from newlywed interactions. J Marriage Fam 60:5–22, 1998

Greenberg LS, Watson JC, Lietaer G (eds): Handbook of Experiential Psychotherapy. New York, Guilford, 1998

Greene BL (ed): The Psychotherapies of Marital Disharmony. New York, Free Press, 1965

Gurman AS: Brief integrative marital therapy: a depth-behavioral approach, in Clinical Handbook of Couple Therapy, 3rd Edition. Edited by Gurman AS, Jacobson NS. New York, Guilford, 2002, pp 180–220

Gurman AS, Fraenkel P: The history of couple therapy: a millennial review. Fam Process 41:199–260, 2002

Jacobson NS: Behavioral couple therapy: a new beginning. Behav Ther 23:493–506, 1992

Jacobson NS, Addis ME: Couples therapy: what do we know and where are we going? J Consult Clin Psychol 61:85–93, 1993

Jacobson NS, Christensen A: Integrative Couple Therapy: Promoting Acceptance and Change. New York, WW Norton, 1996

Jacobson NS, Gurman AS (eds): Clinical Handbook of Couple Therapy, 2nd Edition. New York, Guilford, 1995

Johnson SM: The Practice of Emotionally Focused Couple Therapy: Creating Connection. New York, Brunner/Routledge, 2004

Johnson SM, Denton W: Emotionally focused couple therapy: creating secure connections, in Clinical Handbook of Couple Therapy, 3rd Edition. Edited by Gurman AS, Jacobson NS. New York, Guilford, 2002, pp 221–250

Johnson SM, Lebow J: The "coming of age" of couple therapy: a decade review. J Marital Fam Ther 26:23–38, 2000

Johnson SM, Hunsley J, Greenberg L, et al: Emotionally focused couples therapy: status and challenges. Clinical Psychology: Science and Practice 6:67–79, 1999

Kluwer ES, Heesink JAM, Van De Vliert E: The marital dynamics of conflict over the division of labor. Journal of Marriage and the Family 59:635–653, 1997

Krokoff LJ, Gottman JM, Hass SD: Validation of a global rapid couples interaction scoring system. Behav Assess 11:65–79, 1989

Lebow JL: Open-ended therapy: termination in marital and family therapy, in Integrating Family Therapy: Handbook of Family Psychology and Systems Theory. Edited by Mikesell RH, Lusterman D-D, McDaniel SH. Washington, DC, American Psychological Association, 1995, pp 73–86

Lebow JL: Building a science of couple relationships: comments on two articles by Gottman and Levenson. Fam Process 38:167–173, 1999

Lebow JL: Integrative approaches to couple and family therapy, in Handbook of Family Therapy: The Science and Practice of Working With Families and Couples. Edited by Sexton T. New York, Brunner-Routledge, 2003, pp 201–225

Lebow JL, Gurman AS: Research assessing couple and family therapy. Annu Rev Psychol 46:27–57, 1995

Leiblum S: Principles and Practice of Sex Therapy. New York, Guilford, 2007

Margolin G: Ethical and legal considerations in marital and family therapy. Am Psychol 37:788–801, 1982

Markman HJ, Renick MJ, Floyd FJ, et al: Preventing marital distress through communication and conflict management training: a 4- and 5-year follow-up. J Consult Clin Psychol 61:70–77, 1993

Michaelson R: An analysis of the changing focus of marriage counseling. Unpublished doctoral dissertation, University of Southern California, Los Angeles, CA, 1963

Orlinsky DE, Ronnestad MH: Current development: growth and depletion, in How Psychotherapists Develop: A Study of Therapeutic Work and Professional Growth. Edited by Orlinsky DE, Ronnestad MH. Washington, DC, American Psychological Association, 2005, pp 117–129

Pinsof WM: Integrative problem-centered therapy: toward the synthesis of family and individual psychotherapies. J Marital Fam Ther 9:19–35, 1983

Pinsof WM: Integrative Problem-Centered Therapy: A Synthesis of Family, Individual, and Biological Therapies. New York, Basic Books, 1995

Pinsof WM: Integrative problem-centered therapy, in Comprehensive Handbook of Psychotherapy, Vol 4: Integrative/Eclectic. Edited by Lebow JL (Kaslow FW, series ed). Hoboken, NJ, Wiley, 2002, pp 341–366

Rampage C: Working with gender in couple therapy, in Clinical Handbook of Couple Therapy, 3rd Edition. Edited by Gurman AS, Jacobson NS. New York, Guilford, 2002, pp 533–545

Roberts LJ, Krokoff LJ: A time-series analysis of withdrawal, hostility and displeasure in satisfied and unsatisfied marriages. Journal of Marriage and the Family 52:95–105, 1990

Rogers CR: Client-Centered Therapy. Boston, MA, Houghton Mifflin, 1951

Ronnestad MH, Orlinsky DE: Comparative cohort development: novice to senior therapists, in How Psychotherapists Develop: A Study of Therapeutic Work and Professional Growth. Edited by Orlinsky DE, Ronnestad MH. Washington, DC, American Psychological Association, 2005, pp 143–157

Scharff DE, de Varela Y: Object relations couple therapy, in Handbook of Couples Therapy. Edited by Harway M. Hoboken, NJ, Wiley, 2005, pp 141–156

Scharff JS, Bagnini C: Object relations couple therapy, in Clinical Handbook of Couple Therapy, 3rd Edition. Edited by Gurman AS, Jacobson NS. New York, Guilford, 2002, pp 59–85

Snyder DK, Aikman GG: Marital Satisfaction Inventory—Revised, in The Use of Psychological Testing for Treatment Planning and Outcomes Assessment, 2nd Edition. Edited by Maruish ME. Mahwah, NJ, Erlbaum, 1999, pp 1173–1210

Snyder DK, Schneider WJ: Affective reconstruction: a pluralistic, developmental approach, in Clinical Handbook of Couple Therapy, 3rd Edition. Edited by Gurman AS, Jacobson NS. New York, Guilford, 2002, pp 59–85

Snyder DK, Whisman MA: Understanding psychopathology and couple dysfunction: implications for clinical practice, training, and research, in Treating Difficult Couples: Helping Clients With Coexisting Mental and Relationship Disorders. Edited by Snyder DK, Whisman MA. New York, Guilford, 2003, pp 419–438

Snyder DK, Wills RM: Behavioral versus insight-oriented marital therapy: effects on individual and interspousal functioning. J Consult Clin Psychol 57:39–46, 1989

Snyder DK, Castellani AM, Whisman MA: Current status and future directions in couple therapy. Annu Rev Psychol 57:317–344, 2006

Spanier GB: Measuring dyadic adjustment: new scales for assessing the quality of marriage and similar dyads. Journal of Marriage and the Family 38:15–28, 1976

Sperry L (ed): Assessment of Couples and Families: Contemporary and Cutting-Edge Strategies. New York, Brunner-Routledge, 2004

Sprenkle DH (ed): Effectiveness Research in Marriage and Family Therapy. Alexandria, VA, American Association for Marriage and Family Therapy, 2002

Stanley S, Markman HJ, Peters S, et al: Strengthening marriages and preventing divorce: new directions in prevention research. Fam Relat 44:392–401, 1995

Stith SM, Rosen KH, McCollum EE: Developing a manualized couples treatment for domestic violence: overcoming challenges. J Marital Fam Ther 28:21–25, 2002

Straus MA, Hamby SL, Boney-McCoy S, et al: The revised Conflict Tactics Scales (CTS2): development and preliminary psychometric data. J Fam Issues 17:283–316, 1996

Thibaut JW, Kelley HH: The Social Psychology of Groups. New York, Wiley, 1959

Weiss RL, Cerreto MC: The Marital Status Inventory: development of a measure of dissolution potential. Am J Fam Ther 8:80–85, 1980

Weiss RL, Heyman RE: Marital distress, in International Handbook of Behavior Modification and Therapy, 2nd Edition. Edited by Bellack AS, Hersen M, Kazdin AE. New York, Plenum, 1990, pp 475–501

Whisman MA: Marital dissatisfaction and psychiatric disorders: results from the National Comorbidity Survey. J Abnorm Psychol 108:701–706, 1999

Whisman MA, McClelland GH: Designing, testing, and interpreting interactions and moderator effects in family research. J Fam Psychol 19:111–120, 2005

Whisman MA, Uebelacker LA: Impairment and distress associated with relationship discord in a national sample of married or cohabiting adults. J Fam Psychol 20:369–377, 2006

Wood BL, Miller BD: A biopsychosocial approach to child health, in Comprehensive Handbook of Psychotherapy, Vol 4: Integrative/Eclectic. Edited by Lebow JL (Kaslow FW, series ed). Hoboken, NJ, Wiley, 2002, pp 59–80

Suggested Readings

Christensen A, Jacobson NS: Reconcilable Differences. New York, Guilford, 2000

Gottman JM: The Marriage Clinic: A Scientifically Based Marital Therapy. New York, WW Norton, 1999

Gottman JM, Silver N: The Seven Principles for Making Marriage Work: A Practical Guide From the Country's Foremost Relationship Expert. New York, Three Rivers Press, 1999

Gurman AS, Jacobson NS (eds): Clinical Handbook of Couple Therapy, 3rd Edition. New York, Guilford, 2002

Johnson SM: The Practice of Emotionally Focused Couple Therapy: Creating Connection. New York, Brunner/Routledge, 2004

Snyder DK, Whisman MA (eds): Treating Difficult Couples: Helping Clients With Coexisting Mental and Relationship Disorders. New York, Guilford, 2003

Snyder DK, Baucom DH, Gordon KC: Getting Past the Affair: A Program to Help You Cope, Heal, and Move On—Together or Apart. New York, Guilford, 2007

Chapter 20

Emotionally Focused Couples Therapy

An Attachment-Based Treatment

Susan Johnson, Ed.D.
Scott R. Woolley, Ph.D.

The field of couples therapy is undergoing a sea change. It is becoming more and more feasible to help a couple go from

> **Wife:** You are always the same—cold, distant, hostile—you are an emotional cripple—I have never felt so miserable. I should have left you years ago, and if you don't smarten up I'll do it.
>
> **Husband:** You are so difficult to live with—maybe we would be better apart. All we do is fight. I don't see the point.

to

> **Husband:** I do shut down—I am so devastated when you get so angry with me—me—the Big Disappointment. I want you to stop hammering me so I can come out of my shell and we can be close again. I don't want to lose you. Please don't tell me that you are leaving.

Wife: I just get so scared—so I need your reassurance that you do love me—even if we get stuck in these fights. It's hard for me to admit how much I need you, but I'm not leaving. I want us to be together.

The context for the transformation in couples therapy is the recent expansion of what might be called the "science of everyday life." The couples therapist can now refer to a body of literature on key variables such as the nature and significance of emotion (Ekman 2003), the nature of marital distress and satisfaction (Gottman 1994), and most significantly, the nature of adult love (Johnson 2003). As long as love was viewed as a random and mysterious process, it was almost impossible for couples therapy to evolve into a viable discipline that might successfully address the quality of couple relationships. Indeed, this therapy modality has often been accused of being simply a set of techniques in search of a theory. It has also traditionally been very much on the sidelines of psychotherapy, the key players being individual therapy and family therapy. Family therapists have always acknowledged that the couple relationship is the foundation of the family but have focused on parent–child interactions. Individual therapists focusing on intrapsychic variables most often miss the power of the client's present interpersonal context and how this context continually defines the self and shapes affect regulation strategies. But now, at last, it is possible to ground couple intervention on a scientific basis so that it may become a powerful discipline in its own right. In fact, it is fast evolving into a major mental health intervention with the potential not only to heal our most precious relationships but to create relationships that heal. Emotionally focused couples therapy (EFT) is at the forefront of this new discipline.

The Nature of Emotionally Focused Therapy

EFT is an empirically validated, brief, systemic approach to changing distressed couples' rigid interaction patterns and emotional responses and promoting the development of a secure bond between partners (Johnson 2004; Johnson and Denton 2002). This approach targets absorbing affect states that organize "stuck" patterns of interaction in distressed relationships (Gottman et al. 2002). These patterns become self-reinforcing, often taking the form of critical pursuit followed by distance and defensiveness. EFT combines an experiential, intrapsychic focus on the ongoing construction of inner experience with a systemic focus on interactional responses and ensuing cyclical patterns. Key elements of experience, such as attachment needs and fears, are unfolded and crystallized in therapy sessions, and new positive interactions are structured and enacted.

In a typical EFT session, an observer would see the therapist reflecting and distilling the patterns in the process of interaction between partners. Because emotion is viewed as the main organizer of key interactions, the therapist would then focus on particular emotional responses and the link between these emotions and key interactional moves. The therapist works to deepen and expand these responses—for example, by expanding reactive anger into expressions of hurt or fear—and then uses the resulting expressions to shape new kinds of interactions. In a snapshot of therapy, an observer might hear the therapist make the following kinds of comments:

> So, could you help me? It appears that this dance here is what happens very often between the two of you. Marie, you become very "upset," as you put it, when David turns his head away and says that you are too difficult, and David, you turn away and shrug your shoulders, almost as if you are giving up here. Is this right? And Marie, the more upset and "difficult" you become, the more you, David, turn away and shut down. This pattern leaves you both anguished and alone. Is that right?

> What is it like for you, David, to talk about this right now? How do you feel as you say to Marie, "You are just too difficult to talk to"? Could you help me understand "difficult?"

> When you use this word, you push away with your hands and I notice your face changes. It is almost like a sadness creeps over your face. Is that right?

> Yes, I understand. It is sad to feel you are giving up begin able to reach your partner. So you move away and shut down. And then Marie feels "shut out," as she put it, and both of you are alone and unhappy. But is it too hard to stay here and talk?

David then talks of how he is filled with sadness and a sense of hopelessness.

> Do you think you could help your wife understand these feelings? Can you tell her, please, "I do give up and move away. It just feels so hopeless. I don't know how to talk with you."

The therapist then explores Marie's response to this message and how it might shift her perception of her partner and expand her view of their negative pattern.

EFT integrates key elements of experiential therapy (Elliott et al. 2004; Rogers 1951) with general systems theory principles as implemented in structural family therapy (Minuchin and Fishman 1981). Attachment theory (Bowlby 1969, 1988) provides EFT with a developmental, nonpathologizing theoretical framework for understanding the importance of emotional bonds, interdependency, and adult love.

The "client" in couple EFT is the relationship between partners. EFT is systemic in that it emphasizes the power of present interactional sequences and feedback loops to define the relationship and to direct individual behavior. The therapist is active and directive, using such interventions as reframing and creating enactments between partners or family members (EFT is also used with families) to explicate negative patterns and to shape new positive ones. The EFT focus on emotion and the inclusion of the concept of self, however, differs from the focus of pure systemic models. Emotion, often thought of as a "within" rather than "between" phenomenon, is not addressed in traditional versions of systems theory. Systems theorists have relied on the mechanistic concept of homeostasis to explain how interactions become structured into patterns. Ludwig von Bertalanffy, the father of systems theory, hated this application, believing it reduced a living organism to the level of a robotic machine (Nichols and Schwartz 2005). EFT views emotion as linking self and system; emotion is the primary signaling system that organizes key interactions in couple and family systems. These interactions then in turn shape and color each partner's inner realities.

Because EFT is an experiential therapy, the therapist uses advanced empathy to immerse himself or herself in the client's immediate experience and expand that experience. Clients are continually led to more fully experience, become aware of, and process their emotions. The therapist explicates the order inherent in each partner's emotional experience and validates this experience. The session has to be a safe, validating place where each partner has a genuine positive relationship with the therapist for this to occur. Emotions are seen as powerful, healthy, and informative, telling partners what it is they need and how to engage with each other (Johnson 2004). Expressions of emotion—the music of the dance between partners—pull for particular responses from others. As one partner, for example, angrily insists that his partner dismisses and neglects him, his partner braces and withdraws in self-protection. Later, however, when the former moves through his anger and expresses the emotions of hurt and fear, his partner is drawn toward him. Generally, the distortion and disowning of emotion and attachment needs is viewed as problematic. However, at times, intense emotion is also contained in EFT, especially in work with trauma survivors (Johnson 2002). Human beings are viewed as generally healthy and oriented toward growth, with healthy needs and desires.

Research on Emotionally Focused Therapy for Couples

EFT has been established as an empirically validated approach to couples therapy (Baucom et al. 1998; Johnson et al. 1999), and other research apart from that of the originators of the approach has demonstrated efficacy (Denton et al. 2000). Recognized as one of only two systematically tested couple interventions, the other being behavioral couples therapy (BCT), EFT is a meta-analytically supported treatment (Sprenkle 2002) and appears to obtain larger effect sizes than BCT.

EFT is empirically supported not only in terms of outcomes but also in terms of the focus of therapy, change processes, and theory of relatedness. The critical importance of the targets of the EFT change processes—namely, negative interaction patterns and constrained emotional responsiveness—is supported by empirical research linking these factors to marital happiness and distress (Gottman 1994; Huston et al. 2001). Attachment theory as applied to adults has spawned an enormous amount of creative research in the last two decades, much of which has direct relevance for the couples therapist (Johnson 2003; Simpson and Rholes 1994). The EFT process of change has also been studied, and there is support for the key mechanisms of change in EFT; for example, deepening emotional experience in sessions appears to lead to better outcomes (Johnson and Greenberg 1988).

In terms of outcome, a meta-analysis of the four most rigorous EFT outcome studies demonstrated a 70%–73% recovery rate in couples treated for relationship distress and 86% significant improvement (Johnson et al. 1999). Positive changes made in treatment also appear to be stable, with little evidence of relapse even in vulnerable populations (Cloutier et al. 2002).

EFT also continues to evolve and expand. Evidence for this can be seen in the expansion of EFT to address issues of forgiveness and the renewal of trust (Johnson et al. 2001; Makinen and Johnson 2006) and the outlining of key therapist interventions utilized in key change events (Bradley and Furrow 2004). There is a growing base of treatment applications with diverse populations: couples suffering from trauma (Johnson 2002; Macintosh and Johnson, in press), depression (Dessaulles et al. 2003), or chronic illness such as heart disease or breast cancer (Kowal et al. 2003); and same-gender couples (Josephson 2003). EFT is used across cultures with reported clinical success. For example, it is used in European countries such as Finland, in Australia, and in more collectivist cultures such as Japan, Korea, and China. Although a focus on the universals of emotion and attachment allows EFT to address the universal elements of couple relationships, the humanistic stance and focus on the moment-to-moment process of emotional regulation and interaction allows it to be sensitive to unique individual differences. The key predictors of success in EFT appear to be engagement in the therapy process and the woman partner's level of trust that her partner loves her; the initial level of distress that the couple displays on entering therapy is not a significant predictor (Johnson 2004).

The EFT Theory of Love: Love as an Attachment Bond

As Yogi Berra stated, "If you don't know where you are going, you will wind up somewhere else." Attachment theory provides the EFT therapist with a map to the drama of distress and primary emotions and needs, a language for effective dependency, a direction and a focus for therapy, and a guide to the key moves and moments that define an adult love relationship. This allows the EFT therapist to zero in and help couples create not just a less aversive relationship with less conflict but a more secure emotional bond. Attachment theory offers the therapist a broad explanatory theory of relatedness, but it also has the depth and specificity to guide the moment-to-moment change process.

Many strands in recent scientific studies are beginning to converge and provide support for the basic assumptions of attachment theory in ways that are empowering for the couples therapist. A recent study (Coan et al. 2006) considered the impact of hand holding on stress response. Women were placed in a magnetic resonance imaging machine. When a small light came on, they occasionally received a mild shock on their feet. Researchers watched how being alone, holding the hand of a stranger, and holding their loved one's hand changed how their brains responded to this stress. Being alone heightened the stress response, and their pain affected the brain in a particular way. In contrast, holding the partner's hand, especially when the couple had a very positive marriage, "calmed jittery neurons," which led to a gearing down of the areas in the brain that had become charged in response to the threat, and a lowering of the level of physical pain reported after shocks. This would seem to be a clear example of how, as attachment theory predicts, "proximity to an attachment figure tranquilizes the nervous system" (Schore 1994). Attachment figures are emerging as hidden regulators of an individual's physiological reality. Evidence of this can also be seen in the literature on recovery from heart attack, in which it has been demonstrated that recovery is significantly affected by the intimate relationship of the victim (Coan et al. 2006).

Attachment theory, originally formulated by Bowlby (1969, 1988) and applied to adult love by researchers such as Cassidy and Shaver (1999), sets out how default modes of affect regulation and models of self and other create habitual ways of engaging loved ones. These modes and models can either become rigid and constraining in close relationships or remain flexible and open to revision, as in the following case:

> A client named John views all needs and softer emotions as a sign of weakness and failure. For him, others are mostly potential judges. Emotional ex-

perience such as vulnerability and longing and emotional engagement with others are then dangerous and to be avoided. When he fights with his wife, Judy, or when she expresses disappointment with him, he tends to numb out and shut down. In this process, he shuts his wife out. She then becomes more anxious and isolated and criticizes him more. Her anger confirms his fears and increases his tendency to avoid emotional engagement. Attachment theory elucidates how habitual individual emotional responses build feedback loops with attachment figures that then confirm or revise these habitual responses.

Attachment theory fits very well, then, with a systemic approach to couples therapy that focuses on patterns of interaction in a relationship. It also fits with a normalizing, experiential approach to relationship problems. Bowlby (1979, p. 23) believed that all responses, even extreme anxiety, anger, avoidance, or a sense of shameful worthlessness, are "perfectly reasonable constructions" if one understands the interactional context and the attachment dilemmas of the relationship partners.

What are the basic premises of this theory of love? In brief, attachment theory postulates the following:

- Seeking and maintaining contact with a few significant others is an innate primary motivation in human beings from the cradle to the grave. Disconnection and isolation are inherently traumatizing; in fact, some emotion theorists suggest that these induce "primal panic" (Panksepp 1998). Closeness to others is the ultimate resource when we encounter existential anxiety. The couples therapist sees this deep need for connection in sessions when partners speak in life-and-death terms about their relationship and the intolerable pain of loss of connection. For example, Cathy says, "I just can't seem to reach him. That is why I get so mad. I feel so alone all the time. I can't bear it."

- Secure dependence complements autonomy and is associated with a more coherent, articulated, and positive sense of self (Mikulincer 1995). Systemic therapies have generally neglected the dimension of nurturance in favor of a focus on issues of power, autonomy, and control. Attachment theory challenges the pathologizing of dependence and speaks of effective dependency in which connection makes partners stronger, more confident, and more able to be themselves. For example, Tony says at the end of therapy, "I feel stronger, knowing that we are together again and that she loves me. And now I can tell her when I don't like things— and I feel more sure of myself."

- Attachment offers a safe haven—a retreat from the world by which comfort, security, and a buffer against stress and anxiety are provided. Attachment also offers a secure base—a bridge to the world that promotes exploration and openness to new information. Securely attached children can reach for parents for reassurance, express their needs, take in comfort, and then sail forth into the world to play, explore, and learn. For example, Sarah says, "Now when the fear that the cancer will come back rears up, I don't just get irritable or overwhelmed. I can go to him and get a hug, and it makes all the difference in the world. He is there for me. I can count on him."

- Emotional accessibility and responsiveness is the essence of secure connection. As Bowlby noted, a loved one can be physically present but emotionally absent. If there is no emotional responsiveness, the message from the attachment figure reads as "Your signals do not matter to me and there is no connection between us." Emotion is central to attachment, and emotional signals organize attachment interactions. Interventions such as the creation of insight or the building of skill sequences usually miss this dimension of emotional responsiveness that is so essential to secure bonding. The EFT therapist gradually structures dialogues in which the partner can express attachment emotions and needs in a way that pulls the other partner toward him or her and in which the other partner can engage on a deeper emotional level. We can see this need for responsiveness in the beginning of therapy when, for example, Marie says, "I poke him and poke him. I know I do. Anything to get a response out of him."

- When emotional connection with an attachment figure is lost, a predictable process of separation distress follows. This begins with angry protest. In secure, positive relationships protest is heard and accepted and then results in reconnection. If this protest, first full of hope, turns into desperate despair, negative cycles of demand and distancing often ensue in the relationship. If the protesting partner cannot get the other to respond reassuringly, clinging, depression, and finally detachment follow. This picture fits with the findings on marital distress and the power of cycles, such as angry demanding followed by defensive withdrawal, in predicting divorce.

  Research has found that happy couples often can ask for their needs to be met in a softer, more vulnerable way and can stay emotionally engaged even when the other partner is demanding or distressed. The attachment perspective offers an explanatory frame for these findings, telling us that the plot underneath these response patterns is all about separation distress and unmet attachment needs. Researchers such as Gottman (1994) note that stonewalling, a complete lack of emotional response, is toxic for marriage. Attachment theory tells us why it is toxic and exactly how this toxicity undermines relationships. In a similar vein, other researchers find that direct support—the offering of advice and problem-solving help—is often aversive for partners (Cutrona et al. 1990; Finch et al. 1997). Indirect support—the offering of emotional recognition and emotional contact, as in "This is so hard for you, but I know you can do it and I am here"—is much more effective. Partners talk in sessions of how their loved one habitually offers them problem solving, when what they want is his or her emotional presence.

As a couples therapist, it is essential that the therapist understand the basic needs and emotional realities behind a couple's dramatic conflict in order to intervene effectively. The therapist might say to Al, "So, Al, I think I am hearing your wife say that she is hurling herself against your wall—not to demolish you but to get past your barriers—to reach you. But you see her as just trying to criticize you, and you withdraw. She is lighting a signal fire saying, "Here I am—where are you?" but you see her as trying to burn the house down." Couples find this way of viewing their negative interactions enormously relevant. This way of understanding love and translating the meaning of responses and interactions speaks to people and is perhaps why we have so very few dropouts in EFT studies and clinical practice.

- When connection is lost or uncertain, there are very few ways to regulate attachment emotions and respond. Attachment research with children and adults has identified three basic patterns of responses. Some partners become anxiously attached and hyperactivate the attachment system. They become flooded with anxiety and swing between angry coerciveness, demands, and an obsessive pursuit of reassurance. This often results in driving their loved one farther away. Jealous partners, for example, find evidence of betrayal in minor details and continually test their partner as to his or her dependability. Some partners become avoidantly attached and try to deactivate the attachment system. They have learned to minimize attachment needs and emotions and to numb out and focus on external tasks. They do not acknowledge attachment needs and do not ask for connection. Unfortunately, this often induces anxiety and deprivation in the other partner. As attachment research demonstrates, these avoidant partners are in fact highly physiologically aroused but are protecting themselves from anticipated rejection or abandonment (Dozier and Kobak 1992; Johnson 2004). Once a therapist understands this, it is easier to reach such clients and help them connect with their partner.

Research on EFT suggests that EFT is effective with spouses described as inexpressive by their partners and with traditional avoidant male partners. Some partners integrate both anxious pursuit and fearful avoidance of closeness. This is exceedingly confusing to their spouses because it usually presents as a form of "I need you desperately—don't you touch me." These are usually partners who have been violated by attachment figures and so are caught in a dilemma in which the other is a longed for source of comfort and a dreaded source of danger. Again, once the therapist understands this dilemma, it is possible to clarify this dilemma and work toward expanding this response (Johnson 2002).

Some attachment literature speaks of these three response patterns as styles, almost as personality traits. As a couples therapist it seems more appropriate to view them as habitual strategies or ways of engaging others. These strategies become more extreme, rigid, and difficult to revise when negative patterns of interaction constantly confirm attachment fears and reinforce these coping strategies.

- Finally, attachment theory outlines the cognitive representations that are distilled from repetitious patterns of interaction. Working models of self and other, especially those concerning the worthiness of self and the reliability of the other, are formed and then become expectations and biases that influence perception in new interactions. These models are procedural scripts for relationships; they are formed and maintained, and can be revised, through emotional communication. Couples therapy here enters the realm of helping to redefine the self of partners. As Nancy, for example, says, "I will not ask for help. I decided a long time ago that I wasn't going to need anyone. People just let you down. And anyway [weeping], I just can't do it. I don't know how—even if he does want to be there for me." In adult attachment, partners use representations as safe havens. For example, soldiers might look at pictures of their partner and speak to this picture before leaving on a mission in order to calm themselves down. Compared with attachment in children, adult attachment is more reciprocal, representational, and integrated with sexuality.

The EFT therapist uses attachment theory, the most potent theory of love we have, to understand emotions, needs, and interactions and to find a systematic way to transform key love relationships. Most importantly, attachment informs the therapist as to the key moves and moments in a couple's ever moving multilayered dance. The therapist then can focus on and work with negative moments that define the relationship as insecure and can structure key moments of emotional engagement and responsiveness that promote more secure bonds. Secure attachment predicts numerous positive aspects of relationship functioning, such as greater commitment, trust and satisfaction; greater intimacy; less aggression; more appropriate caregiving; and greater ability to reflect on and meta-communicate about patterns in relationship interactions (Johnson 2003).

The EFT Treatment Process

In clinical practice, EFT is usually completed in 10–20 sessions; however, treatment may be longer if other problems, such as clinical depression or symptoms of posttraumatic stress disorder (PTSD), are present. The therapist has to be able to create a safe haven for the couple in the therapy session; if this is not possible—because, for example, there is ongoing abuse or serious drug addiction in the relationship—EFT is contraindicated. The EFT therapist is a process consultant rather than an expert who offers advice or teaches skills. The alliance in EFT is collaborative and based on Rogerian principles of genuine connection, positive respect, and transparency.

As a model of intervention based on attachment theory, EFT is characterized by the following:

- A focus on and validation of attachment needs and fears, and the promotion of safe emotional engagement, comfort, and support
- A privileging of emotional responses and communication, and direct addressing of attachment vulnerabilities and fears so as to foster emotional attunement and responsiveness
- The creation of a respectful collaborative alliance so that the therapy session itself may be a safe haven and a secure base
- An explicit shaping of responsiveness and accessibility so that withdrawn partners will become reengaged and blaming partners will soften, promoting the creation of bonding events that offer an antidote to negative cycles and insecurity
- A focus on how the self is defined and can be redefined in emotional communication with attachment figures
- An explicit shaping of pivotal attachment interactions that redefine a relationship, and an addressing of attachment injuries that block relationship repair

The process of change in EFT occurs in three stages that are described in the literature in nine steps (Johnson 2004):

1. *De-escalation*—the de-escalation of negative cycles, such as demand-withdraw, that maintain attachment insecurity and block safe emotional responsiveness. Naming these cycles and understanding their impact help the couple to see the cycles, rather than each other, as the enemy. Each partner is also helped to deepen his or her emotional experience, unpacking the softer, more vulnerable emotions that lie beneath reactive secondary responses such as reactive rage or numbing dismissal of problems. Feeney (2004) suggests that the emotion of hurt is essentially a soup of sadness, anger, and fear. Most people start by expressing anger,

but the more core emotion is grief and fear of rejection or abandonment. New emotions evoke new responses from partners, and at the end of this stage couples are friendlier and less reactive. The EFT therapist assumes that if therapy stops at this point, relapse is extremely likely.

2. *Restructuring*—the shaping of new cycles of responsiveness and accessibility. First, withdrawn partners take a more involved and active stance and state their needs and fears. The therapist helps the other partner hear, integrate, and respond to this statement. More critical, pursuing partners can then begin to ask for their needs to be met in ways that foster compassion and contact. Once both partners are accessible and responsive, powerful bonding events can occur that offer a new emotional experience of connection.

3. *Consolidation*—the consolidation of gains and the integration of the process of change into the couple's model of the relationship and each partner's sense of self. The EFT therapist is always concerned with three therapeutic tasks: creating and maintaining an empathic therapeutic alliance with both partners, helping clients reprocess key emotions, and gradually modifying interaction patterns to create key moments of safe emotional engagement and bonding.

EFT Interventions

Reflecting Present Emotional Experience

To address and reformulate key emotions, the therapist tracks and attunes to each client's relational experience and reflects the essential elements in this experience. Emotion theorists note that there are only six or so basic emotions that can be recognized from facial expressions by people of all cultures (Ekman 2003; Plutchik 2000). The EFT therapist is happy to deal with positive emotions such as joy and surprise but is usually working with anger, sadness, and shame, and most of all with fear and helplessness. The therapist privileges emotional responses and places them in the context of attachment realities and interactional cycles. The therapist also acknowledges conflicting emotions, recognizing, for example, that a client may long to risk reaching for the partner but is too afraid to do so. As in other experiential therapies, an attuned empathic reflection orders and clarifies responses. The therapist focuses on the most poignant, vivid aspect of emotional experience that is salient in terms of attachment and on a partner's position in the interactional dance. Attachment offers an invaluable guide to the core meaning of the couple's powerful emotions.

A therapist might say, "So I think I am hearing you say that you show the frustrated angry side of you to your husband but that in the more hidden part of you there is a great fear that he does not need you. But it is too hard to talk to him about this fear? You don't feel safe enough to do that?"

Validation

The therapist's acceptance and affirmation of the nature of each partner's experience act as antidotes to anxiety and the climate of disqualification and defensiveness that characterize distressed couples. The therapist legitimizes attachment needs and fears and so encourages exploration of them. A therapist might say, "I understand that it is too hard for you to show your feelings to her right now. In other relationships you had to be careful and stay very silent—that was the only way to survive. It saved your life. So now this conversation is very hard indeed."

Evocative Responding

The therapist can expand emotional responses or interactional positions by using open questions. When addressing emotion, the therapist can ask about the stimulus, bodily response, associated desires, and meanings or action tendencies implicit in emotions. The therapist then helps the client to clarify experience, access marginalized experience, engage more deeply in emotions, and so gradually reorganize them.

The therapist might say, "What's happening right now, as you say that?" "What's that like for you?" "I notice that as you say you feel nothing your hand is hitting at your leg. What is happening for you when you hit your leg like that?" "Can you help me, how do you 'turn off,' as you put it?" or "When do you get this 'shattered' feeling you talk about so much?"

Heightening

Heightening involves the use of repetition, images, metaphors, or structured enactments to intensify and distill clients' experience and encourage engagement in that experience. The therapist's nonverbal behaviors are important here. A soft, slow voice and simple words, preferably the client's own words repeated, are most effective. At key moments, when a therapist is asking a client to share a new emotion or experiment with a new response to a spouse, heightening is crucial to prepare for key enactments that create new positive cycles of secure bonding.

A therapist might say, "So could you say that again directly please: 'I do turn away. I do shut you out. I feel so unsafe, like there is no ground under my feet'" or "Is this one of those times when you feel like that small child you spoke about? So small. This is the helplessness that you vowed you would never feel again?"

Empathic Conjecture or Interpretation

The therapist here goes to the edge of the client's experience and one small step further. These interpretations are close to the client's experience and are offered tentatively. The therapist might say, "So when you feel this way, this 'upset,' as you call it, my sense is that this is a kind of scary feeling—like you don't know what is going to happen and you have no real control. Is that right?"

Tracking, Reflecting, and Replaying Interactions

The therapist holds up a mirror to specific interactions and patterns to outline negative cycles or positive exceptions to these cycles so that they can be noted and explored. The therapist then slows down and clarifies steps in the interactional dance and replays key sequences so they can be restructured. The therapist might say, "What just happened here? You turned to him and said, 'You never talk to me. It's a waste of time trying to relate to you.' And then you sighed and turned your chair away and stayed silent. Is this the way it usually goes between you? This is the dance of frustrated accusing and silent withdrawal we talked about. This dance really takes over here—and it leaves you both alone and hurting."

Reframing in the Context of the Cycle and Attachment Processes

The therapist here reframes each partner's behavior in the context of the negative cycle, the pull of the other's responses, underlying vulnerabilities, and the quality of the attachment in the relationship. Reframing is used to shift highly charged emotional meanings. The therapist might say,

> It seems like he is "hiding," as you put it, not because you do not have any impact on him but because you have so much. He cannot risk a negative response from you. But you see his moving away as indifference.

or

> The problem here is not that he is less verbal than you, or that he does not care, or that you are just a blaming kind of person. The problem seems to be that this dance of push/prod followed by stay still/respond less has taken over the relationship. This dance has taken over your relationship. It is now the problem. You cannot defeat this dance unless you help each other get unstuck here.

Restructuring and Shaping Interactions

Restructuring and shaping interactions involves enacting present positions so they can be explicated and owned, enacting new behaviors based on new emotional responses, and choreographing specific reparative sequences in the restructuring phase of therapy, when partners are able to ask for their attachment needs to be met. The therapist might say, "Can you tell him what you just said to me? 'I do blame him. I do it to get a reaction, any reaction. I won't let him hurt me like this. I refuse to be so helpless,'" or "You have just spoken about being sad. Could you tell him right now about that sadness?" or "Can you just stay with these scary feelings and stay with the longings and ask him for what you need right now?"

Therapists who are learning EFT often have doubts about setting up these enactments in situations of emotional intensity. If distressed partners are to have a corrective emotional experience, however, they cannot simply listen to each other talk through the therapist; they must risk and experience new kinds of interactions. Enactments can become negative, and interventions to allow the therapist to contain negative messages and "catch the bullet" are outlined in the EFT literature (Johnson 2004). These interventions are discussed in more detail elsewhere, together with markers or cues as to when specific interventions are used, and descriptions of the process partners engage in as a result of each intervention (Johnson and Denton 2002; Johnson et al. 2005). The key change events that lead to mutual accessibility and responsiveness—withdrawer reengagement and blamer softening—are also described in detail in the EFT literature.

Recent Developments in EFT

Recent work in EFT has begun to address specific kinds of impasses in therapy, such as the recently formulated attachment injury (Johnson et al. 2001), and the nature of the forgiveness process (Makinen and Johnson 2006). Developments in EFT also illustrate how the couples therapist is able to treat effectively complex forms of relationship insecurity and distress that occur in tandem with mental health problems and physical health problems, such as those found in the relationships of trauma survivors (Macintosh and Johnson, in press) and breast cancer survivors (Naaman and Johnson 2006). Couples therapy is more and more being viewed as a potential healing environment in which individual problems can be treated in the relational context in which they occur. The resources of a client's primary relationship can then be marshaled to cope more effectively with a particular partner's health problems. The process of change in EFT is also becoming more delineated, with researchers moving from a focus on the exact moves a client makes in a specific change event to identifying the therapist interventions that contribute to positive change.

Once the efficacy of EFT was established, the question then arose as to what blocks recovery from distress in EFT. Clinicians agreed that in the restructuring stage of EFT, some partners would begin to engage in key change events only to suddenly pull back, refuse to risk, and retreat into defensiveness. At such times, partners would bring up past hurtful incidents in an emotionally charged way and refuse to risk depending on their partner again. Attachment theorists have pointed out that incidents in which one partner responds or fails to respond at times of urgent need seem to disproportionately influence the quality of an attachment relationship (Simpson and Rholes 1994). Such incidents either shatter or confirm a partner's assumptions about attachment relationships and the dependability of his or her partner. Negative attachment-related events, particularly abandonments and betrayal at key moments of vulnerability, often cause seemingly irreparable damage to close relationships. Many partners who enter therapy are in general distress but also have the specific goal of bringing closure to such events and so restoring lost intimacy and trust. During the therapy process, these events, even if they are long past, often reemerge in an intensely emotional manner, much like a traumatic flashback, and overwhelm the injured partner, creating an impasse and hindering the process of change. These incidents usually occur in the context of life transitions, loss, or physical danger or uncertainty—for example, at a time of miscarriage or medical diagnosis, when attachment needs are most salient and compelling. These incidents can be considered relationship traumas rather than general hurts. These traumas are often compounded by the offending partner's continued attempts to discount or dismiss the significance of the injury. Attachment theory offers an explanation of why certain painful events, such as specific abandonments, become pivotal in a relationship, as well as an understanding of what the key features of such events will be, how they will affect a particular couple's relationship, and how such events can be optimally resolved. Indeed, these injuries must be resolved if the partners are to repair their bond and create lasting change in their relationship. For example, Kerry says to her husband, "I think we are better now—as friends. But I don't want to do this—this final leap into trusting you. Every time I think of it I have an image of that night. You drove me to the hospital, asked how long the labor would be, and then went off to clinch your important deal. I was so scared. And where were you? I had the baby by myself. Something shut down in me that night, and for years you would never even talk about it. You just told me to get over it."

The steps in the successful resolution of these relationship traumas appear to be as follows:

- After de-escalation, in the restructuring stage of therapy, the injured spouse is encouraged to stay in touch with the injury. He or she then begins to articulate its impact and its attachment significance. New emotions frequently emerge at this point. Anger evolves into coherent expressions of hurt, helplessness, fear, and shame. The connection of the injury to present negative cycles in the relationship becomes clear.
- The partner begins to hear and understand the significance of the injurious event and to view it in attachment terms as a reflection of his or her importance to the injured spouse rather than as a reflection of his or her personal inadequacies. This partner then acknowledges the injured partner's pain and suffering and elaborates on how the event evolved for him or her. The point of this elaboration is not to justify one's actions but to enhance one's predictability to the offended partner.
- The injured partner then tentatively moves toward a more integrated and complete articulation of the injury and expresses grief at the loss involved in it and fear concerning the specific loss of the attachment bond. This partner allows the other to witness his or her vulnerability.
- The offending partner becomes more emotionally engaged and acknowledges responsibility for his or her part in the injury and expresses empathy, regret, or remorse.
- The injured spouse then risks asking for the comfort and caring from the partner that were unavailable at the time of the injurious event.
- The other spouse responds in a caring manner that acts as an antidote to the traumatic experience of the attachment injury. The partners are together then able to construct a new narrative of the event.

Once the attachment injury is resolved, the therapist can more effectively foster the growth of trust and the beginning of positive cycles of bonding and connection. Recent research (Makinen and Johnson 2006) suggests that EFT enabled distressed couples to resolve these injuries when a single injury had occurred. However, when trust levels were lower and multiple attachment injuries had occurred, the couples had more trouble reaching resolution, and they uniformly commented that they needed more sessions to reach resolution, although the pain associated with the incident had diminished. The gains seen among couples who had experienced a single injury in terms of trust, injury resolution, and improvement in relationship distress were maintained at 3-year follow-up. As postulated in EFT protocols, positive results were associated with deeper levels of emotional experiencing during the processing of the injury, and, as expected, more affiliative responses were seen in key enactments.

Preliminary research is also complete on the effectiveness of a 20-session course of EFT on PTSD symptoms and marital distress in a sample of sexual abuse survivors with complex PTSD. Although this sample included a number of dual-trauma couples and partners with chronic problems and many comorbidities, the results were promising (Macintosh and Johnson, in press). The study generally confirmed clinical formulations of the necessary modifications to EFT for such a population (Johnson 2002)—for example, treatment is longer, emotional risks have to be sliced thinner, and emotions have to be contained as well as heightened. EFT has been used for many years with other kinds of survivors, including firefighters, war veterans, and motor vehicle accident victims.

Attachment theory helps to link specific qualities in a primary relationship to individual problems such as depression and PTSD. If couples therapists can help traumatized partners create a more secure bond, they also create a potent healing environment in which such trauma can be addressed and trust in self and others restored. An attachment-based couples therapy offers the possibility of helping the couple create the secure connection with a loved one that is the "primary protection against feelings of helplessness and meaninglessness" (McFarlane and van der Kolk 1996, p. 24).

Finally, the process of change in EFT is becoming clearer and more substantiated. The study of change is crucial, as demonstrated by the research finding that improvement in BCT is not in fact related to the proposed key elements in this approach, communication skills and more positive cognitions (Halford et al. 1993). EFT process research has linked the softening change event, in which a previously blaming spouse is able to risk asking for attachment needs to be met from a position of vulnerability, to positive outcome. Successful softening is also characterized by deeper emotional experiencing and more affiliative responses to the other spouse in EFT (Johnson and Greenberg 1988). The steps that constitute this event also have been mapped out. The final step in this kind of process research is to delineate the specific therapist interventions that foster a specific change event. Research (Bradley and Furrow 2004) has confirmed, as expected, that the effective EFT therapist uses evocative responding, reframing in terms of attachment, and heightening before choreographing an enactment in which one spouse confides in the other. However, those therapists who were successful in helping couples complete these events had given partners a picture of what a secure attachment response might look like while at the same time validating how hard it would be to make such responses. The therapist might have said, "So you could never, never turn and ask for reassurance, just turn and say how afraid you are and how much you long for his soothing? That would be too hard for you right now." This intervention seemed to offer partners an image of an alternative response while encouraging them to acknowledge blocks to this response. This kind of intervention might be especially appropriate for traumatized couples, who may never have experienced any kind of safe attachment and who need to begin by acknowledging how almost impossible it is to risk this kind of interaction.

Case Example

Mike and Annika had been married for 25 years when Mike called for therapy. He said he wanted therapy for "PTSD due to Vietnam combat." In the phone interview, he indicated his wife had just moved out of the home, their two daughters were both away at college, and he had to work on himself or "I am going to lose Annika." The therapist asked if Annika could come in with him for the first session, but he said he had to come alone—the therapist would understand once he explained the situation.

In the first session Mike revealed that he and Annika had not had any sexual engagement in 20 years. The last time they had sexual intercourse was when they conceived their second daughter, who was now 19 years old. In a voice full of shame, he explained that he did not know why he did not want to be sexually intimate but "I am the problem and I don't know how to change." He did not masturbate or use pornography, and he had not had an affair. He was not taking any medication, and a recent physical indicated he was in excellent physical shape. He showed some signs of depression but no other obvious symptoms.

The therapist again discussed how it would be helpful if Annika was at the session, and he agreed to ask her. Annika attended the second session and said, "I am here to help my husband; I am not the problem! I moved out, and I am not sure things can change." She then said she had been in therapy on and off for over 20 years because of depression and trauma related to her childhood and her feelings of rejection because her husband was not attracted to her. She talked of having been raised by a mentally ill mother, going in and out of homelessness and foster care, and trying to protect her two younger sisters. As an adult she had struggled with depression and deep feelings of inadequacy and rejection. However, she said she had "dealt with all that, and I am fine now, but I am angry that Mike has not been willing to get help for his problems. I am tired of trying to get him to see me and being rejected. It is better to live alone than to live with him and constantly feel rejected."

As the couple interacted, the therapist observed Annika subtly criticize her husband. Mike's response was either to ignore her or to stop talking. The therapist worked to reflect the pursue–distance cycle they were caught in and to access and validate how painful and lonely it had been for both of them over the years. The therapist was also able to access Mike's deep sadness and shame around his beliefs that he was "not a good husband" and had "failed Annika."

Mike's sexual history did not reveal sexual trauma. He was raised Catholic and believed sex was special and should be reserved for the one you love and were going to marry. The first time he had sexual intercourse was with Annika after they were deeply in love and planning marriage. They lived together for about a month before they married, and their sexual life was active and positive during that month. For Mike, it all changed the day they got married. Annika reported he did not seem interested in sex on their honeymoon, and although they had intercourse infrequently, mostly at her initiation, after 5 years it completely stopped. He said he had no idea what had changed the day they got married or why he eventually stopped. He suspected it had to do with the trauma of his Vietnam combat experiences, which he said he had never "worked through."

Mike was a college student who was "in love with science" when he was drafted into the infantry and shipped to Vietnam. Most of the soldiers he went over with were killed, many right in front of him in brutal combat. He was wounded twice and received several combat medals. Although he talked some about his war experiences when he came home, given society's hostile attitude about Vietnam solders, he mainly tried to forget about Vietnam and go on. The therapist spent the third, fourth, and fifth sessions on processing the trauma, terror, pain, and sadness of his war experiences. He gradually moved from a cold, analytical analysis of his experiences to accessing and processing powerful feelings of fear, terror, horror, grief, and sadness. He reported that talking about the traumas of Vietnam exhausted him and that it took "3 days to recover" from each of those sessions.

As Mike expressed his intense combat-related emotions, Annika, who was initially cool and distant, began to warm up. The therapist worked to reframe her occasional blaming remarks and connect them to her attachment longing to connect and her profound feelings of hurt and rejection. She talked about how powerful it was for her to see him emotionally open after being shut down for so many years, and she expressed her deep attachment-related longings to connect with him. As she did so, he responded by saying he loved her and wanted to be there for her. During these sessions, she started spending time in the home and even slept there on occasion, although there was no intimate contact.

At the end of the fifth session, he said, "As traumatic as Vietnam was— I have been thinking—I didn't realize it before, but I don't think Vietnam was nearly as traumatic as my mother's death." The therapist followed up on this at the beginning of the sixth session, and Mike said that at age 18, in his first semester away at college, his father called one morning and said his mother (whom Mike described as very warm, nurturing, and ideal) had died in a car accident that morning. Mike's world shattered. He became angry at God—so angry, he could not look in the coffin to say good-bye to her at the funeral. He went back to school, stopped going to church (which had been a central part of his life growing up), and felt alone and angry. His father became depressed and withdrawn. Mike and his only sibling became distant and did not talk about the loss. Shortly thereafter he was drafted, he went to Vietnam, and death became a part of his daily life.

As Mike talked about this shattering loss, the therapist worked with Annika to facilitate her engagement. She accessed and expressed her own grief over her history, his history, and the challenges in their marriage. Mike, with the therapist's support, responded with understanding and warmth. The therapist frequently had them talk with each other (enactments) in order to create direct engagement and bonding. At the end of the sixth session, with the help of the therapist, Annika said, "I know this is difficult for you, but you being open like this is exactly what I need. It doesn't always need to be this intense, but I need to know you are there and you understand me. This helps me know that you get me." With the therapist's help, she then went on to say in a low, vulnerable, gentle voice, "I need you, I need to be with you, I need your comfort, I need to know you get me—it feels like you do." Mike responded, "I want to be there for you," and he reached out and held her.

In the seventh session, in a response to the therapist's probe, Mike said, "Annika reminded me of my mother and everything that was good about my childhood. The day we got married, I felt I had regained everything that was good in my life, everything I had lost when my mother died." As the therapist focused on Mike's emotions the day of their marriage, Mike said, "Once I had Annika, I became terrified that I would lose her—that day I became terrified." He said he didn't feel afraid before because "I didn't really have her until we were married, so I couldn't lose her. Once we were married, I really had her and then I could lose her." As the therapist explored a possible connection between his fear of losing Annika and sexual intimacy, the following dialogue occurred:

Mike: I felt I wasn't good enough in bed. She had been involved with two other men before me, one for 2 years, and she was so much more sexually experienced than I was.

Therapist: Do you feel that way now? That you aren't good enough in bed because she had had sex with two other men and was more sexually experienced?

Mike [*looking down in shame*]: Yes. It is worse now. The last 20 years—all the suffering I have put her through—I am sure she wishes she had married one of those other men.

Therapist: You think because you haven't had sex in 20 years and she has suffered so much—feeling undesirable and rejected and lonely—that she wishes she had married one of those other men?

Mike [*looking down and in a low voice*]: Yes, I think so. How could she want me after all this?

Therapist: Have you ever asked her?

Mike [*still looking down*]: No.

Therapist: Could you ask her? [*Therapist makes a hand gesture toward Annika.*]

Mike [*Looking up at the therapist*]: Right here? Right now????

Therapist: Yes. Right here. Right now. [*Therapist gestures again toward Annika and moves back away from the couple. Mike looks down and after a while takes a deep breath and looks over at Annika.*]

Mike [*slowly in a voice filled with shame and fear*]: Well, ah, ah, ah...Do you wish you had married one of them? [*Mike looks back down immediately.*]

Annika [*looking right at Mike, leaning toward him*]: Of course not. They don't compare to you. Yes, the last 20 years have been rough, but you are so much better than either of them. I wish I hadn't lived with either of them.

Mike [*with relief washing over his face, looking up*]: Hold on—really?

Annika: YES, of course. I love you. I don't want to be married to anyone else—that is why it has hurt so much—I do love you.

Mike [*speaking slowing*]: Wow. That is very important; that is very significant. Wow—you really mean it!

Annika: Yes, of course I do!

Therapist [*slowly—after a pause—looking at Mike*]: So, that sounded like you just faced your greatest fear in this relationship and you found out that she, even after all these years and the troubles and the difficulties, she is still glad she married you. She still cares deeply about you. Am I getting that right?

Mike: Boy, are you—yes. That makes a big difference. Wow—that is really important.

The next week both came in smiling. The therapist asked how they were doing, and both giggled. After some small talk, they reported that she was sleeping at home in their bed again and that twice that week they had had sexual intercourse, with him initiating the first time and both initiating the second time. He said everything worked with his body the way it was supposed to (he was afraid that after so many years he might not have the ability). She also reported that he was far more open emotionally and that she was thrilled with their new emotional and sexual intimacy. In the following session, he reported he had had a "spiritual reawakening," felt a connection with God for the first time since his mother's death, and was going back to church again. He was very happy and reported feeling things were better in his life than ever before. He said he was "very excited" about life and the future with Annika.

The couple did several more weekly sessions to work through and talk about their newfound connection and intimacy, during which time she completely moved back into the home and gave up her apartment. The therapist made explicit how Mike had shut down emotionally in response to the horrors of Vietnam and the loss of his mother, and how his terror of losing Annika after their marriage and his fear of not being as good as her previous sexual partners led to his sexual shutdown. With Mike, the therapist heightened how when he faced his fears and reached out for comfort and connection, she was there for him and their relationship fundamentally changed. With Annika, the therapist emphasized how when she asked for connection in ways that he would find safe, he responded by engaging with her.

They came in for what they called "maintenance" once a month for the following year because, as Mike said, "We have made such major changes. I just want to make sure we maintain them." Twice in the next year, as he got stressed with work problems, he started to pull away emotionally and sexually. Each time, after giving him some space, Annika asked him directly and gently about it, expressed her love, and asked him for connection. Each time, he said he was sorry, that he wanted to be there for her, and that he was used to withdrawing when stressed rather than engaging. He then went on to open himself back up. At an 18-month follow-up from the initial weekly sessions, they were still having regular sexual intercourse, and both reported that the relationship had fundamentally changed and that they were happier than at any time in their marriage.

Much of the early work in this case centered around helping Mike reengage and process his trauma experiences and on helping Annika soften and engage in a more vulnerable, direct manner. This work was critical to making it safe enough for Mike to face his powerful attachment fears and sense of inadequacy and led to the key enactment in which Mike faced his deepest fears and Annika responded with warm reassurance and love.

Not all EFT trauma cases go this well or this quickly, but this case illustrates the power of focusing on attachment-related affect and creating safe engagement. It also demonstrates how what may appear to be intractable problems (20 years of no sex and a couple who are physically separated, with one person planning to divorce) can be changed in a relatively short period of time by using attachment emotions to heal the relationship and create a relationship that heals.

Conclusion

Couples therapy is a powerful arena for change. In this arena, partners inevitably demonstrate key elements of their personality: that is, their basic strategies for the regulation of emotion; the key cognitions that make up their sense of self; the habitual manner in which they view others; and how they engage others at significant moments in their lives. If the therapist has a clear and scientific understanding of love relationships and a systematic way to move partners into positive, attuned bonding interactions with each other, the potential for intrapsychic and interpersonal change is enormous. Many individual problems are also difficult to change unless a client's everyday interactions with his or her most significant other are taken into account. Interventions such as emotionally focused couples therapy appear to have the ability not only to build positive connection between partners, and so impact the quality of love relationships, but also to encourage partners to use this positive connection in the service of personal healing and growth.

Key Points

- Emotionally focused couples therapy (EFT) is an empirically based and validated, brief approach to changing distressed couples' rigid interaction patterns and emotional responses and promoting the development of a secure bond between partners. Research consistently indicates that the majority of couples recover from couple distress with EFT (Johnson et al. 1999) and that results are stable, even with vulnerable populations (Makinen and Johnson 2006).

- EFT targets absorbing affect states that organize "stuck" patterns of interaction in distressed relationships (Gottman et al. 2002). These patterns become self-reinforcing, often taking the form of critical pursuit followed by distance and defensiveness.

- EFT combines an experiential, intrapsychic focus on the ongoing construction of inner experience, with a systemic focus on present interactional responses and ensuing cyclical patterns.

- In EFT, key elements of experience, such as attachment needs and fears, are unfolded and crystallized in therapy sessions, and new positive interactions are structured and enacted to create secure bonds.

- Emotions are seen as powerful, healthy, and informative, indicating to clients what it is they need and how to engage with a partner (Johnson 2004). Expressions of emotion—the music of the dance between partners—elicit particular responses from others.

- The EFT therapist uses advanced empathy to immerse himself or herself in the client's immediate experience and expand that experience. Clients are continually led to more fully experience, become aware of, and *process* their emotions.

- Attachment theory serves as an adult theory of love that provides the EFT therapist with a map to the drama of distress and primary emotions and needs, a language for effective dependency, a direction and a focus for therapy, and a guide to the key moves and moments that define an adult love relationship. The EFT therapist is thereby allowed to zero in and help couples create not just a less aversive relationship with less conflict but a more secure emotional bond.

- EFT can be conceptualized as occurring in three stages—de-escalation, restructuring, consolidation—involving nine steps and clear, specific interventions.

- EFT is increasingly being used throughout the world and continues to be researched and developed in order to help a growing number of couples with a variety of presenting problems.

References

Baucom D, Shoham V, Mueser K, et al: Empirically supported couple and family interventions for marital distress and mental health problems. J Consult Clin Psychol 66:53–88, 1998

Bowlby J: Attachment and Loss, Vol 1: Attachment. New York, Basic Books, 1969

Bowlby J: The Making and Breaking of Affectional Bonds. London, Tavistock, 1979

Bowlby J: A Secure Base: Parent-Child Attachment and Healthy Human Development. New York, Basic Books, 1988

Bradley B, Furrow J: Toward a mini-theory of the blamer softening event: tracking the moment-by-moment process. J Marital Fam Ther 30:233–246, 2004

Cassidy J, Shaver P (eds): Handbook of Attachment: Theory, Research and Clinical Applications. New York, Guilford, 1999

Cloutier PF, Manion I, Walker JG, et al: Emotionally focused interventions for couples with chronically ill children: a 2-year follow-up. J Marital Fam Ther 28:391–398, 2002

Coan J, Schaefer H, Davidson RJ: Lending a hand: social regulation of the neural response to threat. J Soc Clin Psychol 16:323–342, 2006

Cutrona C, Cohen B, Ingram S: Contextual determinants of the perceived supportiveness of helping behaviors. J Soc Pers Relat 7:553–562, 1990

Denton WH, Burleson BR, Clark TE, et al: A randomized trial of emotion focused therapy for couples in a training clinic. J Marital Fam Ther 26:65–78, 2000

Dessaulles A, Johnson SM, Denton WH: Emotion-focused therapy for couples in the treatment of depression: a pilot study. Am J Fam Ther 31:345–353, 2003

Dozier M, Kobak RR: Psychophysiology in attachment interviews: converging evidence for deactivating strategies. Child Dev 63:1473–1480, 1992

Ekman P: Emotions Revealed: Recognizing Faces and Feelings to Improve Communication and Emotional Life. New York, Times Books/Henry Holt, 2003

Elliott R, Watson J, Goldman R, et al: Learning Emotion-Focused Therapy: The Process-Experiential Approach to Change. Washington, DC, American Psychological Association, 2004

Feeney JA: Hurt feelings in couple relationships: toward integrative models of the negative effects of hurtful events. J Soc Pers Relat 21:487–508, 2004

Finch J, Barrera M Jr, Okun M, et al: The factor structure of received social support. J Soc Clin Psychol 16:323–342, 1997

Gottman J: What Predicts Divorce? Hillsdale, NJ, Erlbaum, 1994

Gottman JM, Driver J, Tabares A: Building the sound marital house: an empirically derived couple therapy, in Clinical Handbook of Couple Therapy, 3rd Edition. Edited by Gurman AS, Jacobson NS. New York, Guilford, 2002, pp 373–399

Halford WK, Sanders MR, Behrens BC: A comparison of the generalization of behavioral marital therapy and enhanced behavioral marital therapy. J Consult Clin Psychol 61:51–60, 1993

Huston TL, Caughlin JP, Houts RM, et al: The connubial crucible: newlywed years as predictors of marital delight, distress, and divorce. J Pers Soc Psychol 80:237–252, 2001

Johnson SM: Emotionally Focused Couple Therapy With Trauma Survivors: Strengthening Attachment Bonds. New York, Guilford, 2002

Johnson SM: Attachment processes in couple and family therapy, in Introduction to Attachment: A Therapist's Guide to Primary Relationships and Their Renewal. Edited by Johnson SM, Whiffen V. New York, Guilford, 2003, pp 3–17

Johnson SM: The Practice of Emotionally Focused Couple Therapy: Creating Connection. New York, Brunner/Routledge, 2004

Johnson SM, Denton W: Emotionally focused couple therapy: creating secure connections, in Clinical Handbook of Couple Therapy, 3rd Edition. Edited by Gurman AS, Jacobson NS. New York, Guilford, 2002, pp 221–250

Johnson SM, Greenberg L: Relating process to outcome in marital therapy. J Marital Fam Ther 14:175–183, 1988

Johnson SM, Hunsley J, Greenberg L, et al: Emotionally focused couples therapy: status and challenges. Clinical Psychology: Science and Practice 6:67–79, 1999

Johnson SM, Makinen J, Millikin J: Attachment injuries in couple relationships: a new perspective on impasses in couples therapy. J Marital Fam Ther 27:145–155, 2001

Johnson SM, Bradley B, Furrow J, et al: Becoming an Emotionally Focused Couple Therapist: The Workbook. New York, Brunner-Routledge, 2005

Josephson G: Using an attachment based intervention with same sex couples, in Attachment Processes in Couple and Family Therapy. Edited by Johnson SE, Whiffen V. New York, Guilford, 2003, pp 300–320

Kowal J, Johnson SM, Lee A: Chronic illness in couples: a case for emotionally focused therapy. J Marital Fam Ther 29:299–310, 2003

Macintosh H, Johnson SM: Emotionally focused therapy for couples facing heart disease, in Handbook of Clinical Psychology and Heart Disease. Edited by Molinari E. New York, Springer (in press)

Makinen JA, Johnson SM: Resolving attachment injuries in couples using emotionally focused therapy: steps toward forgiveness and reconciliation. J Consult Clin Psychol 74:1055–1064, 2006

McFarlane AC, van der Kolk BA: Trauma and its challenge to society, in Traumatic Stress. Edited by van der Kolk BA, McFarlane AC, Weisaeth L. New York, Guilford, 1996, pp 24–45

Mikulincer M: Attachment style and the mental representation of the self. J Pers Soc Psychol 69:1203–1215, 1995

Minuchin S, Fishman CH: Family Therapy Techniques. Cambridge, MA, Harvard University Press, 1981

Naaman S, Johnson S: Emotionally focused couples therapy with second stage breast cancer survivors and their partners: an outcome study. Unpublished doctoral dissertation, University of Ottawa, Ontario, Canada, 2006

Nichols M, Schwartz R: Family Therapy: Concepts and Methods, 7th Edition. Needham Heights, MA, Allyn & Bacon, 2005

Panksepp J: Affective Neuroscience: The Foundations of Human and Animal Emotions. New York, Oxford University Press, 1998

Plutchik R: Emotions in the Practice of Psychotherapy. Washington, DC, American Psychological Association, 2000

Rogers CR: Client Centered Therapy. Boston, MA, Houghton Mifflin, 1951

Schore A: Affect Regulation and the Origin of the Self: The Neurobiology of Emotional Development. Hillsdale, NJ, Erlbaum, 1994

Simpson JA, Rholes WS: Stress and secure base relationships in adulthood, in Advances in Personal Relationships, Vol 5: Attachment Processes in Adulthood. Edited by Bartholomew K, Perlman J. London, Jessica Kingsley, 1994, pp 181–204

Sprenkle DH: Editor's introduction, in Effectiveness Research in Marriage and Family Therapy. Edited by Sprenkle DH. Alexandria, VA, American Association for Marriage and Family Therapy, 2002, pp 9–25

Suggested Readings

See http://www.eft.ca for numerous training resources and complete references for EFT.

Cassidy J, Shaver P (eds): Handbook of Attachment: Theory, Research and Clinical Applications. New York, Guilford, 1999

Johnson SM: Emotionally Focused Couple Therapy With Trauma Survivors: Strengthening Attachment Bonds. New York, Guilford, 2002

Johnson SM: The Practice of Emotionally Focused Marital Therapy: Creating Connection. New York, Brunner/Mazel, 2004

Johnson SM: Hold Me Tight: Seven Conversations for a Lifetime of Love. New York, Little, Brown, 2008

Johnson SM, Whiffen VE (eds): Attachment Processes in Couple and Family Therapy. New York, Guilford, 2003

Johnson SM, Bradley B, Furrow J, et al: Becoming an Emotionally Focused Couple Therapist: The Workbook. New York, Brunner/Routledge, 2005

Karen R: Becoming Attached: First Relationships and How They Shape Our Capacity to Love. New York, Oxford University Press, 1994

Chapter 21

Psychodynamic Couples Therapy

An Object Relations Approach

John Zinner, M.D.

Object relations couples therapy is a psychoanalytically based method of couple treatment that integrates past with present, conscious with unconscious, and the intrapsychic with the interpersonal. The object relations approach helps couples discern how past life experiences as individuals can limit their possibilities in the present as a couple. It clarifies how unconscious processes can promote conflict and disappointment. It helps partners take ownership for how their individual perceptions, fears, and motivations may be shaping their interactions as a couple. What follows is an explication of an object relations theory of the couple relationship and the implications of this theory for couple treatment.

Practitioners of couples therapy are likely to agree that the most difficult aspect of this work is posed by partners' intractable blaming of each other. We are all too familiar with the polarizations that occur within the session in which each partner clings to an unambivalent point of view that is in exact opposition to that of the other. In the following example from a marital session, I examine how our psychoanalytic approach informs a particular understanding of and intervention in such an argument.

Clinical Illustration: Conflict as a Safe Haven

For Alice and Jack, after years of emotional distancing and conflict, a more friendly relation had gradually evolved during 1½ years of marital therapy. Physical intimacy, however, remained a remote and improbable goal. On the surface, Jack appeared to be the spouse who sought a sexual connection whereas Alice disavowed any desire. She blamed her lack of interest on the many ways she felt that Jack disappointed her. He attributed his lack of sexual initiative to her episodes of hostility. In the session to be described, the couple opened with what appeared to be a regressive, angry argument, recalling to me the early months of our work. All the old familiar bones of contention were resurrected. Alice "ragged" on Jack for his failure to take good care of her by seeking out a higher-paying job. Jack criticized Alice for neglecting the needs of the children and letting the housekeeping go. I soon discovered that the weekend before this fight began the couple had had "good family-together time," and that, more precisely, the retrograde conflict began shortly after the couple had "cuddled in bed." Jack had drawn close to Alice and she had responded. This degree of physical closeness had not occurred in ages. As the discussion deepened, I learned that, uncharacteristically, Alice had gone to bed, that night, nude. Jack said that Alice is a "toaster bear" when she is naked in bed and he had asked to come close to her. To my query, Alice admitted that she liked this "cuddling…but it also made me mad" because Jack, she thought, would wrongly conclude she had forgiven him for all his transgressions. Then Alice laughed, saying, "I knew this [cuddling] would come up in the session and maybe it *is* the reason [for the fight]." She admitted to me, "I knew you would say that it was, so I didn't want to come today." Internalizing more and more, Alice revealed that she had recently experienced an awakening sexual desire for Jack and had asked him to "kiss and hug." She joked that she was afraid to have sex because she would have to talk about it in couples therapy. Alice said she was reluctant to relinquish her "survival mode"—that is, her determination to depend only on herself and not to allow herself to rely on and come close to Jack. Earlier that evening she told herself that she was going to bed naked because she had been painting the kitchen and had streaked paint on her clothes. She took them off and did not put on anything else because "it was too dark to see." She laughed, however, as she revealed her fantasy that I would think this was an excuse for her wanting, in fact, to sleep naked with Jack. Thus, in the transference, I became, through projective identification, the embodiment of her own sexual motivations. For Jack's part, he admitted that he felt anxious when the couple hugged and kissed at Alice's request. She perceived this as a subtle sense of his distancing after their physical contact. Jack then associated to his fear of being dependent on Alice and to the death of both his parents when he was quite young.

There is an apparent paradox, here, in which these seemingly warring adversaries are, in fact, sharing a common internal ambivalence over closeness, dependency, and intimacy. Their ordinary, consistent way of relating involves maintaining a distance, often hostile, which keeps at bay, for each of them, the anxieties that would emerge from a more intimate connection. When they "cuddled in bed," Jack was aware of anxiety, whereas Alice found herself getting angry at him. With their usual equilibrium destabilized by the sexual contact, shared anxiety led them to dig up the familiar bones of contention and to restore, through arguing, their costly but safer distance.

The object relations couples therapist looks beyond the manifest content of an argument to understand the unconscious factors that may have triggered the conflict in this instance. Every marriage or intimate couple relationship is likely to have significant unresolved issues, bones of contention, which may be managed by compromise or simply tolerated and accepted as a difference, as in "we agreed to disagree." When these "bones" suddenly get reactivated in the relationship, as with Alice and Jack, we look for the possible triggers of this current conflict and focus on developing understanding of the underlying issues, in this case, fantasies about the dangers of sexual intimacy. This approach is quite different from those couples therapies that focus entirely on the manifest content of the conflict—for example, with Alice and Jack, the therapist attending to complaints about poor housekeeping or not seeking more financial security with a higher-paying job.

Projective Identification

What then is the object relations understanding of the origins of significant couple conflict? Fundamentally, our view is that interpersonal conflict reflects the transposition of intrapsychic conflict within each partner on to the couple relationship. The mental mechanism that is responsible for this transformation is *projective identification*, the core concept of the object relations approach (Zinner 1976).

Melanie Klein (1946, p. 110) defined *projective identification* as "a combination of splitting off parts of the self and projecting them onto another person," later describing it as "the feeling of identification with other people because one has attributed qualities or attributes of one's own to them" (Klein 1955, p. 57). Klein saw this as a defensive mode evolving from an early infantile developmental stage in which anxiety is warded off by experiencing intolerable affects, especially aggression, as if they resided in a space external to the self. This defensive "splitting" thereby creates the first "me–not me boundary." As the infant matures, and a self–object boundary develops, the preobject "not me" realm fuses with the object world, and what is projected is now directed into the mental image of the other.

What is projected, however, are not only the disavowed aspects of the self but also those aspects that are cherished. Decades before Melanie Klein's naming of the phenomenon, Sigmund Freud (1921) provided an example of projective identification in characterizing the "falsification of judgment" that accompanies the idealization of loved objects, what we refer to as falling "head over heels" in love:

> The tendency that falsifies judgment in this respect is that of idealization, but now it is easier for us to find our bearings. We see that the object is being treated in the same way as our own ego, so that when we are in love a considerable amount of narcissistic libido overflows onto the object. It is even obvious, in many forms of love choice, that the object serves as a substitute for some unattained ego ideal of our own ego, and which we should now like to procure in this roundabout way as a means of satisfying our narcissism. (p. 112)

In a more modern and comprehensive view (Zinner 2001), we can say that projective identification is our universal way of perceiving and comprehending others. When we are interacting with another person, our behavior toward that other is determined by our mental image of him or her. Our consequent behavior impinges on and affects that other person, but the person we are relating to exists only within our mind as a construct. This created mental image of the other is built from sensory stimuli coming from the outside that are then processed by our own mental apparatus. We never truly know the other person and what he or she feels. We can only approximate the actuality and subjectivity of the external object by drawing on our own experience and attempting to match it with what our senses are receiving from the outside. We unconsciously regard the actual object as the embodiment of our mental construct and treat him or her accordingly. This unconscious recognition of a projected aspect of our self in the object is the identification process in the mechanism of projective identification. Thus, in this definition, both projection *and* identification occur within the mind of one person, the subject. There appears to be, perhaps, a wired-in propensity to distance oneself from emotional pain by placing its source outside of the self, a generic process we refer to as *externalization*. When our effort to form a realistic picture of the other is burdened by a simultaneous need to expel a part of our self, the image of the other is thus tainted and distorted by our own defensive requirements.

Projective identification, as a mechanism, occurs along a developmental continuum. It is a reflection of psychological maturity to be able to consciously discern a sense of separateness and uniqueness both within one's self and concerning another person. This refined capacity is the result of a gradual evolution originating out of the earliest phase of infancy, in which there is no ability to delineate cognitively and experientially between the self and the mother, who is the infant's primary other. Those individuals who continue to maintain insufficiently developed self–object boundaries do not acquire the capacity to monitor the disparity between what the external stimuli inform them about the object and what their inner imperatives are directing them to put into the mental image of the object. Thus, individuals with significant blurring of self–object boundaries are prone to distort the image of others to a greater degree, at the extreme end, creating a delusional percept of the other. At higher developmental levels, the self–object boundary is progressively more distinct, so that in neurotic individuals there appears to be less global disparity between the actuality of the external object and the internal image of that object. The boundary is firmer in a relative sense only. Neurotic individuals do distort the image of the other through projective identification, but there is an increasing ability to become aware of and modify the distortion at higher developmental levels.

Empathy is the highest-level transformation of projective identification (Klein 1955). Here, defensive needs to externalize are no longer significantly influencing the construction of the image of the other. The subject is, in a probing fashion, temporarily loosening the self–object boundary in an effort to find a resonance in the subject's own experience with what his or her senses are telling the subject about the external object. Firming up the boundaries, again, the empathic individual asks himself or herself, "Now, is this what *she [he]* is feeling, or am I putting this in to *her [him]?*" Empathy is a form of projective identification that includes an explicit or implicit ongoing examination in an effort to approximate the actuality of the other. Empathy involves an openness and curiosity about the nature and subjectivity of the other as well as a willingness to alter one's perceptions depending on fresh impressions communicated by the other. One hallmark of defensive projective identification is the sense of certainty that the subject has of the nature of the other and the inflexibility of the subject's perceptions regardless of what the other may be communicating that may differ from these perceptions. Thus, in our understanding of the interaction of the couple, we ask ourselves not *whether* projective identification is occurring but rather to what degree it is serving defensive or empathic functions. Bear in mind that when we say that one is projecting his or her feelings onto another, we should consider this a form of verbal shorthand for the following: the subject is attaching his or her own feelings on to his or her mental picture of the other and behaving toward the real-world object accordingly. Thus, projections do not fly through the air mysteriously to penetrate and take control of the mind of the recipient. Rather, fantasies influenced by

projection are communicated to the actual object through the subject's behavior. The recipient of these behaviors infers either implicitly or explicitly
how he or she is being perceived by the subject.

When projective identification is serving the defensive economy of the
subject by projecting a conflicted aspect of the self, then what was previously an intrapsychic process between warring parts of the self has become
an interpersonal conflict—for example, among partners in a couple. In intimate relationships, behavior generated by projective identification may
have a coercive quality that is very likely to evoke in the recipient an experience of himself or herself that resonates with the way the projecting
spouse is behaving toward him or her. A loving glance can evoke in the partner a feeling of being lovable. Conversely, a contemptuous sneer from a
husband, one of a pattern of such behaviors, is likely to evoke in the wife a
sense of being disgusting and contemptible. Because both partners are
viewing each other through the filter of projective identification, we can view
the entire relationship as a nexus of interlocking projective identifications
generated by both partners, in which the experience of the self is strongly
affected by the way one is perceived and treated. Rather than there being a
randomness to all these projections, when they are serving a defensive function, the projections tend to be organized around certain problematic intrapsychic issues that both partners share. Participants in close relationships
are often in collusion to sustain their mutual projections—that is, to support
each other's defensive operations and to provide experiences through which
the other can participate vicariously. It is the subject's unconscious identification with the recipient of his or her projections that allows for this vicarious experience of living through the other.

For projective identification to function effectively as a defense, the true
nature of the relationship between the self and its projected part must remain unconscious, although the individual may feel an ill-defined bond or
kinship with the recipient of his or her projections. The disinheriting of the
projected part is not so complete that the subject loses his or her capacity to
experience vicariously a wide range of the object's feelings, including those
which the subject has himself or herself evoked. These vicarious experiences contain features associated not only with gratification but with punishment and deprivation as well.

In the case of Alice and Jack, each experienced considerable unconscious inner conflict over sexual intimacy and its threatening consequence
of emotional dependency. As a way of warding off anxiety, both partners
colluded in parceling out the elements of their own ambivalence into roles
each would assume. Thus, Jack spoke in behalf of their shared desire for sex,
whereas Alice represented their fear of physical intimacy. In this manner,
the intrapsychic conflict of each was transformed into interpersonal conflict

within their relationship. It does appear that conflict between partners is often more bearable than conflict within oneself. This is vividly articulated in the statement of one wife, "Of course! I would much rather he hate me than I hate myself!" When Alice reversed roles with Jack and initiated sexual contact, their distant but stable equilibrium dissolved. Each became anxious and managed to restore the sexual distance by regenerating conflict in digging up the familiar bones of contention.

Differing Definitions of Projective Identification

The mental mechanism that Melanie Klein defined as projective identification has been widely observed in a number of clinical contexts, and, especially since the beginning of interest in an interpersonal and family psychology, a variety of terminology has arisen to describe the same phenomenon. To name a few: Anna Freud (1936) wrote of "identification with the aggressor," whereas Martin Wangh (1962) characterized the "evocation of a proxy." In the family therapy literature we find "scapegoating" (Vogel and Bell 1960), "trading of dissociations" (Wynne 1965), "family projection processes" (Bowen 1965), and "irrational role assignments" (Framo 1970), among many others.

Even among those who use the term *projective identification*, two competing definitions have evolved, and this has led to considerable confusion among those who are trying to understand the process. Proponents of each of these differing denotations agree that the mental phenomenon exists but ascribe contradictory meanings to the word *identification* as it applies to projective identification. Meissner (1987) labels these two views as the "one-body context" in distinction to the "two-or-more-body context." In the former, as explained previously, and in Klein's (1946) original definition, both projection and identification take place in one mind. It was Bion (1962) who first recharacterized Klein's (1946, 1955) individual intrapsychic concept of projective identification as an interpersonal event. He described a rich, transformative, highly reciprocal interplay of projections and introjections occurring between mother and infant. This reconceptualization paved the way for others (Ogden 1982; Scharff 1992) to embrace a "two-body" definition in which the *identification* in projective identification now occurred in the object rather than in the subject. In the two-body view the subject projects, whereas it is the object who identifies with what the subject has projected onto him or her. That is, it takes two individuals to fulfill the definition of projective identification. This two-body view does serve to emphasize the coercive power of the subject's projections in shaping the recipient's subjective experience, in that the latter is pressured into actually feeling that he or she has become the person the subject has perceived him or her to be. Certainly this is true in intimate relationships in which the object's self-perception is heavily influenced by the way that he or she is seen and therefore treated by his or her partner.

There are, however, many situations in which the person who is the object of another's projective perceptions is not even aware he or she is on the mind of the subject, no less on the receiving end of the subject's behavior. In walking down a dark and empty street at night, I see a group of youths gathered at some distance on the next corner. Imagining them to be a potential threat, I cross over to the other side of the road and continue on my journey. In the one-body view, this qualifies as projective identification, whereas in the two-body view it does not, because the youths have not even observed me and therefore are not affected by my projective perception. Yet the mechanism operating in *my* mind is the same as if the objects of my fear had been directly affected by my behavior. For this reason, this author prefers to break the sequence of events into two separate steps by adopting the one-body definition. In the first step, the subject projectively identifies. In the second phase, the object may or may not identify with—that is, internalize—the way he or she is being perceived. This one-body view allows for a closer examination of the possible permutations in the interaction of partners and the degree to which one is reactive to the perceptions and behavior of the other. Both the one-body and the two-body definitions explain the powerful influence that partners' perceptions of one another have on the nature of their relationship as well as their individual self-experience.

It may be asked, why not use the simple word *projection* when the object is not affected by the subject's perceptions and behavior, as in the nighttime crossing of the street described above? The term *projective identification* could then be reserved for only those situations in which the object was actually affected by how he or she was perceived and treated by the subject. For those of us who adhere to the one-body view, however, all of what we tend to call projection is, in fact, projective identification. There is no distinction between the two, because the activity in the mind of the subject always involves the fantasy of an object, whether the actual object is present, absent, or even exists. This effort to be precise about what the mind is doing is increasingly important as we attempt to employ the methods of neuroscience to enhance our understanding of the relationship between mind and brain.

Transference, strictly speaking, is one form of projective identification, as it appears in the psychotherapeutic setting. The term, however, has been expanded to be almost synonymous with *projective identification* by including many situations in which " a normal person's perceptions and affective responses vis-à-vis the self and others are heavily influenced by the activation of significant relationship representations from the past" (Gerber and

Peterson 2006, p. 1320). As of this writing, researchers such as Gerber and Peterson are employing functional magnetic resonance imaging methods to "compare brain activation when subjects are engaged in a transference situation…and when they are not." In these kinds of studies, the one-body view promises a higher yield because it postulates consistency in the mind of the perceiving and behaving subject independent of the presence or even existence of a real-world other. The most parsimonious expectation would be that there would be a single pattern of brain activity also independent of the location of the actual object.

The operation of projective identification within marriage, however, is more than a matter of externalization of disavowed or cherished traits. We find that in the defensive mode, the contents of the projected material contain highly conflicted elements of the spouse's object relationships with his or her own family of origin. Although it is commonplace to think of a husband selecting a mate who is "just like the girl who married dear old dad," we are here referring to the unconscious striving to reenact conflictful parent–child relations through such an object choice. Highly fluid role attributions occur in which a husband, for example, may parentify his spouse, or, on the other hand, infantilize her by experiencing the wife as the child he once was. The externalization of aspects of old nuclear relationships may serve not only a defensive need but also a restorative one, to bring back to life, in the form of the spouse, the individual's lost infantile objects, both good and bad. The perception of the partner colored by the image of a beloved deceased parent may be salutary, heightening affection for the spouse. On the other hand, it may also be constraining on the object of the perception insofar as it detracts from her individuality and may lead to conflict when she does not conform to the parental image. Thus, recognizing the restorative function of these projective identifications may lead the therapist to fruitful exploration of unresolved grief over the death of the parent or other important person.

Our understanding of the impact of projective identification on couple relationships has profound implications for our therapeutic approach. For working with couples, many therapists utilize some form of a focal problem-solving approach, often cognitive-behavioral in style, with a primary focus on the manifest content of the conflict and perhaps an elaboration of dynamic patterns across conflicts. According to these methods, a couple enters therapy with its disputes, and the therapist seeks to resolve the conflict through identifying strengths, making behavioral contracts, conducting conflict resolution, assigning paradoxical interventions, or promoting fair fighting techniques, among other similar interventions. When a couple's conflict, however, is deeply anchored in interlocking processes of mutual projective identification, it can be very difficult, if not impossible, to make progress with most problem-solving strategies. This follows from our understanding that in these situations, interpersonal conflict is serving the intrapsychic defense of each partner so that there is a strong unconscious motivation for sustaining the couple's disharmony in order to preserve each partner's internal equanimity.

The object relations therapeutic approach is indicated for just these kinds of refractory couple discord. Our theory informs us that the manifest conflict and anger are not the primary targets of our efforts, but rather we seek to uncover the sources of pain within both partners that have caused them to use the relationship as a repository for disavowed aspects of their own selves. When successful, our exploration of the underpinnings of the manifest conflict reveals a more poignant subtext in which each partner is able to become aware of the emotional pain that led to the expulsion of the distress, appearing as anger, into the interpersonal space. Insofar as the therapist's efforts lead to a shift from blame to internalization of conflict within the individual partners, there is a diminution of anger and an increased capacity for empathy, compassion, and respect for one another that was not possible when each spouse was the target or perpetrator of criticism and rage.

The following description of a marital therapy session with Ted and Debra illustrates the ebb and flow of externalizing and internalizing processes in the relationship, with concomitant shifts between anger and sadness.

Clinical Illustration: Conflict as a Defense Against Fear of Loss

Debra began with a wisecrack, after I again reminded her I could not schedule their sessions to an earlier time. She quipped, "Don't *any* of your patients get better?" This response reflected her sense of continued bickering with Ted recently, although not at the level of several weeks ago.

They described a typical fight in which the two of them ended up snapping at each other in front of Rachel (their 3-year-old daughter) after the child fell and hurt herself. Each blamed the other for not keeping a watchful eye on the little girl as she was playing on their bed. I heard this as a typical instance of their taking out their shared anxiety on one another and polarizing over who would bear all the worry. One scene during this altercation involved Debra panicking when she noticed some blood in Rachel's mouth and then shouting at Ted to "get off the fucking phone" while he was taking his time, casually conversing with his son. *She* had actually handed the phone to Ted earlier when he had followed the crying Rachel into the room as he moaned, "Oh my gosh! Oh my gosh!" Debra commented that after this blowup, both felt "heartsick" at the way they had dealt with Rachel's injury.

They reported several other bickers during which Debra was nagging Ted while he was dragging his feet on a project because he felt again that giving in to Debra was being "euchred," which is his expression for being "led by the nose." Their fight seemed to be over the proper height of the wall they were building in the basement. Debra wanted a higher wall than Ted, and they couldn't agree. I commented that in recent weeks they have been erecting a wall between them such that they're not pulling together as a team under stress and, as Debra put it earlier, "It's like we're having all our old fights all over again." I inquired about the deeper layer of concern underlying the wall, and Debra teared up, saying, "It's because when I need him he's not there. I can't count on him being here." Hearing the reference to Ted's absence, I asked Debra if she had been concerned about Ted's health lately. Ted is considerably older than her and not scrupulous about his health habits. At this she nodded affirmatively and began to cry. The conflict seemed to start while he was away so much recently working so hard on a contract that he, incidentally, just informed me he had successfully completed. She felt like a "single parent" then and imagined him dying and how much worse it would be if he did. She worried about his knees, his hearing, and, above all, about his weight and his drinking. She revealed she carries a fantasy that at any time he could have a heart attack and die. Then she would be all alone with Rachel and unable to remain in their house, because she couldn't afford it even for 6 months. In this recent concern she pleaded to Ted to draw up an accounting of how much she would be left with, and he did. Of course, he was unaware of the poignant aspect of her request and how frightened she was at the prospect of losing him.

The night before, Debra arrived home late from work to find Ted devouring a 12-ounce steak. This upset her considerably although she did not mention it to Ted. To her this was an example of his self-neglect. Ordinarily, when she is home and cooking dinner, she prepares meals that are suitable for a man with heart disease, such as beans and rice. She was angry at him in the session for his "not letting yourself use me as a resource," because she is able to prepare for him foods that are tasty and healthful. "Instead, you act like I'm your enemy," she says when she admonishes him for eating foods that are unhealthful for him.

At a neighborhood Halloween parade the previous week, Debra had felt "sad" for Ted because he was not able to walk the distance of the parade with Rachel and her because of the pain in his knees. She imagined him in a wheelchair, unable to walk.

Reflecting on this session, we see that this couple has recently been bickering again: as Debra said, "It's like we're having all our old fights all over again." She is referring to the bones of contention—"our old fights"—unique to this couple. Her guilty perception of their backsliding into conflict is transformed into a wisecracked projective identification in which she blames me, in the transference, for not getting "*any* of [my] patients...better." Rather than eliciting the manifest content of their recent bickering, I search for the precipitant of this current round of conflict. Hearing her critical reference to Ted—"I can't count on him being here"—I associate to the possibility of her losing him and ask if she is concerned about his health. This question reveals the source of their recent tensions, as Debra begins to cry and tell how, in the face of Ted's recent prolonged absence, she worries that he might die and leave her and their daughter, Rachel. In their relationship, the fear of death and loss is parceled out by projective identification. Ted is cavalier in his dismissal of the dangers to his health from his very casual attitudes about his eating, drinking, and lack of exercise. Debra, on the other hand, carries all the worry for the couple about the consequences of his health habits. Because he does not internalize his own concern about dying prematurely, Ted runs the risk of fulfilling that grim prophecy by, for example, gorging on a 12-ounce steak the night before the session. Interestingly, this behavior may be his way of expressing his own feeling of abandonment by Debra, who came home too late to cook a healthful dinner for him. These interactions illustrate a fundamental consequence when a couple uses their relationship as a repository of disavowed and devalued projections. They are unable to work as a team because their polarization causes them to pull in opposite directions. In distinction, when each partner in a couple is able to internalize intrapsychic conflict and tolerate anxiety, ambiguity, or sadness, the pair can function as a team and benefit from its joint and collaborative efforts. In this connection, Debra lamented to Ted that "You are not letting me use you as a resource."

Their failure to share anxiety and guilt following Rachel's fall is another example of how defensive projective identification leads to couple conflict and dysfunction. The role of the worrier switched during the interaction so that at first, Ted was moaning "Oh my gosh! Oh my gosh!" while Debra handed him the phone so that he could speak with his son, a nonurgent matter. He was bearing the anxiety for both of them. Spotting a small amount of blood in Rachel's mouth, Debra panicked, as the defense against her anxiety crumbled. At that point *she* became the worrier and raged at Ted for being on the very phone she had handed him moments before. Because of the work that they had previously done in therapy about their flawed handling of anxiety connected with Rachel, both recognized their return to an old pattern of blaming and felt "heartsick" about what they had allowed to happen.

During their conflict over Rachel's fall, however, we can see that what remained constant was the polarization of attitudes. In an intimate couple, who reflects which attitude at a given moment may fluctuate. We will recall from our earlier couple how Jack became anxious and distanced himself when Alice, uncharacteristically, reversed roles and spoke for their sexual desire.

Another important feature of object relations couples therapy is to listen for the symbolic and metaphoric quality of the content of marital conflict. In the session with Ted and Debra we hear that a significant and emotionally charged argument persists over how high to build a wall within their basement. When such an intensity of feeling arises over what would appear to be a manageable difference of opinion, we as therapists look for the metaphoric meaning of what is contested. In this case, in recent weeks a "wall" was being erected as the couple distanced itself through "having all of our old fights" after Ted's return from his travels.

A primary goal of object relations couples therapy is to help each partner reinternalize what he or she has projected into the interpersonal sphere in a way that has burdened the relationship. The conflicted internal relationships can only be resolved intrapsychically. When such reinternalization occurs, there is a striking shift from anger and polarization within the couple toward sadness, tenderness, and poignancy in each partner. This transition is evident in the session with Ted and Debra as they finally share the "heartsick" feeling at how they divided and fought over Rachel's fall. Similarly, their arguments over the wall and their old fights are ameliorated when they become aware of their concerns about abandonment and death. Following the successful reinternalization of projected elements, there can be considerable individual intrapsychic work done in the course of the couple sessions. What often does occur, however, is that the partners seek out individual psychotherapy with a different therapist as a complement to the couple treatment. Both Ted and Debra had been in individual therapy before the couples work began and continued with that synergistic combination.

Use of Transference in Couples Therapy

According to the object relations approach, the world of internalized object relationships is transposed onto the world of actual interpersonal relations through the mechanism of projective identification. This transposition occurs in a variety of spheres, not just within the couple relationship. Interactions with children, friends, employers, colleagues, and others are governed by the same psychological mechanism. Transference is the form projective identification takes in the therapeutic relationship. In couples therapy, transference feelings and marital issues are often inextricably interwoven threads of the same interpersonal fabric. Because the couples therapy is a three-person relationship, there is an increase in the permutations the forms of this transference may take in contrast with individual psychotherapy.

First, as in individual work, there is the focused transference that each partner feels toward the therapist based on that partner's internal object world. Second, there is a very common triangular transference configuration in which each partner is seeking to be the one preferred by the therapist at the expense of the other. This threesome interaction often reenacts sibling experiences in competition for the favor of their parent. More often than not, each partner enters couple treatment with the fantasy hope that the therapist will validate his or her point of view and work to change his or her partner's wrongful attitudes and behavior. Many of the early efforts by the therapist are devoted to helping the couple understand that each partner is contributing to the problematic interactions in their relationship. This requires that the therapist actually be able to rise above, in attitude and behavior, the drumbeat of blaming and fault-finding that so frequently take place in an adversarial couple situation. Evenhandedness and neutrality in the therapist are greatly aided by his or her understanding of the complex and complementary interplay of the internal object world of the partners as it is transposed onto their current relationship.

Third, there is a complex transference that encompasses the experience of the entire three-person group in interaction. One such instance is the shared fantasy within the couple that the couple treatment is in itself a danger to the integrity of the relationship and the safety of individual members, rather than a resource for help, healing, and growth. Especially where words have been used as instruments of aggression rather than of understanding and support, there may be a great fear of becoming open and vulnerable in the session, with a consequent constriction of communication and a perception of the therapist as an agent of harm. It is therefore an early priority that the therapist recognize and explore this shared fantasy that talking is dangerous because language, the very vehicle for healing in therapy, is seen paradoxically as the greatest threat to the safety and security of the couple. Because of the emotional power inherent in a group, strong countertransference experiences are to be expected in couples therapy, and it is often a challenge to convert these feelings into stimuli for constructive therapeutic reflection and intervention, in contrast to internalizing them so that they color the therapist's self experience in a way that helps no one in the threesome.

This attitude that the treatment situation is one of harm rather than of help is often discovered through the therapist's own countertransference experiences in a variety of ways. For example, the therapist may find himself or herself, in the face of the couple's silence and constricted communication, feeling the need to energize the interaction with frequent superficial interventions. In the absence of the therapist's forced efforts the group feels lifeless and defeated, and the therapist's sense of himself or herself as helpful and competent may suffer. It is useful for the therapist to be aware of such personal reactions because they serve as a signal that there is some problematic fantasy operating within the threesome that requires explicit exploration. In this instance, the therapist can use his or her sense of ineffectiveness to ask directly about the couple's experience of the therapy and the therapist, and what their fears are of saying what is on their mind in the session.

The elucidation of transference by the therapist offers the valuable opportunity to examine the marital relationship in the here and now of the session. This in-the-moment examination is often more highly affectively charged than the couple's rehashing of the more remote then-and-there events of the previous week. Working in the here and now is especially helpful to the therapist, as he or she has the opportunity to experience and learn from his or her countertransference reactions as the drama unfolds in the session. It is also necessary to address problematic negative transference issues that might lead to acting out or an interruption of treatment if ignored.

Work in the transference is illustrated in the couple treatment of Tom and Trish. The session occurs soon after a difficult summer interruption, involving a lengthy unanticipated absence by the female therapist and the death of Tom's mother. The hour opens with an extended silence and downcast expressions:

> **Trish:** I feel so bad. Everything's falling apart. I'm too angry, hurting.
> **Therapist:** Your relationship is falling apart?
> **Trish:** Yeah, and between me and myself.
> **Tom:** It's also a hard time for me. I'm feeling very alone. I'm not through feeling the loss of my mother. I'm feeling alone with Trish, too, feeling there's not much room for me. I'm not sure what to do about that.
> **Therapist:** You look quite sad.
> **Tom:** I've had pretty sad days. I wrote all the thank-you notes for people who helped a lot. I'm feeling pretty bad, pretty sad. Yesterday, I spent time going back through things…greeting cards…business stuff. I felt pretty sad, pretty alone.
> **Therapist:** You feel alone in your grieving or without your mother?
> **Tom:** Both…[*Tom recounts how he called his uncle and aunt, who were close to his mother*]…it's a sad thing.
> **Therapist:** Right now you seem very closed in, inside your grief.
> **Tom:** Yeah.
> **Therapist:** Is your grief complicated? I had the impression your relationship with your mother was not satisfying for you, which would complicate your grief.
> **Tom:** The last few years she tried to reach out and we worked through a lot of stuff. She was a critical person, not easy to talk to. I was always feeling I'd be criticized.

Tom and the therapist engage in a discussion in which the therapist especially questions him about his relationship with his mother. Throughout, Trish remains utterly silent, often staring out into space. Tom is responsive to the therapist's interventions. He begins to cry, concluding, "No matter how bad things were, she loved me and now she's gone."

Tom: All these feelings are overwhelming. I don't know how to be with Trish when she's having all these feelings, too. Somehow it feels like it has to be either her or me. I don't know how to work it so that we can both be depressed or sad or both be mourning.

Therapist: You have the idea that Trish is feeling cut out because I'm talking to you and drawing you out?

Tom: Yeah, I do. And feeling she's resenting it a lot…[*silence*]…I know part of the problem is I want somebody to take care of me…to be kind…and I know that's not fair…to expect…of her. It took me a lot to get to the point where I could recognize that. I just don't know how things are supposed to be anymore.

During the course of the session thus far, the therapist has been acutely aware of Trish's conspicuous silence and lack of involvement. The therapist found herself irritated at Trish and was determined to keep the channel of communication open with Tom by ignoring Trish's efforts to undermine it. This countertransference experience was familiar to her in working with this couple. She had frequently felt as if she were compelled to make a choice between devoting attention to one spouse or the other. The partner not receiving the therapist's attention at the moment would remain silent and sullen. Thus, the interaction had a quality of taking turns rather than of give and take. Aware that she was acting out her own countertransference irritation, the therapist decided to shift to interpretation.

Tom: I've been feeling I have to have something to help me get through this. I don't have Trish. I just don't know how to get to her…without her feeling resentful. It's like I have to totally be on my own or I have to rely on Trish—those two things—the dependency I want isn't good, isn't healthy, but I still want it…and I feel like there must be some appropriate halfway point, but I don't know how to get there.

Therapist: You do both look as though if either of you were to want anything from the other you'd be very disappointed. Is that what breaks down so fast, Trish? Fall apart very quickly, you said. [*Silence.*]

Trish: Sitting here while you've been talking to Tom has been very difficult. I find myself resenting a couple of things you said. I resent the time you're spending with him—I feel very small.

Therapist: When I'm talking to Tom it doesn't feel like you're both getting something because if he's getting something, then you're not.

Trish: Yeah.

Therapist: That makes you feel very small.

Trish: Well, he's got this enormous grief to deal with and he needs a lot. I shouldn't get mad when you're helping him.

Therapist: It's such a deep loss and both of you have a need for an abiding presence that's just for you. That need is very strong.

> You're both talking about how you're struggling with the fact that it's not there—a very reliable, immediate, understanding presence—how much you each need it and how much it's not there either from each other or from anyone, really.
>
> **Trish:** That's a lot of what happens to me. It's not there. I don't think I ever really had it. Sometimes I feel I have it, but then I lose it, which I do, then I can't…I can get through a session with Myra [Trish's individual therapist], and then I can do what I need to do with Tom, except then when something comes up between us, then I can't hold on to it. If I don't have it, then I don't want to deal with all his stuff. But I can't adjust. If I can't have it, then I'm through.…Sometimes it feels really good, but there's an awful lot of pain with it, all that pain around therapy this summer, I can't get away from it.
>
> **Therapist:** You mean my absence and the effect it had on everything?
>
> **Trish:** Yeah. I was afraid, really afraid. I felt badly. I was a little weird. I didn't notice it was a pattern. When I was supposed to see you and I didn't, I'd get weird, but I didn't connect it.
>
> **Therapist:** Maybe now with things settling down, seeing me for a couple of weeks, maybe now it will be possible to understand these feelings, not just to have to endure them.
>
> **Trish:** Yeah.

This excerpt reveals a highly interwoven blend of transference, countertransference, and marital issues. A triangular configuration is evident, but it is, however, a pre-oedipal, or oral, triangle in which there is a competition not for a sexual relationship with the parent of the opposite sex but rather for the basic supplies of emotional survival.

The raw data for the therapist's grasp of the marital unconscious assumption come from several sources. She reflects on the manifest behavior in the session, which is characterized by the lack of give and take, and the sullen silence of each spouse when the therapist is attending to the other. She contemplates the manifest verbal content—for example, Tom's regret that "It has to be her or me" but not both who can be sad or mourning. The therapist includes in her consideration Tom's story of a mother who was not warm, but a "critical person, not easy to talk to." A crucial part of the mix is the tension within the therapist over the competition for her attention and her own irritated determination to defy Trish's envy to the point of ignoring her.

Out of her experience in the here and now, the therapist is able to formulate for herself an unconscious assumption governing the marital relationship. That is, that resources for a basic sense of worth and for psychological survival are limited and only sufficient for one partner. Whatever sustenance is received from the good object, couple, or individual therapist is ephemeral. There is a tenuous capacity for one spouse to give to the other without experiencing envy for what the other is getting and rage at what one is giving up. The couple *shares* this fantasy and, in the session, the transference vision of the therapist as the central source of sustenance. The specific transference feeling of each spouse toward the therapist at any given moment is different, determined by whether the therapist is seen as attending to or ignoring Tom or Trish.

In this excerpt, the therapist's capacity to grasp the here-and-now situation inclusive of both transference *and* marital dynamics allows her to focus her intervention on the issue that carries the highest affective charge of the moment. Therapeutic interventions are most effective when directed toward issues linked to strong affects. In the absence of an affectively toned area, interpretations are received with intellectualization and little emotional impact. In couples therapy, we see this latter phenomenon in the all-too-frequent retrospective bland analyses of the marital fight of the previous week.

The Frame of Object Relations Couples Therapy

What are the nuts and bolts of conducting object relations couples therapy? The frame of the couples treatment and the nature of the therapist's activity follow from the object relations theory that has been elaborated here. Sessions are held once or more times weekly at a set time. The length of treatment is open-ended, and termination evolves naturally out of completion of the task. Meetings take place only when both partners are able to be present and begin when both have arrived. Concurrent individual psychotherapy can act in synergy with the couples work, in which the partners each have their own individual therapist who is not also the couples therapist. It is advisable that the couple's therapist not do both forms of treatment. When one partner meets with the couples therapist in the absence of the other partner, there is the risk that the therapist will learn something that would disturb the absent mate should he or she become aware of this information. Thus, the therapist is left with the dilemma of having to protect the confidentiality of the spouse with whom he or she met alone and therefore having to hold a secret that cannot be shared with the absent partner. This is an untenable position for the therapist, whose responsibility is to the couple as a whole and not to only one spouse. In addition, when the therapist wears both hats in doing the individual and couples work, jealousy and destructive competition can arise, and this only serves to compound the adversarial relationship that existed in the first place. With separate individual and couples therapists, either the patient can transmit understanding gained across the boundary of the two therapies, or both therapists can confer as needed with permission. The couples therapist's responsibility is to the couple as a unit, and his or her stance should be one of evenhandedness in the presence of conflict. Primarily, the therapist serves as an observer, listener, active formulator, and interpreter of the forces that shape the couple's interaction. Active behavioral interventions mainly involve encouraging the partners to use direct and attentive communication with each other in the session rather than to speak to each other through the therapist by referring to the spouse as "he" or "she." Homework, such as experimentation with physical intimacy, is a creative product of the couple's imagination rather than a generic exercise determined by the therapist.

Object relations couples therapy attends to both the interpersonal and the intrapsychic simultaneously. It is a flexible approach tailored to the nature of the relational difficulty and to the developmental level of each partner. Thus, the treatment is an approach to formulating and intervening rather than a prescription of specific interventions and tasks that could apply to all couples. What is constant, however, in the object relations approach is the attention to the way in which the world of early internalized relationships has unconsciously come to life again in the current life of the couple.

Key Points

- The central concept of object relations couples therapy is the transposition of the internalized object world of each partner into the interpersonal sphere of the relationship.

- The mental mechanism that transforms the intrapsychic into the interpersonal is projective identification.

- Unconscious forces are paramount in choosing intimate partners as well as in guiding the interaction of the couple.

- The relationship of the couple, in its most refined form, can make possible empathic and collaborative efforts in which the whole is greater than the sum of its parts. In contrast, for defensive purposes, the couple relationship may become the repository of devalued aspects of each partner, leading to conflict, polarization, and dysfunction.

- Interpersonal conflict may be more tolerable than intrapsychic distress, leading partners to resist efforts to reduce the level of interpersonal conflict.

- The primary goal of object relations couples therapy is to foster reinternalization of projected devalued aspects of each partner, leading to a reduction in couple conflict, enhanced empathy, but an increase in individual emotional pain.

- Those devalued aspects of the self that have become reinternalized are now available for intrapsychic resolution, which may take place as part of the couples therapy as well as in concurrent individual therapy with another therapist.

- The couples therapist seeks the underlying issues that precipitate conflict rather than focusing on resolving the manifest content of the conflict. Anger is seen as reactive to hurt and emotional pain within the individual partners.

- Use of transference–countertransference phenomena in the here and now of the couple session may provide access to affectively charged and workable dynamics that are central to the couple relationship itself.

References

Bion WR: Learning From Experience. London, Heinemann, 1962

Bowen M: Family psychotherapy with schizophrenia in the hospital and in private practice, in Intensive Family Therapy. Edited by Boszormeny-Nagy I, Framo JL. New York, Hoeber, 1965, pp 213–244

Framo JL: Symptoms from a family transactional viewpoint, in Family Therapy in Transition. Edited by Ackerman NW. Boston, MA, Little, Brown, 1970, pp 125–171

Freud A: The ego and the mechanisms of defense (1936), in The Writings of Anna Freud, Vol 2. New York, International Universities Press, 1966

Freud S: Group psychology and the analysis of the ego (1921), in The Standard Edition of the Complete Psychological Works of Sigmund Freud, Vol 18. Translated and edited by Strachey J. London, Hogarth Press, 1955, pp 65–143

Gerber AJ, Peterson BS: Measuring transference phenomena with fMRI. J Am Psychoanal Assoc 54:1319–1325, 2006

Klein M: Notes on some schizoid mechanisms. Int J Psychoanal 27:99–110, 1946

Klein M: On identification (1955), in Our Adult World and Other Essays. New York, Basic Books, 1963, pp 55–98

Meissner WW: Projection and projective identification, in Projection, Identification, Projective Identification. Edited by Sandler J. Madison, CT, International Universities Press, 1987, pp 27–49

Ogden TH: Projective Identification and Psychotherapeutic Technique. New York, Jason Aronson, 1982

Scharff JS: Projective and Introjective Identification and the Use of the Therapist's Self. Northvale, NJ, Jason Aronson, 1992

Vogel EF, Bell NW: The emotionally disturbed child as the family scapegoat, in A Modern Introduction to the Family. Edited by Bell NW, Vogel EF. Glencoe, IL, Free Press, 1960, pp 412–447

Wangh M: The evocation of a proxy: a psychological maneuver, its use as a defense, its purpose and genesis. Psychoanal Study Child 17:451–469, 1962

Wynne LC: Some indications for exploratory family therapy, in Intensive Family Therapy. Edited by Boszormeny-Nagy I, Framo JL. New York, Hoeber, 1965

Zinner J: The implications of projective identification for marital interaction, in Contemporary Marriage: Structure, Dynamics and Therapy. Edited by Grunebaum H, Christ J. Boston, MA, Little, Brown, 1976, pp 293–308

Zinner J: A developmental spectrum of projective identification, in Proceedings of the International Conference of the Society of Psychoanalytical Marital Psychotherapists. Oxford, UK, Society of Psychoanalytical Marital Psychotherapists, 2001, pp 28–34

Suggested Readings

Dicks HV: Marital Tensions: Clinical Studies Towards a Psychological Theory of Interaction. New York, Basic Books, 1967

Ruszczynski S (ed): Psychotherapy With Couples: Theory and Practice at the Tavistock Institute of Marital Studies. London, Karnac Books, 1993

Ruszczynski S, Fisher J (eds): Intrusiveness and Intimacy in the Couple. London, Karnac Books, 1995

Scharff DE, Scharff JS: Object Relations Couple Therapy. Northvale, NJ, Jason Aronson, 1991

Zinner J: The implications of projective identification for marital interaction, in Contemporary Marriage: Structure, Dynamics and Therapy. Edited by Grunebaum H, Christ J. Boston, MA, Little Brown, 1976, pp 293–308

[Reprinted in Scharff JS (ed): Foundations of Object Relations Family Therapy. Northvale, NJ, Jason Aronson, 1989, pp 155–173]

Chapter 22

Behavioral Couples Therapy

Andrew Christensen, Ph.D.
Meghan McGinn, M.A.
Katherine J. Williams, M.A.

For the last 35 years, behaviorally oriented clinicians have adapted principles of behavior therapy to the problems of couples. They have carefully assessed couples and documented the success of their therapeutic interventions. As a result, there is a large body of evidence on the effectiveness of behavioral couples therapy (BCT). Dozens of randomized clinical trials have shown that BCT is better than no treatment or placebo treatment. These studies are summarized in major reviews (Baucom et al. 1998; Christensen and Heavey 1999; Snyder et al. 2006) and meta-analytic studies (Baucom et al. 2003; Shadish and Baldwin 2005). In the most recent of these meta-analytic studies, Shadish and Baldwin (2005) concluded that BCT "might be viewed as a mature therapy, with relatively fewer questions left to research compared with these newer therapies" (p. 11).

The original name for this treatment was behavioral marital therapy because the initial focus was on married couples. Although that remains the most common focus of the approach, some clinicians have applied the treatment to unmarried heterosexual couples and to gay and lesbian couples (e.g., Martell et al. 2004). To be more inclusive in their focus, most now refer to the approach as BCT.

The strategies of BCT have been applied as a preventive and enhancement intervention for couples early in their relationship and prior to the development of serious distress. The Prevention and Relationship Enhancement Program (PREP) developed by Markman, Stanley, and colleagues is the best example (e.g., Markman et al. 1994). These strategies have also been applied to established couples who are not yet distressed but who may be at risk for marital distress (Cordova et al. 2001). In this chapter, we focus only on the use of behavioral strategies in couples therapy—namely, those procedures that are applied to couples who are generally dissatisfied or distressed in their relationship. That distress is usually assessed with widely used measures of marital satisfaction, such as the Dyadic Adjustment Scale (Spanier 1976), Marital Adjustment Test (Locke and Wallace 1959), and Marital Satisfaction Inventory—Revised (Snyder 1997), all of which have normative data on them. Often, one standard deviation in the direction of distress on a normative distribution is defined as a cutoff score for distress; some version of these cutoff scores is often used to define distressed couples who can be included in the clinical trials of the approach.

Not all couples who are distressed in their relationship are appropriate for couples therapy. Couples who are separating, who are seriously violent, who persist in ongoing affairs, or who have certain mental disorders may not be appropriate for typical couples therapy. Because the goal of couples therapy is improvement in the relationship, couples who have decided to separate and divorce are not appropriate for this therapy but instead may consider seeking separation counseling or mediation. A majority of couples who present for therapy are likely to have some level of violence (Simpson et al. 2007). If that violence is serious, causing injury and/or intimidation, then couples therapy is not appropriate. The sessions themselves might arouse strong emotions that are later expressed in violence (e.g., a husband beats up his wife for what she said in therapy). Also, couples therapy assumes joint responsibility for relationship problems, whereas therapeutic approaches for domestic violence require the perpetrator of violence to take responsibility for his or her actions and are usually conducted separately for perpetrators and for victims. Couples therapy can, however, be effective in couples with mild to moderate levels of violence (Simpson et al. 2008) but does require attention to that violence, even if mild. Couples in which a partner is having an ongoing, secret affair and refuses to end it or reveal it to his or her partner are usually considered inappropriate for couples therapy. The emotional involvement in the affair prevents full commitment to the relationship, yet the ongoing affair cannot be a focus of discussion in the session. Finally, certain types of mental disorder, such as substance abuse and dependence, psychosis, and suicidal depression, when present in one or both spouses, require primary therapeutic attention to that disorder, with later or secondary attention to the couple problems. As an adjunct to the primary treatment, couples therapy can be quite useful, often enhancing the couple relationship as well as the treatment for the mental disorder. For example, Fals-Stewart and O'Farrell have shown that addition of BCT improves the effectiveness of treatment for substance use disorders (Fals-Stewart and O'Farrell 2003; O'Farrell and Fals-Stewart 2006).

In this chapter, we discuss three major types of behavioral couples therapy: traditional BCT, cognitive-behavioral couples therapy (CBCT), and integrative behavioral couples therapy (IBCT). In the original behavioral couples therapy, BCT, the focus was on making positive changes in behavior. For CBCT, an emphasis on cognitive restructuring was added to the behavioral techniques of BCT. Finally, IBCT integrated strategies for changing behavior with strategies for promoting acceptance of the partner. Although each of these approaches is derived from behavioral principles and thus is appropriately described as "behavioral," each emphasizes different principles and incorporates different techniques. More importantly, each has a separate body of empirical literature supporting its efficacy.

We describe each of these approaches and their supporting evidence later in this chapter, but we now focus on several commonalities. First, all three approaches start with a separate assessment phase that consists of several sessions, usually involving an individual session (or half session) with each partner as well as joint sessions with both. The problems that brought the couple to therapy, as well as their relationship strengths, are assessed. Questionnaire data are collected during this phase and usually consist of a measure of relationship satisfaction, such as one of those mentioned previously, a measure of relationship violence such as the Conflict Tactics Scale (Straus et al. 1996), and measures particular to the specific behavioral approach. During the assessment phase, particularly during the individual interviews, the therapist assesses violence in the relationship, commitment to the relationship, and the presence of affairs. Second, the assessment phase is followed by a feedback session in which the therapist goes over the findings from the assessment, including results from the questionnaires. The therapist emphasizes the strengths as well as the problems in the couple's relationship and discusses how therapy will attempt to help them. Third, the feedback session is followed by an active phase of therapy in which the therapist and the couple work together to improve the relationship. The therapist tends to take an active rather than merely a reflective role, attempting to alter how the partners communicate with each other, how they interpret each other's behavior, and how they emotionally react to each other. Sessions usually take place weekly for about an hour but can last longer or occur more or less frequently. Finally, therapists often taper sessions toward the end of therapy. If sessions have been weekly, the couple may come in every other week for a few sessions to see how they fare on their own before terminating therapy. Typically, BCT is short-term treatment. During the clinical trials of BCT, the number of sessions usually ranges from 8 to 25 sessions.

Traditional Behavioral Couples Therapy

Traditional BCT developed out of the behavioral and social learning movement of the 1960s and 1970s in which operant conditioning techniques were being adapted to address a range of problems, such as child externalizing behaviors. In 1969, Stuart published the first case study to apply a behavioral technique, a token economy, to a couple's relationship issues. Around the same time, researchers led by Robert Weiss and Jerry Patterson began applying behavioral change techniques that included an emphasis on skills training to treat marital distress (Weiss et al. 1973). Interest spread to other researchers, and in 1979 Jacobson and Margolin published their treatment manual of behavioral techniques titled *Marital Therapy: Strategies Based on Social Learning and Behavior Exchange Principles.* BCT soon became the most widely studied intervention for couples.

Behavior therapy is based on the premise that behaviors do not occur in isolation but rather are contingent on environmental antecedents and consequences. Environmental consequences that increase the likelihood of particular behaviors are reinforcers, whereas consequences that decrease the likelihood of particular behaviors are punishers. Stimuli that cue one to the likely occurrence of a reinforcer or punisher, dependent on appropriate behavior, are discriminative stimuli. When couples' problems are being addressed, particularly relevant reinforcers and punishers are the behaviors of one's partner. Early research summarized by Jacobson and Margolin (1979) suggested that distressed couples lacked positive reinforcing behaviors, had an abundance of punishing behaviors, or had an unfortunate combination of the two. The focus of BCT, therefore, is to alter the contingencies by increasing positive and decreasing negative behaviors.

Assessment

BCT begins with an assessment period aimed at identifying the current punishing behaviors and the desired but missing reinforcing behaviors that are contributing to the couple's distress. The conceptual model for assessment is the *functional analysis of behavior*, in which the antecedent and consequent stimuli of important target behaviors are examined. For example, a functional analysis might determine that both partners often ignore or reject affectionate gestures by the other even though both indicate a desire for greater affection. The initial assessment is completed over a period of 3–4 weeks and ideally culminates in the adoption of a treatment plan based on the assessment results. Information is gathered in a variety of ways, including interviews with the couple together and with each partner separately, self-report measures, and observation of couple communication. During this time, the therapist attempts to transform broad, general complaints such as complaints that "he doesn't show any love toward me" or "she never supports me" into specific, concrete behaviors. This behavioral pinpointing process creates concrete behavioral goals for therapy. The therapist also works to create an empathic alliance with each partner and to develop a shared conceptualization of the relationship based on both partners' experience. After the initial assessment, the therapist meets with the couple to present the findings of the assessment and make recommendations for treatment. Although the initial assessment has concluded at this point, behavioral assessment continues for couples who accept the treatment recommendations throughout the course of therapy in order to provide feedback to the clients and therapist.

For couples to be successful in BCT, it is necessary that they accept the behavioral model of change and adopt a collaborative set. Therefore, the therapist is responsible for establishing the credibility of the model and treatment program, for providing a clear understanding of how he or she views the couple's relationship within the model's framework, and for increasing the couple's positive expectancies about the potential benefits of treatment. To accomplish these goals, the therapist should begin assessment by outlining and describing the rationale for all assessment procedures, and should emphasize positive aspects of the relationship in addition to problems during assessment feedback while expressing a level of optimism about the potential for improvement (Jacobson and Margolin 1979). To promote a collaborative set, the therapist may explain the concept of mutual causality in relationships, may ask each partner what he or she can do individually to improve the relationship, and may advance the notion that the way toward a better relationship is for each one to focus on the other's needs rather than his or her own needs.

BCT comprises three main components: behavioral exchange, communication training, and problem-solving training. The behavioral exchange component is meant to provide immediate, short-term gains for the couple and to increase their willingness to collaborate, whereas the communication and problem-solving training seek to address the couple's presenting problems but, more importantly, arm them with skills for dealing with issues in the future.

Behavioral Exchange

The goal of behavioral exchange techniques is to identify behaviors that are positively reinforcing for each partner and to increase the occurrence of these behaviors. Because behavioral exchange occurs in the early stages of treatment and the couple may not yet have a collaborative set in place, the behaviors should be relatively low cost and easy to implement.

One common option for implementing behavioral exchange is for each partner to create a list of behaviors that he or she could perform that might be pleasing to the other. The list is then analyzed by the couple to identify benefits to the receiver and costs to the giver, and each partner is then able to choose behaviors that maximize benefit and minimize cost. Each partner is encouraged to engage in the identified behaviors on a special "caring day" or to simply increase them as possible throughout the week. At the next session, the therapist debriefs their experience, acknowledging the effort that each has made and perhaps revising the list of behaviors as appropriate.

Behavioral exchange techniques capitalize on the fact that although distressed couples do not frequently engage in positive exchanges with each other, they still have great potential for reinforcing each other. Behavioral exchange usually results in short-term increases in relationship satisfaction, setting couples up for the more intensive, collaborative work of the communication and problem-solving phase of treatment.

Communication Training

The goal of communication training is to facilitate the ability of couples to discuss difficult or problematic issues in ways that do not lead to argument but instead lead to greater understanding. Speaker skills as well as listener skills are taught. Speakers are encouraged to describe potential problems in the relationship by using "I statements," which describe the speaker's emotional reactions to specific behavior by the partner in a particular context. The model is "I feel X when you do Y in situation Z." By using this model the speaker avoids accusatory comments, character assassinations, and overgeneralizations. For example, rather than saying, "You are so thoughtless," the speaker might say, "I felt upset and embarrassed when you told that story about my mother to our friends." Such a comment communicates the speaker's dissatisfaction and the reason for it clearly; the listener is more likely to understand the speaker's comments, even if he or she does not agree. Listeners are taught to demonstrate behaviorally that they have heard the speaker by summarizing the main points of the speaker to the speaker's satisfaction before they state their own points. For example, the listener in the previous example would paraphrase or summarize the speaker's upset about the story of the mother before describing his or her own position. In addition to these general skills, the therapist may teach skills that are specific to each partner's abilities and deficits. For example, the therapist might teach greater eye contact in a partner who frequently looks down or away during conversation.

Problem-Solving Training

Although communication training may lead to greater understanding between partners, it may not correct a repeated problem. Problem-solving training allows couples to resolve their presenting problems as well as acquire the skills necessary to deal with future issues. The techniques are focused on changing the process by which couples communicate regarding conflicts in their relationships, and do not explicitly deal with the content of the conflicts themselves. A primary focus is to teach the couple the difference between arguing and problem solving. In arguing, the goal is often to win the discussion by having the other partner concede to one's points, whereas in problem solving, the goal is to reach a mutually agreed-on solution to the problem. Although angry or emotional exchanges are unlikely to be eliminated from the relationship, it is important that the couple recognize that unlike a problem-solving discussion, such exchanges will not lead to positive behavioral change. Couples who find themselves in an argument may therefore agree to put off the discussion for their next problem-solving session rather than allowing the argument to escalate.

Problem solving is broken down into two distinct, nonoverlapping phases. The first phase, problem definition, requires the couple to precisely define the problem and each partner to acknowledge his or her role in the problem. The second phase, problem solution, focuses on reaching an agreement that is acceptable to both partners.

The problem definition phase should be relatively brief and follow these three steps:

1. One partner states the problem. The problem definition should be confined to include one issue only, regardless of how the issue may interact with other issues in the relationship. When stating the problem, the partner is instructed to begin with something positive, to define the problem in specific behavioral terms, and to use feeling expressions.
2. The other partner paraphrases the problem definition, summarizing the points of his or her partner's statement. The partner must be careful not

to react defensively to the problem definition by trying to justify his or her behavior. Rather, the purpose of paraphrasing is to ensure that the partners carefully listen to each other and refrain from interrupting and to clear up any misinterpretations of the problem definition. Up to this point, the problem definition phase relies heavily on what is taught above in communication training.

3. As a final step, each of the partners expands on the problem definition by acknowledging his or her role in the problem. This does not mean that partners are agreeing to change their behaviors; behavioral change is something to be explored in the problem solution phase. However, each should be able to admit that he or she engages in behaviors that are upsetting the partner or may contribute to the maintenance of those behaviors.

Once these steps have been successfully completed, the couple is ready to move on to the problem solution phase. This phase, too, can be completed in three steps:

1. Couples engage in a brainstorming session in which they generate and verbalize possible solutions without taking time to evaluate them. The therapist may model this step by suggesting solutions to a sample problem and including humorous or absurd solutions to emphasize the non-evaluative nature of brainstorming.

2. Couples evaluate the costs and benefits involved in each of the potential solutions and decide whether to include these solutions in the final change agreement.

3. Couples put the final change agreement into writing. Included are specifics such as the frequency and duration of the agreed-on behaviors and the conditions under which the behaviors should occur.

The partners practice the problem-definition and problem-solution steps during therapy sessions, but an important goal is for the couple to generalize this experience to their home environment and future issues. To facilitate this, the therapist may become less active and directive as therapy continues, allowing couples to do more of the work on their own. Likewise, termination should occur gradually, with less frequent sessions and occasional "booster sessions" as needed, allowing the couple to slowly become accustomed to handling problem solving on their own.

BCT, which includes behavioral exchange and communication and problem-solving training, has consistently outperformed no treatment or control conditions in ameliorating relationship distress (Hahlweg and Markman 1988; Markman and Hahlweg 1993) and has been shown to improve communication skills and enhance couples' positive interactions and satisfaction (Halford et al. 1993). Meta-analyses estimate a treatment effect size of around 0.95 (Byrne et al. 2004; Dunn and Schwebel 1995). However, despite the large effect size, researchers have noted that around a quarter to a third of couples do not significantly improve with BCT, and another quarter to a third of couples improve but do not reach a nondistressed level (Halford et al. 1993; Jacobson 1989). Even those couples helped initially by BCT may be prone to relapse (Jacobson et al. 1987). These statistics have led a number of researchers to search for ways of improving on BCT so that it might help a wider range of couples. Two newer approaches, cognitive-behavioral couples therapy and integrative behavioral couples therapy, are described below.

Cognitive-Behavioral Couples Therapy

CBCT was developed in the 1980s as part of the cognitive revolution that was taking place in psychology. CBCT, which combines elements of Beck's (1970) cognitive therapy with BCT, is based on the assumption that relationship distress includes cognitive, behavioral, and affective components, which influence relationship distress and one another. CBCT extends the treatment strategies of BCT by examining partners' interpretation of each other's behavior as well as that behavior itself. CBCT therapists assume that changes in partners' thoughts will ultimately lead to changes in behavior and emotion, and vice versa. Thus, they advocate an examination of all three aspects of behavior but give greater causal credence to thoughts. The book by Baucom and Epstein (1990) has often served as the treatment manual for studies of CBCT.

Assessment

Like BCT, CBCT includes a several-session assessment phase. The distinctive aspect is that assessment focuses on the cognitive as well as behavioral and affective factors that play a role in the couple's distress. In assessing the cognitions of each partner, the therapist explores perceptions, attributions, expectancies, assumptions, and standards (Baucom and Epstein 1990). Partners' perceptions of themselves, the other, and the relationship are evaluated to determine whether their views are skewed by a focus on negative events and an exclusion of positive events. CBCT therapists also evaluate the attributions, or explanations, that partners make for their own and their partner's behavior using instruments such as the Marital Attitude Survey (J.L. Pretzer, N. Epstein, B. Fleming, "The Marital Attitude Survey: A Measure of Dysfunctional Attributions and Expectancies," unpublished manuscript, 1985), which evaluates the reporter's attributions of relationship problems to the partner's (or his or her own) behavior or personality, to the partner's lack of love, or to malicious intent of the partner. Primarily through observation of communication, therapists evaluate partners' predictions of the other's behavior (expectancies) that could hinder their working on solutions to problems. The therapist focuses on the clinical interview for information about partners' assumptions about the other or the relationship, with an eye toward incorrect assumptions. Finally, the therapist evaluates standards in the relationship—what partners report in the interview or during communication that they think the other *should* do. The therapist attends to unrealistic standards partners have in this evaluation. Across cognitions, the therapist seeks to recognize those that are distorted and may be problematic for the relationship. In the assessment of affect, the therapist examines the rate and intensity of positive and negative affect, partners' awareness and insight relating to their emotions, emotions that are dysfunctional, and the extent to which emotions disrupt couple functioning (Baucom and Epstein 1990).

Cognitive Interventions

In addition to the behavioral interventions of BCT, CBCT therapists specifically focus on biased or distorted cognitions and attempt to alter them with cognitive restructuring strategies. The goals of cognitive restructuring are to increase partners' ability "to identify their cognitions that are associated with marital discord, to test the validity or appropriateness of those cognitions, and to modify dysfunctional cognitions" (Baucom et al. 1995, p. 80). CBCT therapists first provide psychoeducation about the cognitive model, describing what cognitive distortions are and giving examples of common distortions. One example is selective abstraction, a perceptual distortion in which a person focuses on only certain parts of a situation in drawing conclusions. In distressed couples this could be problematic if one partner focuses more attention on the negative aspects of the behavior of his or her partner (e.g., a partner coming home late one night a week) than on the positive aspects (a partner having more time for the relationship over the weekend), yielding an inaccurate conclusion (the partner cares more for work than for the relationship).

CBCT therapists typically present the different types of cognitions that are the focus in CBCT (perceptions, attributions, expectancies, assumptions, and standards) and help partners identify, test, and modify problematic cognitions in these areas through logical analysis, "behavioral experiments," and other evidence gathering (Baucom and Epstein 1990). Through the use of logical analysis of previous events, partners are taught to consider alternative explanations for events. Therapists often use Socratic questioning to help partners see their inaccurate or illogical thoughts about situations in their relationship.

In behavioral experiments, partners work with the therapist to plan an experiment that will actually test the cognitions of focus. For example, for the couple that has concluded they cannot spend an evening together without arguing, the therapist might help them plan a positive evening, discuss how they will avoid conflictual discussions, and test their hypothesis by the couple's spending the planned evening together. If the evening goes without an argument, they will have contradicted their conclusion that they are unable to spend an evening without arguing.

Affective Interventions

In addition to the behavioral interventions of BCT and the cognitive interventions described previously, CBCT therapists use strategies to target dysfunctional emotions. Partners are taught emotion regulation strategies such as recognizing and labeling emotions, appropriately expressing emotions, and changing certain high-intensity negative emotions. Often the therapist will use emotional expressiveness training (EET), a type of communication training that focuses on adequately expressing emotions and related thoughts to one's partner. In EET, as in communication training, the therapist provides the couple with guidelines for expressing emotions ("expresser skills") and receiving a partner's expression empathically ("empathic listener skills"). EET includes expresser skills such as being subjective, stating positives when realistic, and being specific. Empathic listener skills include summary, reflection, and demonstration of acceptance. Typically the therapist will role-play these skills with each partner before coaching the partners in the practice of the skills. For high-intensity negative emotions, couples will often need additional interventions that may include individual therapy.

The order of the CBCT interventions depends on the couple; there is no specific sequence of interventions that should be implemented in treatment. CBCT therapists begin treatment with interventions that target the specific skills deficits presented by the couple (typically behavioral or affective interventions). For example, a couple that does not effectively communicate their feelings about problems in the relationship would begin treatment with EET and other affective interventions. Once these skills are acquired, the couple can more effectively engage in behavioral and cognitive interventions. If the couple does not seem to have a specific skills deficit but struggles with behavioral interventions, the therapist might shift to cognitive interventions to explore whether cognitive distortions are keeping the couple from progressing with behavioral strategies. Over the course of therapy, CBCT therapists will almost always use each of the three types of interventions to target problems in each respective area. The therapist and couple work together to determine when each type of intervention is most beneficial for the couple.

Empirical research has documented the efficacy of CBCT in the treatment of distressed couples. CBCT was found to be efficacious relative to wait-list control groups (Baucom and Lester 1986; Baucom et al. 1990) and as efficacious as BCT in increasing relationship adjustment, although it was not found to be more efficacious (e.g., Halford et al. 1993).

Enhanced Cognitive-Behavioral Couples Therapy

Since its initial development and testing, Epstein and Baucom (2002) have revised CBCT to develop what they call the *enhanced cognitive-behavioral couples therapy* (ECBCT) approach. The enhanced treatment focuses more on general themes in relationships rather than on specific behavioral, cognitive, or affective events. The enhanced treatment extends the cognitive model by going beyond the dyad, focusing on contextual factors relevant to the relationship (e.g., family and cultural context) and focusing on the contribution of the individual partners such as their psychopathology, personality styles, and unresolved individual issues that have the potential to affect the relationship. Finally, ECBCT involves an adaptation model of couple functioning that acknowledges changes in the relationship and the individual partners to which the couple must adapt. Individual factors (e.g., psychopathology), dyadic factors (e.g., interaction patterns), and environmental factors (e.g., family of origin) are discussed during assessment in ECBCT and are targeted in treatment. Although the outcome research to date has focused on the efficacy of CBCT, not ECBCT, the enhanced model extends the CBCT model to factors outside the couple that affect relationship functioning and likely play a role in relationship enhancement or deterioration (see Baucom et al. 2002 for a summary of ECBCT).

Integrative Behavioral Couples Therapy

IBCT was developed by Andrew Christensen and the late Neil S. Jacobson (Christensen and Jacobson 2000; Christensen et al. 1995; Jacobson and Christensen 1998) in an effort to enhance the power of BCT. Several theoretical principles distinguish IBCT from both BCT and CBCT. First, IBCT assumes that most marital problems are caused not just by the presence of problematic behavior (and the absence of constructive behavior) by one or both partners but by their emotional reactions to those behaviors. Because of this emphasis on reactions as well as actions, IBCT integrates strategies for promoting emotional acceptance with those for promoting behavioral change. Second, IBCT focuses on broad classes of behavior or themes in partners' concerns. Although IBCT values behavioral specificity in illustrating these themes, it assumes that the theme is never fully captured by a group of specific behaviors. Third, IBCT represents a return to the central assessment technique of the functional analysis of behavior in which the therapist examines the antecedent and consequent contextual factors that causally influence targeted behavior. Although both BCT and CBCT purportedly rely on a functional analysis of behavior, Christensen and Jacobson (Jacobson and Christensen 1998) suggest that these approaches often apply standard treatments such as communication training in BCT and cognitive restructuring in CBCT, whether or not those behaviors were implicated in a functional analysis of the couple's distress. Finally, IBCT distinguishes between treatment strategies that bring about change through deliberate strategies, such as when partners are given guidelines for communicating differently or thinking differently, and evocative strategies, such as when partners behave differently as a result of new emotional experiences or new insights discovered in treatment. Although IBCT employs both types of strategies, it emphasizes evocative strategies, assuming that those will lead to more durable change. In contrast, BCT and CBCT focus primarily on deliberate change strategies.

Assessment

The distinctive aspect of assessment in IBCT is its focus on the conflictual theme in a couple's interactions and a conceptual formulation about that theme that is shared with the couple. *Conflictual theme* refers to a class of behaviors that are the focus of struggle within a couple. For example, many couples struggle around the theme of closeness-independence, with one partner pushing for a more connected relationship and the other pushing for more autonomy. In order to generate a formulation about this theme, IBCT therapists examine vulnerabilities in each partner that make this theme so emotionally distressing for them. For example, perhaps the closeness seeker did not feel special to loved ones in the past and now is seeking, desperately, that special feeling within the couple. Similarly, perhaps the independence seeker often felt in past family relationships that he or she never got the freedom to explore and was always under the watchful and judgmental eye of a parent. Thus, both partners may be especially sensitive to issues around closeness-independence. Despite the importance of historical material to the formulation, current interactional patterns are even more important than past behavior to the maintenance of problematic behavior and thus to the formulation about this behavior. Our couple with the theme of closeness-autonomy may be engaging in a self-perpetuating cycle of interaction in which the more that one seeks closeness, the more the other seeks autonomy. In this vicious cycle of interaction, each partner's efforts to achieve his or her own goals serve to push the partner in a direction counter to those goals. During the feedback stage immediately after assessment, IBCT therapists share with couples their formulation of the couples' problems in an effort to bring them to a dyadic understanding of their difficulties that emphasizes the ways in which each partner contributes to the problem, as opposed to an individual understanding in which blame is imputed primarily to one partner.

Strategies for Promoting Emotion Acceptance

After the assessment and feedback stage, active treatment begins. The focus during treatment is normally on emotionally salient material that the couple brings to the treatment session. A recent negative or positive incident relevant to the formulation is a common focus in therapy. For example, if the couple earlier who were struggling with the theme of closeness–independence had a distressing conflict in which the independence seeker wanted to spend an evening with friends or a gratifying incident in which they felt particularly close to each other, both events could be material for the session. Upcoming events as well as recent events can be the focus of the session. For example, an anticipated family visit may create anxieties about spending time alone with family versus together with the spouse. Finally, broader issues not related to any specific incident can be a focus of therapeutic attention, as when the pair talks about the ways in which they feel close to one another or the ways in which they feel free and independent. Sometimes the most emotionally salient material is what happens right in the session. Couples typically enact their problems in the session, and the IBCT therapist focuses on those events as ideal material for discussion. For example, the independence seeker might be withdrawn in the session as the closeness seeker voices his or her needs.

In dealing with this emotionally salient material, IBCT therapists use three major strategies to promote emotional acceptance and positive behavior change: empathic joining around the problem, unified detachment from the problem, and tolerance building. All three strategies try to use the struggles of the partners to bring about greater intimacy between them. All three strategies are evocative rather than deliberate change strategies in that the couple is not told that they should accept any particular behavior or that they should change any particular behavior. However, the strategies often lead to important changes in emotional reactions and conflictual behaviors.

The first two strategies, empathic joining and unified detachment, are conceptually as well as technically different. *Empathic joining* is an emotionally evocative process in which the therapist elicits emotional disclosures by each that may lead to more sympathetic responding by the other. In contrast, *unified detachment* involves emotional distance from the conflict at hand. The therapist assists couples in looking at their problems from a distant, more objective observer stance.

The first step in empathic joining often occurs during the feedback session. As IBCT therapists provide a formulation of their couples' problems, they discuss the emotional vulnerabilities that each partner may experience that make these conflicts so upsetting for him or her. During the active treatment phase, IBCT therapists use the daily incidents and issues that are the focus of therapy as material for eliciting further emotional material. Usually couples discuss their conflictual incidents and issues with blame and express "hard" emotions such as anger, frustration, and resentment, which portray the self aggressively. The combination of blame and hard emotions typically pushes the partner away, who responds with his or her own level of blame, defensiveness, and hard emotion. During empathic joining, the therapist moves the discussion away from blame by shifting the focus from the responsibility and motives of the partner who did some upsetting behavior to the emotional reactions of the partner who received that behavior. Furthermore, the therapist, in an effort to move away from the hard emotions that are usually expressed, probes for softer emotions such as hurt, disappointment, and feelings of neglect or rejection. When executed successfully, empathic joining can lead to partners experiencing greater emotional intimacy with each other in the context of a problem discussion. It also can lead to subtle changes in their emotional reactions to one another (acceptance) and in their behavior toward one another (behavior change).

The first step in unified detachment also occurs during the formulation phase of the feedback session. IBCT therapists often describe the vicious cycle of interaction in which couples get stuck, such that each partner's behavior triggers undesired behavior in the other and leads to a polarization in their positions. By portraying their problems as a reciprocal negative interaction, the therapist invites the couple to step back from their usual stance in which they are caught up in conflict to a stance where they can look at the problem as an observer. They can begin to see the problem as an "it" rather than as a "you."

During the active treatment phase, IBCT therapists continue their efforts at unified detachment by encouraging a mindful attitude toward the couple's interaction in which the partners can observe and describe it nonjudgmentally. When the couple describes a positive or negative incident relevant to their theme, the therapist may enlist them in a nonjudgmental description of the important sequence of acts between them that, in the case of a negative incident, serves to escalate the conflict or, in the case of a positive incident, prevents escalation and allows them an enjoyable encounter. The therapist may help the couple catalogue a list of "triggering events" that serve to turn disagreements into arguments. The therapist may engage couples in a comparative analysis of two similar incidents that had different emotional impacts so they can speculate about what might have made for the different effects. The therapist may encourage couples to create a descriptive or humorous name for their pattern of interaction, the repeated dance that they do. For example, the couple with the closeness-independence problem might name one of their behavioral patterns the cat-and-mouse game, as the closeness seeker (the cat) chases after the forever-hidden independence seeker (the mouse). When an acceptable name can be generated, it helps the couple label an unpleasant incident ("Oh, we got into our usual cat-and-mouse game again"), contain that incident, and recover from it more quickly.

Tolerance building includes a variety of strategies that serve to increase partners' acceptance of one another, even though the offending behavior may still bother them. Tolerance interventions do not bring the couple together as successful empathic joining and unified detachment interventions do. However, they do reduce the tension associated with partners' actions. There are a number of tolerance interventions, but space permits a discussion of only one of them here.

During the feedback session or early in the treatment, IBCT therapists may discuss the positive features that are part of what each partner sees as the negative features of the other. For example, a couple may include one member who is easygoing and carefree and another who is ambitious and goal directed. It is easy to discuss the positive features of each (e.g., the carefree partner adds relaxation; the ambitious partner keeps them on target to complete needed tasks) as well as the negative features of each (e.g., the carefree partner may not follow through; the ambitious partner may take things too seriously) as well as discuss the possible balance that could be achieved between their different strengths. Such a discussion can lead partners to be more accepting of what each brings to the relationship and can counteract their tendency to polarize (so the carefree partner becomes irresponsible and the goal-directed partner becomes compulsive in reaction to each other).

In addition to these three interventions for promoting acceptance between partners (empathic joining, unified detachment, and tolerance building), IBCT therapists can also use the direct change interventions of BCT, such as behavioral exchange, communication training, and problem-solving training. Typically, IBCT therapists start off therapy with acceptance interventions and turn to direct change interventions only as needed. Also, these interventions are often done in a less rule-governed way, adapting them to the couple as needed. For example, in teaching communication training, IBCT therapists would be less rigid about encouraging couples to follow the "I statement" model of "I feel X when you do Y in situation Z" and might encourage each partner to talk more about his or her own emotional reactions and less about the partner's possible motives in doing the behavior.

Three separate clinical trials have documented the efficacy of IBCT. In his dissertation, Wimberly (1998) randomly assigned 8 couples to a group format of IBCT and 9 couples to a wait-list control group and found superior results for the IBCT couples. Jacobson and Christensen and colleagues (Jacobson et al. 2000) randomly assigned 21 couples to BCT or IBCT and found greater support for IBCT than for BCT. A large two-site clinical trial of 134 chronically and seriously distressed couples randomly assigned to IBCT or BCT found positive results for both treatments at termination (Christensen et al. 2004) and at 2-year follow-up (Christensen et al. 2006), with results favoring IBCT. A study of therapeutic processes supported the putative change mechanisms in both treatments (Doss et al. 2005).

Conclusion

In this chapter we have described three behavioral approaches to couples therapy. Each has several clinical trials supporting the efficacy of the approach. Although there is some evidence for the superiority of integrative behavioral couples therapy over behavioral couples therapy, none of these treatments has clearly and unequivocally indicated its superiority over the others. All represent viable approaches for improving couple relationships. Furthermore, there is evidence that couples therapy can be beneficial not just for improving a couple's relationship but for assisting partners with diagnosable disorders as well. For example, couples therapy is useful in treating substance abuse and dependence (Fals-Stewart and O'Farrell 2003), depression (O'Leary and Beach 1990), and agoraphobia (Craske and Zoellner 1995). Thus, couples therapy represents a well-validated treatment for relationship problems and an adjunct for certain individual disorders.

Key Points

- Numerous clinical trials have demonstrated the efficacy of behavioral approaches to couples therapy.
- Typical, stand-alone couples therapy is not appropriate for seriously violent couples, couples in which one or both persist in undisclosed affairs, and couples in which one or both partners have a serious mental disorder requiring primary attention.

- Behavioral couples therapy (BCT) usually begins with 1–3 evaluation sessions in which partners are seen alone and together, followed by a therapy feedback session and active treatment sessions in which partners are normally seen conjointly.

- Sessions are typically conducted weekly for almost an hour for a total of 8–25 sessions.

- Evidence supports the efficacy of three approaches to behavioral couples therapy: traditional behavioral couples therapy (BCT), cognitive-behavioral couples therapy (CBCT), and integrative behavioral couples therapy (IBCT).

- BCT consists of procedures designed to increase the frequency of positive behavior and to teach constructive communication and problem solving.

- CBCT adds strategies of cognitive restructuring to BCT.

- IBCT includes strategies to promote emotional acceptance and mindfulness so there is a balance between acceptance and change.

References

Baucom DH, Epstein N: Cognitive-Behavioral Marital Therapy. New York, Brunner/Mazel, 1990

Baucom DH, Lester GW: The usefulness of cognitive restructuring as an adjunct to behavioral marital therapy. Behav Ther 17:385–403, 1986

Baucom DH, Sayers SL, Sher TG: Supplementing behavioral marital therapy with cognitive restructuring and emotional expressiveness training: an outcome investigation. J Consult Clin Psychol 58:636–645, 1990

Baucom DH, Epstein N, Rankin LA: Cognitive aspects of cognitive-behavioral marital therapy, in Clinical Handbook of Couple Therapy, 2nd Edition. Edited by Jacobson NS, Gurman AS. New York, Guilford, 1995, pp 65–90

Baucom DH, Shoham V, Mueser KT, et al: Empirically supported couple and family therapies for adult problems. J Consult Clin Psychol 66:53–88, 1998

Baucom DH, Epstein N, LaTillade JJ: Cognitive-behavioral couple therapy, in Clinical Handbook of Couple Therapy, 3rd Edition. Edited by Gurman AS, Jacobson NS. New York, Guilford, 2002, pp 26–59

Baucom DH, Hahlweg K, Kuschel A: Are waiting-list control groups needed in future marital therapy outcome research? Behav Ther 34:179–188, 2003

Beck AT: Cognitive therapy: nature in relation to behavior therapy. Behav Ther 1:184–200, 1970

Byrne M, Carr A, Clark M: The efficacy of behavioural couples therapy and emotionally focused therapy for couple distress. Contemporary Family Therapy: An International Journal 26:361–387, 2004

Christensen A, Heavey CL: Interventions for couples. Annu Rev Psychol 50:165–190, 1999

Christensen A, Jacobson NS: Reconcilable Differences. New York, Guilford, 2000

Christensen A, Jacobson NS, Babcock JC: Integrative behavioral couple therapy, in Clinical Handbook of Marital Therapy, 2nd Edition. Edited by Jacobson NS, Gurman AS. New York, Guilford, 1995, pp 31–64

Christensen A, Atkins DC, Berns S, et al: Traditional versus integrative behavioral couple therapy for significantly and chronically distressed married couples. J Consult Clin Psychol 72:176–191, 2004

Christensen A, Atkins DC, Yi J, et al: Couple and individual adjustment for two years following a randomized clinical trial comparing traditional versus integrative behavioral couple therapy. J Consult Clin Psychol 74:1180–1191, 2006

Cordova JV, Warren LZ, Gee CB: Motivational interviewing with couples: an intervention for at-risk couples. J Marital Fam Ther 27:315–326, 2001

Craske MG, Zoellner LA: Anxiety disorders: the role of marital therapy, in Clinical Handbook of Marital Therapy, 2nd Edition. Edited by Jacobson NS, Gurman AS. New York, Guilford, 1995, pp 394–410

Doss BD, Thum YM, Sevier M, et al: Improving relationships: mechanisms of change in couple therapy. J Consult Clin Psychol 73:624–633, 2005

Dunn RL, Schwebel AI: Meta-analytic review of marital therapy outcome research. J Fam Psychol 9:58–68, 1995

Epstein N, Baucom DH: Enhanced Cognitive-Behavioral Therapy for Couples: A Contextual Approach. Washington, DC, American Psychological Association, 2002

Fals-Stewart W, O'Farrell TJ: Behavioral family counseling and naltrexone for male opioid-dependent patients. J Consult Clin Psychol 71:432–442, 2003

Hahlweg K, Markman MJ: Effectiveness of behavioral marital therapy: empirical status of behavioral techniques in preventing and alleviating marital distress. J Consult Clin Psychol 56:440–447, 1988

Halford WK, Sanders MR, Behrens BC: A comparison of the generalization of behavioral marital therapy and enhanced behavioral marital therapy. J Consult Clin Psychol 61:51–60, 1993

Jacobson NS: The maintenance of treatment gains following social learning-based marital therapy. Behav Ther 20:325–336, 1989

Jacobson NS, Christensen A: Acceptance and Change in Couple Therapy: A Therapist's Guide to Transforming Relationships. New York, WW Norton, 1998

Jacobson NS, Margolin G: Marital Therapy: Strategies Based on Social Learning and Behavior Exchange Principles. New York, Brunner/Mazel, 1979

Jacobson NS, Schmaling KB, Holtzworth-Munrow A: Component analysis of behavioral martial therapy: two-year follow-up and prediction of relapse. J Marital Fam Ther 13:187–195, 1987

Jacobson NS, Christensen A, Prince SE, et al: Integrative behavioral couple therapy: an acceptance-based, promising new treatment for couple discord. J Consult Clin Psychol 68:351–355, 2000

Locke HJ, Wallace KM: Short marital-adjustment and prediction tests: their reliability and validity. Marriage Fam Living 21:251–255, 1959

Markman HJ, Hahlweg K: The prediction and prevention of marital distress: an international perspective. Clin Psychol Rev 13:29–43, 1993

Markman HJ, Stanley SM, Blumber SL: Fighting For Your Marriage: Positive Steps for Preventing Divorce and Preserving Lasting Love. San Francisco, CA, Jossey-Bass, 1994

Martell CR, Safren SA, Prince SE: Cognitive-Behavioral Therapies With Lesbian, Gay, and Bisexual Clients. New York, Guilford, 2004

O'Farrell TJ, Fals-Stewart W: Behavioral Couples Therapy for Alcoholism and Drug Abuse. New York, Guilford, 2006

O'Leary KD, Beach SRH: Marital therapy: a viable treatment for depression and marital discord. Am J Psychiatry 147:183–186, 1990

Shadish WR, Baldwin SA: Effects of behavioral marital therapy: a meta-analysis of randomized controlled trials. J Consult Clin Psychol 73:6–14, 2005

Simpson LE, Doss BD, Wheeler J, et al: Relationship violence among couples seeking therapy: common couple violence or battering? J Marital Fam Ther 33:270–283, 2007

Simpson LE, Atkins DC, Gattis KS, et al: Low-level relationship aggression and couple therapy outcomes. J Fam Psychol 22:102–111, 2008

Snyder DK: Marital Satisfaction Inventory—Revised (MSI-R) Manual. Los Angeles, CA, Western Psychological Services, 1997

Snyder DK, Castellani AM, Whisman MA: Current status and future directions in couple therapy. Annu Rev Psychol 57:317–344, 2006

Spanier GB: Measuring dyadic adjustment: new scales for assessing the quality of marriage and similar dyads. J Marriage Fam 38:15–28, 1976

Straus MA, Hamby SL, Boney-McCoy S, et al: The Revised Conflict Tactics Scales (CTS2): development and preliminary psychometric data. J Fam Issues 17:283–316, 1996

Stuart RB: Operant-interpersonal treatment for marital discord. J Consult Clin Psychol 33:675–682, 1969

Weiss RL, Hops H, Patterson GR: A framework for conceptualizing marital conflict, technology for altering it, some data for evaluating it, in Behavior Change: Methodology, Concepts, and Practice. Edited by Hamerlynck LA, Handy LC, Mash EJ. Champaign, IL, Research Press, 1973, pp 309–342

Wimberly JD: An outcome study of integrative couples therapy delivered in a group format. Dissertation Abstracts 58:6832, 1998

Suggested Readings

Treatment Manuals for Therapists

Cognitive-Behavioral Couples Therapy

Epstein N, Baucom DH: Enhanced Cognitive-Behavioral Therapy for Couples: A Contextual Approach. Washington, DC, American Psychological Association, 2002

Integrative Behavioral Couples Therapy

Jacobson NS, Christensen A: Acceptance and Change in Couple Therapy: A Therapist's Guide to Transforming Relationships. New York, WW Norton, 1998

Traditional Behavioral Couples Therapy

Jacobson NS, Margolin G: Marital Therapy: Strategies Based on Social Learning and Behavior Exchange Principles. New York, Brunner/Mazel, 1979

Guides for Couples

Christensen A, Jacobson NS: Reconcilable Differences. New York, Guilford, 2000
Integrative Behavioral Couple Therapy (http://ibct.psych.ucla.edu/home.htm)

Research Papers

Research Reviews

Christensen A, Heavey CL: Interventions for couples. Annu Rev Psychol 50:165–190, 1999
Snyder DK, Castellani AM, Whisman MA: Current status and future directions in couple therapy. Annu Rev Psychol 57:317–344, 2006

Clinical Trials (Examples)

Christensen A, Atkins DC, Berns S, et al: Traditional versus integrative behavioral couple therapy for significantly and chronically distressed married couples. J Consult Clin Psychol 72:176–191, 2004
Christensen A, Atkins DC, Yi J, et al: Couple and individual adjustment for two years following a randomized clinical trial comparing traditional versus integrative behavioral couple therapy. J Consult Clin Psychol 74:1180–1191, 2006

Chapter 23

Psychodynamic Group Therapy

Hillel I. Swiller, M.D., D.L.F.A.P.A., F.A.G.P.A.

The patient in long-term psychodynamic group psychotherapy is a participant in the work of a laboratory of interpersonal relationships. Each patient has the opportunity to experience his or her problems within the psychotherapy itself. Those problems are the interpersonal manifestations of whatever psychological problems the group member has. In individual therapy, the patient is the focus of concentrated attention by a dedicated individual who attempts to minimize the effect of his or her own agenda. That in itself is an extraordinary state of affairs—one that is encountered in ordinary life rarely, if ever. Perhaps the healthy parent of a newborn attempts to create such a one-sided relationship, but nowhere else in life will the other equivalently ignore his or her own needs and desires. Life is with people, ordinary people

An earlier version of much of the material in this chapter (Swiller HI: "Introduction to Group Psychotherapy") appeared in *The Psychiatric Times*, Volume XII, No. 12, December 1995.

who all want to have their own requirements met. That is the situation that is achieved in the psychodynamic therapy group. Consequently, the group member experiences a setting far closer to the one in which he or she lives than is otherwise available in therapy. That immediate experience of collaborating and contending with others to have one's needs met is the hallmark of psychodynamic group psychotherapy and leads ineluctably to the crucial principle that underlies the work of the therapist in leading such a group. The primary principle of technique is to use this microcosm of the interpersonal world—the group—to the fullest extent possible.

Therapeutic Factors

Therapeutic factors include, first and foremost, hope (Yalom 1995). Without hope, there is no treatment of any sort. Therefore, an underlying belief in the efficacy of treatment must be communicated to the group members. Early in the life of a therapy group, this is the responsibility of the therapist; in a well-functioning ongoing group, this will be a major theme during the absorption of a new member. Affiliation is also of the utmost importance. People who have emotional and mental difficulties invariably have the additional anguish of feeling isolated and alienated. The ability to reconnect to the human race afforded patients in a therapy group is of tremendous importance. The belief that "I am alone" adds anguish to any difficulty, and the experience "only connect" (Forster 1910)—the experience of being part of the human community—is almost invariably an experience of relief. Feedback is available in group therapy in a way that it is rarely, if ever, available in any other context.

> Mr. A, an articulate, attractive, heterosexual 40-year-old man, had never been able to sustain a relationship with a woman. Ms. B, a fellow group member, liked and admired him. His initial responses to her compliments and her attempts to flirt with him were criticisms and even attacks on her. No woman he had pursued socially had stuck around long enough for him to understand this, and he was unaware that this was his pattern until the group was able, over time, to help him identify and begin to modify this behavior.

The feedback comes, as it does in life, from people responding primarily subjectively. Group members receive candid and multifaceted views of how they are experienced by others. Members also see how other group members deal with specific kinds of interactions; new behaviors are modeled, and multiple techniques are demonstrated. If a model seems useful, the patient can then experiment with the model and, if the experiments are successful, practice the new behavior within the group. This leads to an increase in coping skills.

A unique therapeutic factor of group therapy is altruism.

> Mr. C entered group therapy, as patients with alexithymia almost always do, at the insistence of his wife (Swiller 1988). His ability to experience subtle gradations of feelings, to empathize, and to communicate intimately was limited, in stark contrast to his high intelligence and notable professional achievement. Over time in group, he greatly increased his capacity to experience and understand a wide range of emotions and his ability to be empathic. When Mr. D, new to therapy and severely alexithymic, joined the group, it was Mr. C's understanding and compassion that were most helpful to him. Mr. C's helpfulness not only was most useful to Mr. D but also substantially bolstered Mr. C's own self-esteem.

Psychiatrists are well aware that one of our most powerful motivations for doing this difficult work is the psychic benefit to be gained from the opportunity to be helpful to other people. For the most part, patients in individual psychotherapy have little opportunity within the therapy to be helpful. In long-term psychodynamic group psychotherapy, patients have multiple opportunities to be helpful to one another. This leads, for patients as it does for therapists, to increased feelings of self-esteem. Insight is enhanced through interpretations made not primarily by the group leader but by group members, who may be more in touch with one another's unconscious conflicts than even the most skillful leader would be. Finally, in long-term group psychotherapy, group members have the opportunity to work through their conflicts over time. Correction, repetition, practice, and encouragement lead to progress in therapy as in any other field of endeavor.

Group Norms

A well-functioning psychotherapy group is characterized by its norms of behavior (Alonso 1989; Alonso and Swiller 1993). Five norms are of particular importance:

- *Honesty.* Group members assume the obligation to respond to one another with maximum candor, and the consequent discussions are spontaneous and emotionally rich.
- *Respect.* The honest expression of feelings does not mean self-indulgence; civility has its place. Communication is exclusively verbal, and impulses to act are expressed verbally, never enacted.

> Discussing the recent death of her father, Ms. E began to weep. Ms. F, seated next to her, reached over to take her hand. Ms. F was encouraged to put her feelings into words rather than action, and this led, for the first time, to her expression of loss when her father, following her parents' divorce when she was 7, lost contact with the family.

- *Industry.* Industry involves doing the work of therapy in the psychotherapy group itself. The expression of thoughts and feelings is not an end in itself but forms the data set for meaningful and probing inspection.
- *Responsibility.* Each member must do his or her fair share. Every member has the responsibility to participate with appropriate frequency and to interact with every other group member.
- *Application.* The gains acquired in the group experience must be used outside the group in one's everyday life. Although the process of group discussion is most fruitful when focused on the here and now of group, some report of the effect of new knowledge and skills in one's outside life can enhance the relevance of the work.

Patient Selection

Exclusion criteria are straightforward and fall into three general categories. The first is related to diagnosis. Patients who are acutely psychotic or acutely suicidal require far more intensive help than is available in the ordinary once-a-week long-term psychodynamic group. No one should be added to an ongoing group in such a state. There is reasonable debate among group therapists as to including old members who have fallen into such dangerous psychological states in regular group meetings while they are at their most ill. There are both advantages and disadvantages to doing so, and each situation must be judged on its individual merits, with consideration given to the welfare of the group as well as to the long-term welfare of the individual. Patients who have gotten through the crisis of psychosis or suicidality, once they have been stabilized, almost always can be productive members of such groups.

Severe sociopathy is a contraindication to participation in a heterogeneous group. Patients with severe antisocial personality traits may take advantage of other group members and must be excluded for their protection.

> Mr. G was given an ultimatum that he go into therapy by the woman with whom he had been living for several years, who was no longer willing to tolerate his unwillingness to work and his parasitic financial dependence. The degree of his sociopathy was underestimated by the group therapist, who was taken in by his charm and superficial despondency. So, unfortunately, was a vulnerable, single, and lonely female member of the group. Within a few weeks, Mr. G had seduced her, dropped out of the group, and moved into her apartment. He lived off her for the next 2 years.

Note, however, that patients with severe sociopathy are often best treated in a group setting. That is, within a homogeneous group, in which the other members share their pathology. Such a group is usually conducted in a structured setting. Sociopathic patients are generally far more attuned to and able to understand and confront fellow sociopathic patients than are either nonsociopathic group members or even the best-trained group leaders.

Patients with extremely poor impulse control also must be excluded, for the protection of themselves and others. Patients with moderate to severe organic brain syndrome will have difficulty in a heterogeneous group. Their experiences often will be more humiliating than productive. In a homogeneous group, modified to fit their needs, they can do extremely well.

The second major exclusion criterion is associated with the ability to tolerate anxiety. For some individuals, the anxiety of being a participant in a group—any group—is overwhelming. Until that anxiety can be moderated, they cannot tolerate the experience.

The third category of exclusion criteria relates to the circumstances of the individual's life. Any factor that would create an inability to fulfill the treatment contract, such as a professional obligation to travel frequently and miss many sessions, contraindicates this form of group therapy. Similarly, secrets that the patient feels unable to discuss, even after he or she knows and trusts the other members, will have a destructive effect on the group therapy process. Although it is understood that almost everyone enters group with something "I could never talk about," part of the treatment contract usually should include working toward detoxifying such a "secret" and making it available to the therapy.

The inclusion criteria follow simply after the exclusion criteria. Everyone else who can benefit from psychotherapy is a good candidate for long-term psychodynamic group psychotherapy. For some patients, group therapy—either alone or combined with appropriately spaced individual sessions—is the treatment of choice. Among these people are those who have repetitive interpersonal difficulties (such as a lack of intimacy or low self-confidence) or who are involved in stereotypical ungratifying relationships (characterized by repetitive power struggles or approach/avoidance).

Patients with low self-awareness and those who are socially inept are often best treated in group. Individuals with moderate to severe alexithymia are almost always best treated in long-term psychodynamic group therapy combined with individual psychotherapy (Swiller 1988).

In forming a psychotherapy group, it is important to allow for a mix of diagnostic categories. (A group composed exclusively of depressed patients will soon have a depressed leader; a group composed exclusively of highly histrionic patients will rarely bore its leader but may offer little benefit to its members.) It is also important, however, that patients have approximately the same degree of psychopathology. Issues such as social class, race, and sexual orientation are rarely, if ever, relevant factors in the composition of a long-term psychodynamic group.

Dropouts must always be expected in group therapy practice. The absence of any dropouts over an extended period suggests that exclusion criteria are being applied too rigorously and patients who are high-risk/high-gain (i.e., patients who are most likely to drop out but who could benefit substantially from the experience) are not being offered the opportunities to benefit from the group experience. Psychotherapists tend to view dropouts from therapy as indications of failure on the part of either an unsophisticated and unworthy patient or an easily blamed, masochistically inclined therapist. It is quite possible that neither is the main issue: group therapy is demanding, and if all who could benefit are given the opportunity to participate in group therapy, some will not be able to use it. A group therapist should be willing to extend the possibility of a good experience in group to those who may, for whatever reason (not among exclusion criteria), not be able to continue their participation to completion.

Group Structure

Most groups meet weekly for 90 minutes. These groups are generally composed of approximately eight members, although the therapist just starting a group should not hesitate to begin with fewer members. Groups of small size tend to produce more self-disclosure and interaction, whereas larger groups tend to produce more leader-centered behavior.

Therapist Resistance to Group Therapy

Many therapists with much experience and skill in individual psychodynamic psychotherapy resist working as group therapists. In the past, this was often the legacy of training as a psychotherapist in an era when classical psychoanalysis was seen as the best possible treatment for every nonpsychotic psychiatric condition. This legacy led to a lack of training and supervision and to a prejudice against group psychotherapy. Some therapists, often more recently trained ones, rely too exclusively on biological therapies, neglecting the psychosocial aspects inherent to every psychiatric condition. Other therapists who have overcome these prejudices hesitate to use group therapy because they are concerned about insufficient referrals. The development of an adequate referral stream often requires an investment in the education of possible referral sources about the unique benefits of group therapy. Writing, lecturing, participation in conferences, and individual discussions all have their place. A more profound resistance may be a result of the therapist's unconscious fears of the primal horde (Halperin 1989). Some therapists also may fear their own exhibitionist impulses and attempt to minimize the inappropriate expression of these impulses by avoiding a venue in which they could be gratified.

Major Approaches to Psychodynamic Group Psychotherapy

Three major approaches to psychodynamic group psychotherapy exist. The first uses the group as the setting for therapy (Wolf 1949; Wolf and Schwartz 1962). Although patients are treated within a group, they are treated as individuals, and the therapist essentially makes rounds in the group, working one-on-one with patients. When psychoanalysis was at its zenith, this approach was common. Many gestalt (Perls et al. 1965) and hypnotherapy (Haley 1986) therapists also used this approach. The second approach uses the group as the object of the treatment itself (Agazarian 1997; Winnicott 1958). This approach is based on the theory that a group transference neurosis forms from the joint unconscious of all members of the group, the resolution of which will aid all members of the group. The most widely applied approach uses the group as the therapeutic agent, and the discussion of technique that follows is based primarily on this approach (Rutan et al. 2007; Yalom 1995).

Interpersonal learning is a valuable aspect of such groups. Unfortunately, interpersonal learning is often seen as a far more complicated subject than it is. It can be thought of as relating to a few simple questions: How am I seen? What am I doing? Why am I doing it? Where does it come from? Developing new and more profound answers to these and related questions constitutes much of the content of the group process. Working-through in group therapy consists of the repetition and elaboration within the group of new ways of understanding and responding to interpersonal interactions.

Underlying Psychodynamic Principles

Five basic psychodynamic principles form the foundation of all psychodynamic psychotherapies (Alonso 1989):

1. Psychological determinism (i.e., psychic states have psychic causes)
2. Existence of unconscious processes
3. Dynamic motivation (i.e., thoughts, feelings, and behavior are driven by the desire to gratify a variety of basic instincts)
4. Epigenetic development (i.e., new psychological developments do not displace old ones but are layered on top of them, and the old patterns and complexes continue to exist)
5. Existence of persistent mental structures with aspects of thoughts, feelings, and behavior that tend to be mobilized in their entirety

Transference and its varied manifestations in the therapeutic process underlie psychodynamic group therapy. It is important to note that transferences in group therapy can be to the leader, to individual members of the group, to subgroups within the group, and to the group as a whole. Often, all of these are in operation simultaneously. As with any other psychodynamic therapy, there has to be at least a minimal positive transference that allows for the development of a therapeutic alliance. Initially, this transference is toward the therapist. Over time, the basic positive transference or the therapeutic alliance with the group itself forms. Just as transference exists on several levels, so does countertransference. Group therapists have countertransferences to individual members, to subgroups, and to the group as a whole.

All of the major schools of psychoanalytic theory—ego psychology, object relations, and self psychology—have made their contributions to the current state of knowledge and practice of long-term psychodynamically oriented group psychotherapy.

Patient Preparation and the Group Contract

Appropriate preparation of patients for group therapy is essential. The all-too-common clinical practice of having one therapist screen and prepare patients while others lead the group creates a difficult complication. Inadequate preparation is perhaps the single leading cause of unnecessary and avoidable dropping out. A therapeutic alliance with the leader must be established. Leader and potential group member must negotiate appropriate goals for the therapy. Patients should be given guidelines for using the group therapy experience to best advantage. Nobody knows how to be a successful patient in any psychotherapy without a certain amount of instruction. Most patients are anxious about joining a therapy group, and it is important to allay some of their anxiety. Mutual agreement must be reached on a therapeutic contract. The formulation of this contract should be done explicitly and in detail. Patient responsibilities in the group therapy contract include being there on a regular and continuous basis. Each group member agrees to work toward the individual goals negotiated in the original discussions with the therapist. As therapy proceeds, it should be understood that important new goals may evolve.

Candid and spontaneous interaction, which is exclusively verbal, is an essential patient responsibility. The patient, however, has no responsibility to be constant or to be correct in the opinions, emotions, and thoughts that he or she voices in the group. The primary corollary to candid and spontaneous speech is to listen and to consider what is said to oneself by others. That does not mean that the group member has to accept everything said to him or her, but such feedback has to be thoughtfully considered.

In most psychodynamic long-term groups, there is no outside contact among group members. This minimizes both vitiation of transferences and formation of fixed person-based subgroups. It is essential that all members understand that everything discussed in the group is kept confidential and is never the subject of discussion with a nongroup member (other than an individual therapist). Group members also agree to stay until their work is done and to regularly and promptly pay the agreed-on fee for their therapy. All members of a group usually pay the same fee, regardless of differences in economic resources, but at the discretion of the leader, special circumstances may lead to a modification of an individual's fee.

The therapist's responsibilities in the group therapy contract include appropriate patient selection and preparation, enforcement of the contract, attendance to group norms previously enumerated, availability (which is in no way inferior to the availability one has to patients in individual therapy), communication as necessary with individual therapists, record keeping, and insurance claim filing. Usually, if the group therapist is also managing a member's medications, this is done in individual sessions. The ability to observe the group members on an ongoing basis often means that medication management can be accomplished with relatively infrequent and brief meetings. For a group composed homogeneously of more seriously ill members, this approach to medication management can be modified, and the group can serve as the setting for the prescribing of medications (Brook 1993).

Developmental Stages

Long-term psychodynamic therapy groups are organic entities and go through a developmental process. A developmental scheme that is simple but quite useful includes four stages. The first stage, that of *engagement or group formation*, is characterized by patients coming together through problem sharing with an emphasis on similarities. Aggression tends to be muted, although competition for time and attention may be obvious. During the second stage, that of *differentiation and individuation*, patients establish their individual identities within the group; differences are established, and appropriate aggression emerges. This leads to the third stage, that of the *working group*, which is characterized by intimacy. Here affiliation and group cohesion are at a maximum. Members who were initially skeptical about their ability "to talk to a bunch of strangers" find themselves looking forward to the next meeting with unexpected force. Stages two and three frequently blend into each other and are difficult (and unnecessary) to tease apart. Fourth is the stage of *termination or disengagement*. Although long-term groups may continue for years, all of these stages are routinely seen as events affect the group. For example, anticipation of an extended vacation, or the graduation of a valued group member, leads to manifestations of termination phenomena. Similarly, the introduction of a new member or members brings the group back to the stage of group formation. (A test of how well the group is functioning is how rapidly the group reemerges from this stage. A well-functioning group can bring a new member up to speed in a remarkably short time.)

As noted earlier, dropouts are an inevitable part of group therapy, and a zero drop-out rate is not an appropriate goal. People drop out mostly for a few simple reasons. These include inappropriate selection (with a level of pathology, function, or sophistication that is not sufficiently similar to that of other members of the group). Fear of confrontation or of self-disclosure also leads members to drop out, as do feelings of humiliation following premature self-disclosure or the emergence of conflicted material that the patient is inadequately able to process. Generally, such dropouts take place early in the group members' participation in the group.

Leadership Technique

The most important task of the group therapist operating primarily with the approach of group as an agent of therapeutic change is to help the group do its work. General principles of technique for such a group therapist are enumerated in Table 23–1 (after Yalom 1995).

Early in the development of the group, technique is characterized by the creation of an atmosphere of hope. Group formation is encouraged through an awareness of universality and of the commonalities of the group, by the limitation of premature conflict, and by guarding against excessive self-disclosure. In the middle stages of group therapy leadership technique is responsive primarily to phenomena related to resistance. Often it is sufficient simply to identify the resistance and allow the well-trained group to overcome it without further help. Subgrouping is an invariable part of the life of any group and is not necessarily antitherapeutic. The group leader must assess the nature of the subgrouping. If subgroups form and reform in a fluid manner as new issues are taken up and old ones dropped, the subgrouping is appropriate. If subgroups are rigidly adhered to and alliance becomes more important than the issue under discussion, then the leader must intervene. Such subgrouping is antitherapeutic. The end stage of subgrouping is the subgroup of one, the scapegoat, which is invariably an antitherapeutic phenomenon requiring intervention of the leader. Essentially the therapist promotes appropriate interaction between group members to enhance the expression of individuality and to keep people moving toward their goals, including the new ones that have developed. In the late or termination stage, the leader attends to the issues of termination and mourning within the group.

The level of therapist activity and other aspects of style are determined by the needs of the group as well as by the therapist's personality (Figure 23–1) (Rutan and Stone 1993).

TABLE 23–1. Principles of technique for group therapists

Hope	Establish an atmosphere of optimism and productivity.
Enhanced affiliation	Build group cohesiveness and culture.
Protection of boundaries	Ensure adherence to the contract and maintain respect for boundaries to enhance group cohesion.
Appropriate activity	Intervene only when the group needs help to do its work.
Purposeful interventions	Frame all comments with a desired modification in the group process as a goal.
Group as the basic resource	Direct comments first and foremost to enhancing the group interactions; individual interpretations are of secondary value.
Productive group norms	Enhance honesty, respect, industry, responsibility, and application.
Shifting alliances	Accept subgrouping (which will inevitably occur) on issues rather than on individuals, and ensure that it is mutable rather than fixed.
Process over content	Focus primarily on the productive flow of material rather than on the material itself.
Level of intervention	Generally keep comments close to the psychological surface.
Timing	Remember that the essence of the art of group therapy is timing.
Attend to termination	Allow the group to mourn losses.

Source. Adapted from Yalom 1995.

When the group is working well, the therapist should be comfortable limiting his or her participation to careful listening. When the group work is blocked by any sort of impediment, the therapist intervenes actively to enable the group to move forward. Such impediments may include monopolization, repetitive dyadic interactions, fixed subgrouping, excessive out-of-group material, and intellectualization. All interventions must be purposeful, and most are based on the principle that group is the basic resource. This means that the most common interventions bring to bear the resources of the group on the issue under discussion. Both general and specifically relevant member interactions are encouraged. The therapist

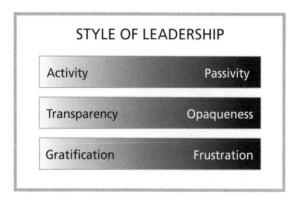

FIGURE 23–1. Style of leadership.

attends to the nurture of productive group norms of honesty, respect, industry, responsibility, and application. He or she protects the boundaries of the group, helps enhance affiliation within the group, and helps individuals keep in mind their own specific goals. The therapist attends to process more than to content, and interventions are made primarily about process rather than content, with the aim of helping the group itself to work on the content. The level of interpretation varies with the therapist's formulation of the needs of the group at a particular time, but most interventions are made close to the psychological surface. Figure 23–2 (Rutan and Stone 1993) presents several continua along which interventions can be located to help the therapist respond accurately to the immediate needs of the group.

Combined Group and Individual Therapy

Many experienced group therapists find that an ideal way of working is combined individual and group therapy. This extends and deepens the therapeutic field. The group component provides powerful emotional material that may be further explored in individual sessions. Usually, the therapist starts with individual sessions and adds group therapy when the patient is sufficiently involved and a therapeutic alliance has been established. Problems that may never surface in the focused, concerned, and supportive atmosphere of individual therapy will arise in group therapy because every member has his or her own needs, agenda, and distortions. Conversely, the individual meetings provide the opportunity for extensive cognitive processing of such issues over as much time as necessary without sacrificing attention to other group members.

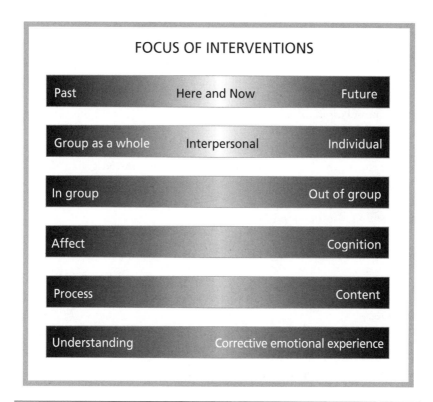

FIGURE 23–2. Focus of interventions.

Often, the same therapist is not available to conduct both modalities of the therapy. Although this situation is not ideal, this compromise can work quite well if both therapists are respectful of the work of the other and if the patient and the therapists operate within a team perspective working toward mutual goals. Thus, the two therapists must be able to communicate about the treatment as they see fit and must be aware of issues of split transferences.

Modifications

Time-limited group therapy requires a constant focus on the theme around which the group has been formed (e.g., divorce, bereavement) and attention to the time-limited nature of the experience, with termination being acknowledged from the outset and explicitly addressed for at least the last several sessions.

Special populations have the advantage (and disadvantage) of shared concerns. The group members are far more expert in their common issues than is the ordinary leader, but the leader can be most helpful by encouraging maximum group participation.

Group psychotherapy is an essential part of the psychiatrist's therapeutic armamentarium. This remains true whether group therapy is used in combination with individual sessions or as the sole psychotherapeutic modality, involves working with a special population or a heterogeneous outpatient population, or is carried out in a time-limited or a time-unlimited setting.

Principles developed in long-term psychodynamic group psychotherapy can be applied with modifications to time-limited group therapy (MacKenzie 1990) and to therapy for specialized populations (Alonso and Swiller 1993; Halperin 1989). Figure 23–1 will help the leader find the most useful style for leadership in these situations.

Key Points

- The immediate experience of collaborating with and contending with others to have one's needs met is the hallmark of psychodynamic group therapy.

- Therapeutic factors in group therapy include instillation of hope, affiliation with group members, feedback from group members, and altruism.

- A well-functioning group requires that group members follow five norms for behavior within the group: honesty, respect, industry, responsibility, and application of gains from the group to everyday life.

- Patients who should be excluded from a weekly psychodynamic psychotherapy group include patients who are acutely psychotic or suicidal, who show sociopathy, who are unable to control impulses or tolerate anxiety, or who are unable to fulfill the treatment contract. All other patients may be usefully considered for group therapy.

- A psychodynamic group functions best when its members represent a mix of diagnostic categories.

- Most psychodynamic groups meet for 90 minutes weekly and consist of approximately eight members.

- Groups of small size tend to produce more self-disclosure and interaction, whereas larger groups tend to produce more leader-centered behavior.

- Patients entering a group should be prepared for the experience beforehand. This includes establishing a therapeutic alliance with the leader, discussing guidelines for using the group therapeutically, and reaching mutual and explicit agreement about a treatment contract.

- A group therapy contract typically establishes expectations that a patient will speak candidly and spontaneously, there will be no contact among group members outside the group, all material discussed within the group will be kept confidential, each group member will agree to stay until his or her work is done, and each member will pay his or her fee (usually the same fee).

- The group therapist has responsibility for appropriate patient selection and preparation, enforcement of the contract, attendance to group norms, availability to each patient, communication with group members' individual therapists, record keeping, and insurance filing. Medications usually are managed in individual sessions.

- The typical developmental stages for a group are engagement, differentiation and individuation, intimacy and the working group, and termination or disengagement.

References

Agazarian YM: Systems-Centered Therapy for Groups. New York, Guilford, 1997

Alonso A: The psychodynamic approach, in Outpatient Psychiatry: Diagnosis & Treatment. Edited by Lazare A. Baltimore, MD, Williams & Wilkins, 1989, pp 37–58

Alonso A, Swiller H (eds): Group Therapy in Clinical Practice. Washington, DC, American Psychiatric Press, 1993

Brook DW: Medication groups, in Group Therapy in Clinical Practice. Edited by Alonso A, Swiller H. Washington, DC, American Psychiatric Press, 1993, pp 155–170

Forster EM: Howard's End. London, Edward Arnold, 1910

Haley J: Uncommon Therapy: The Psychiatric Techniques of Milton H Erickson, MD. New York, WW Norton, 1986

Halperin D: Group Therapy: New Paradigms and New Perspectives. Chicago, IL, Year Book Medical, 1989

MacKenzie KR: Time-Limited Group Psychotherapy. Washington, DC, American Psychiatric Press, 1990

Perls FS, Hefferline R, Goodman P: Gestalt Therapy. New York, Dell, 1965

Rutan S, Stone W: Psychodynamic Group Psychotherapy, 2nd Edition. New York, Guilford, 1993

Rutan JS, Stone WN, Shay J: Psychodynamic Group Psychotherapy, 4th Edition. New York, Guilford, 2007

Swiller HI: Alexithymia: treatment utilizing combined individual and group psychotherapy. Int J Group Psychother 38:47–61, 1988

Winnicott DW: Collected Papers. London, Tavistock, 1958

Wolf A: The psychoanalysis of groups. Am J Psychother 3:525, 1949

Wolf A, Schwartz M: Psychoanalysis in Groups. New York, Grune & Stratton, 1962

Yalom I: The Theory and Practice of Group Psychotherapy, 4th Edition. New York, Basic Books, 1995

Suggested Readings

The material presented in this chapter draws on the work of many scholars. Much more detail and references to the original contributions of specific authors may be found in the following textbooks, which, taken together, form a good foundation for a library of group psychotherapy.

Alonso A, Swiller H (eds): Group Therapy in Clinical Practice. Washington, DC, American Psychiatric Press, 1993

Bernard H, MacKenzie R: Basics of Group Psychotherapy. New York, Guilford, 1994

Rutan S, Stone W: Psychodynamic Group Psychotherapy, 2nd Edition. New York, Guilford, 1993

Yalom I: The Theory and Practice of Group Psychotherapy, 4th Edition. New York, Basic Books, 1995

Chapter 24

Family Intervention for Psychotic and Severe Mood Disorders

William R. McFarlane, M.D.

Family intervention for the severe psychiatric syndromes—psychotic and severe mood disorders—has been established as one of the most effective treatments available, complementing but nearly doubling the treatment effects of medication. Often subsumed under the term *family psychoeducation*, it is a method for incorporating a patient's family members, other caregivers, and friends into the acute and ongoing treatment and rehabilitation process. The descriptor *psychoeducation* can be misleading: family psychoeducation includes many cognitive, behavioral, and supportive therapeutic elements; often uses a consultative framework; and shares characteristics with some types of family therapy. On the basis of a family–patient–professional partnership, the most effective models are essentially cognitive-behavioral therapy with consistent inclusion of family members as collaborators. Family psychoeducation can include any layperson or paraprofessional person who is providing support to persons with a severe mental illness. It combines providing clear and accurate education for family members about the psychobiology of the major disorders with training and ongoing guidance in problem-solving, communication, and coping skills, while providing and developing social support. The goals are both to markedly improve clinical and functional outcomes and quality of life for the patient and to reduce family stress and strain as an indispensable means of achieving those outcomes. Family psychoeducation combines the complementary expertise and experience of family members, patients, and professionals.

Family psychoeducation has been empirically shown to improve outcomes in schizophrenia and bipolar disorder to the same degree as, or to a greater degree than, medication in numerous research studies. Family intervention is particularly beneficial in the early years of the course of a mental illness, when improvements can have a dramatic and long-term effect and while family members are still involved, open to participation and change in attitude and interaction with the patient. Patients who experience frequent hospitalizations or prolonged unemployment and families who are especially exasperated, confused, and hostile about the illness benefit substantially and often dramatically. When a family member is available, psychoeducation should be applied as widely and as routinely as medication.

Family psychoeducation originated from several sources in the late 1970s. Perhaps the leading influence was the growing realization that conventional family therapy, in which family dysfunction is assumed and becomes the target of intervention for the alleviation of symptoms, proved to be, at least, ineffective and perhaps damaging to patient and family well-being. Awareness also grew, especially among family members themselves and their rapidly growing advocacy organizations, that living with an illness such as schizophrenia is difficult and confusing for patients and families alike. The resulting stresses on families often lead to interactions and persisting patterns of interaction that can have equally devastating effects on the patient and the course of the disorder over time. It became increasingly clear that to adapt under these circumstances, the family must possess the available knowledge about the illness itself and coping skills specific to a particular disorder, skills that are counterintuitive to most families. It became clear that it was unrealistic to expect families to understand such mystifying disorders and to know what to do about them independent of professional guidance. The most adaptive family was increasingly seen to be the one that had access to information, with the implication that clinicians are a crucial source of that information.

Families develop methods of dealing with positive, negative, and mood symptoms; cognitive deficits; functional disabilities; and the desperation of their ill relative through painful trial and error. These successes, however, are rare. Another critical need is that families have access to one another to learn of other families' successes and failures and to establish a repertoire of clinically effective coping strategies that are closely tailored to the disorder and to the individual person. Furthermore, family members and significant others often provide emotional and instrumental support, case management functions, financial assistance, advocacy, and housing to their relative with mental illness. Doing so can be rewarding but poses considerable burdens. Family members often find that access to needed resources and information is lacking. Too often, the end result is a family that is sufficiently anxious, confused, or even hostile that their interactions with the patient become risk factors for relapse, functional deficits, and eventually deterioration. Given that perspective, clinical investigators began to recognize the crucial supportive role families play in outcome after an acute episode of schizophrenia and endeavored to engage families collaboratively, sharing illness information, suggesting behaviors that promote recuperation, and teaching coping strategies that reduce their sense of burden. The group of interventions that emerged became known as *family psychoeducation.*

These approaches recognize that schizophrenia and mood disorders are brain disorders that are only partially remediable by medication and that families can have a significant effect on their relative's recovery. Functional deficits and behavior changes induced by these disorders are often the most confusing and burdensome for family members because the family members usually do not identify them as part of the disorder, but they nevertheless find themselves supporting the affected member to compensate for those deficits. The psychoeducational approach shifted the focus away from attempting to get families to change their "disturbed" communication patterns toward educating and persuading families that their interactions with the patient can facilitate recovery by compensating for deficits and sensitivities specific to the various disorders. For example, a family might interfere with recuperation if in their natural enthusiasm to promote and support progress, they create unreasonable demands and expectations, but the same family could have a dramatically positive effect on recovery by gradually increasing expectations and supporting an incremental return of functioning.

Research conducted over the last three decades has supported evidence-based practice guidelines for addressing family members' needs for information, clinical guidance, and ongoing support. This research has found that altering key types of negative interaction, while meeting the needs of family members, dramatically improves patient outcomes and family well-being. Several models have evolved to address the needs of family members: individual family consultation (Wynne 1994); professionally led family psychoeducation (Anderson et al. 1986; Falloon 1984) in single-family and multifamily group formats (McFarlane 2002); modified forms of more traditional family therapies (Marsh 2001); and a range of professionally led models of short-term family education (sometimes referred to as *therapeutic education*) (Amenson 1998). Family-led information and support classes or groups such as those of the National Alliance on Mental Illness (NAMI) are also available (Pickett-Schenk et al. 2000). Of these models, professionally led family psychoeducation has a deep enough research and dissemination base to be considered an evidence-based clinical practice (Dixon and Lehman 1995; Dixon et al. 2001; Lehman et al. 1995; McFarlane et al. 2002).

Professionally led psychoeducational models are offered as part of a treatment plan for the patient and are usually diagnosis-specific. The models differ in format (multiple-family, single-family, relatives only, combined), structure (involvement or exclusion of the patient), duration and intensity of treatment, and setting (hospital, clinic, home). They place variable emphasis on didactic, emotional, cognitive-behavioral, clinical, rehabilitative, and systemic techniques. Most have aimed to achieve clinical and functional patient outcomes, although family understanding and well-being are assumed to be necessary to achieve those outcomes. All focus on family resiliency and strengths. Described here are the theoretical background for this treatment model, evidence of its effectiveness, and its major components and technical features.

Empirical and Theoretical Foundations

Although the scientific evidence is increasingly strong that the major psychotic disorders are based in genetic or neurodevelopmental defects involving brain function and structure, abundant evidence indicates that the final development of psychotic or severe mood symptoms and relapse are the result of psychosocial stress. The diathesis–stress or vulnerability–stress model provides a widely accepted, empirically supported, and useful framework for describing the relations among provoking agents (stressors), vulnerability and symptom formation (diathesis), and outcome (Zubin et al. 1992). Thus, a genetically or developmentally vulnerable person, whose inborn tolerance for stress is incompatible with exposure to either excessive internally or externally generated stimulation, may experience an episode of psychotic illness. This principle underlies the biosocial theory, which states that major psychotic and mood disorders are the result of the continual interaction of specific biological disorders of the brain with specific psychosocial and other environmental factors. These psychosocial factors are the proximal causes of relapse in established cases and of the initial psychotic episode. Specifically, episodes are induced in biologically vulnerable individuals by major stresses imposed by role transitions and other life events, social isolation, family expressed emotion (EE), conflict and exasperation, separation from family of origin, and experienced stigma (see Table 24–1). This causal biosocial theory yields an interactive, feedback-based model for the final stages of onset and relapse, as compared with a simpler linear-causal model. In this conceptual framework, subtle symptoms and behavioral changes induce anxiety, anger, social rejection, confusion, and other reactions in family members, which exacerbate those very symptoms by inducing psychological and ultimately physiological stress reactions in the vulnerable person. The end result is a spiraling deterioration of both the patient and the family.

Family Interaction Prior to Onset: Prospective Studies

Goldstein (1985) and his colleagues, and subsequently Tienari and his colleagues (2004), reported in two landmark prospective studies that family EE and communication deviance, especially negativity directed toward the at-risk young person, predict onset of psychosis, interacting with genetic (having a biological mother with schizophrenia) or psychiatric (already having nonpsychotic symptoms and behavioral difficulties) risk. In support of the stress (environmental risk) part of the biosocial theory, Goldstein showed that onset of schizophrenia in disturbed adolescents seeking psychological treatment could be predicted by in vivo assessment of negative family affective style (a directly observed form of EE) and difficulties in clarity and structure of communication (communication deviance). The Finnish Adoption Study (Tienari et al. 2004) rigorously combined and tested both psychosocial and genetic risk factors and their interaction in a developmentally sensitive design. This study provided the first compelling evidence for a gene–environment interaction for schizophrenia spectrum disorders. The results indicated that risk for development of schizophrenia spectrum disorders was much higher only among genetically at-risk adoptees reared in families in which higher levels of negativity, family constrictedness (flat affect, lack of humor), and family boundary problems (e.g., generational enmeshment, chaotic family structure, unusual communication) were present. No increase in the incidence of schizophrenia spectrum disorders was seen among genetically at-risk adoptees reared in less distressed families. Thus, not only were certain types of common family dynamics implicated in triggering the onset of schizophrenia in genetically vulnerable children, but also healthier family dynamics played a protective role (i.e., preventing an illness in genetically predisposed individuals).

These studies led to a more complex model of etiology, but one that is far more precise and therefore clinically useful. In essence, negative family interactional patterns are as potent and indispensable factors in onset as are genetic and neurodevelopmental factors, but only when those predisposing factors are themselves present. This model joins a now large literature that documents gene–family interaction as a mutually causal process in both mental and physical health disorders (Reiss et al. 2000; Repetti et al. 2002).

TABLE 24–1. **Empirically derived stressors in major psychotic disorders**

The core problem is a biologically based heightened sensitivity to

Sensory stimulation

Prolonged stress and strenuous demands

Rapid change, complexity

Social disruption

Illicit drug and alcohol use

Negative emotional experience

The current conclusion based on empirical, rather than ideological or theoretical, foundations is that severe psychiatric and medical disorders are the result of (negative family) nurture acting on (genetically or developmentally abnormal) nature, specifically defined in each disorder but heavily and equally dependent on both sets of influences. In that empirical context, family intervention targets one of the two fundamental etiological domains in major psychiatric disorders.

Expressed Emotion

High levels of criticism and emotional overinvolvement are strongly predictive of exacerbation or relapse of symptoms (Brown et al. 1972). In an extensive meta-analysis, Bebbington and Kuipers (1994) cited the overwhelming evidence from 25 studies representing 1,346 patients in 12 different countries for a predictive relation between high levels of EE and relapse of schizophrenia and bipolar disorder. Inclusive reciprocal models have been proposed to increase the accuracy of the construct. For example, Cook et al. (1989), Strachan et al. (1989), and Goldstein et al. (1994) found that EE among key relatives is a reflection of transactional processes between the patient and the family, supporting the conclusion that family functioning is strongly and negatively affected by aspects of the illness in the patient-relative, as well as the converse.

Studies have provided support for an ongoing interaction between symptoms and family responses, reflected in data on EE at different phases. Several studies suggested that EE is less pronounced in the earliest phases of psychosis and increases over time. Hooley and Richters (1995) found that criticism and hostility rates rose rapidly in the first few years of the course of illness: beginning at 14% of the families with less than 1 year of illness, rising to 35% within 1–3 years of onset, and peaking at 50% of the sample after

5 years. My study (McFarlane 2006; McFarlane and Cook 2007) compared components of EE (rejection, warmth, protectiveness, and fusion) across chronic and prodromal samples. Parental scores for rejecting attitudes and emotional overinvolvement were all but identical in the established-disorder samples but were markedly higher than scores in the prodromal sample (McFarlane 2006; McFarlane and Cook 2007). Findings from these studies strongly suggested that EE is largely reactive to cognitive deterioration and emerging negative behavior manifested by the young person developing a psychotic disorder.

Attribution—the relatives' beliefs about the causes of illness-related behavior—also has been associated with EE. Relatives described as critical or hostile misperceived the patient as somehow responsible for unpleasant, symptomatic behavior, whereas more accepting relatives saw identical behaviors as characteristic of the illness itself (Brewin et al. 1991). Relatives have special difficulty in distinguishing negative symptoms, especially amotivation and anergia, from simple laziness, personality disorder, or outright oppositional or manipulative behavior. For that reason, they often do not experience the kind of empathy that might protect them from exasperation, on the one hand, or resentment and hostility, on the other. This is an especially acute risk in the prodromal phase and in the first episode, during which symptoms and deficits often develop gradually, sometimes imperceptibly, appearing to reflect emerging personality or behavioral faults. A patient who slowly becomes cognitively impaired—denying illness and becoming paranoid, hostile, affectively labile, socially withdrawn, or anhedonic—will be much less available to receive the support needed to function at an optimal level (McFarlane and Lukens 1998). If family members confronted by such symptoms in a loved one have little formal knowledge of the illness, they are likely to respond with increased involvement, emotional intensity, criticism, or even hostility.

Stigma

Stigma is often associated with a withdrawal of social support, demoralization, and loss of self-esteem and can have far-reaching effects on daily functioning, particularly in the workplace. As Link and colleagues (1991) have observed, stigma has a strong continuing negative effect on well-being, even though proper diagnoses and treatment improve symptoms and levels of functioning over time. Stigma affects the family as well. Withdrawal and isolation on the part of family members as a result of stigma are associated with a decrease in social network size and emotional support, increased burden, diminished quality of life, and exacerbations of medical disorders. Self-imposed stigma tends to reduce the likelihood that early signs will be addressed and treatment sought and accepted, especially during the first episode (Phelan et al. 1998).

Communication Deviance

Communication deviance, a measure of distracted or vague conversational style, has been consistently associated with schizophrenia. It was the other factor, along with affective style/EE, in the prospective long-term outcome study that predicted the onset of schizophrenic psychosis in families of disturbed, but nonpsychotic, adolescents (Goldstein 1985). Studies have found that communication deviance is correlated with cognitive dysfunction in the relatives, which is of the same type as, but of lower severity than, that seen in patients with schizophrenia (Wagener et al. 1986). This suggests that some family members have inherent—probably genetically derived—difficulty holding a focus of attention, with important implications for treatment design. The result is that a child with subtle cognitive deficiencies may learn to converse in a communication milieu that is less able to compensate and correct.

Social Isolation

The available evidence across several severe and chronic illnesses indicates that ongoing access to social contact and support prevents the deterioration of such conditions and improves their course (Penninx et al. 1996). Family members of the most severely ill patients seem to be isolated, preoccupied with the patient, and burdened by the patient. Brown et al. (1972) showed that 90% of the families with high EE were small in size and socially isolated. In addition, social support buffers the effect of adverse life events (Lin and Ensel 1984) and is one of the key factors predicting medication compliance (Fenton et al. 1997), behavior toward treatment in general, schizophrenic relapse, quality of life (Becker et al. 1998), and subjective burden experienced by relatives (Solomon and Draine 1995). Social network size decreases with increases in the number of episodes, is lower than normal prior to onset, and decreases during the first episode (Anderson et al. 1984).

Effects of Psychosis on the Family

Because so much evidence indicates that some family members of patients share subclinical forms of similar deficits and abnormalities, treatment for psychotic and severe mood disorders must be designed to compensate for some of those difficulties. Those deficits lead to diminished coping ability in some family members, which is required in abundance to provide a stabilizing, let alone therapeutic, influence on the affected family member. Furthermore, the psychotic disorders exact an enormous toll on family members in anxiety, anger, confusion, received stigma, rejection, and exacerbation of medical disorders (Johnson 1990). The organization of most families undergoes a variety of changes, including alienation of siblings; exacerbation, or even initiation, of marital conflict; severe disagreement regarding support versus behavior control; and even divorce. Almost every family undergoes a degree of demoralization and self-blame, which may be inadvertently reinforced by some clinicians.

Reciprocal Causation

These critical family and psychosocial factors lead to onset and relapse of psychosis via 1) a general and constitutional sensitivity to external stimulation and 2) a major discrepancy between stimulus complexity and intensity and cognitive capacity. Cognitive deficits, behavioral changes in the patient, effects of the psychosis on the family, and characteristic family coping styles converge, generating external stresses that induce a spiraling and deteriorating process that ends in a major psychosis or onset of a major mood episode.

These factors are potential targets for family psychoeducation and multifamily groups. Family intervention alters critical environmental influences by

- Reducing ambient social and psychological stresses.
- Reducing stressors from negative and intense family interaction.
- Building barriers to excess stimulation.
- Buffering the effects of negative life events.

The family psychoeducational model defines schizophrenia and other psychotic and mood disorders as disorders of brain function that leave the patient highly and unusually sensitive to the social environment. Thus, this form of treatment is seen as bimodal, influencing both the disease, through medication, and the social environment, through techniques that deliberately reduce stimulation, negativity in interpersonal interaction, rate of change, and environmental and interactional complexity. The approach achieves that goal by providing relevant education, training, and support to family members, friends, and other caregivers—those who provide support, protection, and guidance to the patient.

Family Psychoeducation Outcomes in Schizophrenia and Other Psychiatric Disorders

The cumulative record of efficacy for family intervention, variously termed *family psychoeducation*, *family behavioral management*, or *family work* (but not family therapy), is remarkable. More than 20 controlled clinical trials have documented markedly decreased relapse and rehospitalization rates among patients whose families received psychoeducation compared with those who received standard individual services—20%–50% over 2 years; the larger effects were observed in studies in which the treatment was continued for 12 months or more. At least eight literature reviews have been published in the past decade, all finding a large and significant effect for this model of intervention (Dixon et al. 2000). Since 1978, there has been a steady stream of rigorous validations of the positive effects of this approach on relapse in schizophrenic disorders. Overall, the relapse rate for patients provided family psychoeducation has hovered around 15% per year, compared with a consistent 30%–40% for individual therapy and medication or medication alone (Baucom et al. 1998). This effect size equals or exceeds the reduction in relapse in medicated compared with unmedicated patients in most drug maintenance studies and is universally consistent across well-conducted studies.

McFarlane and colleagues have shown that when rigorously compared, psychoeducational multifamily groups lead to even lower relapse rates and better employment outcomes than does the same intervention in single-family sessions (McFarlane et al. 1995a, 1995b). The simplest explanation is that enhanced social support, inherent in the multifamily format, reduces vulnerability to relapse by further reducing anxiety and general distress (Dyck et al. 2002). In a study of differential effects on schizophrenia of single-family and multifamily group forms of the same psychoeducational treatment method, better outcomes were observed for multifamily groups among those having their first hospitalization (McFarlane et al. 1995b, 1996), including very low relapse rates over 4 years (12.5% per year). For those cases in which full remission was achieved after an index admission (Brief Psychiatric Rating Scale mean item score ≤2), there was no difference in relapse rate between treatment modalities (32.7% in psychoeducational multifamily groups vs. 31.8% in single-family therapy). However, among those who were symptomatic at discharge (Brief Psychiatric Rating Scale score >2), relapse occurred in 19% of the multifamily group cases, compared with 51% of the cases assigned to single-family therapy, a risk of relapse only 28% of that of single-family therapy—a highly significant difference. That is, in the highest-risk subsample, the multifamily group relapse rates were actually lower than in relatively well-stabilized patients, but the opposite effect was observed in single-family treatment. These empirical results strongly suggest a multidimensional effect for the multifamily group format as the explanation for improved clinical outcomes. Subsequent reports have only added to the strong validation of the effects on relapse, particularly because these later studies have been conducted in a variety of international and cultural contexts. Reductions in relapse for family intervention, compared with the control conditions, have been reported in China (Zhao et al. 2000), Spain (Muela Martinez and Godoy Garcia 2001), Scandinavia (Rund et al. 1994), and England (Barrowclough et al. 2001).

These and other studies have reported significant effects on other areas of functioning, going beyond relapse as the main dimension of outcome. In particular, family intervention, especially in the multifamily group format, has resulted in clinically significant reductions in negative symptoms, something not achieved by antipsychotic or any other group of medications. This reflects an observation from the earliest reports of multifamily groups—patients seemed to gradually reemerge from their anergia and social withdrawal and begin to relate more positively to their families and peers in these groups, compared with other forms of therapy and medication. Many patients and their family members are more concerned about the functional aspects of the illness, especially housing, employment, social relationships, dating and marriage, and general morale, than about remission, which tends to be somewhat abstract as a goal. In several of the previously mentioned models, particularly the American versions—those of Falloon, Anderson, and McFarlane—remission (the absence of relapse) is used as both a primary target of intervention and a necessary first step toward rehabilitative goals and recovery. In addition, these models all include major components designed to achieve functional recovery, and the studies have documented major progress in those same domains. Several investigators, including our research team, have extended the aims beyond the clinical to include targeting these more human aspects of illness and life. Other effects have been shown:

- Improved family member well-being (Cuijpers 1999; Falloon and Pederson 1985)
- Increased patient participation in vocational rehabilitation (Falloon et al. 1985)
- Substantially increased employment rates (McFarlane et al. 1996, 2000)
- Decreased psychiatric symptoms, including negative symptoms (Dyck et al. 2000; Zhao et al. 2000)
- Improved social functioning (Montero et al. 2001)
- Decreased family distress (Dyck et al. 2002)
- Reduced costs of care (McFarlane et al. 1995b; Rund et al. 1994)

As a result of the compelling evidence, the Schizophrenia Patient Outcomes Research Team project included family psychoeducation in its set of treatment recommendations. The team recommended that all families in contact with a mentally ill relative be offered a family psychosocial intervention spanning at least 9 months and including education about mental illness, family support, crisis intervention, and problem-solving skills training (Lehman and Steinwachs 1998). Other best practice standards (American Psychiatric Association 1997; Frances et al. 1996) also have recommended that families receive education and support programs. An expert panel that included clinicians from various disciplines, families, patients, and researchers emphasized the importance of engaging families in the treatment and rehabilitation process (Coursey et al. 2000).

It is important to note that most studies evaluated family psychoeducation for schizophrenia or schizoaffective disorder only. However, several controlled studies have supported the effects of family intervention for other psychiatric disorders, including dual diagnosis of schizophrenia and substance abuse (Barrowclough et al. 2001; McFarlane et al. 1995b), bipolar disorder (Miklowitz et al. 2000; Tompson et al. 2000), major depression (Emanuels-Zuurveen and Emmelkamp 1997; Leff et al. 2000), depression in mothers with disruptive children (Sanders and McFarland 2000), mood disorders in children (Fristad et al. 1998), obsessive-compulsive disorder (Van Noppen 1999), anorexia (Geist et al. 2000), alcohol abuse (Loveland-Cherry et al. 1999), Alzheimer's disease (Marriott et al. 2000), suicidal children (Harrington et al. 1998), intellectual impairment (Russell et al. 1999), child molestation (Walker 2000), and borderline personality disorder (Gunderson et al. 1997), including single- and multifamily approaches. Steinglass (1998) has extended this work to deal with the secondary effects of chronic medical illness.

Psychoeducational Multifamily Group Treatment: Methods and Techniques

The psychoeducational multifamily group treatment model described here is designed to assist families in coping with the major burdens and stresses of the psychotic and severe mood disorders. Thus, this approach

- Allays anxiety and exasperation;
- Replaces confusion with knowledge, direct guidance, and problem-solving and coping skills training;
- Reverses social withdrawal and rejection by encouraging participation in a multifamily group that counteracts stigma and demoralization; and
- Reduces anger by providing a more scientific and socially acceptable explanation for symptoms and functional disability.

In short, it relieves the burdens of coping while more fully engaging the family in the treatment and rehabilitation process and compensating for the expected subclinical symptoms that many relatives can be expected to manifest.

Optimally, family intervention should occur as early as possible for those who are experiencing a first episode of psychosis or major mood disorder or during the early course of the disorder. The multifamily group intervention, which incorporates elements of family psychoeducation and family behavioral management, is described briefly here and in detail elsewhere (McFarlane 2002). The intervention model consists of four treatment stages that approximately correspond to the phases of an episode of schizophrenia, from the acute phase through the recuperative and rehabilitation phases. These stages are 1) engagement, 2) education, 3) reentry, and 4) social and vocational rehabilitation (Anderson et al. 1986).

Engagement

Contacts with the families and with the newly admitted individuals are initiated within 48 hours after a hospital admission or onset of psychosis. Initial contacts with the patient are deliberately brief and nonstressful. The young person is included in at least one of the joining sessions, and the caregiving relatives meet alone with the clinician for at least one session. Patients who are actively psychotic are not included in these sessions but are engaged in only a patient–clinician format. The aim is to establish rapport and to gain consent to include the family in the ongoing treatment process. The clinician emphasizes that the goal is to collaborate with the family in helping their relative recover and avoid further deterioration or relapse. The family is asked to join with the clinician in establishing a working alliance or partnership. This phase typically includes three to seven single-family sessions for either the single-family or the multiple-family group format, but in the group approach, more sessions may be required until a sufficient number of families are engaged.

Education

Once the family is engaged and while the patient is still being stabilized, the family is invited to a workshop conducted by the clinicians who will lead the group. These 6-hour sessions are conducted in a formal, classroomlike atmosphere, involving five or six cases. Biological, psychological, and social information about psychotic disorders and their management is presented through a variety of formats, such as videotapes, slide presentations, lectures, discussion, and question-and-answer periods. Information about the way in which the clinicians, patient, and family will continue to work together is presented. The families are also introduced to guidelines for management of the disorder and the underlying vulnerability to stress and information overload (see Table 24–2). Patients attend these workshops if clinically stable, willing, interested, and seemingly able to tolerate the social and informational stress.

TABLE 24–2.   **Guidelines for management of the disorder for patients and families: ways to hasten recovery and to prevent a recurrence**

Believe in your power to affect the outcome: you can.

Make forward steps cautiously, one at a time.

> Go slow. Allow time for recovery. Recovery takes time. Rest is important. Things will get better in their own time. Build yourself up for the next life steps. Anticipate life stresses.

Consider using medication to protect your future.

> A little goes a long way. The medication is working and is necessary even if you feel fine. Work with your doctor to find the right medication and the right dose. Have patience; it takes time. Take medications as they are prescribed. Take only medications that are prescribed.

Try to reduce your responsibilities and stresses, at least for the next 6 months or so.

> Take it easy. Use a personal yardstick. Compare this month with last month rather than last year or next year.

Use the symptoms as indicators.

> If they reappear, slow down, simplify, and look for support and help, quickly. Learn and use your early warning signs and changes in symptoms. Consult with your family clinician or psychiatrist.

Create a protective environment.

Keep it cool.

> Enthusiasm is normal. Tone it down. Disagreement is normal. Tone it down too.

Give each other space.

> Time out is important for everyone. It's okay to reach out. It's okay to say "no."

Set limits.

> Everyone needs to know what the rules are. A few good rules keep things clear.

Ignore what you can't change.

> Let some things slide. Don't ignore violence or concerns about suicide.

Keep it simple.

> Say what you have to say clearly, calmly, and positively.

Carry on business as usual.

> Reestablish family routines as quickly as possible. Stay in touch with family and friends.

Solve problems step by step.

To the extent possible, the clinicians build education and information-sharing on each patient's and family's unique and evolving experience, as assessed during the engagement process. Psychosis is defined as a reversible, treatable condition, like diabetes. The core problem is presented as an unusual sensitivity to sensory stimulation, prolonged stress and strenuous demands, rapid change, complexity, social disruption, illicit drugs and alcohol, and negative emotional experience. As for blame and assigning fault, the clinicians take an important position: neither the patient nor the family caused that sensitivity. Whatever the underlying biological cause might be, it is part of the person's physical personhood, with both advantages and disadvantages. Families are explicitly urged not to blame themselves for this vulnerability.

Reentry

Following the workshop, the clinicians begin meeting twice monthly with the families and patients in the multiple-family group format. The goal of this stage of the treatment is to plan and implement strategies to cope with the vicissitudes of a person recovering from an acute episode of psychosis or to facilitate recovery from the prodromal state. Major content areas include treatment compliance, stress reduction, buffering and avoiding life events, avoiding street drugs and alcohol, lowering of expectations during the period of negative symptoms, and a temporary increase in tolerance for these symptoms. Two special techniques are introduced to participating members as supports to the efforts to follow family guidelines: formal problem solving and communications skills training (Falloon et al. 1984). To facilitate community reentry, the approach maintains stability by systematically applying the group problem-solving method, case by case, to difficulties in implementing the family guidelines and fostering recovery.

Social and Vocational Rehabilitation

The family intervention approaches as a group are designed to accommodate and exploit the natural course of recovery from an acute psychotic episode. That is, because the time course of recovery from negative symptoms can be measured in months to years, rather than days to weeks as in the response of positive symptoms to medication, the family is coached, having initially tempered expectations and demands after the acute episode, to carefully and gradually increase expectations and demands toward the end of the first postepisode year. This strategy, derived from empirical analysis of time courses optimal for recovery (Hogarty and Ulrich 1977), is crucial to the success that family intervention has had in the functional domain (see

Figure 24–1). It is entirely analogous to the strategy currently used to recover successfully from myocardial infarction—initial recuperation followed several months later by a careful increase in exercise and cardiac stress. Thus, approximately 1 year after initiation of treatment for an acute episode, most patients begin to show signs of a return to spontaneity and active engagement with those around them. This is usually an indication that the negative symptoms are diminishing, and the patient can now be challenged more intensively.

The focus of this later phase deals more specifically with his or her rehabilitative needs, addressing the three areas of functioning associated with the most common deficits: social skills, academic challenges, and the ability to obtain and maintain employment. The rehabilitation phase should be initiated by patients who have achieved clinical stability by successfully completing the community reentry phase. The central emphasis during this phase is the involvement of family (and multifamily group) members in helping each patient to begin a gradual, step-by-step resumption of responsibility and socializing. The clinicians continue to use problem solving and brainstorming in the psychoeducational multifamily group to identify and find jobs and social contacts for the patients, to find new ways to enrich their social lives. As stability increases, the multifamily group version of the approach functions in a role unique among psychosocial rehabilitation models: it operates as an auxiliary to the in vivo social and vocational rehabilitation effort being conducted by the clinical team.

Multifamily Group Methods

Multifamily groups address elements of EE, social isolation, stigmatization, and burden directly by education, training, and modeling. Some of this effort focuses on modulating emotional expression and clarifying and simplifying communication. However, much of the effectiveness of the approach results from increasing the size and density of the social network, by reducing the experience of being stigmatized, by providing a forum for mutual aid, and by providing an opportunity to hear similar experiences and mutually to find workable solutions.

Five to seven families, forming a stable membership, meet with two clinicians on a biweekly basis usually for 1–3 years following the onset of an episode of psychosis; all family members would have participated in an educational workshop. Unless psychotic, the patients also attend the group, although the decision to do so is based on the patient's mental status and susceptibility to the amount of stimulation such a group occasionally engenders. Each session lasts for 1.5 hours.

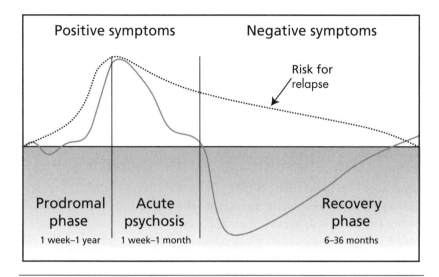

FIGURE 24–1.   Risk for relapse over time in relation to positive and negative symptoms of schizophrenia.

Initial Sessions

The first meeting of the ongoing psychoeducational multifamily group, which follows the workshop by 1–2 weeks, is co-led by the clinicians (usually two) who have engaged the participating families. The format of the sessions is controlled by the clinician, who follows a standard paradigm. From this point forward, patients are strongly encouraged to attend and actively participate. The task of the clinicians, particularly at the beginning, is to adopt a warm, but businesslike, tone and approach that promotes a calm, supportive, and accepting group climate, oriented toward learning new coping skills and engendering hope.

During the first two multifamily group sessions, the goal is to establish a partnership quickly among all participants. The initial sessions are intended to build group identity and a sense of mutual shared interest before going on to discuss clinical and rehabilitation issues. This approach promotes interfamily and interpersonal social support and does *not* promote expressing feelings and usually suppresses negative emotional interactions among group members. Solving problems in the group depends on ideas being shared and accepted across family boundaries, so it is best to proceed slowly and take the time to develop trust and empathy.

People need an opportunity to get to know one another apart from the illness. The first and second group sessions are designed to help the participants and cofacilitators learn about one another and bond as a group. Psychoeducational multifamily group members are encouraged to talk about topics unrelated to the illness, such as their personal likes, dislikes, and daily activities. The first two sessions are especially important in this regard. To succeed, the co-leaders act as a good host or hostess, one who makes introductions, points out common interests, and guides conversations to more personal subjects, such as personal histories, leisure activities, work, and hobbies. The leaders also act as role models; they should be prepared to share a personal story of their own. The guiding principles for this session are validation and positive reinforcement.

The second group session focuses particularly on how the mental illness has changed the lives of the people in the group, and is intended to quickly develop a sense of a common experience of having a major mental illness or having a relative with a major mental illness. The mood of this session is usually less lighthearted than the previous session, but it is the basis for the emergence of a strong group identity and sense of relief. The leaders begin with socializing, encouraging participation by modeling, pointing out connections between people and topics, and asking questions. After socializing, the clinicians proceed to the topic for this meeting. The leaders share as much as possible about their own professional and personal experiences, sharing a story about a friend or family member with mental illness or talking about how they became interested in their work. Some individuals may find it difficult to talk about their experiences, so the leaders strive to point out any similarities among group members' experiences. Compared with the first meeting, the mood of this meeting is often sad, and anger and frustration may be expressed as well. In closing, the leaders also remind group members that during future meetings, everyone will be working on solving problems like the ones expressed in this meeting and that similar issues have been dealt with successfully in previous groups. It is important to be optimistic and send people home with the sense that the group can help them. There should be about 10 minutes to socialize before concluding the group.

Using Problem-Solving Procedures

Problem solving within the context of the psychoeducational multifamily group is the essence of the process and its most potent therapeutic element. In this portion of the group, patients, families, and clinicians begin to make clear gains against the illness in a planned and methodical manner. The goal of the multifamily group is not just to have the group's help to solve problems. Rather, it is to provide individuals and families with an ongoing means to manage the symptoms of the illness beyond the group itself.

The multifamily group's primary working method is to help each family and patient to apply the family guidelines to their specific problems and circumstances. This work proceeds in phases whose timing is linked to the clinical condition of the patients. The actual procedure uses a multifamily group–based problem-solving method adapted from a single-family version by Falloon and Liberman (1983). It is the core of the multifamily group approach, one that is acceptable to families, remarkably effective, and nicely tuned to the low-intensity and deliberate style that is essential to working with the specific sensitivities of people with psychotic disorders.

Each session of the psychoeducational multifamily group begins and ends with a period of social interchange, facilitated by the leaders (see Table 24–3). The purpose is to give patients and even some families the opportunity to recapture and practice any social skills they may have lost as a result of their long isolation and exposure to high levels of stress. Following the socializing, the clinicians specifically inquire as to the status of each family, offering advice based on the family guidelines or direct assistance, when it can be done readily. A single problem that has been identified by any one family is then selected, and the group as a whole participates in problem solving. This problem is the focus of an entire session, during which all members of the group contribute suggestions and ideas.

The affected family then reviews their relative advantages and disadvantages, with some input from other families and clinicians. Typically, the most attractive of the proposed solutions is reformulated as an appropriate task for trying at home and assigned to the family. This step is then followed by a final period of socializing. This group format continues for most of the duration of the work but is sometimes interspersed with presentations by visiting speakers; problem solving focused on generic issues facing several families or patients; and celebrations of steps toward recovery, holidays, and birthdays.

This five-step approach helps breaks down problems into a manageable form, so that a solution can be implemented in stages. One of the clinicians leads the group through the five steps. The other ensures group participation, monitors the overall process, and suggests additional solutions.

Defining the problem. Defining the problem is sometimes viewed as a rather simple process but is often the most difficult step in the psychoeducational multifamily group process. If the problem is not properly defined, individuals, families, and clinicians become frustrated and may be convinced that the problem cannot be solved. Common difficulties that groups experience in this aspect of the process are choosing a problem that is too large or too general, defining the problem in an unacceptable way for a participant, and defining the problem as the person with the problem.

The problem-solving process begins in the "go-around." The leaders address each issue presented individually, avoiding the temptation to combine similar concerns of group members. After each person has had an op-

TABLE 24–3. Session program for ongoing family psychoeducation meetings

		Duration (minutes)	
		Multifamily group	Single-family
1.	Socializing with families and patients	15	10
2.	A go-around, reviewing	20	15
	a. The week's events		
	b. Relevant biosocial information		
	c. Applicable guidelines		
3.	Selection of a single problem	5	5
4.	Formal problem solving	45	25
	a. Problem definition		
	b. Generation of possible solutions		
	c. Weighing pros and cons of each		
	d. Selection of preferred solution		
	e. Delineation of tasks and implementation		
5.	Socializing with families and patients	5	5
	Total	**90**	**60**

portunity to report his or her perceptions of difficulties with the illness, the facilitators review the issues presented to determine which will be the focus of the group's efforts. To decide which problem to work on, the clinicians ask detailed questions to clarify the problem, focusing on behavioral aspects as much as possible. The clinician must talk with the individual who raised this issue to be sure that the group truly understands his or her perception of the issue. The scale of problems, at least in the first few months of the group, is also a factor in selecting the problem. For instance, long-standing or previously intractable problems should be addressed only if they can be broken down into more solvable subproblems. Leaders may choose to select simpler problems early in the group, so that the members learn the method, gain trust in one another, and achieve a few successes.

Once a problem has been defined in a way that is acceptable to each member of the family, the clinician asks the recorder to write it down and read it back to the group. The clinicians need to consider carefully any report of actual or potential exacerbation of symptoms. Areas of particular significance are safety, incorporating the family guidelines, issues concerning medications and substance use, life events, and disagreement among family members as to how to assist the ill member.

Generating possible solutions. The group members are then asked to offer whatever solutions they think may be helpful. The leaders should stress that it is important to resist evaluating or discussing solutions because doing so dramatically reduces the number of solutions presented. After all solutions have been presented, facilitators invite group members to share their thoughts on the efficacy of each solution. Each solution is addressed individually, with the "pros" and "cons" marked after each solution. This allows the group to become active in thinking about possible solutions, even when multiple solutions are already available.

Choosing the best solution. When all solutions have been evaluated, facilitators review the list and stress those with the most positive and fewest negative responses. The entire solution list is then presented to the individuals who provided the issue originally. They are asked to select the solutions they would like to test out over the next 2 weeks. It is important to stress that testing solutions is for the benefit of both the individual and the group because everyone is looking for things that work.

Implementing the chosen solution. Once a solution has been selected, a very detailed, behaviorally oriented plan is developed. Each step is discussed, and a person is assigned responsibility for completion of each step. The greater the detail, the better. Some groups offer the solutions to all group members to try, asking that the group be informed of their efforts, successes, or lack of success, thus increasing the repertoire of knowledge of the group.

Reviewing implementation. The individual is reminded that the facilitators may call during the coming week to check on his or her progress and to offer assistance. The individual is also asked to report at the next group meeting how successful he or she was and any obstacles that were encountered.

Single-Family Psychoeducation

The model described for multifamily group can be readily adapted to work in single-family sessions. Details of the single-family clinical models are to be found in Anderson et al.'s (1986) and Falloon's (1984) books and are summarized here. Both the single-family and the multifamily approaches described here are based on these works and the outcome research conducted by these authors' research groups. Another key source is *Bipolar Disorder: A Family-Focused Treatment Approach*, by Miklowitz and Goldstein (1997), which describes the family behavioral management approach for that disorder. Table 24–3 details the structure of the process in both formats; single-family sessions are usually an hour in length, but the sections of the session are all but identical.

Clinical Methods

As in the psychoeducational multifamily group format, the basic psychoeducational model consists of four stages that correspond approximately to the phases of an episode of schizophrenia, from the acute phase through the slow recuperative and rehabilitation phases.

Engagement

Engagement refers to a way of working with families that is characterized by collaboration in attempting to understand and relate to the family. The joining phase is typically three to five sessions and is the same in both single- and multifamily formats. The goals of this phase are to 1) establish a working alliance with both the family members and the patient, 2) acquaint oneself with any family issues and problems that might contribute to stress either for the patient or for the family, 3) assess and validate the family's strengths and resources in dealing with the illness, 4) instill hope and an orientation toward recovery, and 5) create a contract with mutual and attainable goals.

Engagement, in its most general sense, continues throughout the treatment, because it is always the responsibility of the clinician to remain an available resource for information and guidance for the family as well as their advocate in dealing with any other clinical or rehabilitation services necessitated by the illness of their relative. To foster this relationship, the clinician acknowledges the family's loss and grants them sufficient time to mourn, is available to the family and patient outside of the formal sessions, helps to focus on the current crisis, and serves as a source of information specifically geared to their needs and questions about the illness.

Educational and Training Workshop

The family is invited to attend workshop sessions conducted in a formal, classroomlike atmosphere. If a multifamily workshop is not feasible, information is provided to a single family, tailored to their specific situation and the diagnosis and phase of illness of the patient. Biological, psychological, and social information about schizophrenia (or other disorders, as the case may be) and its management is presented through a variety of formats, such as videotapes, slide presentations, lectures, discussion, and answering specific questions. An advantage of single-family education is that the education can be done in the family's home. Information about the way in which the practitioner and the family will continue to work together is also presented. A multifamily educational workshop is typically 6–8 hours in length, but single-family education can be set up as a series of shorter sessions on a weekly basis. The family is also introduced to the "guidelines" for management of the illness. These consist of a set of behavioral instructions for family members that integrate the biological, psychological, and social aspects of the disorder with recommended responses that help maintain an optimal home environment that minimizes stress (see Table 24–2).

Community Reentry

Regularly scheduled biweekly single-family meetings focus on planning and implementing strategies to cope with the vicissitudes of a person recovering from an acute episode. These working sessions are similar in structure to those described in the multifamily group format. Major content areas include the effects and side effects of medication, common issues about taking medication as prescribed, helping the patient avoid the use of street drugs and alcohol, the general lowering of expectations during the period of negative symptoms, and an increase in tolerance for these symptoms. Two special techniques are introduced to participating members as supports to the efforts to follow family guidelines (Falloon et al. 1984): 1) formal problem solving and 2) communications skills training. The application of either one of these techniques characterizes each session. Furthermore, each session follows a prescribed, task-oriented format or paradigm, designed to enhance family coping effectiveness and to strengthen the alliance among family members, the patient, and the clinician.

The reentry and rehabilitation phases are addressed with formal problem-solving methods and communication skills training. The problem-solving method is described more fully in the section on multifamily groups earlier in this chapter (see subsection "Using Problem-Solving Procedures"). The principal difference is that in single-family sessions, the participants and the recipients of ideas are the same, so that family members most commonly develop new approaches to their problems by brainstorming among themselves.

In the single-family approach, communications skills training is particularly important, whereas in the multifamily group format, the influence of other families tends to improve communication within and among families, so explicit communication skills training usually is not required. Communication skills training was developed to address the cognitive difficulties often experienced by patients with the severe mental illnesses, especially those with a psychotic phase. The core goal is to teach family members and the patient new methods of interacting that acknowledge and hopefully counteract the effects of mental illness on the patient's information-processing abilities and marked sensitivity to negative emotion and stimulation. The key skills include 1) communication of positive feelings for specific positive behavior, 2) communication of negative feelings for specific negative behavior, and 3) attentive listening behavior when discussing problems of other important family issues. The approach involves rehearsing communication skills in the session, often modeled by the clinician, followed by repeated rehearsal, often at home, and then homework to assist in generalizing the skills learned to other contexts, with social reinforcement used throughout the process of training. These skills are especially useful for families whose members are markedly exasperated, manifesting criticism or hostility toward the patient and/or severe anxiety, preoccupation, and intrusiveness as a consequence of disability and symptoms caused by the illness. Often, such reactions by family members are a result of poor treatment response, substance abuse, medication refusal, or expectations that are beyond what the patient is able to achieve at present given the severity of illness.

This process is repeated throughout the community reentry phase and continued as needed through the rehabilitation phase. The focus of this later phase deals specifically with the rehabilitative needs of the patient, addressing the two areas of functioning with the most common deficits: social skills and the ability to obtain and maintain employment. The sessions are used to role-play situations that are likely to cause stress for the patient if entered into unprepared. Family members assist in various aspects of this training endeavor. Additionally, the family is assisted in rebuilding its own network of family and friends, which usually has been weakened as a consequence of the illness. Regular sessions are conducted on a once- or twice-monthly basis, although more contact may be necessary at particularly stressful times.

Conclusion

Family psychoeducation and multifamily groups have shown remarkable outcomes in more than a score of studies, and multifamily groups appear to have a specific efficacy in earlier phases and in more distressed families. Clinical trials and extensive clinical experience have shown that family-oriented, supportive, psychoeducational treatment is acceptable to families and meets many of their needs. Theoretical support exists for the efficacy of these methods, with their strategy of stress avoidance, stress protection, and stress buffering, and the multifamily group format adds an inherent element of social support and network expansion.

Key Points

- Family psychoeducation and multifamily group therapies have shown remarkable outcomes in more than a score of studies, achieving a minimum of 50% reduction in relapse rates beyond medication effects and marked improvements in social and vocational functioning.

- Multifamily groups appear to have a specific efficacy in earlier phases and in more distressed or negative families and are markedly more cost-effective.

- Clinical trials and extensive clinical experience have shown that family-oriented, supportive, psychoeducational treatment is acceptable to families and meets many of their needs.

- Theoretical support exists for the efficacy of these methods, with their strategy of stress avoidance, stress protection, and stress buffering, and the multifamily group format adds an inherent element of social support and network expansion.

- The core elements are as follows:

  - Joining with families and patients to engage them in a mutual partnership to treat and overcome the impairments of severe mental disorders

  - Educating families and patients about the psychobiology of those disorders, their effective treatments, and the strategies that families and patients can use to overcome and cope with those symptoms and impairments

  - Problem-solving specific clinical and functional barriers to recovery by using the perspectives of each family member, the clinician, and—in the multifamily group format—other families

  - Initiating communication skills training to reduce negativity and maximize warmth and clarity

  - Setting limits on self-destructive, threatening, or annoying behavior secondary to the illness

  - Building or providing—in the multifamily group format—social support and validation

- The outcomes consistently observed, such as a 50%–85% reduction in rehospitalization rates, can be achieved only by adhering to well-tested practice guidelines and protocols.

References

Amenson C: Schizophrenia: A Family Education Curriculum. Pasadena, CA, Pacific Clinics Institute, 1998

American Psychiatric Association: Practice Guidelines for the Treatment of Schizophrenia. Washington, DC, American Psychiatric Association, 1997

Anderson CM, Hogarty G, Bayer T, et al: Expressed emotion and social networks of parents of schizophrenic patients. Br J Psychiatry 144:247–255, 1984

Anderson C, Reiss D, Hogarty G: Schizophrenia and the Family: A Practitioner's Guide to Psychoeducation and Management. New York, Guilford, 1986

Barrowclough C, Haddock G, Tarrier N, et al: Randomized controlled trial of motivational interviewing, cognitive behavior therapy, and family intervention for patients with comorbid schizophrenia and substance use disorders. Am J Psychiatry 158:1706–1713, 2001

Baucom DH, Shoham V, Mueser KT, et al: Empirically supported couple and family interventions for marital distress and adult mental health problems. J Consult Clin Psychol 66:53–88, 1998

Bebbington P, Kuipers L: The predictive utility of expressed emotion in schizophrenia: an aggregate analysis. Psychol Med 24:707–718, 1994

Becker T, Leese M, Clarkson P, et al: Links between social network and quality of life: an epidemiologically representative study of psychotic patients in south London. Soc Psychiatry Psychiatr Epidemiol 33:229–304, 1998

Brewin CR, MacCarthy B, Duda K, et al: Attribution and expressed emotion in the relatives of patients with schizophrenia [published erratum appears in J Abnorm Psychol 101:313, 1992]. J Abnorm Psychol 100:546–554, 1991

Brown GW, Birley JL, Wing JK: Influence of family life on the course of schizophrenic disorders: a replication. Br J Psychiatry 121:241–258, 1972

Cook WL, Strachan AM, Goldstein MJ, et al: Expressed emotion and reciprocal affective relationships in families of disturbed adolescents. Fam Process 28:337–348, 1989

Coursey R, Curtis L, Marsh DT, et al: Competencies for direct service staff members who work with adults with severe mental illness in outpatient public mental health managed care systems. Psychiatr Rehabil J 23:370–377, 2000

Cuijpers P: The effects of family interventions on relatives' burden: a meta-analysis. Journal of Mental Health 8:275–285, 1999

Dixon LB, Lehman AF: Family interventions for schizophrenia. Schizophr Bull 21:631–644, 1995

Dixon L, Adams C, Lucksted A: Update on family psychoeducation for schizophrenia. Schizophr Bull 26:5–20, 2000

Dixon L, McFarlane WR, Lefley H, et al: Evidence-based practices for services to families of people with psychiatric disabilities. Psychiatr Serv 52:903–910, 2001

Dyck DG, Short RA, Hendryx MS, et al: Management of negative symptoms among patients with schizophrenia attending multiple-family groups. Psychiatr Serv 51:513–519, 2000

Dyck DG, Hendryx MS, Short RA, et al: Service use among patients with schizophrenia in psychoeducational multiple-family group treatment. Psychiatr Serv 53:749–754, 2002

Emanuels-Zuurveen L, Emmelkamp PM: Spouse-aided therapy with depressed patients. Behav Modif 21:62–77, 1997

Falloon IRH: Family Management of Mental Illness: A Study of Clinical Social and Family Benefits. Baltimore, MD, Johns Hopkins University Press, 1984

Falloon I, Liberman R: Behavioral family interventions in the management of chronic schizophrenia, in Family Therapy in Schizophrenia. Edited by McFarlane WR. New York, Guilford, 1983, pp 141–172

Falloon IRH, Pederson J: Family management in the prevention of morbidity of schizophrenia: the adjustment of the family unit. Br J Psychiatry 147:156–163, 1985

Falloon I, Boyd J, McGill CW: Family Care of Schizophrenia. New York, Guilford, 1984

Falloon IR, Boyd JL, McGill CW, et al: Family management in the prevention of morbidity of schizophrenia: clinical outcome of a two-year longitudinal study. Arch Gen Psychiatry 42:887–896, 1985

Fenton WS, Blyler CR, Heinssen RK: Determinants of medication compliance in schizophrenia: empirical and clinical findings. Schizophr Bull 23:637–651, 1997

Frances A, Docherty J, Kahn D: Expert Consensus Guideline Series: treatment of schizophrenia. J Clin Psychiatry 57 (50, suppl 12B):5–58, 1996

Fristad MA, Gavazzi SM, Soldano KW: Multi-family psychoeducation groups for childhood mood disorders: a program description and preliminary efficacy data. Contemporary Family Therapy 20:385–402, 1998

Geist R, Heinmaa M, Stephens D, et al: Comparison of family therapy and family group psychoeducation in adolescents with anorexia nervosa. Can J Psychiatry 45:173–178, 2000

Goldstein M: Family factors that antedate the onset of schizophrenia and related disorders: the results of a fifteen year prospective longitudinal study. Acta Psychiatr Scand Suppl 319:7–18, 1985

Goldstein MJ, Rosenfarb I, Woo S, et al: Intrafamilial relationships and the course of schizophrenia. Acta Psychiatr Scand Suppl 384:60–66, 1994

Gunderson JG, Berkowitz C, Ruiz-Sancho A: Families of borderline patients: a psychoeducational approach. Bull Menninger Clin 61:446–457, 1997

Harrington R, Kerfoot M, Dyer E, et al: Randomized trial of a home-based family intervention for children who have deliberately poisoned themselves. J Am Acad Child Adolesc Psychiatry 37:512–518, 1998

Hogarty G, Ulrich R: Temporal effects of drug and placebo in delaying relapse in schizophrenic outpatients. Arch Gen Psychiatry 34:297–301, 1977

Hooley J, Richters JE: Expressed emotion: a developmental perspective, in Emotion, Cognition and Representation (Rochester Symposium on Developmental Psychopathology, Vol 6). Edited by Cicchetti D, Toth SL. Rochester, NY, University of Rochester Press, 1995, pp 133–166

Johnson D: The family's experience of living with mental illness, in Families as Allies in Treatment of the Mentally Ill: New Directions for Mental Health Professionals. Edited by Lefley HP, Johnson DL. Washington, DC, American Psychiatric Press, 1990, pp 31–65

Leff J, Vearnals S, Brewin CR, et al: The London Depression Intervention Trial: randomised controlled trial of antidepressants v couple therapy in the treatment and maintenance of people with depression living with a partner: clinical outcome and costs. Br J Psychiatry 177:95–100, 2000 [Published erratum appears in Br J Psychiatry 177:284, 2000]

Lehman AF, Steinwachs DM: Translating research into practice: the Schizophrenia Patient Outcomes Research Team (PORT) treatment recommendations. Schizophr Bull 24:1–10, 1998

Lehman AF, Carpenter WT Jr, Goldman HH, et al: Treatment outcomes in schizophrenia: implications for practice, policy, and research. Schizophr Bull 21:669–675, 1995

Lin N, Ensel W: Depression-mobility and its social etiology: the role of life events and social support. J Health Soc Behav 25:176–188, 1984

Link BG, Mirotznik J, Cullen FT: The effectiveness of stigma coping orientations: can negative consequences of mental illness labeling be avoided? J Health Soc Behav 32:302–320, 1991

Loveland-Cherry CJ, Ross LT, Kaufman SR: Effects of a home-based family intervention on adolescent alcohol use and misuse. J Stud Alcohol Suppl 13:94–102, 1999

Marriott A, Donaldson C, Tarrier N, et al: Effectiveness of cognitive-behavioural family intervention in reducing the burden of care in carers of patients with Alzheimer's disease. Br J Psychiatry 176:557–562, 2000

Marsh D: A Family-Focused Approach to Serious Mental Illness: Empirically Supported Interventions. Sarasota, FL, Professional Resource Press, 2001

McFarlane WR: Multifamily Groups in the Treatment of Severe Psychiatric Disorders. New York, Guilford, 2002

McFarlane WR: Family expressed emotion prior to onset of psychosis, in Relational Processes and DSM-V: Neuroscience, Assessment, Prevention and Treatment. Edited by Beach SRH, Wamboldt MZ, Kaslow NJ, et al. Washington, DC, American Psychiatric Publishing, 2006, pp 77–87

McFarlane WR, Cook WL: Family expressed emotion during onset of psychosis. Fam Process 46:185–198, 2007

McFarlane WR, Lukens EP: Insight, families, and education: an exploration of the role of attribution in clinical outcome, in Insight and Psychosis. Edited by Amador XF, David AS. New York, Oxford University Press, 1998, pp 317–331

McFarlane WR, Link B, Dushay R, et al: Psychoeducational multiple family groups: four-year relapse outcome in schizophrenia. Fam Process 34:127–144, 1995a

McFarlane WR, Lukens E, Link B, et al: Multiple-family groups and psychoeducation in the treatment of schizophrenia. Arch Gen Psychiatry 52:679–687, 1995b

McFarlane WR, Dushay RA, Stastny P, et al: A comparison of two levels of family-aided assertive community treatment. Psychiatr Serv 47:744–750, 1996

McFarlane WR, Dushay RA, Deakins SM, et al: Employment outcomes in family aided assertive community treatment. Am J Orthopsychiatry 70:203–214, 2000

McFarlane WR, Dixon L, Lukens EP, et al: Severe mental illness, in Effectiveness Research in Marriage and Family Therapy. Edited by Sprenkle DH. Alexandria, VA, American Association for Marriage and Family Therapy, 2002, pp 255–288

McFarlane WR, Dixon L, Lukens E, et al: Family psychoeducation and schizophrenia: a review of the literature. J Marital Fam Ther 29:223–245, 2003

Miklowitz DJ, Goldstein MJ: Bipolar Disorder: A Family Focused Treatment Approach. New York, Guilford, 1997

Miklowitz DJ, Simoneau TL, George EL, et al: Family-focused treatment of bipolar disorder: 1-year effects of a psychoeducational program in conjunction with pharmacotherapy. Biol Psychiatry 48:582–592, 2000

Montero I, Asencio A, Hernández I, et al: Two strategies for family intervention in schizophrenia: a randomized trial in a Mediterranean environment. Schizophr Bull 27:661–670, 2001

Muela Martinez JA, Godoy Garcia JF: Family intervention program for schizophrenia: two-year follow-up of the Andalusia Study [in Spanish]. Apuntes de Psicología 19:421–430, 2001

Penninx BWJH, Kriegsman DMW, van Eijk JTM, et al: Differential effect of social support on the course of chronic disease: a criterion-based literature review. Fam Syst Health 14:223–244, 1996

Phelan JC, Bromet EJ, Link BG: Psychiatric illness and family stigma. Schizophr Bull 24:115–126, 1998

Pickett-Schenk SA, Cook JA, Laris A: Journey of Hope program outcomes. Community Ment Health J 36:413–424, 2000

Reiss D, Plomin R, Neiderhiser JM, et al: The Relationship Code: Deciphering Genetic and Social Influences on Adolescent Development. Cambridge, MA, Harvard University Press, 2000

Repetti RL, Taylor SE, Seeman TE: Risky families: family social environments and the mental and physical health of offspring. Psychol Bull 128:330–366, 2002

Rund BR, Moe L, Sollien T, et al: The Psychosis Project: outcome and cost-effectiveness of a psychoeducational treatment programme for schizophrenic adolescents. Acta Psychiatr Scand 89:211–218, 1994

Russell PSS, al John JK, Lakshmanan JL: Family intervention for intellectually disabled children: randomised controlled trial. Br J Psychiatry 174:254–258, 1999

Sanders MR, McFarland M: Treatment of depressed mothers with disruptive children: a controlled evaluation of cognitive behavioral family intervention. Behav Ther 31:89–112, 2000

Solomon P, Draine J: Subjective burden among family members of mentally ill adults: relation to stress, coping, and adaptation. Am J Orthopsychiatry 65:419–427, 1995

Steinglass P: Multiple family discussion groups for patients with chronic medical illness. Fam Syst Health 16:55–70, 1998

Strachan AM, Feingold D, Goldstein MJ, et al: Is expressed emotion an index of a transactional process? II: patient's coping style. Fam Process 28:169–181, 1989

Tienari P, Wynne LC, Sorri A, et al: Genotype-environment interaction in schizophrenia-spectrum disorder: long-term follow-up study of Finnish adoptees. Br J Psychiatry 184:216–222, 2004

Tompson MC, Rea MM, Goldstein MJ, et al: Difficulty in implementing a family intervention for bipolar disorder: the predictive role of patient and family attributes. Fam Process 39:105–120, 2000

Van Noppen B: Multi-family behavioral treatment (MFBT) for OCD. Crisis Intervention and Time-Limited Treatment 5:3–24, 1999

Wagener DK, Hogarty GE, Goldstein MJ, et al: Information processing and communication deviance in schizophrenic patients and their mothers. Psychiatry Res 18:365–377, 1986

Walker DW: The treatment of adult male child molesters through group family intervention. J Psychol Human Sex 11:65–73, 2000

Wynne LC: The rationale for consultation with the families of schizophrenic patients. Acta Psychiatr Scand Suppl 90:125–132, 1994

Zhao B, Shen J, Shi Y, et al: Family intervention of chronic schizophrenics in the community: a follow-up study. Chinese Mental Health Journal 14:283–285, 2000

Zubin J, Steinhauer SR, Condray R: Vulnerability to relapse in schizophrenia. Br J Psychiatry Suppl, October (18):13–18, 1992

Suggested Readings

Several reviews, Web sites, and textbooks have proven useful to clinicians who are embarking on understanding and becoming proficient in family psychoeducation. The books by Anderson, Falloon, Leff, Miklowitz, McFarlane, and their colleagues are particularly useful as clinical guides; several of them are the treatment manuals for their respective outcome research studies. The Web site for the Substance Abuse and Mental Health Services Administration includes a workbook that gives a brief overview of the clinical intervention as a practice model.

Anderson CM, Hogarty GE, Reiss DJ: Schizophrenia and the Family. New York, Guilford, 1986

Dixon LB, Lehman AF: Family interventions for schizophrenia. Schizophr Bull 21:631–644, 1995

Falloon I, Boyd J, McGill CW: Family Care of Schizophrenia. New York, Guilford, 1984

Leff J, Vaughn C: Expressed Emotion in Families: Its Significance for Mental Illness. New York, Guilford, 1985

McFarlane WR: Multifamily Groups in the Treatment of Severe Psychiatric Disorders. New York, Guilford, 2002

McFarlane WR, Dixon L, Lukens E, et al: Family psychoeducation and schizophrenia: a review of the literature. J Marital Fam Ther 29:223–245, 2003

Miklowitz DJ, Goldstein MJ: Bipolar Disorder: A Family Focused Treatment Approach. New York, Guilford, 1997

Substance Abuse and Mental Health Services Administration, National Mental Health Information Center: Evidence-Based Practices: Shaping Mental Health Services Toward Recovery: Family Psychoeducation. Available at: http://mentalhealth.samhsa.gov/cmhs/communitysupport/toolkits/family/default.asp.

Chapter 25

Group Cognitive-Behavioral Therapy for Chronic Pain

Beverly E. Thorn, Ph.D., A.B.P.P.
Melissa C. Kuhajda, Ph.D.
Barbara B. Walker, Ph.D.

Virtually all psychiatric and medical disorders have biological, psychological, and social components, and each of these domains needs to be considered when treating patients. Group cognitive-behavioral therapy (CBT) is an efficient and effective vehicle for addressing each of these domains while treating patients with psychiatric and medical disorders. Group CBT targets the core psychological and social processes that affect illness, and incorporates pharmacological treatments and other biological treatments at the same time. Group CBT interventions can be tailored to unique symptom pathways that characterize a specific disorder.

In this chapter, we use chronic pain as an example to illustrate how group CBT can be used to treat a specific disorder. Most clinical principles and interventions from this chapter are transferable to other psychiatric disorders (e.g., mood, anxiety, psychotic, or personality disorders), with some modifications of the cognitive and behavioral interventions to fit the specific disorder. For example, group CBT approaches have been shown to be efficacious in a variety of psychiatric and biomedical problems, such as decreasing intrusive thoughts and anxiety in women undergoing treatment for breast cancer (Antoni et al. 2006); decreasing frequency of relapse in patients with schizophrenia and stress among their caregivers (Hazel et al. 2004); reducing recurrences, hospitalizations, and the number of hospitalized days in patients with bipolar disorder (Colom et al. 2003); and reducing suicidal behavior, affective distress, and illicit drug use in patients with borderline personality disorder (Binks et al. 2006).

In this chapter, the general principles of group CBT are illustrated as applied to chronic pain, which shares many features with major psychiatric disorders. Like patients with many other chronic conditions, those with chronic pain often suffer privately and in isolation, and there is no "cure" for their problem. Exacerbations are produced both by the burden of stressful life events and by negative cognitive appraisals. The goal is to help patients learn how to improve their overall functioning and quality of life. Because of these shared features, clinical work with chronic pain patients can be generalized to patients with many other psychiatric and medical disorders.

Group psychotherapy has been shown to be an efficient modality for treating patients suffering from chronic pain-related disorders. Although various types of group psychotherapy for chronic pain have been attempted, CBT has received the most empirical support. Numerous randomized controlled trials (RCTs) have demonstrated that group cognitive–behaviorally oriented psychotherapy is an effective intervention for chronic pain.

CBT approaches to pain management (both group and individual) have been shown to be generally efficacious for a variety of pain disorders (Hoffman et al. 2007; Morley et al. 1999; Ostelo et al. 2005). The specific treatment approach covered in this chapter—cognitively focused CBT—was evaluated in an RCT with patients experiencing chronic headache. Compared with wait-listed control subjects, participants reported significant reductions in pain-related catastrophizing and anxiety, and they showed large (and significant) increases in headache management self-efficacy; these changes were maintained at 12-month follow-up. Furthermore, approximately 50% of treated participants showed clinically significant changes in headache indices, including reductions in headache frequency and intensity, and reductions in medication intake (Thorn et al. 2007). Another RCT is currently in progress to compare this cognitively focused CBT approach with pain education in patients with various pain complaints.

This chapter illustrates how group-administered CBT can be used to help patients learn to better manage chronic pain–related disorders. We present the major components of a cognitively focused group CBT intervention. In cognitively focused CBT, a cognitive framework is adopted to motivate and empower patients to engage in pain self-management behaviors (e.g., restore or maintain work and family activities; use the health care system and pain medications appropriately; engage in regular, paced physical activity). Although cognitively focused CBT tends to be more targeted toward patient cognitions (Thorn 2004), it does not ignore patient behaviors. It is thought that the cognitive components of CBT serve as the catalysts to promote the necessary behavior change in pain self-management.

General Considerations of Group Treatment for Pain Management

Rationale for Group Cognitive-Behavioral Therapy

Efficacy of Group Treatment

First appearing in the pain management literature in the early 1980s, group treatment has become a common method of administering CBT for chronic pain (Keefe et al. 2002). RCTs have established the efficacy of group CBT compared with a variety of control conditions, including education groups, relaxation groups, medical treatment as usual, and wait-list controls. These RCTs have shown group CBT to be efficacious in patients with a variety of chronic pain problems, including mixed chronic pain conditions (Ersek et al. 2003; Puder 1988; Subramanian 1991), low back pain (Basler et al. 1997; Cole 1998; Turner et al. 1990), arthritis (Bradley et al. 1985), fibromyalgia (Keel et al. 1998), headache (Figueroa 1982; James et al. 1993; Johnson and Thorn 1989; Kneebone and Martin 1992; Kropp et al. 1997; Scharff and Marcus 1994; Thorn et al. 2007), irritable bowel syndrome (van Dulmen et al. 1996), and pain related to metastatic breast cancer (Goodwin et al. 2001).

Lack of Outcome Differences in Group Versus Individual Treatment

Although many studies have demonstrated that group CBT is more effective than a variety of control conditions, there is a dearth of research directly comparing the efficacy of group-administered and individually administered CBT for chronic pain. The few studies that have been published demonstrate a consistent *lack* of difference in treatment outcome (Frettlöh and Kröner-Herwig 1999; Johnson and Thorn 1989; Spence 1989, 1991; Turner-Stokes et al. 2003). In one study, researchers noted that although there were no overall differences in treatment outcome between individual and group modalities, effect sizes in improvement at follow-up suggested that group treatment was superior to individual treatment (Frettlöh and Kröner-Herwig 1999). Similarly, Spence (1991) reported minimal overall differences between individual treatment and group treatment. Post hoc analyses revealed that immediately following treatment, individual treatment was more effective than group treatment in improving self-reported coping strategies, but at follow-up, those in group treatment reported less pain-related interference than individually treated patients. Turner-Stokes et al. (2003) compared outpatient group therapy and individual therapy for 113 chronic pain patients and reported that both treatments resulted in improvements on measures of depression, anxiety, medication consumption, general activity, and pain severity. It is interesting to note that those treated via the group modality showed greater initial gains than individually treated patients, but those treatment differences did not hold up over time. The individually treated patients showed slower gains but ended with the same benefits in outcome as those who were treated in a group. Furthermore, the treatment gains made by individually treated patients were less likely to drift back toward baseline over time. These differences notwithstanding, the authors concluded that there were very few meaningful differences between group-administered and individually administered treatments. Given the lack of difference in treatment outcomes between group and individual CBT, it could be argued that group treatment is a more efficient modality of therapy for chronic pain disorders. A distinct practical advantage of group CBT may be that it is more cost-effective than individual therapy for both patients and practitioners.

Advantages of Group Treatment

There are several other advantages to using a group modality with patients who have chronic pain–related conditions. First, a group approach provides social proximity to and a sense of support from other people who share common distressing experiences. Individuals struggling with chronic pain often feel isolated and misunderstood. Disclosing thoughts and feelings to others in similar circumstances offers patients a greater sense of legitimacy. Examination of anecdotal remarks following group treatment of headache patients suggests that patients in group treatment feel they have the opportunity to express their thoughts and feelings openly with other members who understand their situation (Johnson and Thorn 1989). A qualitative study of previously treated group members confirmed that being listened to, understood, accepted, tolerated, and affirmed by the therapist(s) and other group members were highly valued perceived benefits of the group approach for pain management (Steihaug et al. 2002).

Second, studies have shown group CBT to be superior to group relaxation sessions (Turner 1982) and group discussion sessions (Larsson et al. 1987), both of which offer the type of social support received in group CBT. In addition, Maunder and Esplen (2001) reported that a supportive-expressive group for patients with inflammatory bowel disease did not improve symptoms of gastrointestinal distress/pain, patient quality of life, anxiety, or depression, and they concluded that at least for this population, supportive-expressive group therapy alone is not efficacious.

Third, group treatment provides clinicians with multiple examples to discuss during group sessions. This increases the likelihood that patients will understand the intervention and implement it in their lives.

Fourth, group treatment emphasizes the importance of a collaborative approach to treatment between patient and practitioner. Early in the group process, the leader establishes the expectation that patients will actively participate in group discussions, self-monitor their activities, and complete homework assignments. Through selective reinforcement of patients who actively engage in their treatment through group participation, the leader is likely to increase active coping in all of the group's members. A qualitative study of group CBT treatment with women suffering from chronic pelvic pain revealed that this collaborative approach facilitates a therapeutic progression, beginning with developing self-knowledge, followed by assuming responsibility for self-management, and ending with increasing self-control and personal mastery of emotions (Albert 1999).

A final potential advantage of group treatment is the use of group process to facilitate treatment gains (i.e., utilizing the interpersonal exchange between group members in addition to the exchange between therapist and patient). A group of patients provides an opportunity to capitalize on the moment-by-moment interchanges among group members as well as the interpersonal relationships that develop over time. It is noteworthy that group members will often take feedback from a group member better than the same feedback from the group leader. This may be due not only to the feeling of being more understood by a fellow patient (someone who has "walked in my shoes") but also to the power of the interpersonal process that occurs in group settings.

Patient Considerations in Group Treatment

Group Composition, Size, and Type

Almost anyone deemed appropriate for individual CBT for pain management is also suitable for group treatment, but there are a few exceptions. Patients with moderate to advanced dementia or other cognitive impairment, psychosis, or a history of chronic interpersonal relationship problems are inappropriate candidates for group treatment. Clearly, if a patient expresses a strong preference for individual treatment or if his or her schedule prohibits involvement at a prescribed group time, individual approaches will need to be employed.

Group size and type are also important when this treatment option is being considered. We favor five group members because that number is sufficient to facilitate interaction among group members, accommodate the absence of a member without jeopardizing group cohesiveness, and provide enough time to work briefly with each patient during each session. However, we have successfully managed groups with as few as three and as many as nine individuals. Most CBT groups will have more women than men because women have more chronic pain problems, present more frequently for pain treatment than men (Unruh 1996), and may be more receptive to group interventions based on their tendency to cope via a communal support process (Lyons et al. 1998). Although groups have often been formed to help patients manage pain associated with one particular diagnosis (e.g., arthritis, fibromyalgia), it does not appear necessary to segregate different types of pain patients in this way. One possible exception might be separating those with chronic nonmalignant pain from those with other forms of pain (e.g., pain related to cancer or HIV), because there is some evidence that psychosocial issues differ for these populations (Wheeler 2005). Differences in age, ethnicity, and cultural background do not appear to jeopardize the group process, perhaps because chronic pain serves as a unifying factor, making other potentially divisive issues less important.

The practical constraints of organizing people who are willing to participate in multisession group treatment at a designated common time require taking a somewhat liberal approach to group composition. Unless the patient is likely to interfere with the group process or is unable to keep pace with the group, we err on the side of inclusion even if we question his or her potential *optimal* utilization of the treatment.

Ongoing Versus Time-Limited Groups

Another factor to consider is whether the group will be ongoing or time-limited. Because we use a structured CBT approach (with a manual; see Thorn 2004), we limit the group to 10 sessions, although there is the option to be flexible. We have found that patients invariably want the group to extend beyond the 10 sessions, which is acceptable if planned for in advance but probably is inappropriate if the group began with the understanding that patients would meet for 10 sessions. From a clinical perspective, we have found it preferable to run a "closed group," in which all members start (and end) group treatment at the same time. From a practical perspective, however, running closed groups can prove difficult in some settings because new patients may have to wait up to 10 weeks to enter a group. In response to this issue, one of the authors of this chapter (Walker) has experimented with a hybrid model that allows new patients to enter an ongoing group the first week of each month. The advantage to this model is that no patient has to wait more than 3 weeks to enter group treatment; the disadvantage is that the group leader faces additional challenges. With this hybrid model, group dynamics change each month, and the leader needs to present material each week in a manner that will enable both new and former members of the group to participate.

Assumptions of a Cognitively Focused Cognitive-Behavioral Therapy Approach to Pain Management

Pain Is Real

In group CBT, the assumption that each patient's pain is real is critical and should be made explicit at the outset. This is particularly important to patients who have been referred to mental health practitioners for pain management. Such referrals often carry the implication that patients' pain is "in their head." Reassuring patients that their pain is real may remove some resistance to a psychosocial or cognitive-behavioral approach.

Pain Is Stress-Related

Another important assumption in group CBT is that pain is related to stress. In CBT, pain itself is conceptualized as a stressor; in addition, various physical and environmental stressors trigger and exacerbate pain. The assumption that pain is related to stress allows patients to consider the impact of stress on their pain (and vice versa) without requiring them to concede a psychogenic or psychosomatic basis for their pain.

Pain Is a Biopsychosocial Phenomenon

The biomedical model assumes that physiological pathology causes pain, and treatment therefore focuses first on finding the physiological cause of the pain and then on eliminating the pain by removing the cause (a curative approach). This approach is in stark contrast to the biopsychosocial model on which the CBT approach is based. In the biopsychosocial model, pain is conceptualized as a multidimensional phenomenon involving psychological, biological, and social factors. This concept is a key assumption underlying group CBT for pain and is emphasized throughout treatment.

Theoretical Framework

The theoretical foundation for CBT pain intervention is based on Aaron Beck's (1976) cognitive model, which promotes the idea that thoughts influence feelings, behaviors, and physiological responses. The structural foundation of CBT for chronic pain is based on an adaptation of Lazarus and Folkman's (1984) transactional model of stress. The stress-appraisal-coping model of pain (Thorn 2004) suggests that patients' cognitions predict their adjustment to chronic pain through their appraisal of the pain and related stressors, their beliefs about their ability to exert control over the pain situation, and their choice of coping options. The research foundation for this program also suggests that cognitive variables are a critical component in successful CBT for chronic pain (see Thorn 2004 for a review of the relevant literature).

Aims of a Cognitively Focused Cognitive-Behavioral Therapy Approach to Pain Management

Enhancing Pain Self-Management

Because chronic pain conditions are rarely curable, the focus of CBT is not on eliminating the pain but on helping patients to enhance their quality of life and minimize the impact of pain on their lives (i.e., to improve function). This treatment focus presents its own challenges because a downward spiral of disability often accompanies chronic pain, with pain leading to distress, withdrawal, and inactivity, which then lead to further dysfunction and eventual disability, promoting even further pain, distress, and so on. Helping patients to maintain their level of functioning or to change their behavior to regain function is a difficult but attainable goal. Appropriate pain self-management behaviors (also referred to as *coping behaviors*) include restoring or maintaining work and family activities, using the health care system and pain medications appropriately, and engaging in regular, paced physical activity. It is interesting to note that although pain reduction is not a primary aim of CBT, patients often report reductions in pain following treatment (Hoffman et al. 2007; Ostelo et al. 2005; Rains et al. 2005).

Changing Behavior by Focusing on Thoughts

The CBT approach is based on strong evidence that thoughts influence emotions and behavior, which is particularly true with regard to the experience of pain. A patient's highly negative cognitions regarding his or her pain and its sequelae are predictive of poor coping with chronic pain (Sullivan et al. 2001). For example, negative pain-related cognitions have been shown to be a robust predictor of higher perceived pain intensity, lower tolerance of painful procedures, greater psychological distress and psychosocial dysfunction, higher analgesic use, and greater pain interference, disability, and inability to work (Jacobsen and Butler 1996; Keefe et al. 1989; Sullivan et al. 2004). In addition, negative cognitions are a better predictor of poor coping (and therefore poor adaptive outcome) than disease severity, perceived pain intensity ratings, age, sex, depression, or anxiety (Flor et al. 1993; Geisser et al. 1994; Gil et al. 1993; Jacobsen and Butler 1996; Keefe et al. 1989; Martin et al. 1996; Robinson et al. 1997; Sullivan and Neish 1999; Sullivan et al. 1997). Given this evidence, the basis of cognitively focused CBT for pain is on helping patients become aware of, examine, and gain control over the thoughts that influence their feelings, coping behavior, and physiology. (Table 25–1 lists examples of pain-related thoughts and beliefs leading to subsequent maladaptive coping behaviors.)

Treatment Specifics of Cognitively Focused Group CBT for Chronic Pain

Overview of Standard Session Format

All group sessions (except the first) begin with a pre-session process check and end with a post-session process check (see Figure 25–1). The pre-session

TABLE 25–1. Examples of negative patient pain-related thoughts and beliefs, and subsequent maladaptive behaviors

Thoughts	Behaviors
My spine is disintegrating.	Avoidance of physical activity for fear of (re)injury
I'm no good to anybody anymore.	Withdrawal from social interaction
The only thing that can help is strong pain medicines.	Taking more than the prescribed dose of analgesic medication; mixing medications
Anything I try to do makes the pain worse.	Staying in bed all day
My life is ruined.	Angry outbursts at family and health care workers
There is only one way out of this.	Suicidal behavior

process check serves several purposes. First, it encourages participants to think about and practice material learned in the session throughout the week, and it sets an explicit expectation that participants will have done so. Second, it provides an opportunity for the practitioner to determine which concepts taught during the previous week need further clarification. The next session task is to review concepts learned and homework assigned in the previous session. Following homework review, the current session's treatment objectives are presented in the form of brief "mini-lectures," which include pertinent examples. Toward the end of the session, a worksheet is introduced to clarify treatment objectives. As group members begin to work together on the activities covered in the worksheet, each patient is encouraged to provide a relevant example. Following the interactive worksheet activity, the new homework assignment is introduced and discussed. Typically, the worksheet begun in the current session is incorporated into the homework assignment due the following week. Therapists must repeatedly highlight the importance of homework completion so that patients practice the CBT skills and implement them in everyday life. At the end of the session, patients are asked to list ways they could use the current session's material to think and behave differently during the ensuing week. The therapist then uses this post-session process check to determine if individuals understood and were able to apply the major concepts discussed during that session.

Main Objectives of Individual Sessions

The major objectives of each of the 10 cognitively focused CBT sessions are listed in Table 25–2. A complete description of each session is beyond the scope of this chapter, but a detailed discussion of each session, along with a step-by-step manualized guide to treatment, is available (Thorn 2004). Incorporated in the 10 sessions are four core components that are critical to the cognitively focused CBT process: the stress-appraisal-pain connection, pain-related automatic thoughts, pain-related intermediate beliefs, and pain-related core beliefs. Below we introduce each of these core components and illustrate with a brief case vignette, about Alice, and associated worksheets used during treatment.

Understanding the Stress-Appraisal-Pain Connection

The first core component involves introducing the group to the importance of understanding the stress-appraisal-coping model of pain. Group leaders help patients understand that pain produces stress, stress increases pain, and managing stress reduces the negative impact of pain on one's life. Moreover, stress itself can trigger and/or exacerbate pain. Thus, it is crucial that pa-

Pre- and Post-session Process Check

Pre-session process check

1. List the main point of last week's session.

2. List one thing you did or thought differently following last week's session.

3. Was there anything said during last week's session that confused or troubled you?

4. Do you have any questions from last week's session?

Post-session process check

1. List the main point of this week's session.

2. List one thing you can do or think differently during the next week as a result of this week's session.

3. Was there anything said during this week's session that confused or troubled you?

4. Do you have any questions from this week's session?

FIGURE 25–1. **Pre-session and post-session process check.**

TABLE 25–2. **Major objectives of the 10 cognitively focused group cognitive-behavioral therapy sessions**

Session	Major objectives
1	Build rapport among group members; discuss therapy rationale, goals, format, and rules; discuss the stress–pain connection; and introduce the stress-appraisal connection
2	Discuss the stress–appraisal–coping model of pain; begin identification of automatic thoughts or images
3	Evaluate automatic thoughts for accuracy; identify sources of distorted thoughts; recognize connection between automatic thoughts and emotional/physical shifts
4	Challenge negative, distorted automatic thoughts; construct realistic alternative responses
5	Identify general underlying belief systems; challenge negative distorted beliefs; construct new beliefs
6	Identify pain-related intermediate and core beliefs; challenge negative, distorted pain-related beliefs; construct new, more adaptive beliefs
7	Learn passive relaxation exercise; construct and use positive coping self-statements; incorporate coping self-statements into relaxation
8	Learn and practice expressive writing or verbal narration of expressive writing exercise
9	Learn about assertive communication; plan an assertive communication
10	Review concepts and skills learned; provide feedback about helpful and challenging aspects of the treatment; continue to practice and use skills in everyday life

tients with chronic pain learn about stress and how to manage stressors more effectively.

After surveying some of the physiological mechanisms of the stress response, group leaders introduce the notion that a person's judgments about and reactions to situations are more important than the actual situations themselves, and that stressors are typically appraised as threats, losses, or challenges. The concept of "appraisal" is introduced as a determinant of "coping," which comprises thoughts, feelings, and behavior. Group leaders share a vignette that involves a couple experiencing infertility. The group is asked to consider how this hypothetical couple would think, feel, and act differently depending on whether they judged the situation as a threat, a loss, or a challenge. This vignette helps group members to understand the connection between the appraisal and the subsequent thoughts, feelings, and actions. We believe it is useful to begin with a case example that is not directly associated with pain so as to help patients identify with the task without the added complication of overidentification with the stressor. Following this exercise, group members are asked to generate a list of stressors that are both pain related and non–pain related and then share them with the group.

Initial skepticism from group members regarding the power of "mere thoughts" over biological processes is to be expected, and the practitioner's response should aim toward acceptance and a lack of dogmatism:

> We wish we could tell you that you can think your pain away, but this treatment is not a magic bullet. We think that you will quickly recognize, though, that your judgments and thoughts about any situation, including pain, can shape what you think, feel, and do about it.

Most group members are quite aware that pain produces stress, and they are not particularly surprised that stress increases pain. They show less certainty, however, when presented with evidence demonstrating that one's judgment about a situation involving a pain exacerbation can affect one's thoughts, emotions, and behavior.

As a daily homework assignment to be completed throughout the week, group members are asked to add to their list of pain-related and non-pain-related stressful situations. Beside each stressor, they are asked to record the type of appraisal (threat, loss, or challenge), and then to note how their appraisal of those stressors influenced their coping (thoughts, images, feelings, behaviors, and pain).

Case Example

Alice, a 58-year-old divorced school librarian, continues to work full-time despite her pain conditions of fibromyalgia, chronic fatigue, and occasional migraine headaches. As is common, Alice has a primary pain condition (i.e., fibromyalgia), but she has more than one type of pain. Alice has a 40-year history of migraine headaches (since the onset of menses), but pain related to fibromyalgia was not a problem until her mid-40s. Alice takes the following prescribed medications: pregabalin 150 mg/day for fibromyalgia;

sumatriptan 50-mg tablets as needed (up to 200 mg/day) for migraine; and ibuprofen 200 mg twice a day or as needed every 4–5 hours for relief of pain, tenderness, and swelling.

During the group session, and as homework subsequent to the session, Alice filled out the Stress-Pain Connection Worksheet, which helps patients identify their specific stressors and their appraisals of those stressors (see Figure 25–2). This worksheet also introduces patients to the concept of thoughts and images associated with their stressors. [For those readers familiar with the specifics of cognitive therapy, this task will be recognized as a prelude to introducing patients to the concept of automatic thoughts.]

Like many patients, Alice readily understood the connection between stress and pain. She was less convinced, though, that her thoughts and beliefs could influence her experience of pain. During the group, Alice wondered aloud how her situation (having to travel to her son's wedding) could be judged as anything other than a threat, given the fact that travel always caused her pain to worsen. It was another group member who helped Alice turn the corner on this issue by reminding her how thinking about her son's out-of-state wedding as a challenge (instead of a threat or loss) got her to start problem-solving and actively making preparations rather than catastrophizing on the couch. In response to the other group member, Alice added, "And not only that, but when I sit and worry about what I might not be able to do at the wedding, I get uptight, which makes my pain worse!"

Recognizing, Evaluating, and Changing Automatic, Pain-Related Thoughts

The second core component teaches patients to recognize, challenge, and then reconstruct maladaptive automatic thoughts. Group members are taught that automatic thoughts are the ongoing, stream-of-consciousness, internal dialogue that often occurs just below one's immediate level of awareness.

The first step in this phase of treatment involves helping patients learn to recognize their own automatic, pain-related thoughts, especially those that are negative and/or irrational. To accomplish this, we ask group members to consider thoughts or images that run through their mind when their mood or sense of well-being worsens. For example, in response to a worsening of pain while standing at work, a patient might have the automatic thought "I might as well apply for disability because I can't work the way I used to." Patients are often surprised at the volume of negative and irrational thoughts that occur just outside of their immediate awareness. Group leaders explain that these thoughts have a powerful impact on a patient's emotions, behaviors, and other thoughts, whether the individual is aware of them or not. Bringing these thoughts into one's awareness provides greater control over the thoughts because once one is aware of a thought, one can evaluate it. We emphasize that all thoughts contain at least a grain of truth,

Stress–Pain Connection Worksheet

Stressful Situation	Appraisal Category (threat, loss, challenge)	Impact on Emotions, Thoughts, Behavior	Any Specific Thoughts Associated With Stressful Situation? can also be an image	Comments/ Other Notes to Self
My son is getting married, and I will have to travel out of state. Traveling triggers pain flare-ups.	Threat	*Emotions:* Fear, increased depression *Thoughts:* Worry *Behavior:* More vegetative	*Thoughts:* What if I can't walk with my son down the aisle?! Oh, God, I'll look like a fool! *Image:* I am walking arm in arm with my son down the aisle when sudden fatigue overcomes me. I fall to the ground, bringing my son down with me! The congregation "Ahhs" and "Oohs" as I'm carried out on a stretcher.	These thoughts are not helping me prepare for this happy family event. Also, the thought that I'm "losing" my son is creating more stress. If I see this situation as a challenge—I feel more determination and less fear. Challenge appraisal will get me more active instead of paralyzed on the couch.

FIGURE 25–2. **Stress–Pain Connection Worksheet.**

and some are completely true, but many thoughts are distorted. These distorted thoughts, especially negative ones, coincide with negative emotions and can lead to or exacerbate feelings of helplessness and hopelessness. Once group members learn to identify common cognitive distortions, they can begin to recognize how their own negative, distorted automatic thoughts influence their moods, behavior, and pain.

Next, group members are guided through a process of Socratic questioning to help determine whether their distorted thoughts are completely true, partially true, or not at all true. Specifically, Socratic questioning is a "tell me more" technique by which patients are taught to ask themselves a series of questions that will ultimately guide them to the answer. In the case of automatic thoughts, patients ask themselves, "What are the facts that support this thought?" and "What are the facts that do not support this thought?" Evaluating the rationality of their distorted automatic thoughts provides a segue into learning to construct alternative thoughts that are more realistic and adaptive. The point of focusing on distorted thoughts is not so much to change the content of the thought as it is to uncouple the emotion from the thought. The thought becomes "just a thought" by removing the power of "truth" from it.

Case Example *(continued)*

Over time Alice learned better pain self-management by evaluating, challenging and altering her negatively distorted pain-related and non-pain-related thoughts. She became aware that she had the tendency to focus on, as she put it, "the negative side of situations, sometimes making them more negative than they actually were. No wonder my kids tell me I need to lighten up!" Alice and other group members commented frequently on how amazed they were that they could actually change their thoughts. "I had just accepted my thoughts as the truth. In fact, I wasn't even aware I was having these thoughts so much of the time." When providing feedback about her group experience, Alice admitted that the most challenging concept was "figuring out how to make my thoughts more realistic and positive."

Figure 25–3 provides an example of how Alice used the Automatic Thoughts Worksheet to become aware of her pain-related automatic thoughts, evaluate their rationality, and come up with alternative (more adaptive) automatic thoughts.

Identifying and Evaluating Intermediate Pain-Related Beliefs

The third core component of treatment teaches group members to identify and evaluate intermediate pain-related beliefs. They begin to recognize thought processes such as underlying beliefs that are more deeply ingrained than situation-specific automatic thoughts. Patients are taught that their pain-related intermediate beliefs are those beliefs related to the cause of pain (e.g., "This pain just came out of nowhere"), beliefs about appropriate treatment of their pain (e.g., "A competent doctor should be able to find the causes of this pain and eliminate it"), and beliefs about their ability to influence their pain (e.g., "The only thing that can help my pain is strong pain medication"). Intermediate beliefs are often represented by rules and assumptions that patients make about the way things "should," "must," or "ought to be" in the situations in which they find themselves. It is thought that intermediate beliefs give rise to automatic thoughts (J.S. Beck 1995).

To help patients recognize these attitudes and beliefs about pain and the way it should be treated, group leaders first ask patients to identify key automatic thoughts (ones that come up repeatedly) and then explain to patients that these thoughts may be linked to underlying beliefs. Using the downward arrow technique described by Burns (1999), the group leaders ask the group members to consider, "If that (automatic) thought is true, what does it mean to you?" Patients often need help identifying the underlying belief systems that are driving their irrational automatic thoughts. Intermediate beliefs may be harder to identify than automatic thoughts because the former are not as easily recognized as irrational by the patient. For example, a patient's automatic thought that "I might as well apply for disability, because I can't work the way I used to" could be driven by the belief that "I should be able to lift the same amount of freight that I could before the accident, in the same way, in the same amount of time." The self-expectation held by this particular patient feels completely true to the patient when he first identifies his belief. Using a process of Socratic questioning similar to that used to examine automatic thoughts (e.g., "What are the facts supporting this belief?"; "What are the facts not supporting this belief?"), group leaders can help patients begin to question these attitudes and assumptions about the way they (and the world) "should" be.

In many cases, patients' intermediate beliefs promote the attitude of passive patients receiving a diagnosis, treatment, and cure. The group process can be used to the group leaders' great advantage in helping patients understand how their attitudes and beliefs about the cause and treatment of their pain can impact what they choose to do (or not do) to help themselves. For example, with very little therapist intervention, one group member can open the door to considering alternative beliefs by saying something like "So, none of our surgeries and none of the medicines have worked to cure our pain, and we've all been trying different things for years. Maybe it's time to try something else." As the group leaders help patients realize that beliefs and attitudes, like automatic thoughts, are also *just thoughts* and not necessarily absolute truths, patients become more receptive to the idea of taking more responsibility for pain self-management behaviors instead of relying

Automatic Thoughts Worksheet

Date/ Time	Stressful Situation	Emotional/ Physical/ Other Change	Automatic Thought or image (How much do you believe it?) 0–100%	Alternative Thought (Use questions below to review the evidence and compose alternative)	Results 1. How much do you now believe original thought? 2. Emotional/behavioral/ physical response to alternative thought
Saturday 8:30 A.M.	Lying in bed noticing how tired and achy I feel	Frustration, anger Pain and fatigue worsen Decide to stay in bed rather than running errands as planned	This pain and fatigue are never going away. It's the weekend—time to do some things I want to do, and I'm hurting too badly to do them! (About 90%)	**What is the evidence that the thought is true?** I seem to hurt all the time. It seems worse on weekends when I could be getting out and about and doing things. **What is the evidence that the thought is not true?** My pain and fatigue do subside some at different times—two weekends ago I shopped all day with my sister. Had a ball! Woke up in morning that day—felt awful. Told myself I had to get my butt out of bed—start moving. Love to shop—didn't want to let my sister down.	**1. Belief in original thought now:** About 20%–30% **2. Emotional/ behavioral/ physical response to alternative thought:** I feel more hopeful and less frustrated. More likely now to get out of bed and get a few things done, and moving around some makes my pain better.

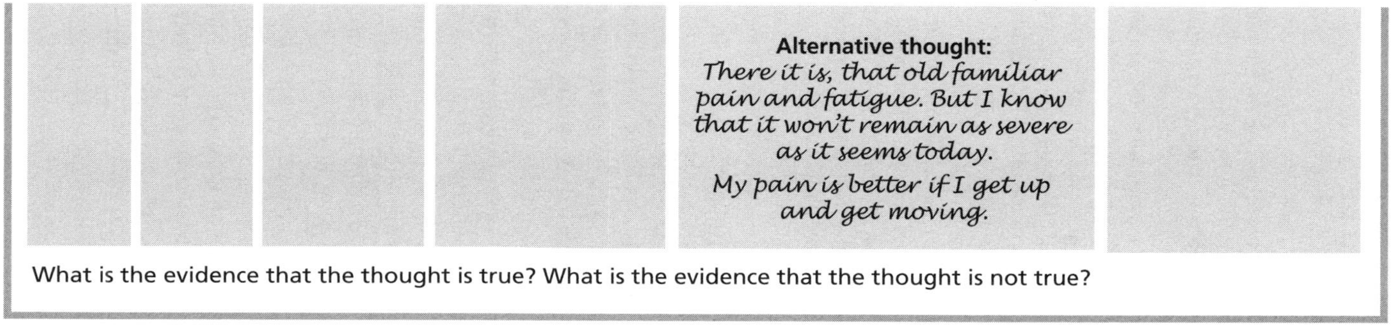

Alternative thought:

There it is, that old familiar pain and fatigue. But I know that it won't remain as severe as it seems today.

My pain is better if I get up and get moving.

What is the evidence that the thought is true? What is the evidence that the thought is not true?

FIGURE 25–3. Automatic Thoughts Worksheet.

on the belief in a cure and the attitude that their health and well-being are in the hands of physicians.

Case Example *(continued)*

Alice filled out the Changing Pain Beliefs Worksheet (Figure 25–4). On the left half of the worksheet, Alice's automatic thought ("I'll be suffering like this for the rest of my life") is connected to her intermediate beliefs about her ability to control the pain ("I am powerless to do anything about the pain") and about the cause of her pain ("I must have done something to deserve this"). Alice was able to identify her pain-related intermediate belief by asking herself, "If my automatic thought (I'll be suffering like this for the rest of my life) were true, what would it mean to me?" Through the process of Socratic questioning, she was able to examine the rationality of her beliefs ("I am powerless; I did something to deserve this") and come up with more adaptive (and realistic) beliefs about her ability to control the pain as well as "deserving" to suffer. Alice recalled that increasing her physical activity and eating a more nutritious diet do indeed positively impact her pain self-management skills. Alice was also able to recognize her belief that she "deserves to suffer" as irrational, and that her best approach would be to discard it as not helpful and to replace it with "Believing that I deserve pain is detrimental to my health! No one deserves pain!"

Identifying and Evaluating Pain-Related Core Beliefs

In the fourth core component of treatment, group members learn that *core beliefs* are rigid, long-held beliefs about one's basic worth or lovability as a human being. Although for most people, negative core beliefs do not predominate over positive core beliefs, it is thought that during times of significant stress (e.g., a pain flare-up), underlying beliefs often become negatively distorted, which in turn negatively impact thoughts, feelings, and behavior (J.S. Beck 1995). Pain-related core beliefs reflect the patient's sense of self as an individual in pain. Unfortunately, with increasing pain duration and mounting associated problems, patients with chronic pain often adopt the pain-related core belief that "I am a disabled chronic pain patient" and assume the role commensurate with such an identity.

Core beliefs are probably the most difficult to change because they are so deeply ingrained and often thought of as indisputable fact. However, building on previous sessions and patient success with mastering automatic thoughts and intermediate beliefs, group leaders teach that core beliefs are not absolute truths, but rather ideas that can be altered. Again using the downward arrow technique (Burns 1999), group leaders ask patients to identify a frequently occurring automatic thought, perhaps stemming from a previously identified intermediate belief. Patients are then asked to consider, "If that automatic thought were true, what would it mean *about* me?"

Building from a previous example, the automatic thought that "I might as well apply for disability," driven by the belief that "I should be able to work the same as I used to," might in turn be driven by the pain-related core belief that "I am a worthless chronic pain patient." It is also sometimes useful to get at pain-related core beliefs by having patients ask, "Why me?" Often patients feel that they are in pain because they deserve some sort of punishment, are basically unlovable anyway, or have always felt unworthy.

Uncovering patient beliefs can be an emotionally intense experience. However, it has been our experience that patients are already quite aware of negative core beliefs—they simply accept them as immutable. Partly to remove the emotional resistance to work on core beliefs, and partly to respect the patients who may feel that core belief work is too intense to tolerate, we tell patients it is not necessary to engage in the core belief work to benefit from treatment. Most patients do the work related to core beliefs, although a small remaining minority simply avoid engaging in this part of the treatment, and an occasional patient engages in the work but becomes so emotionally involved that follow-up individual sessions are useful.

Challenging and changing patients' negative pain-related core beliefs are formidable tasks. The group process is invaluable because patients will more readily accept confrontation about the belief that "I am unlovable because I have chronic pain" from a fellow pain patient than from a group leader. Group work is also useful to help patients examine the disadvantages as well as the advantages of holding on to negative pain-related core beliefs. With help, patients often recognize that adopting their negative core beliefs gives them permission to give up—to no longer try to cope. Patients are often motivated to challenge their beliefs when they come to this recognition. Another tool used to help patients challenge their pain-related core beliefs is to experiment with the "acting as if" exercise (J. S. Beck 1995). In this exercise, group members are asked to consider what specific things they would do differently if they did not hold their pain-related core belief. Ideally, the treatment component examining pain-related core beliefs will ultimately help the patient dissociate pain from both disability and suffering, and thereby adopt a new identity that "I am a well person with pain."

Case Example *(continued)*

As pointed out previously, in the Changing Pain Beliefs Worksheet (Figure 25–4), Alice's automatic thought ("I'll be suffering like this for the rest of my life") is connected to intermediate beliefs about her ability to control the pain ("I am powerless to do anything about the pain") and about the cause of her pain ("I must have done something to deserve this"). Alice's automatic thought ("I'll be suffering like this for the rest of my life") is also connected to her core belief that "I am a disabled chronic pain patient." Alice was able

Changing Pain Beliefs Worksheet

AUTOMATIC THOUGHT (How much do you believe it?) 0–100%	Intermediate Belief (How much do you believe it?) 0–100%	Evidence For/Against Advantages/ Disadvantages	Core Belief (How much do you believe it?) 0–100%	Evidence For/Against Advantages/ Disadvantages	ALTERNATIVE BELIEF (Use questions below to review the evidence and compose alternative)
My pain will never get better. I'll be suffering like this for the rest of my life. 90%	If your automatic thought were true, what would it mean to you? It means I am powerless to do anything about my pain (75%)	**For:** Sometimes meds help, but not usually. Seems like every time I plan something, pain stops me—lie in bed feeling worthless. Maybe I have pain because I didn't stay married. **Against:** I'm not really powerless. Feel better when I get more exercises and eat right. If you get pain from doing	If your automatic thought were true, what would it mean about you? I am a disabled chronic pain patient. 98%	**For:** I am tired and ache all the time. So many doctor appointments. I miss work because of pain and tiredness. **Against:** Really don't miss that much work—I usually tough it out! I think there's a lot of people who could not tolerate the pain and fatigue that I do!	I am not powerless over my pain and fatigue. I'm still working and sometimes getting out evenings and weekends. Labeling myself as a chronic pain patient is not helpful, but rather degrading and depressing. Makes me want to do nothing but lie in bed.

I must have done something in my life to deserve this suffering. 85%

bad things in life; I know people who should be suffering more than I am! Believing that I deserve pain makes me depressed. No one deserves pain!

Advantages:
It's easier this way! I don't have to beat myself up for not being more successful.

Disadvantages:
Giving up on self and life. Feel depressed.

Advantages:
I don't have to try so hard, just give into it—accept it.

Disadvantages:
I feel bad taking on the label of a chronic pain patient. Makes me feel hopeless/ helpless.

and feel sorry for myself. A lot more useful for me to say, "I am a well person with pain!"

What is the evidence that the belief is true? What is the evidence that the belief is not true? What are the advantages and disadvantages of holding this belief? Is the belief still serving you? Is there an alternative belief that can be tested?

FIGURE 25–4. Changing Pain Beliefs Worksheet.

to identify her pain-related core belief by asking herself, "If my automatic thought were true, what would it mean *about* me?" Although she was able to examine the rationality of this belief somewhat, her intermediate belief that "I deserve to suffer" continued to be problematic for her. She was able to follow this group work with some additional individual work on negative core beliefs about unworthiness, and she was ultimately able to abandon the belief that her pain was "payment" for some amorphous transgression. Eventually, she was able to see herself as more of "a well person with pain," and her quality of life improved dramatically.

Conclusion

In this chapter, we delineated the supporting research and illustrated the format for conducting group-administered cognitively focused CBT as an effective treatment to help patients better manage chronic pain conditions. The main assumptions underlying this treatment approach are that 1) chronic pain is real, 2) chronic pain is stress-related, and 3) the experience of pain involves psychological, biological, and social factors. Improving functioning despite the presence of pain is the central goal of group CBT. The theoretical foundation of cognitively focused CBT is based on Aaron Beck's (1976) cognitive model, and its structural foundation is based on Lazarus and Folkman's (1984) transactional model of stress.

The four core cognitively focused components critical to this therapy include the stress-appraisal-pain connection, pain-related automatic thoughts, pain-related intermediate beliefs, and pain-related core beliefs. Patients learning about the stress-appraisal-pain connection discover that stressful situations can be appraised as threats, losses, or challenges, and more importantly, that appraisal of these situations can significantly influence their pain experience, including how they cope with pain. The second core component involves teaching patients to recognize, challenge, and replace their distorted pain-related automatic thoughts with more accurate and rational ones, which in turn can lead to less distress and a greater sense of control over pain. Intermediate pain-related beliefs (e.g., beliefs about the cause of pain and the appropriate treatment for pain) are connected to pain-related automatic thoughts and, therefore, can be evaluated and altered to be more realistic and useful. Pain-related core beliefs (e.g., beliefs about a patient's sense of self as a person in pain) are connected to both pain-related intermediate beliefs and automatic thoughts and, therefore, can also be evaluated and altered to be more accurate and realistic. Although cognitively focused CBT tends to target patient cognitions (Thorn 2004), it does not ignore patient behaviors. The case illustration of Alice, woven throughout this chapter, exemplifies how these four core cognitive components play a role in group therapy sessions.

Cognitively focused group CBT for chronic pain management is not a panacea. However, cognitions are key treatment variables. In this chapter, we have presented evidence that supports the use of cognitively focused group therapy to treat patients with chronic pain, and have illustrated the important underlying assumptions and core concepts using clinical examples. We have presented converging lines of evidence demonstrating that distorted pain-related thoughts and beliefs negatively impact chronic pain, and that successfully changing distorted thinking can help patients better manage their pain, ultimately leading to improvements in quality of life. Our ultimate goal is for our patients to leave the last group session with new skills that they can continue to use, and at least a few steps closer to believing that they are well persons with pain rather than disabled chronic pain patients.

Key Points

- Both group and individual cognitive-behavioral therapy (CBT) for chronic pain have been shown to be efficacious in the treatment of a variety of chronic pain conditions. Group CBT has numerous advantages compared to individual CBT for pain. Advantages include gaining social support from others with pain, modeling of adaptive pain coping from group members, enhancing the ability to illustrate a teaching point with multiple examples, and capitalizing on the power of the group process.

- Main assumptions underlying the group CBT approach to treating pain are that chronic pain is real, chronic pain is stress-related, and the experience of pain involves psychological, biological, and social factors.

- The main goal of group CBT is to improve patients' functioning despite the presence of pain. Cognitively focused CBT targets maladaptive cognitions that are thought to interfere with behaviors that can lead to improved functioning and decreased disability.

- The four core cognitively focused components critical to this treatment approach are the stress-appraisal-pain connection, pain-related automatic thoughts, pain-related intermediate beliefs, and pain-related core beliefs.

- Pain causes stress, stress exacerbates pain, and personal judgments about stressors influence subsequent thoughts, emotions, and behaviors. Stressful situations can be appraised as threats, losses, or challenges, and how one appraises a situation can significantly influence the pain experience, including how one copes with pain.

- Automatic thoughts are those that occur just under the surface of one's immediate awareness, and pain-related automatic thoughts are often negatively distorted in patients experiencing chronic pain. Teaching patients to replace negative, distorted automatic thoughts with more rational, accurate thoughts presumably leads to less distress and a greater sense of control over pain.

- Intermediate pain-related beliefs are beliefs about the cause of the pain, the appropriate treatment for the pain, and the extent of personal control over the pain. Intermediate pain-related beliefs can be evaluated and can then be altered to be more realistic and useful.

- Pain-related core beliefs involve beliefs about an individual's sense of self as a person in pain. Although challenging to overcome, these beliefs can be evaluated for overly negative distortions, which if found can then be altered to be more realistic and useful.

References

Albert H: Psychosomatic group treatment helps women with chronic pelvic pain. J Psychosom Obstet Gynaecol 20:216–225, 1999

Antoni MH, Wimberly SR, Lechner SC, et al: Reduction of cancer-specific thought intrusions and anxiety symptoms with a stress management intervention among women undergoing treatment for breast cancer. Am J Psychiatry 163:1791–1797, 2006

Basler HD, Jäkle C, Kröner-Herwig B: Incorporation of cognitive-behavioral treatment into the medical care of chronic low back patients: a controlled randomized study in German pain treatment centers. Patient Educ Couns 31:113–124, 1997

Beck A: Cognitive Therapy and Emotional Disorders. New York, International Universities Press, 1976

Beck JS: Cognitive Therapy: Basics and Beyond. New York, Guilford, 1995

Binks CA, Fenton M, McCarthy L, et al: Psychological therapies for people with borderline personality disorder. Cochrane Database Syst Rev Issue (1):CD005652. DOI: 10.1002/14651858.CD005652, 2006

Bradley LA, Turner RA, Young LD, et al: Effects of cognitive-behavioral therapy on pain behavior of rheumatoid arthritis (RA) patients: preliminary outcomes. Scandinavian Journal of Behavior Therapy 14:51–64, 1985

Burns DD: Feeling Good: The New Mood Therapy. New York, Avon Books, 1999

Cole JD: Psychotherapy with the chronic pain patient using coping skills development: outcome study. J Occup Health Psychol 3:217–226, 1998

Colom F, Vieta E, Martinez-Aran A, et al: A randomized trial of the efficacy of group psychoeducation in the prophylaxis of recurrences in bipolar patients whose disease is in remission. Arch Gen Psychiatry 60:402–407, 2003

Ersek M, Turner JA, McCurry SM, et al: Efficacy of a self-management group intervention for elderly persons with chronic pain. Clin J Pain 19:56–67, 2003

Figueroa J: Group treatment of chronic tension headaches: a comparative treatment study. Behav Modif 6:229–239, 1982

Flor H, Behle DJ, Birbaumer N: Assessment of pain-related cognitions in chronic pain patients. Behav Res Ther 31:63–73, 1993

Frettlöh J, Kröner-Herwig B: Individual versus group training in the treatment of chronic pain: which is more efficacious? Journal of Clinical Psychology (Germany) 28:256–266, 1999

Geisser ME, Robinson ME, Keefe FJ, et al: Catastrophizing, depression and the sensory, affective and evaluative aspects of chronic pain. Pain 59:79–83, 1994

Gil KM, Williams DA, Keefe FJ, et al: Sickle cell disease pain in children and adolescents: change in pain frequency and coping strategies over time. J Pediatr Psychol 18:621–637, 1993

Goodwin PJ, Leszcz M, Ennis M, et al: The effect of group psychosocial support on survival in metastatic breast cancer. N Engl J Med 345:1719–1726, 2001

Hazel NA, McDonell MG, Short RA, et al: Impact of multiple-family groups for outpatients with schizophrenia on caregivers' distress and resources. Psychiatr Serv 55:35–41, 2004

Hoffman B, Papas RK, Chatkoff DK: Meta-analysis of psychological interventions for chronic low back pain. Health Psychol 26:1–9, 2007

Jacobsen PB, Butler RW: Relation of cognitive coping and catastrophizing to acute pain and analgesic use following breast cancer surgery. J Behav Med 19:17–29, 1996

James LD, Thorn BE, Williams DA: Goal specification in cognitive-behavioral therapy for chronic headache pain. Behav Ther 24:305–320, 1993

Johnson PR, Thorn BE: Cognitive-behavioral treatment of chronic headache: group versus individual treatment format. Headache 29:358–365, 1989

Keefe FJ, Brown GK, Wallston KA, et al: Coping with rheumatoid arthritis: catastrophizing as a maladaptive strategy. Pain 37:51–56, 1989

Keefe FJ, Beaupre PM, Gil KM, et al: Group therapy for patients with chronic pain, in Psychological Approaches to Pain Management: A Practitioner's Handbook, 2nd Edition. Edited by Gatchel RJ, Turk DC. New York, Guilford, 2002, pp 234–255

Keel PJ, Bodoky C, Gerhard U, et al: Comparison of integrated group therapy and group relaxation training for fibromyalgia. Clin J Pain 14:232–238, 1998

Kneebone II, Martin PR: Partner involvement in the treatment of chronic headaches. Behav Change 94:201–215, 1992

Kropp P, Gerber W, Keinath-Specht A, et al: Behavioral treatment in migraine. Cognitive-behavioral therapy and blood-volume-pulse biofeedback: a crossover study with a two-year follow up. Funct Neurol 12:17–24, 1997

Larsson B, Melin L, Lamminen M, et al: A school-based treatment of chronic headaches in adolescents. J Pediatr Psychol 12:553–566, 1987

Lazarus RS, Folkman S: Stress, Appraisal, and Coping. New York, Springer, 1984

Lyons RF, Mickelson KD, Sullivan MJL, et al: Coping as a communal process. J Soc Pers Relat 15:579–605, 1998

Martin MY, Bradley LA, Alexander RW, et al: Coping strategies predict disability in patients with primary fibromyalgia. Pain 68:45–53, 1996

Maunder RG, Esplen MJ: Supportive-expressive group psychotherapy for persons with inflammatory bowel disease. J Soc Pers Relat 46:622–626, 2001

Morley S, Eccleston C, Williams A: Systematic review and meta-analysis of randomized controlled trials of cognitive behaviour therapy and behaviour therapy for chronic pain in adults, excluding headache. Pain 80:1–13, 1999

Ostelo RWJG, van Tulder MW, Vlaeyen JWS, et al: Behavioural treatment for chronic low-back pain. Cochrane Database Syst Rev (2):CD002014 pub2. DOI: 1002/14651858.CD002014, 2005

Puder RS: Age analysis of cognitive-behavioral group therapy for chronic pain outpatients. Psychol Aging 3:204–207, 1988

Rains JC, Penzien DP, McCrory DC, et al: Behavioral headache treatment: history, review of the empirical literature, and methodological critique. Headache 45 (suppl 2):S92–S109, 2005

Robinson ME, Riley JL, Myers CD, et al: The Coping Strategies Questionnaire: a large sample, item level factor analysis. Clin J Pain 13:43–49, 1997

Scharff L, Marcus DA: Interdisciplinary outpatient group treatment of intractable headache. Headache 34:73–78, 1994

Spence SH: Cognitive-behavior therapy in the management of chronic, occupational pain of the upper limbs. Behav Res Ther 27:435–446, 1989

Spence SH: Cognitive-behaviour therapy in the treatment of chronic, occupational pain of the upper limbs: a 2 yr follow-up. Behav Res Ther 29:503–509, 1991

Steihaug S, Ahlsen B, Malterud K: "I am allowed to be myself": women with chronic muscular pain being recognized. Scand J Public Health 30:281–287, 2002

Subramanian K: Structured group work for the management of chronic pain: an experimental investigation. Res Soc Work Pract 1:32–45, 1991

Sullivan MJL, Neish N: The effects of disclosure on pain during dental hygiene treatment: the moderating role of catastrophizing. Pain 79:155–163, 1999

Sullivan MJL, Rouse D, Bishop S, et al: Thought suppression, catastrophizing, and pain. Cognit Ther Res 21:555–568, 1997

Sullivan MJL, Thorn BE, Haythornthwaite J, et al: Theoretical perspectives on the relation between catastrophizing and pain. Clin J Pain 17:52–64, 2001

Sullivan MJL, Adams H, Sullivan M: Communicative dimensions of pain catastrophizing: social cueing effects on pain behavior. Pain 107:220–226, 2004

Thorn BE: Cognitive Therapy for Chronic Pain: A Step-by-Step Guide. New York, Guilford, 2004

Thorn BE, Pence LB, Ward LC, et al: A randomized clinical trial of cognitive behavioral treatment targeted at the reduction of catastrophizing in chronic headache sufferers. J Pain 68:938–949, 2007

Turner JA: Comparison of group progressive-relaxation training and cognitive-behavioral group therapy for chronic low back pain. J Consult Clin Psychol 50:757–765, 1982

Turner JA, Clancy S, McQuade KJ, et al: Effectiveness of behavioral therapy for chronic low back pain: a component analysis. J Consult Clin Psychol 58:573–579, 1990

Turner-Stokes L, Erkeler-Yukset F, Miles A, et al: Outpatient cognitive behavioral pain management programs: a randomized comparison of a group-based multidisciplinary versus an individual therapy model. Arch Phys Med Rehabil 84:781–788, 2003

Unruh A: Gender variations in clinical pain experience. Pain 65:123–167, 1996

van Dulmen AM, Fennis JF, Bleijenberg G: Cognitive-behavioral group therapy for irritable bowel syndrome: effects and long-term follow-up. Psychosom Med 58:508–514, 1996

Wheeler MS: Interviews with patients who have cancer and their family members provide insight for clinicians. Home Healthcare Nurse 23:642–646, 2005

Suggested Readings

Beck JS: Cognitive Therapy: Basics and Beyond. New York, Guilford, 1995

Caudill MA: Managing Pain Before It Manages You, Revised Edition. New York, Guilford, 2002

The Therapy Advisor: Promoting Scientifically Based Psychotherapy (http://www.therapyadvisor.com)

Thorn BE: Cognitive Therapy for Chronic Pain: A Step-by-Step Guide. New York, Guilford, 2004

Turk DC, Winter F: The Pain Survival Guide: How to Reclaim Your Life. Washington, DC, American Psychological Association, 2005

PART 6

Forms of Psychotherapy Integration

Section Editor

Bernard D. Beitman, M.D.

Chapter 26

Theory and Practice of Psychotherapy Integration

Bernard D. Beitman, M.D.
John Manring, M.D.

Psychotherapy integration grew out of increasing dissatisfaction with the continuous creation of new schools of therapy, the demands for accountability by payers, and the confusion of the general public about what psychotherapy is (Prochaska and Norcross 2007). The movement promised several advantages: clarity through recognition of common factors and a common language for the many overlapping concepts and strategies; improved outcomes via selection of the most effective concepts and strategies; and a framework within which new ideas could continue to evolve while simultaneously being tempered by continuing contact with other evolving ideas and the core processes that defined psychotherapy. By attempting to conceptualize psychotherapy as a whole, as an entity itself, the integration movement fostered pragmatic findings that did not fit neatly within specific, school-based theoretical orientations. These findings included the predominance of patient variables in determining outcome, the significant role of personal characteristics of the therapist, the key role of the therapeutic alliance, and the value of focusing on outcome rather than theory and technique.

In this chapter we review the history of the movement to integrate the psychotherapies and some of the reasons it is failing to live up to its initial promise. Then, in an effort to develop a more scientific psychotherapy from this integrative perspective, we list several basic principles of psychotherapy as a whole that do not fit neatly into specific schools. Finally, we describe an approach to psychotherapy that is built on recognizing similarities while utilizing differences, an approach built on the continuous, evidence-based clarification of core processes that define psychotherapy no matter what the theoretical orientation.

A History of Psychotherapy Integration

Psychotherapy continues to evolve within cultural contexts. Similar to most religions, psychotherapy is syncretic—it incorporates apparently useful ideas from the social, political, and religious sources within which it functions. Although the origins of modern psychotherapy are traced back to the early-twentieth-century work of Sigmund Freud, human societies have for millennia developed a variety of relationships between two people for the purpose of healing. Shamans, witch doctors, diviners, priests, rabbis, ministers, imams, holy men and women, dayanim, physicians, and others in their own ways have attempted to utilize emotionally charged relationships with help-seekers to encourage emotional and physical healing.

Freud consciously and unconsciously assimilated ideas from his Viennese-European culture to develop psychoanalysis. Without any direct attribution, he is likely to have applied scholarly Jewish principles to his psychoanalytic work. The Talmud, for example, declares that "a dream unexamined is like a letter unopened." Talmudic interpretations of the five books of Moses (the Pentateuch) may have led Freud to find deeper meanings in the utterances of his patients; the Torah became equivalent to the superficial or explicit meanings, and interpretation explored the hidden meanings (Bakan 1958).

Unlike earlier forms of psychotherapy, Freud's psychoanalysis found widespread and enthusiastic reception in a Western culture ready to begin the process of individual self-exploration. Energized by penetrating insights into human nature as well as intense criticism, psychoanalysis has become a towering intellectual achievement, placing Freud in the company of Karl Marx and Albert Einstein.

After Freud, new forms of psychoanalysis were founded (ego psychology, self psychology, object relations theory), and new schools split off entirely (e.g., Jung's analytical psychology, Adlerian therapy). Still other schools that were developed by psychoanalytically trained theorists (cognitive therapy, behavior therapy, and emotion-focused therapies) seem quite remote from Freud's original conceptions. During the last decades of the twentieth century, therapists expanded into systems concepts involving the family, culture, and spirituality, while also yielding to economic pressures to decrease the number of sessions by developing a variety of brief therapies (Good and Beitman 2006).

Driven also by a data imperative, psychotherapists followed the example of clinical drug trials by pitting their therapies for specific disorders against psychopharmacological treatments as well as against each other. This "horse race" research yielded equivocal results, with the therapy form favored by the principal investigator usually winning. Meta-analyses done several decades apart repeatedly showed little difference in outcomes among the schools of therapy, yet psychotherapy teachers continued to insist that therapists in training must learn the individual "packages" of therapy. These meta-analytic studies have paradoxically diminished emphasis on theory and instead focused researchers on what works (Norcross 2005).

To further demonstrate the questionable nature of treatment packages, Jacobson et al. (1996) deconstructed the basic cognitive-behavioral therapy (CBT) package for depression into three subelements: behavioral activation, focus on automatic thoughts, and focus on underlying schemas. Only experienced CBT therapists were recruited for the study, in which 150 depressed patients were assigned to one of three protocols: behavioral activation exclusively; behavioral activation plus focus on automatic thoughts; or the full therapy with behavioral activation, focus on automatic thoughts, and focus on underlying schemas. The results across the three groups were the same, causing much consternation among those who believed in the necessity of the entire package. The study challenged psychotherapists to define treatment-effective techniques and strategies in a more clear fashion. It is likely that as a result of this debate, optimal techniques and strategies will depend on the therapeutic context of patient, therapist, and their alliance rather than some abstract ideas universally applied based on diagnosis.

Furthermore, reliable surveys of psychiatrists and psychologists tend to show a significant percentage espousing either psychoanalysis (among psychiatrists) or cognitive therapy (among psychologists), whereas a higher percentage of professionals in each field report themselves as "integrationists/eclectics" (Prochaska and Norcross 2007). Most teachers and therapists know that the emperor has no clothes; they know that most therapists evolve their approaches to accommodate the needs of their patients despite the persistent image of psychotherapy as an assortment of conflicting schools. More recently, psychoanalysis has been replaced by cognitive therapy as the "leading school" of psychotherapy in the public mind, despite the relatively few therapists who have been well trained in it.

In 1984 in Annapolis, Maryland, psychologists Marvin Goldfried and Paul Wachtel convened the first annual meeting of the Society for the Exploration of Psychotherapy Integration. The organization grew out of the frustration that many academics and practitioners were feeling about the proliferation of conflicting schools. A journal, now called the *Journal of Psychotherapy Integration*, was soon born. Several types of integration were gradually identified:

- Systematic eclecticism
- Theoretical integration
- Assimilative integration
- Common factors (or core processes)

Therapists who advocate *systematic eclecticism*, exemplified by Lazarus's (1981, 1989) multimodal therapy, rely on "what works" as suggested by research outcome studies, although these therapists must stretch the applicability of research findings to fit the needs of each unique person. Lazarus recommends systematically evaluating patients in seven different categories: Behavior, Affect, Sensation, Imagery, Cognition, Interpersonal relationships, and Drugs (BASIC ID). ("Drugs" actually refers to all things biological, including medications, drugs of abuse, exercise, nutrition, and other physiological inputs.) All research applicable to each of these areas is then applied. For example, if a patient experiences *behavioral* problems such as obsessive-compulsive disorder, the research protocols for obsessive-compulsive disorder are applied. The patient is asked to expose himself or herself to the feared stimulus (e.g., dirt) and then is asked to not wash his or her hands for as long a time as possible. The sequence is called *exposure and response prevention*. For problems with *affect* or emotion, catharsis (full expression of restrained emotion) coupled with examining and owning one's feelings might be used. *Sensation* problems might involve muscle tension, which can be addressed with relaxation training, meditation, or physical exercise. Problematic *images* of oneself or failures to *imagine* success might be discovered and replaced. If the patient shows evidence of faulty thinking (*cognition*) patterns, the therapist encourages using a thought record, a tool used in cognitive therapy to find automatic thoughts and possibly their origins in underlying schemas. If *interpersonal relationship* changes might be helpful, then the therapist might encourage specific ways to alter them. If the person has problems with *drugs* (e.g., alcohol), the therapist recommends several well-studied methods, such as cognitive therapy, Alcoholics Anonymous, and motivational interviewing.

BASIC ID accommodates to individual patients' needs. It is systematic and eclectically borrows from many sources. Then why has this rational, research-based approach not taken over the field? There is very little research support for problems with sensation or imagining, although these brain functions are essential to normal functioning. Experimentally validated therapies often do not translate well into the real world outside the tightly controlled research arena. Also, BASIC ID misses some crucial relationship variables. But perhaps most problematic, Arnold Lazarus, the founder, made it too idiosyncratic, too much in his own image, too much like another "school" of psychotherapy with specific protocols and worksheets and pre-scribed sequences of treatment. Multimodal therapy became a distinctive orientation in 1973 (Wedding and Corsini 1973, p. 330), and that may have limited the influence of this good set of ideas.

Theoretical integration attempts to find overarching principles by which the psychotherapy approaches across the schools can be organized. Pro-chaska and DiClemente (1984) combined three crucial aspects of psycho-therapy that cross schools: readiness to change, processes of change, and levels (or content) of change. Readiness to change can be divided into sev-eral stages: not seeing a problem (precontemplation), recognizing a prob-lem (contemplation), getting ready to change (preparation), changing (ac-tion), and maintaining the change (maintenance). Clients come into therapy usually recognizing the need to do something (contemplation or preparation), but some have no idea that something needs to be changed (precontemplation). Therapists must adjust their responses to fit clients' stages of change. In couples therapy, for example, one member is likely to be less ready to change than the other and must be assisted along the readi-ness-to-change continuum to match the partner who is more ready to change. Change can be initiated via a variety of techniques and methods (processes of change), which include raising self-awareness (consciousness raising), education, emotional release (catharsis), facing fears (countercon-ditioning), choosing, and direct use of the therapeutic relationship.

Prochaska and DiClemente (1984) divided the content of therapy into five levels, from the more superficial to the "deep": 1) symptoms/situational problems, 2) maladaptive cognitions, 3) current maladaptive interpersonal relationships, 4) family/systems problems, and 5) intrapersonal (within the person) problems. Prochaska and DiClemente, like Lazarus (1981, 1989), urged therapists to customize their responses to the patient, rather than at-tempting to fit the patient into the therapist's theoretical mold. They added the important and obvious notion of readiness to change and, like Lazarus, listed the common content and techniques available to therapists.

With *assimilative integration* (Messer 1992), therapists begin with a deep indoctrination into the specific school of therapy that best fits them and then assimilate ideas from different schools into their basic approach. For example, if one begins as a psychoanalytically oriented therapist, one might learn to apply cognitive homework assignments, systems thinking, and behavioral techniques as they seem to fit the needs of patients. All therapists start learning from the base of their own experience. Psychotherapy training, like psychotherapy itself, should be molded to the mind of each trainee.

Common factors, or *core processes*, seek to define what is common to all therapies and build on them (Beitman and Yue 1999a, 1999b, 2004a, 2004b). Psychotherapy has been practiced in varying forms in various cultures throughout human history (Ehrenwald 1976). There exists a single conceptual thing, an archetype, which is psychotherapy. Each school and each relationship are variations of that archetype, just as each person is a variation in body and mind of the human being. There are many different common *factors*, but there are fewer common *processes*. These processes include establishing and maintaining the therapeutic alliance, activating the patient's observing self, searching for maladaptive patterns, initiating and then maintaining change in those patterns, and saying good-bye. Several studies suggest that significantly more of the variance in psychotherapy outcome is a result of common rather than specific factors (Ahn and Wampold 2001; Lambert 2005; Wampold 2001). From his review of the research literature, Lambert (2005) suggested that the largest outcome variable is neither the therapeutic alliance nor the specific therapeutic techniques, but rather the client (called "extratherapeutic change" in Figure 26–1). Accounting for about 40% of the variance in the outcome of psychotherapy, the key client variables include the following: severity of problem, type of problem, readiness to change, helpful and problematic events during the course of therapy (e.g., the person gets a new job or breaks a leg), and degree of support by the social and work networks. Common factors in psychotherapy account for about 30% of outcome, whereas client expectations of success (placebo effects) and specific psychotherapy techniques (schools) each account for about 15% of outcome.

From this array of four general categories of integration—systematic eclecticism, theoretical integration, assimilative integration, and common factors—an astonishing variety of integrative approaches have been developed. Founded on the principle of parsimony in an attempt to reduce the confusing proliferation of schools, the movement to integrate the psychotherapies seems to foster them. Table 26–1 lists a few of the integrative schools, with their acronyms and primary authors.

The proliferation of integrative schools seems to contradict the original intention of the movement, which was to simplify the confusing claims. Like good psychotherapists, integrationists are asking themselves more specific questions about the intent and future of the field. These "meta-looks" at the ever-flowering theories and techniques are yielding fundamental principles by which future developments can be guided (Norcross and Goldfried 2005; Stricker and Gold 2006).

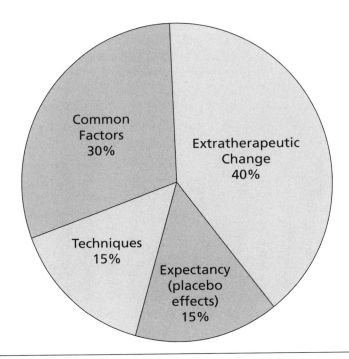

FIGURE 26–1. Variables influencing outcome in psychotherapy.

Source. Reprinted from Norcross JC: "A Primer on Psychotherapy Integration," in *Handbook of Psychotherapy Integration*, 2nd Edition. Edited by Norcross JC, Goldfried MR. New York, Oxford University Press, 2005, pp. 3–24. Reprinted by permission of Basic Books, a member of Perseus Books Group.

Basic Psychotherapeutic Principles

The external reality that we perceive and know is limited by the range of stimuli our brains can process. For example, our eyes and occipital cortices can register only a narrow band of the light spectrum, ranging from infrared to ultraviolet. We cannot register radio waves, although we have at our disposal instruments such as radios to register these waves for us. When we consider complex conceptual processes, we are also limited by the manner in which the brain can organize them. Perhaps we can learn from these limitations and apply the same principles to the social sciences and humanities, as well as psychotherapy.

Evolution seems to have driven the brain to integrate its various components by balancing the two opposing processes of differentiation and linkage. Well-being may grow out of the increasing differentiation of brain parts, with increasing linkages among them (Siegal 2006). Integration of the brain facil-

TABLE 26–1. Various integrative psychotherapies

Psychotherapy (acronym)	Primary author(s)
Acceptance and Commitment Therapy (ACT)	Hayes et al. (2006)
Cognitive-Affective Behavior Therapy	Goldfried (1995)
Cognitive Analytic Therapy (CAT)	Ryle and Kerr (2002)
Cognitive-Behavioral Analysis System of Psychotherapy (CBASP)	McCullough (2000)
Contextual Integrative Psychotherapy	Consoli and Chope (2006)
Cyclical Psychodynamics and Integrative Relational Psychotherapy	Wachtel et al. (2005)
Dialectical Behavioral Therapy (DBT)	Linehan (1993)
Eye-Movement Desensitization and Reprogramming (EMDR)	Shapiro (2001)
Mindfulness-Based Cognitive Therapy (MBCT)	Zindel et al. (2001)
Process-Experiential Therapy (PET)	Greenberg et al. (1998)
Systematic Treatment Selection and Prescriptive Psychotherapy	Beutler and Harwood (2000)
Transtheoretical Approach	Prochaska and DiClemente (1984)

itated adaptation to the environment by simultaneously enhancing flexibility, stability, and coherence. A similar phenomenon occurs with psychotherapy patients and most human beings. The analogy can be used to understand the evolving field of psychotherapy. Applied to psychotherapy, the differentiation (i.e., proliferation) of schools seems likely to continue as new ideas are added to old ones and as culture and social pressures create new combinations and new needs. Linkages may seem less attractive to each of these schools as each one differentiates within the conceptual "skull" of psychotherapy. The term *psychotherapy* binds the schools together. Core processes or common factors help tighten the linkages by reminding therapists that the differentiating concepts share much in common. The continuing differentiation may then shed new light on the core processes that link them, further clarifying and refining them in an ongoing iterative process.

Psychotherapy may be leaving its prescientific state as neuroimaging and specialized electroencephalograms of brain function help to define the neurophysiological bases of psychotherapeutic change. As therapists theorize, their theories will be increasingly testable by concrete brain mapping. Such work will challenge therapists to learn that mind and brain are not separate but are different aspects of the same thing (Beitman et al. 2006).

The scientist of psychotherapy observes psychotherapy from an as unbiased and objective a position as possible. The tendency to establish schools limits this necessary objectivity. Several facts generated by decades of research on psychotherapy are generally avoided by those wishing to emphasize their particular theoretical views. These facts, described in more detail next, are summarized in Table 26–2.

1. *People often make profound psychological changes* without *formal psychotherapy* (Prochaska and Norcross 2007). Individuals use their internal personal resources, family, friends, clergy, bartenders, hairstylists, self-help groups, and self-help books to improve their mood, change their thinking, and modify maladaptive behaviors. In therapy, patients are active participants in the change process, often subconsciously influencing their therapists to provide them with the context and responses to achieve their desired outcomes. Psychotherapy rarely, if ever, is "done to" patients. Instead, the active collaboration with a therapist accelerates the use of available resources within and outside each patient to create change.

2. *Patient variables, rather than theory or technique, most strongly predict outcome.* For example, a 45-year-old, unmarried, unemployed, highly intelligent, very isolated woman was living off the income supplied by her doting 75-year-old parents. They worried about what would happen to their daughter when they died. She pleased them by going to psychotherapy. She rambled on and on about the jobs she had had, the excellent

TABLE 26–2. Basic facts of psychotherapy

People often experience profound psychological changes *without* formal psychotherapy.

Patient variables, rather than the particular theory or technique used, are the strongest predictors of outcome in psychotherapy.

The personal variables of the therapist are far more important predictors of outcome than theory or technique.

Therapists resemble each other in their practice as they mature, despite having different theoretical beginnings.

The strength of the therapeutic relationship is correlated with outcome across schools of psychotherapy.

Effective therapy is customized to the needs of each patient.

Diagnosis limits formulation.

Psychotherapists help patients create new futures for themselves.

Important areas of research on psychotherapy remain underdeveloped (e.g., defining criteria for defining good therapist candidates, determining what makes therapeutic action successful, establishing ways to teach effective timing of interventions).

grades she had maintained in graduate school, the problems with her house, the discourtesy of clerks in supermarkets, and so on. Her therapist was becoming bored. Although patients are not obligated to entertain their therapists, most therapists like to work on something. When the therapist respectfully and urgently inquired what she would do when her parents died, suggesting that she should face that future, the patient became enraged. "I have come here for *you* to listen to *me*. That's all. Goodbye." She never returned. Therapy did not match her expectations.

As this example illustrates, the most important predictor of outcome—the most important variable in the whole formula of psychotherapeutic change—is none other than the patient. What the patient brings to therapy strongly determines what kinds of changes are possible. The more severe the symptoms and the less helpful the social circumstances, the less likely it is that positive gains can be achieved. Think of the cardiac surgeon having to choose between doing a heart transplant on a 56-year-old healthy, athletic man or on a 92-year-old man with emphysema and diabetes. No matter how skilled the surgeon, the first patient is more likely to have a positive outcome. The National Institute of Mental Health's Treatment of Depression Collaborative Research Program showed that matching the patient's basic skills to techniques correlated with outcome:

those people with strong interpersonal skills did better in interpersonal therapy, whereas those with strongly cognitive ways of coping did better in cognitive therapy. The implication clearly is to match the method of therapy to the patient's strengths (Imber et al. 1990).

Patients' expectations of psychotherapy play a crucial role in outcome as well. What do they want? How do they expect to behave in therapy? What do they expect from therapists? What outcome do they seek? How much effort are they willing to put into achieving their outcomes?

3. *The therapist is more important to outcome than theory or technique.* The therapist embodies the practice of psychotherapy and therefore plays a more important role in outcome than do techniques, regardless of how closely the techniques follow a manual (Wampold 2001). Although research has yet to determine which therapist variables seem to be most important, it is possible now to look realistically at therapists and recognize what most people intuitively know: some are more skilled and more effective than others.

4. *Therapists resemble each other in their practice as they mature, despite having different theoretical beginnings.* There are probably as many integrationists as there are therapists because therapists must amalgamate therapy ideas with their own experiences and apply them to the types of clients they serve. Over the past 60 years, three studies have come to the same conclusion about experienced therapists: more experienced therapists, whatever their professed school of therapy, tend to practice similarly (Bandler and Grinder 1975; Blagys and Hilsenroth 2000, 2002). Studies of new versus experienced therapists in different schools of psychotherapy point out how humans tend to resolve (or live with) the tension between theory and practice. They become more like each other with experience. Presumably, they do this without necessarily knowing which kind of integration they have evolved. They integrate new techniques because they perceive that the techniques work for them and their patients on some level (via true practice-based learning, otherwise known as clinical experience).

5. *The strength of the therapeutic relationship is correlated with outcome across schools of psychotherapy.* A remarkably large body of evidence strongly suggests that the working alliance correlates with outcome (Wampold 2001). What makes the working alliance work? Two people in the room interact with each other to create the relationship. The relationship provides a reflective space within which the patient can safely explore his or her mind. The caring, nonjudgmental therapist imagines the inner landscape of the patient's mind and provides impetus and safety to seek problems and then change. The relationship can be healing by providing corrective emotional experiences of acceptance and understanding perhaps rarely experienced by the patient before. The therapist's

warm resonance becomes gradually incorporated into the patient's neuroanatomical circuits. The patient may safely use the therapist as an information coprocessor as the patient's procedural memory becomes altered to create new, more effective responses.

6. *Effective therapy is customized to the needs of each patient.* A quiet research voice is beginning to be heard. Process research does not compare therapy packages but rather examines the correlation between the events of psychotherapy and outcome. Whereas "horse race" research applies different organized or manualized therapies to specific diagnoses, just as do drug trials, process research examines the relationship between and among patient characteristics, the strength of the working alliance, and various common therapeutic strategies such as conveying empathic understanding. The conclusion is that psychotherapy works best if it is customized to the needs of the patient (Norcross 2002). Every successful business knows "the customer is always right." It is time for theory to catch up with reality.

    Norcross (2005) suggested a "four-plus" method for tailoring therapist in-session behavior to patient characteristics based on research findings. The first of the four variables involves asking the patient, "What would your ideal therapist do for you?" and "What is the worst thing a therapist could do to you?" The patient then specifies preferences regarding therapist characteristics—warm versus tepid, active versus passive, informal versus formal, and gender or ethnicity. Although it has not been useful to ask individuals with sociopathic personalities or young children about their preferences in a therapist, matching strong preferences improved outcomes by about 10%, and by more than 30% in gay, lesbian, and transgender patients (Lambert et al. 2003).

    The second variable that Norcross recommended utilizes patient feedback to the therapist's direct questions, asked every three to five sessions, about the patient's 1) progress and improvement, 2) understanding and approval of the treatment methods being used, and 3) perception of the therapy relationship. The questions can be as simple as "How do you think you are doing?" "How do you think the psychotherapy is going?" and "How am I doing in our relationship to help you?" Lambert (2005) adduced a number of studies that show that therapists are not accurate judges of perceived empathy or of progress in therapy. He found that therapists can reduce patient dropout by over 20% by asking these questions every third to fifth session.

    A third variable in Norcross's method for tailoring the therapy relationship involves asking a few questions to determine the patient's stage of change. The therapist begins by asking, "Do you currently have a problem with something?" If the patient answers yes, the therapist asks, "When will you change it?" If the patient answers no, the therapist asks,

"What leads you to say that?" With these simple questions, the therapist can deduce which stage of change the patient is in: precontemplation, contemplation, preparation, action, or maintenance. The therapist can then tailor therapy to the appropriate stage and avoid large mismatches between stage and therapy, such as urging change on someone in the precontemplation stage (Prochaska and DiClemente 1984).

The fourth variable recommended by Norcross for customizing therapy to the individual patient involves the "reactance" or resistance level of the patient. Patients considered to have a low reactance level are those who are compliant with therapy, accept therapist directions, do homework, seek direction, are submissive to authority and nondefensive, and are open to experience. These patients tend to do better with therapist directiveness and less well with paradoxical instructions. Patients with a high reactance level display an intense need for autonomy, are dominant, resist external influences including therapist interventions, and have a history of social and interpersonal conflict. These patients do better with therapists who do not give instructions, emphasize patient self-change, and can utilize paradoxical interventions (Beutler et al. 2002).

The "plus" variable in Norcross's (2005) method of tailoring therapy is a patient's degree of relatedness. This concept is seen in psychoanalytic literature as a patient having one of two interaction styles: 1) an anaclitic or emotionally dependent style of interaction or 2) an introjective or self-definitional style. This distinction is described in cognitive literature as sociotropic versus autonomous style.

Psychotherapy performs a social function for which its practitioners are paid. Psychotherapy is a business. But psychotherapists are not in the psychotherapy business—they are in the business of personal change, of which there are many other forms, including diet, exercise, retreats, and medications. A meta-look at psychotherapy integration and the entire field of psychotherapy includes recognizing that patients want a change and that the goal of psychotherapists is to find the means to help them make a change. Psychotherapists are like the railroad barons of the 1800s who thought they were in the railroad business. They failed to recognize that they were in the transportation business. By neglecting this simple fact, they allowed railroads and their companies to fade from prominence (Miller et al. 2005).

7. *Diagnosis limits formulation.* The National Institute of Mental Health provides funding only for manual-based therapies categorized by diagnoses in DSM (e.g., American Psychiatric Association 2000).

Although this approach has led to an increase in knowledge of particular disorders (e.g., depression, borderline personality disorder), it has also obscured the fact that psychological problems develop and manifest in multiple ways, necessitating that treatments be tailored beyond discrete diagnoses. Furthermore, this reification of discrete disorders hinders the recognition of the extent to which various clinical problems share common processes and symptoms that would respond to similar interventions. (Norcross 2005, p. 505)

8. *Psychotherapists help patients create new futures for themselves.* Within the safety and strength of the therapeutic alliance, patients coimagine with their therapists new, more adaptive scenes containing more effective response sets. These changes take place in the patient's brain, likely in procedural memory. These influences have yet to be understood by the interpersonal biology evolving from the therapist–patient relationship (Beitman et al. 2005).

9. *Important areas of research on psychotherapy remain underdeveloped.* Researchers have not developed effective criteria for selecting good therapist candidates or therapeutic action, and have not determined how to teach effective timing of interventions.

Integration Through Core Process Similarities and Useful Differences Among the Schools

A process is a series of events or activities that occur over time. In psychotherapy, core processes should ideally be linked to subgoals or objectives, and when this occurs, the goals of the relationship are achieved sooner. Therapists first strive to establish a strong therapeutic alliance. Then, as the alliance is being formed, therapists help patients activate their self-awareness and their self-observing capacities. Also as the alliance is being established, therapists usually attempt to define maladaptive patterns in terms that suggest how to change them. Therapists then offer ways to help patients change. In this section, we outline these four primary goals and their related stages (for further detail, see Beitman and Yue 2004b).

Engagement

Establishing and then strengthening a therapeutic alliance is generally the initial goal in any psychotherapy. Many subprocesses may, depending on how well they are carried out, contribute to this process:

1. Defining with the patient his or her expectations regarding the outcomes being sought and the role the therapist and the patient will play in seeking those outcomes
2. Accurately tracking the patient's emotional state through the process of psychotherapy

3. Providing relevant information to the patient
4. Offering effective suggestions to the patient
5. Effectively managing the boundaries of therapy and the therapeutic relationship

Activation of the Self-Observer

Activating and then encouraging the patient's continued self-awareness within a safe, confiding relationship is a second process of psychotherapy. When this process is successfully carried out, patients become less anxious and more able to explore their inner and interpersonal worlds. The increasingly positive therapeutic alliance provides a "reflective space" within which to do such self-exploration. As with any other skill, patients vary in their ability to activate and utilize their observing selves. The increasing utilization of various forms of meditation as part of psychotherapy is aiding this process. Therapists, too, need practice in meditation and other forms of activating self-awareness because exploration of their own inner worlds and their intuitive responses to their patients can play key roles in psychotherapeutic change. There are many names applied to this process in the various schools of psychotherapy: mentalization, mind-sight, mindfulness, insight, recognizing automatic thoughts and schemas, and self-differentiation.

Pattern Search

Defining patterns the patient can change that will lead to a desired goal or subgoal is a third process inherent in psychotherapy. The search for maladaptive patterns relies on a simple formula: examine the unwanted responses (e.g., feelings, thoughts, behaviors), define the events that triggered these responses, and identify the intervening factors that connect the unwanted symptoms to the triggering events (e.g., thoughts, schemas, conflicts, role relationship models). From the specific instances, therapists induce broader patterns that persist over similar situations. Such patterns can be defined at three different levels: personality trait level, psychotherapy school level, and person level.

The *personality trait level* provides a general picture of the client as suggested by the following commonly used labels: submissive, perfectionistic, self-defeating, irresponsible, aggressive, paranoid, borderline, narcissistic, and obsessive. Related general labels include dysfunctional family and maladaptive communication. These terms are used by therapists and the general public in an attempt to categorize, sometimes as a way to blame but rarely as a way to suggest how to change.

At the *school level*, patterns are derived from various theoretical perspectives, each with its own vocabulary. The following are some examples.

Psychodynamic

- Reenactment from past to present
- Unconscious conflicts
- Immature defense mechanisms
- Inadequate mentalization
- Core conflictual relationship themes

Interpersonal

- Role transitions
- Role conflicts
- Unresolved grief
- Interpersonal skill deficits

Behavioral

- Inadequate stimulus control
- Problematic conditioned response
- Problematic modeling
- Neurotic paradox
- Behavioral excesses and deficits

Cognitive

- Dysfunctional automatic thoughts
- Negative cognitive schemas
- Cognitive distortions

Person-Centered

- Conditions of worth and negative self-concept

Existential

- Fear of responsibility and freedom
- Fear of death
- Existential isolation
- Meaninglessness

Emotion-Focused

- Avoidance of emotional awareness
- Conflict splits
- Unfinished business

Family

- Triangulation
- Boundary problems
- Disturbed homeostasis
- Circular causality

Finally, at the *person level*, dysfunctional patterns are defined more concretely in terms that can be observed clinically in daily life. At this level, patterns are defined specifically for individual clients. Consider Iris, for example, who often felt irritated in discussions with others because she felt that they neglected her needs. The therapist discovered that Iris usually assumed that others knew what she needed without her having to make herself sufficiently clear. Thus, her person-level pattern could be stated to her as follows: "You incorrectly assume that you have already communicated your wants and needs. You seem to expect others to read your mind." At the person level, the patient may have a clearer idea about what needs to change.

Change

Psychotherapy does not cure patients; rather, it helps them to change. Cure implies that the problem will never recur—a questionable claim for any helping profession. Therapists help patients decrease symptoms such as anxiety, depression, and substance abuse; increase social functioning at work or school and in relationships; and improve their sense of well-being. Patients "take responsibility for change"; therapists do not change patients. No matter how deeply a therapist may wish to help a patient change, the final decider and implementer is the patient.

Therapeutic objectives can be achieved through many different and often overlapping processes, which include but are not limited to the strategies and techniques offered by the schools of psychotherapy. Some general change strategies are as follows:

- Separating past from present
- Challenging dysfunctional beliefs, behaviors, and emotions
- Generating alternatives
- Deciding what to change
- Exploring the advantages and disadvantages of change
- Suggestions of how and what to change
- Turning stumbling blocks into stepping-stones
- Altering future expectations
- Facing fears

- Reframing
- Resolving conflicts
- Practicing in the session
- Working through
- Positive reinforcement
- Role-playing
- Therapist self-disclosure

School-specific approaches can be organized according to their primary orientation: emotion, cognition, behavior, interpersonal, or systems. Although these target areas are listed as if they are separate discrete entities, they actually are mutually influential. Often but not always, if one element changes, another follows suit. Changes in cognition may lead to changes in emotion and behavior. Therapists become part of each patient's interpersonal system and can influence other people in the patient's world through the patient.

The most straightforward way to select a strategy is to decide which ones are most likely to achieve the goal the patient desires and then, of those, which one the client is most likely to accept. Evidence-based strategies must be considered when making such choices, while keeping in mind that most research findings are based on studies of highly selected, diagnostically homogeneous patients recruited through advertising and willing to follow research protocols. Many therapy dilemmas have escaped research scrutiny, leaving therapists without any guidelines for strategy selection. Therapists are left to follow their own experience and training, as well as lessons learned from previous patients. (For further elaboration of these strategies, see Good and Beitman 2006.)

As the therapist and patient glean patterns from a search of the patient's past, current life, or interaction with the therapist, the discoveries inevitably lead to a new view of the patient's future. The therapist and patient may want to develop stories (narratives) to explain and understand what has happened; they may wish to dive deeply into the present to experience the *now*. But each variation on this past-present theme inevitably contains a search for a better future. The size of the human prefrontal cortex hints at the vast importance of the future. Whatever theoretical framework is used, the therapist is caught up in trying to help the patient develop new ideas, movies, videos of the patient's future. Each time a therapist connects a set of past events with present events, the therapist is implying that this pattern need not be repeated in the future. Each time a therapist comments on a cognitive distortion, the therapist is implying that this reality lens needs adjustment for the future. Psychotherapy is necessarily future oriented. Therapists act as co-imaginers of new ways of being, acting, and thinking (Beitman et al. 2005).

Conclusion: Integrating and Evolving

Rather than talking about psychotherapy integration or different schools or core processes, the field of psychotherapy will benefit from collecting its various selves into a cohesive whole made of each of these parts. The psychotherapy organism, like the human organism, aims for coherence—that is, stability with the flexibility that provides adaptability in a changing environment. Respecting the differences as well as the similarities among psychotherapy schools will ensure their evolution through time. Think of a group of circles, each with its own self-proclaimed identity: "I am cognitive therapy," says one. "I am psychodynamic therapy," says another. "I am an integrationist," say, a third. "I am my own psychotherapy," says yet another. The circles include a brief therapist, a behavior therapist, an emotion-focused therapist, a family therapist, an Adlerian, a Kleinian, a reality therapist. So many different identities. Some are bigger circles, some smaller, each claiming to be different, special, better. Imagine them on a soft, fuzzy, translucent surface that embraces each while permitting each to move on its own. This surface is also alive, vibrating and feeding the circles as they move through time and space. This surface provides the basic energy for the circles. This surface represents the core processes. Imagine the circles reaching tendrils toward each other, connecting with each other and cross-fertilizing each other. The schools influence each other. For example, cognitive therapists pick up the psychoanalytic idea of resistance, and psychodynamic therapists recognize the value of directly addressing cognitions.

Imagine how cultural and technological influences change the functioning of the entire surface and, with those changes, the functioning of each of the circles. Advances in psychopharmacology have dramatically altered the way psychotherapists think about treatment. Where once psychoanalysts claimed that medications would disrupt the therapeutic relationship, now therapists urge patients to seek and maintain useful pills. Therapists must develop ways to adapt psychotherapy to new contexts, new events, new technologies. Just as successfully functioning humans are resilient, so must the field of psychotherapy adapt to new information in a systematic way, minimizing crisis, upheaval, and degradation. Psychotherapy can become one coherent whole, an organization with many components, functioning together in dynamic tension: stable, flexible, and adaptive. It can become an organization resting on a foundation of core processes revealed through experience and research.

Key Points

- Psychotherapy is defined by its core processes, which include engagement, self-awareness activation, pattern search, and change.

- The key outcome variables, in descending order of importance, are the patient (symptom severity and strength of social network), the therapist (personality, skill, and other unquantifiable factors), and the strength of the working alliance.
- Maladaptive patterns are induced from specific instances to the general.
- Patterns are clinically best presented in terms that fit the patient's current concepts and experiences.
- Change strategies may be selected from the range of interventions in which the therapist has confidence, to be fit with the patient's experience with self-change.
- Psychotherapists may talk about the past and the here and now, but therapy primarily attempts to help patients change the ways in which they conceptualize their futures.

References

Ahn H, Wampold BE: Where oh where are the specific ingredients? A meta-analysis of component studies in counseling and psychotherapy. J Couns Psychol 48:251–257, 2001

American Psychiatric Association: Diagnostic and Statistical Manual of Mental Disorders, 4th Edition, Text Revision. Washington, DC, American Psychiatric Association, 2000

Bakan D: Freud and the Jewish Mystical Tradition. New York, Van Nostrand, 1958

Bandler R, Grinder J: The Structure of Magic, Vol 1. Palo Alto, CA, Science & Behavior Books, 1975

Beitman BD, Yue D: Learning Psychotherapy: Leader's Manual. New York, WW Norton, 1999a

Beitman BD, Yue D: Learning Psychotherapy: Trainee's Manual. New York, WW Norton, 1999b

Beitman BD, Yue D: Learning Psychotherapy: Seminar Leader's Manual, 2nd Edition. New York, WW Norton, 2004a

Beitman BD, Yue D: Learning Psychotherapy: Trainee's Manual, 2nd Edition. New York, WW Norton, 2004b

Beitman BD, Soth AM, Bumby NA: The future as an integrating force through the schools of psychotherapy, in Handbook of Psychotherapy Integration, 2nd Edition. Edited by Norcross JC, Goldfried MR. New York, Oxford University Press, 2005, pp 65–84

Beitman BD, Viamontes GI, Soth AM, et al: Toward a neural circuitry of engagement, self-awareness, and pattern search. Psychiatr Ann 36:272–282, 2006

Beutler LE, Harwood TM: Prescriptive Psychotherapy: A Practical Guide to Systemic Treatment Selection. New York, Oxford University Press, 2000

Beutler LE, Moleiro CM, Talebi H: Resistance, in Psychotherapy Relationships That Work: Therapist Contributions and Responsiveness to Patients. Edited by Norcross JC. New York, Oxford University Press, 2002, pp 129–143

Blagys MD, Hilsenroth MJ: Distinctive features of short-term psychodynamic-interpersonal psychotherapy: a review of the comparative psychotherapy process literature. Clinical Psychology: Science and Practice 7:167–188, 2000

Blagys MD, Hilsenroth MJ: Distinctive activities of cognitive-behavioral therapy: a review of the comparative psychotherapy process literature. Clin Psychol Rev 22:671–706, 2002

Consoli AJ, Chope RC: Contextual integrative psychotherapy, in A Casebook of Psychotherapy Integration. Edited by Stricker G, Gold J. Washington, DC, American Psychological Association, 2006, pp 185–199

Corsini RJ, Wedding D: Current Psychotherapies. Itasca, IL, Peacock Press, 2005

Ehrenwald J: The History of Psychotherapy. New York, Jason Aronson, 1976

Goldfried MR: From Cognitive-Behavior Therapy to Psychotherapy Integration: An Evolving View. New York, Springer, 1995

Good GE, Beitman BD: Psychotherapy Essentials. New York, WW Norton, 2006

Greenberg LS, Watson JC, Lietaer G (eds): Handbook of Experiential Psychotherapy. New York, Guilford, 1998

Hayes SC, Luoma JB, Bond FW, et al: Acceptance and commitment therapy: model, processes and outcomes. Behav Res Ther 44:1–25, 2006

Imber SD, Pilkonis PA, Sotsky SM, et al: Mode-specific effects among three treatments for depression. J Consult Clin Psychol 52:352–359, 1990

Jacobson NS, Dobson KS, Truax PA, et al: A component analysis of cognitive-behavioral treatment for depression. J Consult Clin Psychol 64:295–304, 1996

Lambert MJ: Psychotherapy outcome research: implications for integrative and eclectic therapists, in Handbook of Psychotherapy Integration. Edited by Norcross JC, Goldfried MR. New York, Basic Books, 1992, pp 94–129

Lambert MJ: Enhancing psychotherapy outcome through feedback. Journal of Clinical Psychology In Session, 61:165–174, 2005

Lambert MJ, Whipple JL, Hawkins EJ, et al: Is it time for clinicians to routinely track patient outcomes? A meta-analysis. Clinical Psychology: Science and Practice 10:288–301, 2003

Lazarus AA: The Practice of Multimodal Therapy. New York, McGraw-Hill, 1981

Lazarus AA: The Practice of Multimodal Therapy, 2nd Edition. Baltimore, MD, Johns Hopkins University Press, 1989

Linehan MM: Cognitive-Behavioral Treatment of Borderline Personality Disorder. New York, Guilford, 1993

McCullough JP Jr: Treatment for Chronic Depression: Cognitive Behavioral Analysis System of Psychotherapy. New York, Guilford, 2000

Messer SB: A critical examination of belief structures in integrative and eclectic psychotherapy, in Handbook of Psychotherapy Integration. Edited by Norcross JC, Goldfried MR. New York, Basic Books, 1992, pp 130–168

Miller SD, Duncan BL, Hubble MA: Outcome-informed clinical work, in Handbook of Psychotherapy Integration. Edited by Norcross JC, Goldfried MR. New York, Oxford University Press, 2005, pp 84–105

Norcross JC: Psychotherapy Relationships That Work. New York, Oxford University Press, 2002

Norcross JC: A primer on psychotherapy integration, in Handbook of Psychotherapy Integration, 2nd Edition. Edited by Norcross JC, Goldfried MR. New York, Oxford University Press, 2005, pp 3–24

Norcross JC, Goldfried MR: Handbook of Psychotherapy Integration, 2nd Edition. New York, Oxford University Press, 2005

Prochaska JO, DiClemente CC: The Transtheoretical Approach. Homewood, IL, Dow Jones–Irwin, 1984

Prochaska JO, Norcross JC: Systems of Psychotherapy: A Transtheoretical Analysis, 6th Edition. Belmont, CA, Thomson Brooks/Cole, 2007

Ryle A, Kerr IB: Introducing Cognitive Analytic Therapy: Principles and Practice. Hoboken, NJ, Wiley, 2002

Shapiro F: Eye Movement Densensitization and Reprocessing, 2nd Edition. New York, Guilford, 2001

Siegal DJ: An interpersonal neurobiology approach to psychotherapy. Psychiatr Ann 36:248–259, 2006

Stricker G, Gold J (eds): A Casebook of Psychotherapy Integration. Washington, DC, American Psychological Association, 2006

Wachtel PL, Kruk JC, McKinney MK: Cyclical psychodynamics and integrative relational therapy, in Handbook of Psychotherapy Integration, 2nd Edition. Edited by Norcross JC, Goldfried MR. New York, Oxford University Press, 2005, pp 172–195

Wampold BE: The Great Psychotherapy Debate: Models, Methods, and Findings. Mahwah, NJ, Erlbaum, 2001

Wedding D, Corsini RJ: Current Psychotherapies. Itasca, IL, Peacock Press, 1973

Zindel V, Segal J, Williams JMG, et al: Mindfulness-Based Cognitive Therapy for Depression: A New Approach to Preventing Relapse. New York, Guilford, 2001

Suggested Readings

Beitman BD, Good GE: Counseling and Psychotherapy Essentials. New York, WW Norton, 2006

Beitman BD, Yue DM: Learning Psychotherapy, 2nd Edition. New York, WW Norton, 2004

Norcross JC (ed): Psychotherapy Relationships That Work. New York, Oxford University Press, 2002

Norcross JC, Goldfried MR (eds): Handbook of Psychotherapy Integration, 2nd Edition. New York, Oxford University Press, 2005

Stricker G, Gold J (eds): A Casebook of Psychotherapy Integration. Washington, DC, American Psychological Association, 2006

Wampold BE: The Great Psychotherapy Debate: Models, Methods, and Findings. Mahwah, NJ, Erlbaum, 2001

Chapter 27

Theory and Practice of Dialectical Behavioral Therapy

Joan Wheelis, M.D.

The development of a new psychotherapeutic venue defines a clinical problem, a theory of its etiology, and the process and means to change it. Within the climate of managed care and the emphasis on evidence-based treatment, the expectations of clinicians, patients, and insurers alike are increasingly influenced by research efforts to define effective treatment to maximize change.

Research scientist Marsha Linehan developed dialectical behavior therapy (DBT) in an effort to address the particular needs of chronically suicidal women who had a pattern of suicide attempts and/or nonsuicidal self-injury (Linehan 1993a). A radical behaviorist, Linehan initially utilized the more traditional problem-solving approach with these women, but she observed that the treatment was lacking given the multiplicity and complexity of the patients' problems. The primary behavioral focus on change was often experienced by patients as alienating and invalidating, and they often dropped out of treatment. In an effort to test and tease apart the component parts of what proved effective or not in treatment, Linehan reviewed her therapy sessions, which had been videotaped by her research team behind one-way mirrors. In particular, Linehan's addition of acceptance strategies helped patients feel more understood, which in turn helped to improve their relationships with their therapists and to facilitate their progress in treatment. DBT evolved into a treatment for suicidal patients who also met the criteria for borderline personality disorder (BPD). The unique focus of DBT was to develop comprehensive and integrated strategies of acceptance with change. This dialectical tension along with active assessment and problem solving helped teach patients that some suffering was important to accept in addition to the value of changing aversive response patterns and environmental events. Targeting a synthesis of acceptance and change in both therapist behaviors and client behaviors led to calling the treatment *dialectical behavior therapy*. This adaptation of behavioral treatment was unique and especially well suited to the problems faced by patients with borderline personality disorder.

Since its initial development, DBT has been used to treat a variety of problems, including binge eating (Telch et al. 2001) and bulimia (Safer et al. 2001), dissociative disorders (Bohus et al. 2000a), and substance abuse (Linehan et al. 2002; van den Bosch et al. 2002). It has been adapted for use in inpatient services (Barley et al. 1993; Bohus et al. 2004; Kroger et al. 2006; Swenson et al. 2001) and partial programs (Simpson et al. 1998), as well as for use with adolescents (Rathus and Miller 2002), elderly people (Lynch et al. 2003), and couples (Fruzzetti 2006). DBT is indicated for patients with BPD and is covered by some health insurers on the basis of research supporting its efficacy for these patients. DBT is effective for patients with BPD who present with a predominance of serious behavioral dyscontrol, including suicidal behavior and nonsuicidal self-injury.

DBT is for patients who acknowledge their difficulties and are motivated for treatment. Given the enormous flexibility of the model and suitability for modifications, there are no specific contraindications. However, treatment of patients with low IQ, cognitive deficits, active substance abuse problems, or acute psychosis requires modification of the standard DBT model.

Theory

Problems with emotional regulation are believed to be the core dysfunction seen in patients with BPD (Sanislow et al. 2000; Skodol et al. 2002; Stiglmayr et al. 2005). Patterns of behavior highlighting this dysfunction include affective lability, chronic feelings of emptiness, and intense displays of anger. Pervasive *emotional dysregulation* results from high emotional vulnerability and deficits in the ability to regulate emotion (Linehan 1993a). Biological irregularities in temperament and impulse control are thought to lead to emotional vulnerability, characterized by high sensitivity to emotional stimuli, high emotional intensity, and slow return to emotional baseline.

The biosocial theory put forth by Linehan (1993a) highlights the development of BPD as the result of an ongoing transaction between a biological vulnerability to emotional dysregulation and an invalidating environment. An *invalidating environment* is defined as the circumstances by which an individual's emotions, thoughts, and overt actions are interpreted as invalid. A person prone to emotional dysregulation is likely to display intense emotion, which may lead to fear and misunderstanding by those around the person. Typically, these intense, hypersensitive emotional responses are routinely discounted or punished and judged to be inappropriate or socially unacceptable responses. Additionally, such intense displays of emotion may subsequently result in gaining attention, which may reinforce the person's behavior. There are multiple consequences of an invalidating environment (Linehan 1993a), including 1) difficulties recognizing emotions and therefore seeking external cues as information about one's emotional states, 2) oversimplifying problem solving by minimizing or ignoring the validity of one's emotional experience, and 3) vacillating between emotional inhibition and extreme emotionality due to reinforcement of intense emotional responses and invalidation of modulated responses. This transactional process can lead to persistent cycles of invalidation and emotional dysregulation for the person with BPD.

Linehan (1993a) views most dysfunctional behaviors in individuals with BPD as efforts to regulate intense affect or as a consequence of the emotional dysregulation. Such dysfunctional behaviors may include suicide attempts, cutting, burning, and substance abuse. Higher pain thresholds have been noted in patients with BPD who show current self-injurious behavior than in healthy controls (Bohus et al. 2000b; Ludaescher et al. 2007; Russ et al. 1992), and self-inflicted pain may function to normalize neural activity in specific brain regions involved in cognitive and emotional processing (Schmahl et al. 2006). A key assumption in DBT is that suicidal behavior and other dysfunctional behaviors represent attempted solutions to problems. Frequently, it is intense, painful emotion that is the problem. DBT specifically targets the dysfunctional behavior in an effort to identify the precipitating events (thoughts, emotions, overt behavior) and develop more adaptive solutions. Ultimately, the goal of DBT is to develop a life worth living.

DBT, like many other cognitive-behavioral treatments, is based on learning theory, which describes how people and animals learn. Learning is the change in associations via experience, referring to the process by which new behavior is acquired. *Behavior* refers to both overt behaviors (as in events that can be observed by others) and covert or private behaviors (those for which there is no direct access by an observer). This latter category includes thoughts, emotions, conscious memories, fantasies, mental images, urges, and bodily sensations. Behavior is influenced by prior learning and by reinforcing and punishing contingencies. Learning is dependent on memory and its retrieval. When one steps on the accelerator as the traffic light turns green, one is accessing a memory of having learned that a green light means to go. Similarly, if the sight of a bridge stirs up an anxious feeling, one is accessing some prior learning that there is potential danger associated with bridges.

Behavior change, therefore, requires careful and detailed examination of the precipitating events, vulnerability factors (conditions that affect emotional reactivity, such as sleep deprivation), and environmental issues present before (stimulus) and after (response) a problematic behavior has occurred. DBT focuses on revealing the sequences of learning, which relate to the development of problematic behavior, as well as promoting new learning in the service of facilitating more adaptive functioning.

Prominent learning theories include respondent conditioning and operant conditioning. The former, also known as Pavlovian or classical conditioning, is dependent on the antecedent events (e.g., a suicide attempt is preceded by the experience of despair). Generally speaking, operant conditioning, also known as instrumental learning or behavior modification, is dependent on the consequences of behavior. For example, the behavioral treatment of a phobia entails exposing a person repeatedly to the feared stimulus (e.g., going to the bridge where one feels afraid), its memory, or a generalized target (e.g., any bridge or imagining any bridge) in an effort to extinguish the phobic response. *Operant conditioning* refers to the process by which behavior is modified through systems of reinforcing or punishing contingencies. When a patient attempts suicide, a desired hospitalization may reinforce the likelihood of future suicidal behavior. In practice, most behavior is both respondent and operant in that it is influenced by the preceding events as well as the consequences.

Learning new behaviors is central to DBT, and traditional cognitive-behavioral therapy tools (education, skills training, and problem solving) are used toward that end. Specific techniques such as exposure, systematic desensitization, contingency clarification, and cognitive restructuring are employed to unlearn, change, or extinguish dysfunctional behavior and faulty beliefs.

Neurobiological research increasingly reveals underlying biological mechanisms implicated in therapeutic interventions. For example, in Pavlov's experiment of classical conditioning, the dog ceased to salivate when the bell was rung but no food was presented. This phenomenon, in which a conditioned stimulus loses the ability to elicit a conditioned response, is known as extinction. Fear extinction refers to the reduction of fear by repeated exposure to the feared object in the absence of adverse consequences (Barad and Saxena 2005). Research has found that three brain structures play key roles in fear extinction: the amygdala (Garakani et al. 2006), medial prefrontal cortex, and hippocampus (Barad and Saxena 2005). Dysfunction in these circuits may be a neural substrate for anxiety disorders (Barad and Saxena 2005).

An important component of extinction is activation of glutamatergic *N*-methyl-D-aspartate (NMDA) receptors in the amygdala. Partial NMDA agonists, such as D-cycloserine (DCS), have been shown to facilitate extinction. Investigation of the use of DCS in humans with anxiety disorders is already under way (Garakani et al. 2006). Though not a direct anxiolytic, DCS appears to accelerate extinction to fear responses, and has been used with cognitive-behavioral therapy for enhanced effect.

Using Pavlovian conditioning as a model, researchers have clarified the pathophysiology of the fear response over the past several years (Garakani et al. 2006). Brain imaging studies, using functional magnetic resonance imaging and positron emission tomography scanning, have helped to trace the areas of the brain responsible for the unlearning of fear. Extinction is not a passive process of "forgetting" but rather an active "unlearning" process (Medina et al. 2002). Learning requires activation of nerve fibers known as climbing fibers; inhibition of these fibers leads to "unlearning." Molecular and pharmacological studies have implicated a number of neurotransmitter and second messenger systems in extinction learning, offering the possibility of novel approaches to improving treatments for a variety of anxiety disorders (Barad and Saxena 2005).

Overview of Treatment

The three fundamental components of DBT (Linehan 1993a) are problem solving, validation, and dialectics.

Problem Solving

Problem solving involves the detailed analysis of the current problem, followed by evaluation and implementation of alternative solutions. The analysis component of problem solving includes behavioral analysis, didactic strategies, and insight strategies. The change component includes solution analysis, orienting strategies, and commitment strategies.

Validation

Validation is the process by which a patient is given support for his or her experiences that conveys acceptance of a patient's thoughts, feelings, and behavior. Validation is specifically employed to balance the change-based strategies of DBT, provide feedback and reinforcement for clinical progress, model self-validation, and support the therapeutic alliance. Mindfulness, with its emphasis on staying in the present and focusing attention, helps to facilitate both the experience of validation and the tolerance and acceptance of the exigencies of change.

Dialectics

Dialectics serves a dual purpose in DBT. It represents a philosophical view on the nature of reality and it refers to a method of discourse and a manner of relating to a patient. As a philosophical view, dialectical thinking is the middle path between universalistic and relativistic modes of thought. Dialectical thinking refers to a worldview that emphasizes the limitations of linear ideas about causation and emphasizes interrelatedness and change as the fundamental characteristics of reality. It substitutes "both…and" for "either…or" and views truth as an evolving product of the opposition of different views in a transactional process.

With respect to its technical utilization, dialectics offers guidelines to making use of the oppositions inherent in the therapeutic relationship to help the patient and therapist arrive at new possibilities from within old limitations and to search for the deeper essence and a different understanding of problems, which may have been experienced as immutable. This philosophy is particularly pertinent for patients with BPD, for whom the vacillation between extreme emotion and dysfunctional behavior typically forecloses the possibility of new learning. All components of DBT are characterized by an emphasis on dialectical thinking, which serves as an overarching dimension to the entirety of the treatment as well as a particular goal.

The dialectical philosophy leads to the following two assumptions that underlie DBT (Linehan 1993a): 1) patients are functioning as well as they are able and also need to change; and 2) patients may not have caused all of their own problems, but they have to solve them. These assumptions, along with the biosocial theory of pathogenesis, have rescued the BPD diagnosis from a "blame-the-victim tradition," and instead offer a general orientation that is both respectful and nonpejorative. Linehan's work has paved the way to viewing patients with BPD as having understandable responses to the way in which they learned to tolerate their experiences and adapt to their environment. Suicidal or nonsuicidal self-injurious behavior is viewed as problem-solving or communication behavior rather than manipulative behavior.

Structure of Treatment: Functions and Modes

DBT is an empirically supported, manualized psychotherapy. It is a comprehensive and multicomponent approach. It does not, however, provide a session-by-session protocol for the delivery of treatment. DBT is principle driven, emphasizing the *functions* of treatment so as to maximize the versatility of delivery, thereby permitting application across a wide range of clinical settings and for patients with varying degrees of psychopathology (Linehan 1993a).

Although the components of treatment, or *modes*, may need to be condensed or supplemented in various settings, the application of the following five functions of treatment remains constant to each clinical situation (Linehan 1993a): 1) enhancement of patient motivation, 2) development of patient capabilities, 3) generalization of new capabilities to the patient's natural environment, 4) enhancement of therapist capabilities and motivation to treat patients effectively, and 5) structuring of the environment in a manner that will promote and reinforce patient capabilities. These five treatment functions are addressed by the four main modes of standard outpatient DBT: outpatient individual therapy, outpatient group skills training, telephone consultation, and therapist consultation (Linehan 1993a). Ancillary treatments may include pharmacotherapy and acute inpatient psychiatric hospitalization. The typical period of treatment is 1 year, although 2 years is sometimes indicated (Comtois and Linehan 2006).

Individual Therapy

DBT requires that a primary clinician be in charge of a patient's treatment (Linehan 1993a). The primary clinician, who typically meets with the patient for 1–1.5 hours once weekly, is responsible for planning treatment, integrating it across other modes, helping the patient realize his or her target goals, and integrating the patient's acquired competence into daily routines. The primary clinician helps facilitate coordination among treatment team members and provides ongoing consultation and evaluation with the patient to determine what impediments may be interfering with obtaining his or her goals. Often, patients who are referred for DBT already have a primary psychodynamic therapist with whom they meet regularly. Not infrequently, the primary DBT therapist must either recommend that the patient terminate the psychodynamic therapy or, if a patient is opposed to such a change, suggest that the patient consider beginning DBT at another time. Psychodynamic therapists often tolerate dysfunctional behavior in the search for deeper insight into the developmental etiology, whereas the DBT therapist places principal emphasis on utilizing contingencies and teaching skillful behavior to replace the dysfunctional behavior. Psychodynamic psychotherapists traditionally use the structural construct of depth, and behaviorists examine the construct of time as process. Maintaining two primary therapies (intentionally or unintentionally) can be confusing and can often lead to both treatments becoming ineffective.

The DBT therapist is also responsible for reviewing the indications for any ancillary treatment, such as psychopharmacology and couples or family work. Considerable emphasis is placed on consulting to the patient to help them advocate for their needs and to maximize effective interactions with other members of the treatment team, family, friends, and hospital staff.

Group Skills Training

Skills training is typically offered in a highly structured group format and is required concurrently with the individual therapy. The standard group meeting lasts 2.5 hours and is divided between homework review and teaching new skills. Sometimes, due to scheduling conflicts, skills training may be provided on a one-to-one basis by another therapist.

Five major types of skills are taught in a standard outpatient DBT group (Linehan 1993a, 1993b):

1. *Mindfulness:* controlling attention, increasing awareness and acceptance of the present moment
2. *Emotion regulation:* understanding emotions, reducing emotional vulnerability, decreasing emotional suffering, changing by acting opposite to painful emotions
3. *Interpersonal effectiveness:* attending to relationships, balancing priorities versus demands, balancing "wants" versus "shoulds," building mastery and self-respect
4. *Distress tolerance:* crisis survival strategies for tolerating short-term pain and guidelines for accepting reality and tolerating long-term pain
5. *Self-management:* strategies for realistic goal setting, environmental control, and relapse prevention

This variety of skills reflects important dialectical tensions important for successful living as well as effective therapy. There are skills for radical acceptance of things as they are, balanced by assertiveness skills to change them. Distress tolerance skills and emotion regulation skills help to both distract from and face fears. Willingness to try something new is offset by the deliberate consideration of pros and cons before taking action.

Of note, mindfulness must be learned first and continually practiced before patients can become proficient with the other skills, because mindfulness promotes the ability to be aware of and attentive to the present, which are both necessary for new learning. Patients are instructed to participate in their experience of the moment. Simultaneously, they are instructed to notice but not engage in judgment, attachment, or censure of their experience. Linehan (1993b) identifies discrete behavioral skills gained from the practice of mindfulness. Learning to observe, describe, and participate in the moment decreases the patient's proclivity to preoccupations with the past and ruminative worry about the future and helps a patient become able to tolerate emotional pain and suffering without resorting to self-harm. Attention to the present moment allows a patient to observe the natural course of thoughts, feelings, urges, and sensations as transient. As such, mindfulness is an informal exposure to these experiences, which help to develop increasing familiarity and tolerance. Mindfulness promotes facility with dialectical thinking by encouraging a "wise mind," which is the synthesis of reason or logic (reasonable mind) and emotions and intuition (emotion mind) (Linehan 1993b).

Telephone Consultation

Phone coaching is required for clients in treatment as a way to help them utilize specific skills coaching at times when they feel emotionally dysregulated and thus at most risk to engage in maladaptive coping strategies. Phone coaching is typically provided by the individual therapist, but at times, such as during a therapist's vacation, other arrangements for coverage are required.

Therapist Consultation

Therapist consultation, a requirement of DBT, is typically a weekly meeting in which the therapists meet together. The consultation team meeting, which is typically 60–90 minutes long, is intended to 1) help keep the therapists motivated by applying the principles of DBT to the therapists, 2) offer peer supervision, and 3) ensure that treatment is adhering to the model. It is an opportunity for therapists to practice mindfulness and to role-play difficult interactions experienced with their patients or colleagues.

Unique to DBT, the consultation team is an integral part of the treatment, without which, the treatment is not considered adherent to the model. Any venue of DBT without a regularly meeting consultation team should not be implemented. This compelling emphasis on the community of clinicians working together to better understand their patients and their own behavior in therapy helps therapists to stay within the therapeutic frame and to address difficulties as they arise in therapy. The target of the team is to increase each member's adherence to the model. Each member must be committed to the team and understand that one of the team's purposes is peer group therapy. The team calls attention to and addresses members' behaviors, such as making judgmental or defensive comments, being distracted, not holding a dialectical stance, or treating themselves or other members as fragile. Problems regarding personal limits, noncompliance, and burnout are targeted in treatment of the therapist. Team members also practice skills, teaching, and behavioral analysis on one another, and discuss particular treatment problems (Linehan 1993a).

Treatment Planning

The therapist begins with the pretreatment stage of orientation and commitment. The goals are to determine therapist–patient fit, ensure that the patient has made an informed decision to pursue treatment and change, reframe therapy as a learning process, and review treatment expectations.

Following pretreatment, a patient's treatment is organized around the level of the disorder, with each level corresponding to one of four stages of treatment with specific target goals (Linehan 1993a). The four levels of the disorder, and descriptions of the corresponding four stages of treatment, are as follows (Linehan 1993a):

1. *Severe behavioral dyscontrol*. In the first stage of treatment, the therapist seeks to increase behavioral control through helping patients attain basic capacities. The target goals of this stage are listed in Table 27–1.
2. *Quiet desperation*. The intent in this stage is to facilitate emotional experiencing through reducing posttraumatic stress and blocking dissociation. The principal goal of this stage is to block avoidance of emotions and the environmental cues associated with them. In this stage, patients are helped to experience their feelings without avoiding life or experiencing symptoms of posttraumatic stress disorder.
3. *Problematic patterns in living*. The goal of this stage is to achieve ordinary happiness and unhappiness through increasing self-respect and working on problems with relationships and career choices.
4. *Incompleteness*. The goal of the last stage is to develop the patient's capacity for sustained experience of contentment, connection, and freedom.

TABLE 27-1. Stage 1 targets (for severe behavioral dyscontrol) in dialectical behavioral therapy

1. Reduce and eliminate life-threatening behaviors:

   Suicide attempts

   Nonsuicidal self-injury

   Homicidal and assaultive behaviors

2. Reduce and eliminate therapy-interfering behaviors:

   Nonattendance

   Noncollaboration with therapists

   Refusal to complete homework

3.1. Decrease the behaviors that destroy the quality of life:

   Depression, anxiety, eating disorders, and neglect of other medical problems

   Financial difficulties

   Lack of social supports or daily structure

3.2 Increase the behaviors that make a life worth living:

   Relief from depression and anxiety

   Satisfying work and financial comfort

   Having friends

4. Learn skills in order to meet goals

Source. Adapted from Linehan 1993a.

Linehan's treatment manual and the bulk of published research data concern addressing severe behavioral dyscontrol (stage 1 treatment), although research focusing on quiet desperation (stage 2 treatment) is currently under way (Harned and Linehan, in press).

As indicated in Table 27–1, the most pressing task of DBT is to first and foremost reduce the maladaptive overt behaviors (particularly those that are life threatening) and replace them with more effective skillful behaviors. Interestingly, the second target goal of stage 1 is to address any therapy-interfering behaviors, with the therapist highlighting the critical importance of the therapeutic relationship in order for effective treatment to occur. It is understood that change and progression is not linear but rather

TABLE 27–2. **Secondary behavioral targets in dialectical behavioral therapy**

Increase	Decrease
Emotion modulation	Emotional reactivity
Self-validation	Self-invalidation
Realistic decision making	Crisis-generating behaviors
Emotional experiencing	Inhibited grieving
Active problem solving	Active-passivity behaviors
Accurate expression of emotions	Mood-dependent behavior

Source. Adapted from Linehan 1993a.

is a process of shifting between high-priority targets as they appear and lower-priority targets in their absence. Linehan (1993a) describes the "dance" of DBT therapy, referring to the flexibility, light touch, and focus necessary to address multiple agendas simultaneously. While attending to the high-priority behavior and other targets of stage 1, the DBT therapist must also attend to the development of mindfulness and the modeling of a dialectical stance.

It has often been said that the goal of DBT is to develop a dialectical orientation. In describing the behavioral characteristics of BPD, Linehan (1993a) conceived of three dialectical dilemmas frequently associated with BPD. These dilemmas are defined by their opposite poles: emotional vulnerability versus self-invalidation, unrelenting crises versus inhibited grieving, and active passivity (tendency to approach problems passively) versus apparent competence (the unexpected lack of competence in a patient who is typically competent). Typically, patients with BPD vacillate between the two poles of the dialectical dilemmas.

Linehan (1993a) suggests a list of secondary targets related to these dialectical dilemmas that should be addressed to the degree to which they are present and to which attending to them will help facilitate achievement of the primary target goals (see Table 27–2). A secondary behavioral target is addressed only if it is directly related to a primary target goal. If it is considered ancillary to the primary goals, it is not addressed in the first stage of treatment.

TABLE 27–3.   Patient agreements in dialectical behavioral therapy

---

1. Commit to therapy.

2. Attend therapy consistently.

3. Reduce suicidal behavior.

4. Decrease therapy-interfering behavior.

5. Attend skills training.

6. Abide by payment protocols and any research agreements.

Source.   Adapted from Linehan 1993a.

Beginning Treatment

The first task in starting DBT is to develop an initial treatment agreement with the patient. Presentation of the biosocial model is followed by orienting a patient to treatment. Several points concerning DBT philosophy are specified. They include that therapy is supportive, behavioral, and skill oriented; it balances acceptance and change; and it requires a collaborative relationship (Linehan 1993a). The therapist reviews guidelines for phone contact with the patient and discusses the audio- or videotaping of therapy sessions. Orienting the patient's network to treatment is also important. Often, meetings with families, friends, and ancillary services are indicated to review the treatment philosophy and plan and to discuss ways in which these individuals might support or impede therapy. Both patient and therapist make agreements (see Tables 27–3 and 27–4).

TABLE 27–4.   Therapist agreements in dialectical behavioral therapy

---

1. Strive to be effective.

2. Act ethically.

3. Be available to the patient.

4. Show respect for the patient.

5. Maintain confidentiality.

6. Obtain consultation when needed.

Source.   Adapted from Linehan 1993a.

Commitment to treatment—specifically, commitment to treatment goals—is essential. The early sessions of treatment are essentially focused on identifying the particular goals (e.g., to return to school or work, to improve relationships with friends and family), identifying the targeted behavior relevant to the patient's goals (e.g., suicidal behavior, cutting, marijuana smoking, binge eating), and obtaining the patient's commitment to collaborating on these goals. Although it is often easy to obtain a commitment at the beginning of treatment, DBT places particular emphasis on the patient's making a significant emotional commitment. While the DBT therapist asks for a patient commitment of 1 year to refrain from self-injury, the therapist simultaneously (dialectically) challenges the patient that this commitment is not possible. If the patient agrees to make a commitment for 1 year, the DBT therapist might challenge this by drawing attention to the extreme difficulty of doing so (a technique known as *devil's advocate*). The hope is that the patient begins to embrace the rationale for treatment and can then make a more realistic and stronger commitment (e.g., "I can commit to not hurting myself until next week when I next see you"), which can be then repeatedly reinforced. Although no written contract is required for DBT, this type of ongoing extensive assessment of commitment is essential for effective treatment.

Typically, the patient maintains a daily diary card during the first two stages of DBT treatment. (As described in the previous section, "Treatment Planning," the first two stages correspond with patient disorders of level 1, severe behavioral dyscontrol, and level 2, quiet desperation.) The patient records behaviors such as self-injury, alcohol consumption, and illicit drug use, as well as suicidal ideation and affective experience such as degree of misery, shame, or anxiety. The diary card is designed to help therapist and patient to reflect together on the most salient concerns for treatment. Problems are operationalized (i.e., put into behaviorally specific terms such that they can be targeted). In addition, urges are rated on a scale from 0 (indicating the absence of any urge) to 5 (indicating the highest intensity of urges). On the reverse side of the diary card, DBT skills are listed. Patients are asked to circle the ones they have used each day.

It is important for the therapist to make an initial assessment of the patient's emotional state before attending to high-priority topics. Hidden agenda topics suggested by a patient's initial mood or issues not recorded on the diary card are identified at this point. Problematic patient–therapist issues requiring relationship repair should be attended to at least briefly at the start of the session. These might include the therapist's or the patient's emotional experience, misunderstanding, or frustration related to a particular interaction. It is equally important, however, that an extended conversation not occur when there are agenda items of higher priority (e.g., self-injury, substance abuse). Such a lengthy discussion is often a risk, especially if a therapist is nervous or uncomfortable about broaching the high-priority behaviors within the session.

An agenda for each therapy session is set, with the diary card serving as a way to identify the high-priority targets first (i.e., suicidal behavior, nonsuicidal self-injury, and homicidal or assaultive behavior), followed by therapy-interfering behaviors, and then other serious behaviors that interfere with quality of life (e.g., substance abuse), and any other concerns that were identified at the start of the session or other lower-target agenda items a patient may wish to discuss, such as issues related to job opportunities. Organizing the session around a conjoint agenda serves to reinforce the collaborative nature of the patient-therapist relationship as well as to motivate resolution of high-target problems so as to attend to other quality-of-life issues. Checking on a patient's progress in other modes of treatment is an essential function of the primary clinician, in an effort to highlight and consolidate the importance of a treatment plan and the patient's commitment to it. The therapist is also responsible for targeting problems of attendance and cooperation (Linehan 1993a).

Treatment Strategies

Treatment strategies in DBT refer to the procedures and techniques employed by the therapist to help a patient obtain his or her treatment goals. Validation (acceptance strategies) and problem-solving strategies (change strategies) make up the *core strategies* of DBT, which are mediated through the application of the *dialectical strategies* (Linehan 1993a). In addition to the core strategies and dialectical strategies are *stylistic or communication strategies*, which specify the communication and interpersonal styles utilized by the therapist. *Case management strategies*, the fourth category of strategies, include the particular ways in which the therapist engages with the social network in which the patient is involved (Linehan 1993a).

Core Strategies

Behavioral Analysis Strategies

Fundamental to problem solving in DBT is the *behavioral analysis*, which is the collaborative process of identifying and reevaluating over time the sequence of internal and external events that are associated with the problem behavior. Behavioral analysis includes the assessment of multiple chain analyses. Small units (links) of behavior are analyzed with the goal of defining the beginning of the chain, or the antecedents; the middle of the chain, or the problem behavior itself; and the end of the chain, or the consequences of the behavior. Attention is paid to all behaviors, including emotions, bodily sensations, thoughts (explicitly and implicitly as in expectations and assumptions), urges, and overt behaviors. Environmental factors (e.g., a conflictful visit with a relative) and vulnerability factors (e.g., lack of sleep or physical illness) that may affect the behavior are important to ascertain. It is essential to define the problem specifically. Rather than asking questions about causality (e.g., "Why do you think that happened?"), the therapist should ask questions aimed at specifying the antecedents and consequences of the behavior (e.g., "At what point in the day did the thought of suicide enter your mind? What was happening in that moment?"). This information facilitates understanding of typical response patterns to specific stimuli that are germane to the particular behavior.

DBT assumes that eliciting variables tend to be related to intense and typically aversive emotional states and that maladaptive behavior generally is seen as resulting from emotional dysregulation (Linehan 1993a). Because the avoidance of emotional pain is considered a primary motivation, antecedent emotional behaviors are of central importance to be explored. Patterns of environmental events and patient behaviors are instrumental in the maintenance of maladaptive behaviors. Patients commonly have deficits of emotion modulation, self-validation, reasoning and judgment, active problem solving, emotional experiencing, interpersonal effectiveness (especially in conflict resolution), accurate expression of emotion states, and realistic reasoning and judgment. Typically occurring with these deficits are excesses in emotional reactivity, self-invalidation, and crisis-generating behaviors. These deficits and excesses are identified to generate hypotheses about factors controlling behavior. The behavioral analysis is utilized in an effort to identify the salient variables and to verify the insights.

Insight Interpretation Strategies

The insight or interpretation strategies (Linehan 1993a) tend to be particularly effective when they pertain to a patient's behaviors that occur with the therapist. This attention to the therapeutic relationship sets DBT apart from most other behavioral treatments, which tend to focus attention on behavior that occurs between therapy sessions. The therapist offers hypotheses regarding current and observable behaviors so as to highlight recurrent patterns and their functional significance.

Didactic Strategies

Didactic strategies include the dissemination of pertinent information regarding effective methods of behavior change and self-control. Didactic information is intended to help patients understand factors that affect their behavior as well as to serve as information regarding normative emotional, cognitive, and behavioral responses to common problematic situations in which patients may find themselves.

Solution Analysis

DBT, like many other forms of psychotherapy, presumes that insight gained through hypothesis testing of patterns discovered through chain analysis is not sufficient to ensure behavioral change. Behavioral analysis, by which patterns of problematic behavior are understood, must be pursued before developing a road map and plan to effect the desired change.

Identifying the patient's goals, needs, and desires is fundamental to effective solution analysis. Because the suicidal behavior or nonsuicidal self-injury of the patient with BPD is often his or her effort to solve a problem, much of solution analysis requires helping the patient to see that there are other possible solutions than the ones to which he or she gravitates. Helping patients know what they want is dependent on the freedom to choose, and assisting patients to make choices is dependent on facilitating their sense of assertive entitlement.

Solution analysis typically requires generation of multiple solutions, helping patients to consider alternative plans to maximize flexibility and to make accommodations to the inevitable difficulties in solving problems. Sometimes problems can be solved and sometimes they must be tolerated or accepted.

Evaluating solutions and the various difficulties that might occur subsequent to implementing a solution (troubleshooting) allows a patient to prepare and think ahead, thus anticipating more competent ways of handling the unexpected. Role-plays are useful for engaging the patient to consider potential impediments. Problem-solving strategies are typically coordinated with skills training, contingency management, cognitive modification, and exposure-based procedures to help implement new solutions (Linehan 1993a).

Validation

Validation is the process by which a therapist communicates to patients that he or she takes their responses seriously. Validation requires that a therapist seek the validity of a patient's response within the patient's current life situation. It is equally important, however, to validate only what is valid. There are three steps in validating (Linehan 1993a). The first step requires the therapist to be an active observer and listener, communicating alertness and interest in the patient's communication of thoughts, feelings, and action, while letting go of bias and prejudice. The second step requires the therapist to accurately and nonjudgmentally offer understanding of the patient's communication. The third step entails the therapist pointing out the wis-

TABLE 27–5. Levels of therapist validation in dialectical behavioral therapy

1. Showing interest, actively listening
2. Accurately reflecting the client's thoughts, feelings, and behaviors
3. Articulating what is not stated, "mind reading," intuitive understanding of a patient
4. Making the connection between a patient's current experience and past learning or in terms of biological dysfunction
5. Validating the patient in terms of present and normal functioning
6. Showing radical genuineness, treating the patient as someone who is not fragile or unable

Source. Adapted from Linehan 1997.

dom or validity of the patient's response. Behavior is adaptive in the context in which it occurs, and the therapist seeks to find what is reasonable before examining the dysfunctional characteristics. The quest for validity is dialectical, seeking the wisdom and authenticity within the context of the dysfunctional behavior. Linehan identified four types of validation strategies—emotional, behavioral, cognitive, and cheerleading (see Linehan 1993a)—and six levels of validation (see Table 27–5).

Identifying, countering, and accepting the "shoulds" are particularly important behavioral validation strategies. When patients say, "I should have," they convey that they may be placing unrealistic demands on themselves to act differently than they have. This type of thinking can interfere with recognizing preference and with developing a realistic plan for change. The therapist emphasizes that refusing to accept a given reality means that one also cannot act to change it. Wishing reality were different does not change it, and suggesting that something "should not" have happened when it did denies its existence.

Problem-Solving Strategies

The problem-solving strategies discussed below—contingency procedures, behavioral skills training, exposure-based techniques, and cognitive modification—make up the majority of current behavior therapy utilized in DBT. Although these strategies are highly specific with respect to standard behavioral techniques, there is ample room for modification. According to Linehan (1993a), "It is important...that you [the therapist] can and should add any techniques that you believe are effective change procedures or that have been shown in research to be effective" (p. 370).

Contingency procedures. Contingency procedures are based on the premise that the consequences of behavior affect the likelihood of its recurring. *Reinforcement* refers to all contingencies and consequences that increase the probability of behavior. It is worth noting that consequences of behavior do not necessarily prove intention. In addition, 1) much learning is automatic, with no conscious or unconscious intent, and 2) humans construct reasons for their behavior when causes are not apparent. DBT places emphasis on observation and identification of the contingency and favors reinforcement. Although extinction and punishment are both important and sometimes necessary, reinforcement tends to be more effective for new learning to become consolidated. Extinction involves removal of the consequence that has been reinforcing the behavior. For example, if an individual engages in self-injury, which is then reinforced by desired affection and attention from the family, ignoring the self-injury would put it on extinction. Punishment is the pairing of a behavioral response with an aversive consequence. For example, taking away valued privileges to drive the car is punishment.

Because treating patients with BPD can be very stressful, a therapist must be very attentive to the possibility that aversive consequences may arise from his or her own unchecked hostile impulses. The consultation team can be very helpful in assisting a therapist sort out his or her feelings.

Behavioral skills training. There are three types of skills training procedures (Linehan 1993a): skills acquisition, skills strengthening (behavioral rehearsal and feedback), and skills generalization. DBT presumes that patients with BPD have skills deficits rather than a lack of motivation as the primary cause of their problems. Skills are often assessed by role-playing in the office, where one has the opportunity to evaluate whether a particular behavior is within a patient's repertoire. If the behavior does not appear, however, the assumption cannot be made that the skill is absent. It is usually safer for the therapist to work with the patient on *skills acquisition* through instruction and modeling, followed by behavioral rehearsal by the patient, and then reinforcement, feedback and coaching, and generalization.

To promote *skills strengthening*, the therapist provides feedback based on the patient's performance. When feedback is given with interpretations about presumed motivation and intent, helpful feedback is often dismissed by the patient. Feedback needs to be behaviorally specific, referring to identifiable behavior. Suggesting that a patient is manipulating, overreacting, or acting out is not helpful in the absence of any clear behavioral referents for the terms.

Skills generalization refers to the ways in which a patient will be able to access and utilize skills that were learned in treatment during everyday life outside of therapy. In vivo skills coaching is typically conducted by the primary therapist to help the patient apply new behaviors in the context of daily life. Patients are encouraged to call or page their therapist between sessions when they find themselves having difficulty employing skills and are at risk of engaging in dysfunctional behavior. DBT has often been misconstrued as a 24-hour therapy hotline; however, this is not the case, because phone contacts are limited to skills coaching and relationship repair. If a patient calls with a wish to discuss a topic that is not pressing or the patient does not express interest in skills coaching or problem solving, the therapist is advised to end the contact so as not to reinforce phone calling (assuming contact with the therapist is reinforcing to the patient).

If the therapist and patient agree to the use of skills coaching during the phone call, they quickly review the current problematic situation and the skills that the patient has attempted and then generate a new plan to try other skills. This type of phone contact should not last more than 10 minutes and can be enormously helpful in preventing occurrence of self-injury.

Exposure-based procedures.   Exposure-based treatments have historically been used to treat fear-based problems such as panic and have been modified for more informal use in DBT to treat other problems involving emotions of shame, guilt, and anger. Particularly important is that the patient not be exposed to the same cues that will reinforce the anxiety response. Typically, this means choosing cues that are related to but do not re-create the same condition that produced the aversive emotional reaction in the first place. More formal exposure-based treatments are typically utilized in stage 2 treatment to address trauma related to posttraumatic stress disorder.

Cognitive modification.   The cognitive restructuring procedures target four types of thinking (Linehan 1993a): 1) nondialectical thinking (e.g., rigid thinking styles), 2) faulty beliefs or underlying assumptions governing behavior, 3) dysfunctional descriptions (e.g., automatic thoughts, evaluative or judgmental labeling), and 4) dysfunctional allocations of attention. Identification and confrontation of dysfunctional cognitive styles and the generation of more functional thinking are goals of treatment. The four DBT skill sets include interpersonal effectiveness, distress tolerance, mindfulness, and emotion regulation. Specific self-statements are taught in the distress tolerance and interpersonal effectiveness modules. Effectiveness and identifying judgmental descriptions are taught in mindfulness training. Identifying cognitive appraisals related to emotions is part of the emotion regulation skills module (Linehan 1993a).

Dialectical Strategies

Dialectical strategies are woven into the entirety of the DBT treatment. According to Linehan (1993a), the essence of this strategy is "constant attention to combining acceptance and change, flexibility with stability, nurturing with challenging, and a focus on capabilities with a focus on limitations and deficits" (p. 202). Keeping a patient off balance makes it more difficult for him or her to revert to previous patterns of rigid and dysfunctional behavior, and the sensitive back-and-forth of engagement between therapist and patient helps maintain the ongoing treatment integrity. Applying dialectics to the therapeutic relationship is often compared to dancing, in that the "therapist must move quickly from strategy to strategy, alternating acceptance with change, control with letting go, confrontation with support, the carrot with the stick, a hard edge with softness, and so on in rapid succession" (Linehan 1993a, p. 203).

Change involves adjustments and transformations of current capabilities in light of the challenges and limitations of interaction in the therapy relationship, as well as with the environment at large. Mindfulness, with its emphasis on observing, describing, and participating, is balanced with emotion regulation. Interpersonal effectiveness offers possibilities for change, while distress tolerance facilitates acceptance. The presumption is that change is facilitated by emphasizing acceptance and that acceptance is possible when change has been challenged.

In addition to the above general description of dialectical strategies, Linehan (1993a) describes the following specific strategies:

- *Entering the paradox* refers to the ways in which the therapist highlights paradoxical contradictions to stress that an answer can be both yes and no.
- *Using metaphor and story* serves as a means to create alternative meanings and points of reference. Metaphors and stories, especially when tailored to a patient's sensibilities and experiences, are often more compelling and easier for the patient to attend to and remember. They help suggest alternative points of reference to redefine problems and suggest new solutions.
- *Playing the devil's advocate* is a technique in which the therapist makes an extreme propositional statement and then plays devil's advocate to counter attempts by the patient to disprove it. This is a common strategy used in the early phase of treatment to obtain a strong commitment to change. The therapist might argue against change and commitment to therapy (e.g., "I think this therapy is going to be too hard to do; it's going to be so much work and painful and it will take a year"), invoking the patient to take the other side ("No, I can do it; it won't be a problem"). Several rounds of challenge are often indicated ("How is it not going to be a problem?") to approach a more realistic appraisal of the task. In the process of the debate, therapist and patient can arrive at the synthesis (a

thoughtful willingness and informed commitment to treatment, with the understanding that it will be difficult and the patient may likely want to quit).

- *Extending* is a technique by which the therapist takes the patient more literally than the patient takes himself or herself, highlighting the way in which a patient may be exaggerating. For example, to a patient who says, "If you don't see me tomorrow, I will kill myself," the therapist may say, "We must hospitalize you immediately. This is no time to discuss an extra appointment." A small part of a communication is exaggerated to throw the patient off balance. This technique is most effective when the patient does not expect to be taken seriously.

- *Making lemonade out of lemons* is the technique by which the therapist makes use of something problematic to demonstrate how it can offer some new opportunity or benefit (e.g., "You say you had a terrible day— well, this gives us an opportunity to practice acceptance"). It is important that the therapist not be cavalier, as a patient will not feel understood. This technique requires that the patient feel confident of the therapist's compassion and empathy.

- *Allowing natural change* refers to the exposure to change and instability as a therapeutic intervention. A dialectical philosophy presumes that the nature of reality is a developing process of change that is neither arbitrary nor fixed but that evolves.

- *Activating wise mind* is the technique of adding intuitive knowing to emotional experiencing and logical analysis.

Stylistic or Communication Strategies

Communication strategies refers to the style and form of the therapist's communication to the patient. There are two primary communication styles in DBT, the reciprocal and the irreverent. The reciprocal communication style is responsive and genuine, whereas the irreverent style is confrontational and impertinent. These two sets of strategies form the dialectical poles of therapeutic interaction. The therapist is encouraged to employ both, alternating back and forth, ultimately blending the two into a new synthesis.

The two types of reciprocal communication strategies are self-disclosure and genuineness. Self-disclosure is further subdivided into self-involving self-disclosure and personal self-disclosure. In *self-involving self-disclosure*, the therapist reveals his or her feelings toward the patient (this is often referred to as countertransference in dynamic therapies), serving to both validate and challenge. Self-involving self-disclosure functions as contingency management; limits are observed within the therapy relationship so that information on the effect of a patient's behavior on the therapist can be obtained. *Personal self-disclosure*, the second reciprocal communication strategy, allows for modeling of normative responses. Subject to frequent criticism by other traditions of psychotherapy, both genuineness and self-disclosure are utilized in DBT with as much thoughtfulness and rigor as any other technical intervention. Linehan makes very clear that the therapist is always *role* bound but should not be arbitrarily *rule* bound (Gerben 2001). Whatever rules might arise do so as a result of the interaction between therapist and patient as to what is effective for treatment. Linehan suggests that often risk and power are unequally divided by rules established for arbitrary reasons by the therapist, leading to chronic impasses in therapy.

Irreverent communication strategies are unexpected and unorthodox, often resulting in altering the emotional state of the moment. Humorous irreverence can facilitate the examination of the unnoticed assumptions of a patient's behavior by sometimes minimizing and sometimes exaggerating a situation.

Irreverent and reciprocal strategies are effective when woven together. Reciprocity without irreverence is often too saccharine, whereas irreverence alone can run the risk of seeming too mean. Irreverence carries greater risk in the short run of evoking unexpected intense affect but can help facilitate a breakthrough after a long period of little progress. Reciprocity can be riskier in the long run because it can ignore the more urgent nature of a patient's situation (Linehan 1993a).

Case Management Strategies

Case management strategies are aimed at helping patients feel more effective in their necessary interactions in the world. Typically, the DBT therapist consults *to* patients (but not *for* the patients) in an effort to help them become more able to manage their own lives, to increase communication with family and treaters, and to encourage respect for the patients' competence to attend to their treatment needs (e.g., treatment reviews, discussions with psychopharmacologists). Unilateral interventions by the therapist on behalf of the patient are kept to a minimum. Sometimes, however, the therapist must intervene in the environment to protect the patient or change a situation, because the patient does not have the means to do so, as in the case of arranging for hospitalization. For example, acute inpatient hospitalization should be considered when exposure treatment of posttraumatic stress is recommended, when nonresponse to therapy plus severe depression or anxiety are evident, when an overwhelming crisis occurs without an available safe environment, or when there is overwhelming psychosis in the absence of social support. Acute hospitalization for a suicidal patient is

TABLE 27–6.   Reasons for hospitalization in dialectical behavioral therapy

1. Psychotic state along with suicide threats

2. Suicide risk that outweighs risk of inappropriate hospitalization

3. Serious strain in therapeutic relationship that creates a suicide risk or crisis and for which outside consultation seems prudent

4. Need to monitor or change medication when overdose risk is elevated

5. Escalation of operant suicide threats, and aversiveness of the hospitalization

6. Need for the therapist to have a break from the treatment

Source.   Adapted from Linehan 1993a.

worth mentioning here. In general, hospitalization for suicidal patients is not recommended, because it often serves the function of facilitating avoidance of problems and reinforcing suicidal behavior. There is research to suggest that hospitalization of a suicidal patient often produces negative effects (Paris 2004). There are circumstances, however, that warrant hospitalization (see Table 27–6).

Termination From Treatment

DBT has only one formal termination rule: If a patient misses 4 weeks of scheduled individual DBT or skills training, treatment is terminated. Therapists should not reassure patients that termination from treatment will not occur prematurely. Indeed, DBT is viewed as a conditional relationship, with commitment made to resolving therapeutic problems and impasses; if, however, therapists feel that their limits have been pushed beyond their comfort level or believe that effective treatment is not possible, then therapy vacation or termination should be considered and thoughtfully implemented.

Therapist Adherence to Dialectical Behavior Therapy

A 66-item scoring scale has been developed for rating the degree to which a DBT treatment is adherent to the model. The items are grouped into categories that follow the treatment components, including structural strategies, problem assessment strategies, problem solving, skills training, contingency management, exposure-based procedures, cognitive strategies, validation strategies, reciprocal communication strategies, irreverent strategies, dialectical strategies, case management strategies, and protocols. Increasingly, efforts are being made to develop rigorous methods to assess whether practice of DBT is actually true to the model. Toward that end, development of certification and accreditation standards is under way to evaluate both the competence of individuals and of DBT programs in a standardized way.

Research on Dialectical Behavior Therapy

Randomized Controlled Trials

Since 1991, there have been nine randomized controlled trials that have shown the benefits of DBT. In an early study, Linehan et al. (1991) found that the DBT treatment group, in comparison with the treatment as usual in the community (TAU) group, exhibited a reduction in the frequency and medical risk of parasuicidal behavior, an elevated retention rate in therapy, and a decreased number of days of inpatient psychiatric hospitalization. Although the two treatment conditions did not vary in efficacy in terms of improving the patients' depression, hopelessness, suicidal ideation, or reasons for living, Koons et al. (2001) did find such improvement with DBT when studying a cohort of women veterans with BPD against a TAU group. There have been claims that other variables, such as economic status and other confounding factors, lead to statistically significant differences in treatment group outcomes. Researchers, however, refute these claims, arguing that it is the DBT that is driving the results (Linehan and Heard 1993).

Linehan et al. (2006) conducted three 2-year randomized controlled studies to determine the efficacy of DBT compared to a community treatment provided by experts. DBT was found to be uniquely effective for reducing suicide attempts for subjects who had been recently suicidal and engaging in self-injurious behavior. Subjects receiving DBT were half as likely to make a suicide attempt and required fewer psychiatric hospitalizations.

Substance Abuse

For patients with BPD exhibiting comorbid problems of substance abuse, DBT led to greater reduction in severe borderline symptoms than did TAU, although the TAU and DBT groups had similar improvements in substance abuse (van den Bosch et al. 2002). Linehan et al. (1999) found that in addition to decreased attrition rates compared with the TAU group, DBT significantly helped individuals with BPD and substance abuse problems; social and global adjustment was increased and substance abuse reduced at 16-month follow-up. Linehan et al. (2002) compared DBT with the standard 12-step program in a study of opioid-dependent women. Both groups reduced their opioid usage relative to baseline at the end of 4 months. In the last 4 months of treatment, however, the 12-step group increased their usage, while the DBT group maintained the reduced levels.

Eating Disorders

DBT has also been used in treating patients with binge eating disorder. Telch et al. (2001) found that 89% of patients with binge eating disorder had stopped binge eating by the end of treatment. At the 6-month follow-up, over half of the patients still abstained from binge eating.

In another study examining treatment of bulimia nervosa, using a DBT group versus a waiting-list control group, reductions of bulimic symptoms were found in the DBT group. Using emotion regulation techniques, the patients in the DBT group exhibited a decrease in binge-purge behaviors that did not occur in the waiting-list control group (Safer et al. 2001), suggesting that DBT is an effective treatment for individuals with bulimia nervosa.

Depression

DBT has also been shown to play a role in alleviating some of the problems associated with depression. In a study examining the potential benefit of augmenting medication with group psychotherapy, Lynch et al. (2003) divided depressed older individuals into two groups: those given antidepressants only and those treated with antidepressants and DBT. The results showed significant decreases in mean self-rated depression scores only for those patients receiving the combination treatment. Maladaptive coping and significant dependency problems, both of which are believed to contribute to a vulnerability to depression, were significantly ameliorated with the combination treatment.

Nonrandomized Controlled Studies

Although arguably not as reliable as randomized controlled trials, nonrandomized studies have also been conducted to examine the benefits of DBT in various populations. One study of the use of DBT with suicidal adolescents with borderline personality features revealed decreases in suicidal ideation, general psychiatric symptoms, and symptoms of borderline personality, as well as an increase in treatment completion (Rathus and Miller 2002). The application of DBT for patients with BPD within an inpatient setting demonstrated decreased suicidal behavior, hospitalization, and treatment dropout, as well as improved interpersonal functioning and anger management (Swenson et al. 2001). Studies revealed that during hospitalizations, patients with BPD participating in DBT exhibited improvements in ratings of depression, dissociation, anxiety, and global stress (Bohus et al. 2000a). Likewise, use of DBT has led to decreased rates of parasuicide in inpatient settings (Barley et al. 1993; Bohus et al. 2000a). One study, conducted with incarcerated juvenile offenders, revealed decreases in youth behavior problems and use of punitive responses by staff (Trupin et al. 2002). The results of these studies support the efficacy of DBT across a wide range of situations with varying patient types.

Key Points

- The development of borderline personality disorder (BPD) results from an ongoing transaction between a biological vulnerability to emotional dysregulation and an invalidating environment.
- The three fundamental components of DBT are problem solving, validation, and dialectics.
- In DBT, change strategies are balanced by acceptance strategies.
- Modes of therapy include individual psychotherapy, skills training, phone coaching, and therapist consultation.
- Standard individual DBT utilizes a diary card and focuses on behavioral analysis and problem solving.
- The two high-priority targets of stage 1 DBT include decreasing suicidal and nonsuicidal self-injury and addressing any problems in the therapy relationship that threaten the viability of treatment.
- Core skills include mindfulness, emotion regulation, distress tolerance, and interpersonal effectiveness.
- Problem-solving strategies, including contingency management and exposure-based procedures, are central for targeting behavioral change.
- Communication strategies, including irreverent and reciprocal styles, help challenge and validate a patient's experience.
- Primary therapists consult *to* the patient, not *for* the patient.
- An essential component of DBT is the consultation team, whose members meet regularly to help the community of DBT treaters become more effective in treating the patients.
- DBT has been shown to be effective in both randomized and nonrandomized trials.

References

Barad MG, Saxena S: Neurobiology of extinction: a mechanism underlying behav-. ior therapy for human anxiety disorders. Primary Psychiatry 12:45–51, 2005

Barley WD, Buie SE, Peterson EW, et al: The development of an inpatient cognitive-behavioral treatment program for borderline personality disorder. J Personal Disord 7:232–240, 1993

Bohus M, Haaf B, Stiglmayr C, et al: Evaluation of inpatient dialectical-behavioral therapy for borderline personality disorder—a prospective study. Behav Res Ther 38:875–887, 2000a

Bohus M, Limberger MF, Ebner UW, et al: Pain perception during self-reported distress and calmness in patients with borderline personality disorder and self-mutilating behavior. Psychiatry Res 95:251–260, 2000b

Bohus M, Haaf B, Simms T, et al: Effectiveness of inpatient dialectical behavior therapy for borderline personality disorder: a controlled trial. Behav Res Ther 42:487–499, 2004

Comtois K, Linehan MM: Psychosocial treatments of suicidal behaviors: a practice-friendly review. J Clin Psychol 62:161–170, 2006

Fruzzetti A: The High Conflict Couple: A Dialectical Behavior Therapy Guide to Finding Peace, Intimacy, and Validation. Oakland, CA, New Harbinger, 2006

Garakani A, Mathew SJ, Charney DS: Neurobiology of anxiety disorders and implications for treatment. Mt Sinai J Med 73:941–949, 2006

Gerben H: Personalities: Master Clinicians Confront the Treatment of Borderline Personality Disorders. New York, Jason Aronson, 2001

Harned MS, Linehan MM: Integrating dialectical behavior therapy and prolonged exposure to treat co-occurring borderline personality disorder and PTSD: two case studies. Cogn Behav Pract (in press)

Koons CR, Robins CJ, Tweed JL, et al: Efficacy of dialectical behavior therapy in women veterans with borderline personality disorder. Behav Ther 32:371–390, 2001

Kroger C, Schweiger V, Sipos V, et al: Effectiveness of dialectical behavior therapy for borderline personality disorder in an inpatient setting. Behav Res Ther 44:1211–1217, 2006

Linehan MM: Cognitive Behavioral Therapy for Borderline Personality Disorder. New York, Guilford, 1993a

Linehan MM: Skills Training Manual for Treating Borderline Personality Disorder. New York, Guilford, 1993b

Linehan MM: Validation and psychotherapy, in Empathy Reconsidered: New Directions in Psychotherapy. Edited by Bohart AC, Greenberg LS. Washington, DC, American Psychological Association, 1997

Linehan MM, Heard HL: "Impact of treatment accessibility on clinical course of parasuicidal patients": reply. Arch Gen Psychiatry 50:157–158, 1993

Linehan MM, Armstrong HE, Suarez A, et al: Cognitive-behavioral treatment of chronically parasuicidal borderline patients. Arch Gen Psychiatry 48:1060–1064, 1991

Linehan MM, Schmidt H, Dimeff LA, et al: Dialectical behavior therapy for patients with borderline personality disorder and drug-dependence. Am J Addict 8:279–292, 1999

Linehan MM, Dimeff LA, Reynolds SK, et al: Dialectical behavior therapy versus comprehensive validation plus 12-step for the treatment of opioid dependent women meeting criteria for borderline personality disorder. Drug Alcohol Depend 67:13–26, 2002

Linehan MM, Comtois KA, Murray AM, et al: Two-year randomized control trial and follow-up of dialectical behavior therapy vs therapy by experts for suicidal behaviors and borderline personality disorder. Arch Gen Psychiatry 63:757–766, 2006

Ludaescher P, Bohus M, Lieb K, et al: Elevated pain thresholds correlate with dissociation and aversive arousal in patients with borderline personality disorder. Psychiatry Res 149:291–296, 2007

Lynch TR, Morse JQ, Mendelson T, et al: Dialectical behavior therapy for depressed older patients: a randomized pilot study. Am J Geriatr Psychiatry 11:33–45, 2003

Medina JF, Nores WL, Mauk MD: Inhibition of climbing fibres is a signal for the extinction of conditioned eyelid response. Nature 416:330–333, 2002

Paris J: Is hospitalization useful for suicidal patients with borderline personality disorder? J Personal Disord 18:240–247, 2004

Rathus JH, Miller AL: Dialectical behavior therapy adapted for suicidal adolescents. Suicide Life Threat Behav 32:146–157, 2002

Russ MJ, Roth SD, Lerman A, et al: Pain perception in self-injurious patients with borderline personality disorder. Biol Psychiatry 32:501–511, 1992

Safer DL, Telch CF, Agras WS: Dialectical behavior therapy for bulimia nervosa. Am J Psychiatry 158:632–634, 2001

Sanislow CA, Grilo CM, McGlashan TH: Factor analysis of the DSM-III-R borderline personality disorder criteria in psychiatric inpatients. Am J Psychiatry 157:1629–1633, 2000

Schmahl C, Bohus M, Esposito F, et al: Neural correlates of antinociception in borderline personality disorder. Arch Gen Psychiatry 63:659–666, 2006

Simpson EB, Pistorello J, Begin A, et al: Use of dialectical behavior therapy in a partial hospital program for women with borderline personality disorder. Psychiatr Serv 49:669–673, 1998

Skodol AE, Siever LJ, Livesley WJ, et al: The borderline diagnosis II: biology, genetics, and clinical course. Biol Psychiatry 51:951–963, 2002

Stiglmayr CE, Grathwol T, Linehan MM, et al: Aversive tension in patients with borderline personality disorder: a computer-based controlled field study. Acta Psychiatr Scand 111:372–379, 2005

Swenson CR, Sanderson C, Dulit RA, et al: The application of dialectical behavior therapy for patients with borderline personality disorder on inpatient units. Psychiatr Q 72:307–324, 2001

Telch CF, Agras WS, Linehan MM: Dialectical behavior therapy for binge eating disorder. J Consult Clin Psychol 69:1061–1065, 2001

Trupin EW, Stewart DG, Beach B, et al: Effectiveness of a dialectical behaviour therapy program for incarcerated female juvenile offenders. Child and Adolescent Mental Health 7:121–127, 2002

van den Bosch LMC, Verheul R, Schippers GM, et al: Dialectical behavior therapy of borderline patients with and without substance use problems: implementation and long-term effects. Addict Behav 27:911–923, 2002

Suggested Readings

Basseches M: Dialectical Thinking and Adult Development. St Louis, MO, Ablex, 1985

Ben-Porath DD, Koons CR: Telephone coaching in dialectical behavior therapy: a decision-tree model for managing inter-session contact with clients. Cogn Behav Pract 12:448–460, 2005

Butler K: Revolution on the horizon. Psychotherapy Networker, May/June 2001, pp 26–39

Foa EB, Rothbaum BO: Treating the Trauma of Rape: Cognitive Behavioral Therapy for Post-Traumatic Stress Disorder. New York, Guilford Press, 2001

Goldfried ML, Davidson GC: Clinical Behavior Therapy. New York, Wiley, 1994

Kabat-Zinn J: Wherever You Go, There You Are. New York, Hyperion Books, 1995

Linehan MM: An illustration of dialectical behavior therapy. In Session: Psychotherapy in Practice 4:21–44, 1998

Lynch TR, Chapman AL, Rosenthal MZ, et al: Mechanisms of change in dialectical behavior therapy: theoretical and empirical observations. J Clin Psychol 62:459–480, 2006

Pryor K: Don't Shoot the Dog: The New Art of Teaching and Training. New York, Bantam Doubleday Dell, 1999

Chapter 28

Theory and Practice of Mentalization-Based Therapy

Anthony Bateman, M.A., F.R.C.Psych.
Peter Fonagy, Ph.D., F.B.A.
Jon G. Allen, Ph.D.

Mentalization, or better mentalizing, is the process by which we make sense of each other and ourselves, implicitly and explicitly, in terms of subjective states and mental processes. It is a profoundly social construct in the sense that we are attentive to the mental states of those we are with, physically or psychologically. Equally we can temporarily lose awareness of those individuals as "minds" and even momentarily treat them as physical objects (Allen et al. 2008).

A focus on mental states as something uniquely human and as an important area of study seems self-evident for those involved in treating individuals with mental disorder. Yet, even those of us engaged in daily clinical work can all too easily forget that our clients have minds. For example, many biological psychiatrists are happier to think in terms of neurotransmitter imbalance than distorted expectations or self-representation. Parents with children who have psychological problems often prefer to understand these either in terms of genetic predispositions or as direct consequences of the child's social environment, such as the people with whom the child mixes. Even psychotherapists can make unwarranted assumptions about what a patient feels and can lose touch with his or her actual subjective experience.

Understanding other people's behavior in terms of their likely thoughts, feelings, wishes, and desires—that is, what goes on in their minds—is a major developmental achievement that originates, probably biologically, in the context of the attachment relationship. Disruption of this process during development may in part contribute to the development of a number of mental disorders, such as anxiety and depression. Given the generality of the definition of *mentalization*, most mental disorders will inevitably involve some difficulties with mentalization. In fact, most mental disorders can be conceived as the mind misinterpreting its own experience of itself and, therefore, are ultimately disorders of mentalization. However, a key issue is not whether a mental disorder can be redescribed in terms of the functioning of mentalization, but whether the dysfunction of mentalization is core to the disorder and whether a focus on mentalization is heuristically valid— that is, whether such a focus provides an appropriate domain for therapeutic intervention. For example, although mentalizing problems have been described in schizophrenia (Frith 2004), this does not mean that a mentalizing-based intervention will be ultimately useful as a treatment method for schizophrenia. The same applies to conditions such as autism, in which patients have been shown to suffer more or less complete mind-blindness (Baron-Cohen et al. 2000). Again, whether a focus on mentalizing provides an appropriate focus for interventions is currently an open question.

The disorder that has received the most attention in relation to mentalizing is borderline personality disorder (BPD). A fragile mentalizing capacity vulnerable to social and interpersonal interaction is considered a core feature of BPD. This is not an insignificant proposal, because if it is correct, a BPD patient's problems in mentalizing or maintaining a mentalizing capacity will impact directly on the patient's response to treatment; then, if a treatment is to be successful, it must have mentalization as its focus or at the very least stimulate development of mentalizing as an epiphenomenon. Although mentalizing theory is being applied to a number of disorders, including posttraumatic stress disorder (PTSD) (Allen 2001), eating disorders (Skårderud 2007), and depression (Allen et al. 2003), the treatment method is most clearly organized as a therapy for BPD (Bateman and Fonagy 2004). It is only for this condition that clear empirical support with randomized controlled trials (Bateman and Fonagy 1999, 2001) exists, although other studies—for example, investigating mentalizing as a core technique in family therapy and in adolescence (Fearon et al. 2006) and replication of the original studies in BPD by an independent group—are under way. In this chapter, we focus on mentalization-based therapy (MBT) as a treatment for BPD, although aspects of treatment of other conditions will be discussed where relevant.

Mentalizing and Neurobiology

Mentalization is a mostly preconscious, imaginative mental activity. It is imaginative because we have to imagine what other people might be thinking or feeling. It lacks homogeneity because each person's history and capacity to imagine may lead that person to different conclusions about the mental states of others. We may sometimes need to make the same kind of imaginative leap to understand our own experiences, particularly in relation to emotionally charged issues or in trying to understand some of our irrational reactions.

If we are to conceive imaginatively of ourselves and others as having a mind, we require a representational system for mental states. The capacity to represent mind states requires higher cortical processes, and although mentalizing probably involves numerous cortical systems, it is certainly associated with activation in the middle prefrontal areas of the brain, probably the paracingulate area (Gallagher and Frith 2003). It is likely that several brain systems are involved in different aspects of mentalizing, including those underpinning attentional processes and emotional reactions (Fonagy and Bateman 2006a). Brain abnormalities identified in patients with BPD are consistent with the suggestion that a failure of representation of self-states as a key aspect of identity is a key dysfunction in BPD. Lane (2000) proposed that implicit self-representations (i.e., phenomenal self-awareness) can be localized to the dorsal anterior cingulate, whereas explicit self-representations (i.e., reflection) can be localized to the rostral anterior cingulate. In a series of neuroimaging studies, activation of the medial prefrontal cortex was demonstrated in conjunction with a wide range of mentalization inferences, in both visual and verbal domains (Gallagher et al. 2000). It appears that the prefrontal cortex is involved when a person mentalizes interactively in a way that requires implicitly representing the mental states of others.

Social cognitive capacities develop in the context of primary caregiving relationships and, as a result, are relatively vulnerable to environmental disturbance exemplified by severe neglect, abuse, and other forms of maltreatment. Early trauma may cause changes in the neural mechanisms of arousal, leading to a relatively ready triggering of the arousal system underpinning posterior cortical activation in response to relatively mild emotional stimuli.

This triggering simultaneously takes the frontal mentalizing parts of the brain "offline" (Arnsten 1998). Although we think that this process is important in the vulnerability to loss of mentalizing in patients with BPD and some other mental disorders, it is important to remember that there are alternative pathways that lead to failures in the development of social cognitive capacities, many of which may not offer the same chance of remediation. Autism is a case in point: according to the "theory of mind deficit" account, childhood autism is a primary cognitive dysfunction, caused by a genetic defect of the innate "theory of mind" processing that enables the representation of intentional mental states. We envision a spectrum of disturbances, all involving abnormal sensitivities to contingencies. At one extreme is childhood autism, in which individuals fail to move from seeking contingent responses (i.e., sameness) to seeking noncontingent interactions. It is as if the contingency analyzer gets "stuck" forever in its original setting of preferentially seeking out and processing perfectly self-contingent stimuli. As a result, children with autism continue to invest in perfect contingencies (generated by stereotypic self-stimulation or repetitive manipulation of objects) throughout their lives, while showing a lack of interest in the less-than-perfect contingencies provided by their social environment. Our focus on mentalizing as a therapeutic intervention is not meant to imply that it is effective in all conditions showing problems in mentalizing. Effective remediation may be dependent on the underlying cause.

Mentalizing and Emotional Life

Mentalizing is a harsh and ungainly sounding word (Holmes 2006) and has been criticized as implying cognitive rather than emotional processing. This is a misapprehension. Mentalization is procedural, mostly nonconscious, and, for the most part, an intuitive, rapid emotional reaction in response to all the social and personal interactions around us. Feelings within ourselves and our impressions of others' feelings provide us with considerable information about the mental states that underpin behavior, and our experience of the affective tone of an interaction can lead us to relatively complex choices between sets of beliefs. For example, if we experience an individual as threatening, this may lead us to formulate relatively complex theories about his or her hostile intentions.

Mentalizing also helps us to regulate our emotions (Fonagy et al. 2002) by giving them a context. For example, emotions relate directly to our success or failure in achieving specific wishes or desires. Achieving goals or desires will inevitably generate an emotional response. We integrate the emotions with the original belief or desire through the narrative provided by mentalizing, forming a metarepresentation. It is only then that the emotional experience can be given meaning and context. Problems arise if mentalizing fails and emotions cannot be understood, appearing to arise out of the blue and without context. Under these circumstances, people feel distressed and report that they do not know why they feel as they do or that their feelings are all over the place.

It is easy to overlook the nonconscious aspect of mentalizing. For something as simple as maintaining a dialogue, we need to monitor our conversational partner's state of mind. Perceiving and responding fluidly to the other's emotions ensures that our conversation goes smoothly. In an ingenious investigation, Steimer-Krause et al. (1990) demonstrated that we automatically mirror our interlocutors' emotional states, adjusting our posture, facial expressions, and tone of voice in the process. They suggest it is possible to diagnose the characteristic flattened affect of chronic schizophrenia from the facial expressions of a nonschizophrenic person engaged in an ordinary conversation with an individual who has a diagnosis of schizophrenia, even though the nonschizophrenic person is unaware of this diagnosis. Further work is clearly needed in this area.

In general, our awareness of our behavior as driven by mental states—that is, our mentalizing of self and others—gives us the sense of continuity and control that generates the subjective experience of agency or "I-ness" that is at the very core of a sense of identity. And it is identity that is at the core of BPD.

Mentalizing and Development of Borderline Personality Disorder

The mentalizing theory of BPD is rooted in Bowlby's (1988) attachment theory and its elaboration by contemporary developmental psychologists, with attention paid to constitutional vulnerabilities. There is suggestive evidence that patients with BPD have a history of disorganized attachment, which leads to problems in affect regulation, attention, and self-control (Lyons-Ruth et al. 2005; Sroufe et al. 2005). It is our suggestion that these problems are mediated through a failure to develop a robust mentalizing capacity. Although these problems are all central to BPD psychopathology, they are also of significance in other disorders, such as those related to impulse control and those whose primary characteristic is mood disturbance or response to trauma. Most evidence, however, is currently available for the development of BPD (Fonagy and Bateman 2008).

Our understanding of others critically depends on whether as infants our own mental states were adequately understood by caring, attentive, nonthreatening adults. The most important cause of disruption in mentalizing is psychological trauma early or late in childhood, which undermines the capacity to think about mental states or the ability to give narrative accounts of one's past relationships. Building on the accumulating evidence from developmental psychopathology, the mentalization theory of BPD suggests 1) that individuals are constitutionally vulnerable and/or exposed to psychological trauma; 2) that both these factors can undermine the development of social cognitive capacities necessary for mentalization via neglect in early relationships (Battle et al. 2004), especially where the contingency between an individual's emotional experience and the caregiver's mirroring is noncongruent (Crandell et al. 2003); and 3) that these factors lead to the development of an enfeebled ability to represent affect and effortfully control attentional capacity (Posner et al. 2002). Both factors are key components of mentalizing.

The reduced capacity for mentalizing may be speculatively attributed to one or more of at least four processes. First, a child may defensively close down his or her mind in the face of the experience of genuine malevolent intent of others. Second, the child, in "identifying with the aggressor" as a way of gaining illusory control over the abuser, may internalize the intent of the aggressor in an alien (dissociated) part of the self. Although this might offer temporary relief, the destructive intent of the abuser will in this way come to be experienced from within rather than outside of the self, leading to unbearable self-hatred. Third, early excessive, persistent stress may distort the functioning of arousal mechanisms, resulting in an inhibition of activity in the orbitofrontal cortex (arguably the location of one of the neural systems involved in mentalizing) at lower levels of threat than would normally be the case. Finally, any trauma arouses the attachment system, leading to an intensified search for attachment security and a deactivation of reflective capacity. When the attachment relationship is itself traumatizing, such arousal is exacerbated because in seeking proximity to the traumatizing attachment figure, the child may be further traumatized. Such prolonged activation of the attachment system may have specific inhibitory consequences for mentalization.

Given the known continuity of attachment styles over time, residues of attachment problems of childhood might be expected to be apparent in adulthood. The adult attachment literature in relation to BPD has been expertly reviewed by Levy (2005). Nine studies, using the best available assessment of adult attachment (the Adult Attachment Interview), examined attachment patterns in patients diagnosed with BPD; two further studies used rating scales and over a dozen used self-report measures. Although the relationship of BPD diagnosis and specific attachment category is not obvious, there is little doubt that 1) BPD is strongly associated with insecure attachment (only 6%–8% of BPD patients received "secure" ratings), and there are indications of disorganization as a subcategory (ratings of "unresolved attachment" or "cannot classify category of attachment") in interviews; and 2) BPD is associated with fearful avoidant and preoccupied attachment in questionnaire studies. In summaries across several studies (Hamilton 2000; Waters et al. 2000; Weinfield et al. 2000), it appears that early attachment insecurity is a relatively stable characteristic of the individual, particularly in conjunction with subsequent negative life events (Weinfield et al. 2000). Given evidence of the continuity of attachment from early childhood, at least in adverse environments, the extent to which childhood attachment may affect mentalization may be relevant to the development of BPD. The quality of children's primary attachment relationship has been shown in a number of studies to predict mentalizing ability, although a link with emotional understanding aspects of mentalizing rather than theory of mind components is more consistent. Overall, it seems likely that this relationship is mediated within a family via the coherence and mentalizing nature of the general discourse in the home. Certainly, there is considerable indirect evidence to suggest that family environment is important in the genesis of a number of mental disorders, especially BPD.

Family studies have identified a number of factors that may be important in the development of BPD, such as a history of mood disorders and substance misuse, but few of the studies point to the specific features of parenting that create a vulnerability for BPD. Physical, sexual, and emotional abuse all occur in a family context, and high rates are reported in BPD. Zanarini et al. (2000) reported that 84% of patients with BPD retrospectively reported experience of biparental neglect and emotional abuse before the age of 18, with denial by the caretakers of their emotional experiences during childhood being a predictor of BPD, which suggests that these parents were unable to take the experience of the child into account in the context of family interactions. Overall, researchers have concluded that abuse alone is neither necessary nor sufficient for the development of BPD and that predisposing factors and contextual features of the parent–child relationship are likely to be mediating factors in the actual development of BPD. Parental responses play an important role in the pathogenetic effects of abuse: apparently, parental responsiveness (believing the reports, protecting, and not expressing high levels of anger) following reports of abuse promote more rapid adjustment (Everson et al. 1989), whereas lack of emotional responsiveness, low support, and inadequate validation possibly potentiate the effects. Thus, caregiver response to the abuse may be more important than the abuse itself in long-term outcome (Horwitz et al. 2001).

When all this is taken into account, the mentalization approach predicts that it is not the fact of maltreatment but rather the family environment that discourages coherent discourse concerning mental states, and it is this that is likely to predispose the child to BPD. The mentalizing model suggests that individuals with BPD, although able to mentalize, are more likely to abandon the capacity under high emotional arousal (e.g., in response to maltreatment) because mentalization was not well established during the first decade of life, in part as a consequence of early maltreatment and its associated problems.

We consider that the impact of trauma is most likely to be felt as part of a more general failure of consideration of the child's perspective through neglect, rejection, excessive control, unsupportive relationships, incoherence, and confusion, which can devastate the experiential world of the developing child and leave deep scars that are evident in the child's later social-cognitive functioning and behavior. This aspect of our formulation therefore converges with that advanced by Marsha Linehan (1993) and developed further by Alan Fruzzetti et al. (2003, 2005) concerning the assumption of the invalidating family environments. These workers reported that parental invalidation, in part defined as the undermining of self-perceptions of internal states, was associated not only with the young people's reports of family distress, their own distress, and psychological problems, but also with aspects of social cognition, namely their ability to identify and label emotion. Along with other aspects contributing to the complex interaction described as invalidating, this lack of focus on mental states amounts to a systematic undermining of young people's experience of their own mind by the replacement of their mind with another or a failure to encourage discrimination between their own feelings and experiences and those of the caregiver.

Mentalizing and Phenomenology

The phenomenology of BPD is the consequence of this inhibition of mentalization, and of the reemergence of modes of experiencing internal reality that antedate the development of mentalization. Individuals with BPD are "normal" mentalizers except in the context of attachment relationships, when they tend to misread minds, both their own and those of others, while in intense interpersonal encounters, often when emotionally aroused. When this happens, prementalistic modes of organizing subjectivity emerge, which have the power to disorganize these relationships and destroy the coherence of self-experience that normal mentalization sustains through narrative.

Several prementalistic ways of representing subjectivity may come to the fore as mentalizing is lost:

1. *Psychic equivalence* (normally described by clinicians as concreteness of thought). Alternative perspectives cannot be considered; there is no experience of "as if," and everything appears to be "for real."

2. *Pretend mode.* Thoughts and feelings can come to be almost dissociated to the point of near meaninglessness. In this mode, patients can discuss experiences without contextualizing them in any kind of physical or material reality. Attempting psychotherapy with patients who are in pretend mode can lead the therapist to lengthy but inconsequential discussions of internal experience that have no link to genuine experience.
3. *Early modes of conceptualizing action in terms of observable outcomes (teleological)* that can come to dominate motivation. Within these modes, there is a primacy of the physical; experience is only felt to be valid when its consequences are apparent to all. Affection, for example, is only "real" when accompanied by physical expression.

These prementalistic processes may also account for psychopathology found in other conditions, such as PTSD, which may also benefit from treatment providing at least a partial focus on increasing mentalizing skills (Allen 2001). PTSD is a particularly disabling condition. Its victims have experienced sudden frightening events and relive them time and time again in their minds. But the reexperience is not in a normally functioning mind that is able to manage frightening memories. In PTSD, intrusive memories are experienced in psychic equivalence mode, so the individual repeatedly reexperiences the events not as they *were* happening but as though they *are* happening in the moment. For the individual with PTSD, the events happen again and again. The person has to respond in a way she would if the event were happening outside her rather than in her mind. Under these circumstances, it is understandable that an individual suddenly runs away from where she is or sets up avoidance strategies. These are behaviors resulting from nonmentalizing of experience; a sense of representing mental states and differentiating internal from external is temporarily lost, which leads to a wide range of destructive and maladaptive behaviors.

It follows from this understanding of PTSD that the goal of treatment from a mentalizing perspective is to help the patient move from painful and intolerable reliving to bearable remembering. What has been described as desensitization to memories of trauma may, for example, be better considered as helping to turn unmentalized images into mentalized traumatic memories. This becomes the aim of treatment in this condition. Yet, there is a paradox here. If treatment requires a patient to talk about trauma, which in itself will retraumatize him if his mind is functioning in psychic equivalence mode, it seems likely that an expressive treatment might make him worse. Indeed, it has been shown that debriefing soon after traumatic events, when patients are most likely to be functioning in psychic equivalence mode, makes it less likely that patients will recover and may be an intervention that fixes rather than resolves traumatic experiences (Hobbs et al. 1996).

Taking this into account, Allen and Fonagy (2006) have developed a mentalizing approach to treatment of trauma that balances processing the trauma—mentalizing in the form of thinking, feeling, and talking about it—with containment, consisting of a solid treatment frame and therapeutic alliance, supportive elements, and well-rehearsed emotion regulation strategies.

Conceptual Concerns

It is unsurprising that this conceptual view of development of BPD put forward within the model of mentalization-based therapy has led to some questions. Some of the points raised are discussed here.

First, the focus on attachment in the development of BPD is considered as too narrow a focus, and there is some merit in this argument. However, the role of disorganized attachment as an indicator of later psychiatric disturbance is reasonably well recognized (Lyons-Ruth and Jacobovitz 1999). Problems in attachment undermine the felicitous development of higher-level social cognition. Mentalizing theory is particularly concerned that disorganization of the attachment system has two primary consequences: 1) disorganization of the self-system, which normally develops as a mirroring process; and 2) an easily triggered attachment system. New findings from attachment research indicating differences in vulnerabilities to mentalizing are important because they allow further elaboration of the theory and understanding of treatment of BPD and other personality disorders. As mentioned earlier, attachment patterns in patients with BPD have been identified that may be important for treatment. Patients with BPD show higher than normal levels of anxiety but manage their difficulties through either avoidance or approach of others. This provides some support for our suggestion about the use of different techniques for patients with BPD demonstrating different patterns of attachment behavior (Bateman and Fonagy 2006).

The mentalizing perspective is a dynamic developmental view in which the respective capacities of child and parent, and therefore the nature of their contributions to interactions, change as the child matures. While the mentalizing approach considers that contingent mirroring may be the key contribution of the parent in the first year of life, this gives way to more complex interactions centering on language, playfulness, and other developmental processes later on, as long as there is a relative absence of threatening or frightening harsh interactions. In normal development, at each stage, the parent acts optimally within the constraints of the child's capacity to respond appropriately. Thus, contingent mirroring is more difficult with infants whose temperament is harder to manage, but it also appears to be harder for parents with a history of maltreatment, abuse, and borderline symptoms (Crandell et al. 2003).

Second, the concept of the internalization of, for example, the alien self may become confused with the internalization of the split objects of object relations theory. The confusion probably lies in the clash of conceptualizations, because classical psychoanalysis and its structural model are a representational frame of reference, whereas mentalizing is concerned with the construction of a self process rather than a representational structure (i.e., William James's "I" not "me" [James 1890]). What we are attempting to depict with the concept of the alien self is the episodic separation of a sense of ownership or identity with one's own actions or experiences—something that is actually done by "me" but does not feel as if "I" did it, which is a common experience for patients with BPD. The self is manifest through a process, not a mental structure with a location, so we are concerned with how the brain acts and functions as a mind rather than the regions or object relations that are activated.

The emphasis in mentalizing is less on the nature and origins of roles and enactment of object relations than on the dysfunctional use of these (e.g., their rapidly accelerating tempo of intimacy in relationships, the unthinking nature of some of the interpersonal patterns, the massive distortions of others' mental states). This view of internalization certainly has its origins in object relations theory, and although the relationship may be internalized within a secure attachment, we are suggesting that this process is distorted in disorganized attachment. To translate our formulation into the language of psychoanalytic therapy—that is, in the MBT model of BPD—it is not aspects of the caregiver or roles that become represented or internalized within the child, but the understanding the caregiver has of the mind of the child. When this is incongruent or not clearly differentiated, full internalization of roles cannot take place and there is inadequate development of the processing and internalizing ability that develops developmentally via repetitive contrasting of mental states of self and other.

Third, from a mentalizing perspective, role enactments, whatever their origins, lack specificity to BPD, and they are likely to occur in normally developing individuals (although perhaps to a lesser extent) as well as in many different conditions and are therefore not considered core to the difficulty. From a mentalizing perspective, the problem lies in the capacity to process roles and experiences when they are activated within specific contexts. Individuals with a more robust capacity to mentalize are able to manage their minds when confronted with an interaction that stimulates a powerful emotional response that, in turn, may stimulate an equally powerful response from another.

Finally, psychic equivalence and dissociation from feeling may become confused with regressions to earlier modes of function. Mentalization theory does not specifically see psychic equivalence and dissociation from feeling as "regressions." The emphasis is on actual early capacities rather than on how they are imagined by adult analysts to exist in imaginary children's minds. We agree with the skepticism about regression, because regression generally referred to adults behaving in ways that appeared childish to an adult observer. We are attempting to identify mental processes that are actual and not overridden but rather masked by later developments (Fischer et al. 1990). They are, therefore, revealed when mentalizing is lost.

Practice of Mentalization-Based Treatment

To reiterate the developmental perspective since Bowlby's (1988) work, it has generally been agreed that psychotherapy invariably activates the attachment system and thus generates secure-base experience. Accordingly, self-consciously or not, the MBT therapist is necessarily working within an attachment framework. In our view, the attachment context of psychotherapy is essential in creating a context for the recovery of mentalizing capacity and embedding it in a secure-base experience. That is, the MBT therapist provides the patient with the experience of being understood, which generates an experience of security, which in turn facilitates mental exploration. In conducting psychotherapy, the therapist is mentalizing in the sense of engaging the patient in a process of joint attention wherein the patient's mental states typically are the focus of shared attention, and the ultimate therapeutic value of the interchange stems from the joint focus on the patient's subjective experience in the context of one mental content after another. As it does in childhood, this joint attentional process enhances mentalizing capacity and, concomitantly, strengthens the patient's sense of self.

The explicit content of the MBT therapist's intervention will be mentalistic, regardless of theoretical orientation, whether the therapist is principally concerned with transference reactions, automatic negative thoughts, reciprocal roles, or linear thinking. All these approaches entail explicit mentalizing insofar as they succeed in enhancing coherent mental representations of desires, feelings, and beliefs.

The dyadic and interpersonal nature of therapy fosters patients' capacity to generate multiple perspectives. For example, by interpreting transference or challenging belief systems, the MBT therapist is presenting an alternative perspective on a patient's subjective experience. In so doing, the therapist is freeing the patient from being locked into the reality of one view and, accordingly, is enabling the patient to move from the psychic equivalence mode (mind=world) to the mentalizing mode (mind represents world in many different ways). Thus, whatever the therapist construes the mechanisms of therapeutic change to be—creating a coherent narrative, modifying distorted cognitions, providing the emotional experience of a secure base, giving insight, or simply rekindling hope—the effectiveness of the interventions will depend on the patients' capacity to consider their experience of their own mental states alongside the therapist's re-presentations of them (Bateman and Fonagy 2006).

Aims and Limits of Therapy

It follows from the MBT theoretical perspective that the overall aims of MBT are to promote 1) mentalizing about oneself, 2) mentalizing about others, and 3) mentalizing of relationships. To have a chance of success, therapy has to be organized around 1) structure, 2) development of a therapeutic alliance and adequate repair of ruptures, 3) a focus on the interpersonal and social domain, and 4) exploration of the patient–therapist relationship. However, a lot can go wrong in therapy with patients with BPD. These patients are uniquely vulnerable to therapist interventions (Fonagy and Bateman 2006b) and can easily be thrown into pretend mode, in which they take on the perspective of the therapist and use it as part of themselves, or alternatively are thrown into confusion as their mentalizing capacities collapse. A specific formulation too early in therapy runs the risk of inducing pretend mode in vulnerable patients with BPD, and we advise therapists to be alert to such problems, which can be difficult to identify. MBT tries to formulate a process rather than actual relationship patterns in an attempt to reduce the risk of inducing pretend mode.

Nonmentalizing Techniques

Some therapy techniques should be avoided in MBT. First, we suggest that therapists avoid allowing excessive free association, a technique possibly more useful for neurotic patients. Second, we do not encourage active fantasy about the therapist, particularly early in treatment. The use of fantasy and free association is not a major aspect of MBT because the development of insight is not a primary aim of MBT. Working with fantasy is a technique used in insight-oriented therapy as a way of understanding unconscious thinking. MBT is more concerned with preconscious and conscious aspects of mental function within the interpersonal domain. Fantasy itself is too distant from reality, and we therefore do not encourage elaboration of the patient's fantasies about the therapist, because doing so is likely to be iatrogenic and to invoke pretend mode rather than increase elaborated representations linked to reality. Alternatively, fantasy experienced in psychic equivalence mode becomes reality and is experienced as real, losing its "as if" quality. At first sight, this seems to be contradicted by Levy et al.'s (2006) finding that transference-focused psychotherapy, which encourages fantasy development about the therapist, preferentially increases reflective function when compared with behavioral and supportive interventions. Of course, this finding may not be a result of this particular technique, as there were many distinctions between the treatments. However, as we discuss later (see subsection "Mentalizing Interventions"), focusing on mental representations within a current relationship, drawing the patient's attention to distorted perceptions in the immediacy of the moment, and separating the present from the past are interventions that are likely to maintain a mentalizing mode but *only* once it has been reinstated.

We therefore suggest that as treatment progresses and mentalizing becomes more robust in the sessions, stimulation of fantasy about the therapist becomes less likely to induce feelings in the patient of being misunderstood, less likely to stimulate nonmentalizing, and less likely to cause breaks in the therapeutic alliance leading to dropout early in treatment. Our concern about the development of fantasy relates primarily to the patient's current state of mind and to when, within the trajectory of therapy, it is applied as a technique. We caution against use of this technique early in therapy and/or when the patient is functioning within nonmentalizing mode. Further, we suggest not that stimulation of fantasy is automatically harmful, but that it is a high-risk technique. We therefore have tried to identify the risks.

Third, recognizing that patients operate in psychic equivalence mode also implies that their understanding is characterized by a conviction of being right, and that makes entering into Socratic debates mostly unhelpful. Fourth, patients commonly assume that they know what the therapist is thinking. Technical problems for the therapist will arise if he or she claims primacy for introspection (e.g., saying that he knows his own mind better than the patient knows her own mind). This will lead to fruitless debate. Self-exploration of how the patient has come to her conclusions is probably best. Fifth, in contrast to the therapies that actively withhold self-disclosure, MBT encourages therapists to tactfully disclose what they are feeling. This process is the first element of mentalizing the countertransference, in which therapists accept their internal experience as their own and make no attempt initially to interpret the countertransference as representing a patient's own internal experience. Finally, well-meaning therapists need to beware of telling patients what the patients are feeling. Although stimulation by the therapist of a robust process of identifying and contextualizing internal experience is key to mentalizing, the therapist should not take over the process by deciding what a patient's internal emotional experience "really is."

In addition, MBT has concerns that 1) too much identification of patterns, such as that in schema-focused therapy (Young et al. 2003), might reduce the development of the patient's ability to seek his or her own understanding and 2) relationship patterns tend to multiply and, in psychometric terms, have sensitivity without specificity (i.e., they absolutely are there but are not exclusive to the group). Central to MBT are the mental resources that are available to deal with recurrent patterns of behavior and relationships, rather than identification of the patterns themselves. This emphasis is important clinically. Rather than getting involved in discussing the structure or nature of the relationship that the patient brings, mentalizing therapists focus more on the patient's capacity to think about the relationship. For example, the MBT therapist addresses the rigidity of schematic representations or roles rather than the roles or schemas themselves; the MBT therapist tries to enhance and facilitate flexibility and generate alternative perspectives. We suspect that this process may be one effective component of a number of psychotherapeutic approaches: while the focus is ostensibly more on teasing out the actual roles, it is the action of teasing out, rather than the understanding that the patient arrives at as a consequence of the work, that is crucial.

Mentalizing Stance

Taking a mentalizing or inquisitive or not-knowing stance helps the therapist avoid many of the pitfalls mentioned above. The therapist attempts to capture a sense that mental states are opaque and that she can have no more idea of what is in a patient's mind than the patient does and, in fact, probably will have a lot less. The therapist attempts to demonstrate a willingness to find out about the patient, what makes the patient "tick," how the patient feels, and the reasons for the patient's underlying problems. To do this, the not-knowing therapist needs to become an active questioning therapist, discouraging excessive free association by the patient in favor of detailed monitoring and understanding of the interpersonal processes and how they relate to the patient's mental states. Taking a different perspective from that of the patient is encouraged and should be verbalized and explored, with no assumption being made about whose viewpoint has greater validity. The task is to determine the mental processes that have led to alternative viewpoints and to consider each perspective in relation to the other, accepting that diverse outlooks may be acceptable. Where differences are clear and cannot initially be resolved, they should be identified, stated, and accepted until resolution seems possible. As long as the therapist makes the mind of the patient the focus of the therapeutic endeavors, she will be taking a mentalizing stance.

The Focus on Mentalization

Whatever the mechanisms of therapeutic change might be, traditional psychotherapeutic approaches depend for their effectiveness on the capacity of individuals to consider their experience of their own mental state alongside its re-presentation by the psychotherapist. The appreciation of the difference between one's own experience of one's mind and that presented by another person is a key element of interventions in MBT. Hence, the aim of MBT is to increase mentalizing without engendering too many harmful effects (Fonagy and Bateman 2006b). What we hope of another with whom we interact in therapy is not that the other will go through some gyrations that we have already planned in detail, but that the other will make some contributions to moving forward the joint and cooperative enterprise in which we are both, more or less explicitly, engaged.

The therapist's ability to stimulate a mentalizing process as a core aspect of interacting with others and thinking about oneself inevitably will act in part through a process of identification in which the therapist's ability to use his mind and to demonstrate delight in changing his mind when presented with alternative views and better understanding will be internalized by the patient, who then becomes better able to reappraise herself and her understanding of others. In addition, the continual reworking of perspectives and the understanding of oneself and others in the context of stimulation of the attachment system and within different contexts are key to a change process, as is the necessity to work within current rather than past experience. The therapist's task is to maintain mentalizing and/or to reinstate it in both himself and the patient while simultaneously ensuring that emotional states are active and meaningful. Excess emotional arousal will reduce mentalizing and potentially lead to action, whereas inadequate emphasis on the relationship will allow avoidance of emotional states and a narrowing of contexts within which the patient can function interpersonally and socially. The addition of group therapy to individual sessions increases dramatically the contexts in which this process can take place; therefore, MBT is practiced in both individual and group modes.

Careful assessment of mentalizing and its vicissitudes is made at the outset of treatment. Detailed evaluation of mentalizing vulnerabilities takes place within the first few sessions. Patterns of mentalizing failure and success are identified explicitly with the patient and incorporated into a written formulation that represents the therapist's understanding of the patient's problems in developmental and mentalizing terms. In light of the teleological understanding encountered in the majority of patients with BPD, this formulation is given to the patient in writing (the physical world) and continually reworked with the patient as the patient questions it, challenges the therapist's view, or simply corrects factual inaccuracies. This is an example of explicit mentalizing work in which the representation of the patient as held in the mind of the therapist is presented to the patient, who in turn represents his view of himself to the therapist, who then demonstrates the ability to reappraise her understanding of the patient. The important issue here is stimulation of the interactional mentalizing process and not the accuracy of the formulation. In MBT, interventions serve the function of reinstating or stimulating further the process of mentalizing in different emotional states and a variety of contexts. Insight and accuracy are not the primary objectives.

Mentalizing Interventions

Interventions are organized according to the patient's level of mentalizing capacity as assessed by the therapist at any given time. As a rule of thumb, because mentalizing capacity decreases as emotional states increase, less complex interventions—that is, supportive and empathic interventions, which do not require the patient to consider more than her own state of mind—should be given when the patient is aroused. Figure 28–1 shows the hierarchy of interventions, which increase in level of complexity from surface to depth. At surface, the patient does not have to work on both her own mind and the therapist's state of mind, but at depth the patient has to hold both representations. Therapists are advised to use depth interventions only when the patient's mentalizing capacity is intact and emotional arousal is moderate. Detail of the interventions can be found elsewhere (Bateman and Fonagy 2004, 2006), but some general aspects are discussed here.

Capacities vary considerably within sessions and over time, so the mentalizing therapist has to constantly monitor the patient's state of mind and give interventions accordingly. The clinician should monitor several parameters in relation to the quality of mentalization, including the patient's level of emotional arousal, intensity of attachment, and need to avoid a perceived threat (e.g., from the therapist who is experienced by the patient as hostile or unable to understand). In accordance with MBT's focus on the detail of attachment patterns, a detached attachment pattern requires more therapeutic work to be done within the patient–therapist relationship using mentalizing transference interactions, whereas the enmeshed pattern needs careful titration of the emotional state and intensity of the relationship and typically greater use of validating and empathic techniques.

The primary focus for the therapist has to be the patient's current state of mind, and we therefore place considerable emphasis in MBT on understanding the patient's perspective within a validating context and have structured interventions accordingly. Observing and reflection—two aspects of valida-

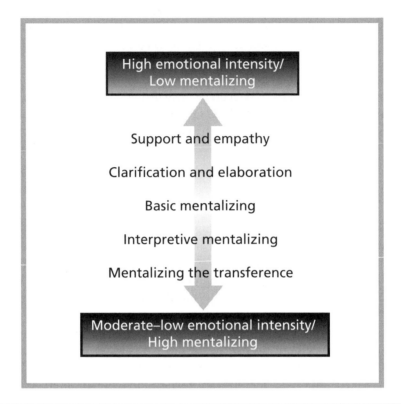

FIGURE 28–1. Levels of mentalizing intervention indicating surface and depth.

Therapists are recommended to link level with patient's emotional intensity and mentalizing capacity.

tion—are common to every therapy and are essential in MBT. However, in promoting validation, we are not suggesting a simple confirmation of the patient's experience and contingent response as being understandable in a specific context, although this must be the first part of any intervention. The patient's experience is rooted in the reality of psychic equivalence, in which alternative perspectives are not possible, and it is the stimulation of alternatives that is at the heart of the mentalizing process. To stimulate this, immediate challenge by the therapist is likely to be futile, and the initial focus instead is on exploration and on elaborating a multifaceted representation based on current experience, particularly with the therapist. Therefore, validation of patient experience moves gradually toward exploration in the current therapeutic relationship, but first the therapist must demonstrate understanding of the patient's experience as real and justified. Only when that is established can alternative perspectives be placed into the dialogue. Even then, in keeping with the "not-knowing" or inquisitive stance of the therapist, this process is understood as impressionistic and the therapist contribution is considered as having no more or less validity than that of the patient—together they should arrive at an understanding, but it is likely to be the therapist who teases out an alternative perspective. It is this teasing out of an alternative perspective that forms the core of mentalizing the transference.

We use the phrase "mentalizing the transference" to differentiate our approach from other ways of using transference, such as interpretive work that places a premium on genetic reconstructions. Nonetheless, we recognize that careful interpretive work can be effective in the treatment of patients with BPD; such work is exemplified by transference-focused psychotherapy (Clarkin et al. 1999). From our point of view, transference interventions in transference-focused psychotherapy are effective by virtue of being conducted in a way that helps patients to remain in the mentalizing mode. Specifically, these interventions place a premium on clarity, recurrently bring the patient's attention back to central themes, carefully link behavior to a hypothetical model of the patient's mind, maintain an interpersonal focus, and move systematically from clarifications to interpretations. Hence, albeit focused more on mental contents than mental processes, such interventions have the potential not only to maintain mentalizing but also to improve mentalizing capacity.

To reiterate, interpretive interventions have the potential to promote mentalizing in patients who are able to remain in the mentalizing mode and to hold multiple perspectives in mind in the face of strong affects. Focusing on mental representations, such interpretive work usually bolsters mentalizing in the sense of drawing patients' attention to distorted perceptions and interpretations of present interactions in the context of understanding the basis of these distortions in past relationships. Indeed, one of the hallmarks of mentalizing is separating the present from the past—as is critical in patients who are prone to reexperiencing trauma in PTSD, for example. As discussed earlier, such traumatized patients are liable to be operating in the psychic equivalence mode, in which case bringing them back to the mentalizing mode is the first priority before any other work can be done.

The major difficulty in conveying the distinctiveness of our approach boils down to our understanding of the term *transference*. We are often asked if we use transference, and MBT has been characterized as "a dynamic psychotherapy that specifically eschews transference interpretation" (Gabbard 2006). Here we need a clarification: When asked if we use transference, our standard reply is, "It all depends on what you mean by 'transference.'" Do we focus on the therapist–patient relationship in the hope that discussion concerning this relationship will contribute to the patient's well-being? In that case, the answer is a most emphatic yes. Do we use the transference to provide an explanation of present behavior as based on unconscious repetition of past behavior? Then the answer is an almost equally emphatic no. Although we might well point to similarities among the therapy relationship, current attachment relationships, and childhood attachment relationships, we do not aim to provide patients with an explanation (insight) that they might be able to use to control their behavior pattern, and we have already mentioned our concern about a focus on delineation of patterns of relationships. Rather, transference provides an opportunity to address how the patient's mind is working with the therapist in the room. Fundamentally, we hope to evoke the patient's curiosity in considering relationship patterns as just one of many other puzzling phenomena that require thought and contemplation as part of our general inquisitive, not-knowing stance aimed to facilitate the recovery of mentalizing.

Thus, "mentalizing the transference" is a shorthand phrase for encouraging patients to think about the relationship they are in at the current moment. We aim to focus patients' attention on another mind, the mind of a therapist, and to assist the patients in the task of contrasting their own perception of themselves with how they are perceived by others—by the therapist or indeed by other members of a psychotherapy group. We emphasize using the transference to show patients how the same behavior may be experienced differently and thought about differently by different minds. For example, a patient's experience of the therapist as persecutory and demanding, destructive and cruelly critical, is one perception among many others. It may be a valid perception, given the therapist's behavior, but there may be alternative ways of construing the therapist's behavior. Once again, the aim is not to give insight to patients as to why they are distorting their perception of the therapist in a specific way, but rather to engender curiosity as to why, given the ambiguity of interpersonal situations, they choose and stick to a specific version. In encouraging them to wonder why they might be doing this, we hope to help them recover the capacity to mentalize and, in so doing, to give up the rigid, schematic, psychic equivalence mode of interpreting their subjectivity and others' behavior.

Once an alternative perspective about an interaction is identified, the therapist must monitor not only his or her own reaction but that of the patient. The joint reaction then becomes the focus of the session, and so the process moves on. It is especially important to note again that the aim is not to increase insight and understanding—for example, about the contribution of the past to the present—but to repair a current break in the self-structure and to facilitate mentalizing within the context of an emotional interaction. The process of therapy becomes more important than the content.

Conclusion

Overall, therapists and therapies should be modest both in their aims and in their claims. Although it may be clear from this chapter that we consider, perhaps rather grandiosely, mentalizing to be the best theoretical concept to describe the mental process that makes us human, we hope that it is also clear that we equally consider there to be little new in mentalizing therapy itself. MBT is a refocusing of therapy rather than a new therapy. Our primary claim is to have brought together the developmental processes that enhance or undermine mentalizing and translated them into therapeutic practice. We do not wish to present a false modesty about this achievement, and we are aware of how little we know and how much more there is to learn about mentalizing as a theoretical construct and as a treatment focus. It is this that makes it such an exciting area. We hope that others will enjoy mentalizing as much as we do but will at times, like us, occasionally take satisfaction from not mentalizing.

Key Points

- Mentalizing is a unifying process of many psychotherapies.

- Disruption in mentalizing contributes to the development of a number of mental disorders, including borderline personality disorder (BPD), post-traumatic stress disorder, eating disorders, and depression.

- A core problem in BPD is a fragile mentalizing capacity.

- Treatment of BPD has to focus on engendering a mentalizing process while stimulating the attachment relationship between patient and therapist.

- Therapists should be aware that psychotherapy may have harmful as well as beneficial effects. Harmful effects tend to be mediated through stimulation of a nonmentalizing process.

- Therapists must ensure that interventions take into account the patient's level of mentalizing capacity.

References

Allen JG: Traumatic Relationships and Serious Mental Disorders. Chichester, England, Wiley, 2001

Allen JG, Fonagy P (eds): Handbook of Mentalization-Based Treatment. Chichester, England, Wiley, 2006

Allen JG, Bleiberg E, Haslam-Hopwood T: Mentalizing as a compass for treatment. Bull Menninger Clin 67:1–11, 2003

Allen JG, Fonagy P, Bateman A: Mentalizing in Clinical Practice. Washington, DC, American Psychiatric Publishing, 2008

Arnsten AF: The biology of being frazzled. Science 280:1711–1712, 1998

Baron-Cohen S, Tager-Flusberg H, Cohen DJ: Understanding Other Minds: Perspectives From Autism and Developmental Cognitive Neuroscience. Oxford, England, Oxford University Press, 2000

Bateman A, Fonagy P: The effectiveness of partial hospitalization in the treatment of borderline personality disorder—a randomized controlled trial. Am J Psychiatry 156:1563–1569, 1999

Bateman A, Fonagy P: Treatment of borderline personality disorder with psychoanalytically oriented partial hospitalization: an 18-month follow-up. Am J Psychiatry 158:36–42, 2001

Bateman A, Fonagy P: Psychotherapy for Borderline Personality Disorder: Mentalization-Based Treatment. Oxford, England, Oxford University Press, 2004

Bateman A, Fonagy P: Mentalization-Based Treatment for Borderline Personality Disorder: A Practical Guide. Oxford, England, Oxford University Press, 2006

Battle CL, Shea MT, Johnson DM, et al: Childhood maltreatment associated with adult personality disorder: findings from the Collaborative Longitudinal Personality Disorders Study. J Personal Disord 18:193–211, 2004

Bowlby J: A Secure Base: Clinical Applications of Attachment Theory. London, Routledge & Kegan Paul, 1988

Clarkin JF, Kernberg OF, Yeomans F: Transference-Focused Psychotherapy for Borderline Personality Disorder Patients. New York, Guilford, 1999

Crandell L, Patrick M, Hobson RF: "Still-face" interactions between mothers with borderline personality disorder and their 2-month-old infants. Br J Psychiatry 183:239–247, 2003

Everson MD, Hunter WM, Runyon DK, et al: Maternal support following disclosure of incest. Am J Orthopsychiatry 59:197–207, 1989

Fearon P, Target M, Fonagy P, et al: Short-term mentalization and relational therapy (SMART): an integrative family therapy for children and adolescents, in Handbook of Mentalization-Based Treatment. Edited by Allen JG, Fonagy P. Chichester, England, Wiley, 2006, pp 201–222

Fischer KW, Kenny SL, Pipp SL: How cognitive processes and environmental conditions organize discontinuities in the development of abstractions, in Higher Stages of Development. Edited by Alexander CN, Langer EJ, Oetzel RM. Oxford, England, Oxford University Press, 1990, pp 162–187

Fonagy P, Bateman A: Mechanisms of change in mentalization-based treatment of BPD. J Clin Psychol 62:411–430, 2006a

Fonagy P, Bateman A: Progress in the treatment of borderline personality disorder (editorial). Br J Psychiatry 188:1–3, 2006b

Fonagy P, Bateman A: The development of borderline personality disorder—a mentalizing model. J Personal Disord 22:4–21, 2008

Fonagy P, Target M, Gergely G, et al: Affect Regulation, Mentalization, and the Development of Self. London, Other Press, 2002

Frith CD: Schizophrenia and theory of mind. Psychol Med 34:385–389, 2004

Fruzzetti AE, Shenk C, Lowry K, et al: Emotion regulation, in Cognitive Behavior Therapy: Applying Empirically Supported Techniques in Your Practice. Edited by O'Donohue WT, Fisher JE, Hayes SC. New York, Wiley, 2003, pp 152–159

Fruzzetti AE, Shenk C, Hoffman PD: Family interaction and the development of borderline personality disorder: a transactional model. Dev Psychopathol 17:1007–1030, 2005

Gabbard G: When is transference work useful in dynamic psychotherapy? Am J Psychiatry 163:1667–1669, 2006

Gallagher HL, Frith CD: Functional imaging of "theory of mind." Trends Cogn Sci 7:77–83, 2003

Gallagher HL, Happe F, Brunswick N, et al: Reading the mind in cartoons and stories: an fMRI study of "theory of mind" in verbal and nonverbal tasks. Neuropsychologia 38:11–21, 2000

Hamilton CE: Continuity and discontinuity of attachment from infancy through adolescence. Child Dev 71:690–694, 2000

Hobbs M, Mayou R, Harrison B, et al: A randomised controlled trial of psychological debriefing for victims of road traffic accidents. BMJ 313:1438–1439, 1996

Holmes J: Mentalizing from a psychoanalytic perspective: what's new? in Handbook of Mentalization-Based Treatment. Edited by Allen JG, Fonagy P. Chichester, England, Wiley, 2006, pp 31–39

Horwitz AV, Widom CS, McLaughlin J, et al: The impact of childhood abuse and neglect on adult mental health: a prospective study. J Health Soc Behav 42:184–201, 2001

James W: The Principles of Psychology (1890). Cambridge, MA, Harvard University Press, 1983

Lane RD: Neural correlates of conscious emotional experience, in Cognitive Neuroscience of Emotion. Edited by Lane RD, Nadel L. New York, Oxford University Press, 2000, pp 345–370

Levy KN: The implications of attachment theory and research for understanding borderline personality disorder. Dev Psychopathol 17:959–986, 2005

Levy KN, Meehan KB, Kelly KM, et al: Change in attachment patterns and reflective function in a randomized control trial of transference-focused psychotherapy for borderline personality disorder. J Consult Clin Psychol 74:1027–1040, 2006

Linehan MM: Cognitive-Behavioral Treatment of Borderline Personality Disorder. New York, Guilford, 1993

Lyons-Ruth K, Jacobovitz D: Attachment disorganization: unresolved loss, relational violence and lapses in behavioral and attentional strategies, in Handbook of Attachment Theory and Research. Edited by Cassidy J, Shaver PR. New York, Guilford, 1999, pp 520–554

Lyons-Ruth K, Yellin C, Melnick S, et al: Expanding the concept of unresolved mental states: hostile/helpless states of mind on the Adult Attachment Interview are associated with disrupted mother-infant communication and infant disorganization. Dev Psychopathol 17:1–23, 2005

Posner MI, Rothbart MK, Vizueta N, et al: Attentional mechanisms of borderline personality disorder. Proc Natl Acad Sci USA 99:16366–16370, 2002

Skårderud F: Eating one's words, Part III: mentalisation-based psychotherapy for anorexia nervosa—an outline for a treatment and training manual. Eur Eat Disord Rev 15:323–339, 2007

Sroufe LA, Egeland B, Carlson E, et al: The Development of the Person: The Minnesota Study of Risk and Adaptation From Birth to Adulthood. New York, Guilford, 2005

Steimer-Krause E, Krause IB, Watson C: Interaction regulations used by schizophrenics and psychosomatic patients. Psychiatry 53:209–228, 1990

Waters E, Merrick SK, Treboux D, et al: Attachment security from infancy to early adulthood. Child Dev 71:684–689, 2000

Weinfield N, Sroufe LA, Egeland B: Attachment from infancy to early adulthood in a high risk sample: continuity, discontinuity and their correlates. Child Dev 71:695–702, 2000

Young JE, Klosko JS, Weishaar ME: Schema Therapy: A Practitioner's Guide. New York, Guilford, 2003

Zanarini MC, Frankenburg FR, Reich DB, et al: Biparental failure in the childhood experiences of borderline patients. J Personal Disord 14:264–273, 2000

Suggested Readings

Allen JG, Fonagy P (eds): Handbook of Mentalization-Based Treatment. Chichester, England, Wiley, 2006

Allen JG, Fonagy P, Bateman AW: Mentalizing in Clinical Practice. Washington, DC, American Psychiatric Publishing, 2008

Bateman A, Fonagy P: Psychotherapy for Borderline Personality Disorder: Mentalization-Based Treatment. Oxford, England, Oxford University Press, 2004

Fonagy P, Bateman A: Mechanisms of change in mentalization-based treatment of BPD. J Clin Psychol 62:411–430, 2006

Fonagy P, Bateman A: Progress in the treatment of borderline personality disorder (editorial). Br J Psychiatry 188:1–3, 2006

Gunderson JG, Hoffman PD (eds): Understanding and Treating Borderline Personality Disorder: A Guide for Professionals and Families. Washington, DC, American Psychiatric Publishing, 2005

Kernberg O, Clarkin JF, Yeomans FE: A Primer of Transference Focused Psychotherapy for the Borderline Patient. New York, Jason Aronson, 2002

Krawitz R, Watson C: Borderline Personality Disorder: A Practical Guide to Treatment. Oxford, England, Oxford University Press, 2003

Chapter 29

Brain Processes Informing Psychotherapy

George I. Viamontes, M.D., Ph.D.
Bernard D. Beitman, M.D.

Successful psychotherapy is correlated with discrete brain changes (Etkin et al. 2005; Roffman et al. 2005) because psychotherapy, like medication, ultimately targets neuroanatomical structures and modulates their function. Early evidence suggests that concepts such as extinction, free association, cognitive restructuring, and repression can be mapped onto the brain (Roffman et al. 2005). Because of the direct correspondence of therapeutic processes to specific neural phenomena, and the power that knowing the details of these phenomena can provide, we argue that psychotherapists should learn the brain. The rationale that supports our opinion is presented in the first section of this chapter, "Reasons for Developing a Neurobiology of Psychotherapy."

Many psychotherapists challenge the need to learn neurobiology, claiming that knowledge of psychotherapeutic theory and technique is sufficient for successful outcomes. Clinicians sometimes argue that there is too much to learn about the brain while, at the same time, knowledge about psychotherapy theory and technique continues to expand. Fears of information overload are therefore not uncommon. To address these concerns, the field must attempt to define a cohesive set of neurobiological concepts that apply specifically to psychotherapy. In the second section of the chapter, we begin this process by presenting some of the basic neuroanatomy that underlies the brain-mind phenomena of engagement, self-observation, and pattern search. We also explore some of the brain correlates of classical psychotherapeutic concepts.

More than these correlates, however, are needed for a successful adaptation of neurobiology to psychotherapy. Clinicians need practical concepts that bridge mind and brain—ideas that encourage them to seek greater knowledge of neurobiology so they can understand how their thoughts, words, and nonverbal behaviors can physically influence the brain of the other. In the third section, "Neurobiological Empathy," we engage in disciplined speculation from current knowledge with an eye toward clinical utility. The ideas presented are not restricted to either "mind" or "brain"; instead, they bridge the Cartesian dualism that isolates psychotherapy from its biological underpinnings by creating mind–brain conceptualizations for the targets of psychotherapeutic change. We use the term *neurobiological empathy* to describe these attempts to know the mind-brain of our patients. It is an objective process that provides special insight into a patient's mental processes through an understanding of the neural deficits that are causing the patient's psychopathology.

In the chapter's next section we address *mirror neurons*, an exciting discovery in neurobiology that has direct applications to psychotherapy. Mirror neurons are specialized circuits in the brains of primates that map the perceived actions of others for the purpose of determining their meaning. Therapists affect the mirror neurons of patients, and vice versa; therefore, the meaning that each participant derives from therapeutic interactions is a synthesis of observations, internal representations, and innate pattern recognition. This complicates communication but at the same time provides an opportunity for uncovering problems in the representational and pattern-matching processes of patients. Mirror neurons provide a neurobiological explanation for a variety of psychotherapeutic phenomena, including some aspects of transference and countertransference.

We conclude the chapter with a review of functional imaging studies that define the neural activation patterns that characterize common psychiatric illnesses and the changes brought about by psychotherapy. It is clear that psychiatric illnesses affect a variety of neural circuits at both cortical and subcortical levels, and that psychotherapy has measurable effects on the functioning of these circuits. Although the complexity of neural circuitry and the lack of uniformity among studies have made it difficult to draw definitive conclusions, a number of trends have emerged that are helpful in understanding how psychotherapy restores the working capacity of malfunctioning neural circuits.

Reasons for Developing a Neurobiology of Psychotherapy

As discussed at the opening of this chapter, we believe it is important for psychotherapists to learn the brain. We enumerate here six reasons why this knowledge is valuable:

1. *Psychotherapy theory is in conceptual disarray.* There are too many schools, too many theories, and too many strategies and techniques. A brain-based infrastructure promises to provide solid grounding for basic psychotherapeutic concepts. This conceptual solidity will help to organize the disparate orientations and allow nonpsychotherapists to grasp more firmly the unique and helpful mechanisms of psychotherapeutic action.

2. *Payers are confused.* Customers, including patients, businesses, the government, and managed care companies, want positive outcomes, not theoretical debates. They want empirically based descriptions of the interpersonal technology of psychotherapy, as well as clarity about the roles of the participants. They want to know more accurately what psychotherapy does.

3. *Brain circuitry is the final common pathway for the ever-expanding set of methods that can be used to alleviate psychological distress.* In addition to psychotherapy, these include such divergent processes as meditation, prayer, friendship, and psychoactive substances, both legal and illegal. It can be productive to visualize our role as therapists in a wider context and think of ourselves as change agents who rely primarily on psychotherapeutic methods. An approach to psychotherapy informed by both mind and brain will sharpen technical, strategic, and theoretical foci by insisting that all theoretical constructs can be mapped onto discrete brain functions.

4. *Brain-informed psychotherapy will confirm the validity of many existing concepts and techniques, as well as disconfirm less empirically based ideas that may seem useful on the surface but actually have little connection to brain function.* Eye movement desensitization and reprocessing (EMDR), for example, is a widely practiced treatment for posttraumatic stress disorder. Yet, the neurobiological underpinnings of EMDR remain unknown and continue to elicit wide debate. It is entirely possible that when the neurobiology of the process is clarified, the eye movements that characterize the technique might not actually be an essential therapeutic element.

On the other hand, if the importance of eye movements in delivering the benefits of EMDR were to be scientifically proven, then the EMDR process could serve to clarify the function of important brain circuits.

5. *Brain-informed psychotherapy can help to simplify psychotherapeutic language.* For example, most therapies include instruction to keep doing that which seems helpful but use a variety of terms for this concept, including "practice," "working through," and "behavioral rehearsal." Psychotherapeutic change is actually based on increasing the probability of triggering adaptive rather than maladaptive pathways within the brain. When adaptive pathways do not exist, psychotherapy will be more difficult because these pathways will have to be created. To increase the probability of triggering adaptive pathways, they must be more firmly instantiated in the brain than less preferable ones. Here, the language of change could be simplified to describe the brain changes that maximize the probability of firing more adaptive circuits.

6. *By knowing how the phenomena that underlie core psychotherapeutic concepts and processes are generated in brain circuits, psychotherapists will become clearer about their psychotherapeutic intentions, more empirical in their understanding of illness, and more confident in their techniques.* It will eventually be possible to visualize the neurobiological targets for producing behavioral change, as well as the neural mechanisms by which psychotherapeutic interventions exert their effects.

The ultimate goal of this chapter is to introduce neurobiology that is relevant to psychotherapy, with the hope of encouraging therapists to learn more (for expansion of these ideas, see Viamontes et al. 2005). We would like to awaken interest in how the brain works during psychotherapy's basic processes, as outlined in the following section. With a deeper appreciation of the underlying neurobiology, therapists may be stimulated to put flesh on the bones of their own therapeutic processes in the context of functional neuroanatomy.

Neural Correlates of Basic Psychotherapeutic Processes

As was suggested in Chapter 26 ("Theory and Practice of Psychotherapy Integration"), numerous reviews (Lambert and Bergin 1994; Lambert et al. 1986) and meta-analyses (Ahn and Wampold 2001; Prochaska and Norcross 2003) have demonstrated that no psychotherapy is inherently superior to any other, although all are superior to no treatment. These bodies of research also suggest that a core set of features shared by all therapies accounts for a significant portion of client symptomatic improvement.

Psychotherapy has a basic structure defined by a set of core processes (Beitman and Yue 2004), among which are engagement (the establishment of the working alliance), self-awareness, pattern search, change, termination, transference, countertransference, and resistance. This definition of core processes aids the task of mapping psychotherapy onto the brain by simplifying the wide variety of professional terms currently used to describe the psychotherapeutic process. We begin the task of linking core psychotherapeutic processes to specific circuits in the brain by describing some of the neural substrates that support the critical functions of engagement, self-observation, and pattern search.

Engagement

The strength of the working alliance has been the most studied process variable, and it has been shown to correlate positively with psychotherapeutic outcome (Krupnick et al. 1996; Wampold 2001). In fact, the working alliance—"the collaborative and affective bond between therapist and patient"—may be considered the therapeutic "quintessential integrative variable" (Wolfe and Goldfried 1988, p. 250).

When a therapist first encounters a patient, he or she immediately infers the patient's emotional state by observing facial expression, verbal output, and bodily demeanor. Work by Rizzolatti et al. (2001) showed that a critical neural processing step must occur prior to the transformation of observation to inference. Before the meaning of bodily movements and emotional expressions can be understood, these observations must be modeled in the therapist's brain (Rizzolatti et al. 2001). An array of mirror neurons found in the primate premotor region and in the parietal cortex become activated when the actions and expressions of others are modeled internally (Rizzolatti et al. 2001). The "meaning" of what the therapist senses both physically and emotionally when observing others is therefore an amalgam of actual observations and an internal transformation. The ability to be empathic and to accurately identify what a patient is "feeling" depends completely on the adequacy of the therapist's own limbic and cognitive circuitry. As such, the training of psychotherapists is, in great part, a tuning of brain circuitry to permit the accurate neural modeling of clinical observations and subsequent extraction of their "meaning."

As a therapist considers a patient's brain, the therapist can search for the neural source of the patient's emotional state. Imaging studies suggest that the patient's outward signs of anxiety—sweaty palms, quivering voice, motor agitation—are the result of activation of the neural circuits that detect risk and prepare the body to take appropriate action (Rolls 2005). Risk-detection circuitry is centered in the amygdala and orbitofrontal cortex (Rolls

1999, 2005). Both of these structures contain genetically preprogrammed information about natural "punishers"—that is, sensory perceptions (e.g., bitter tastes or pain) that throughout the evolutionary history of humans have been connected with unpleasant outcomes.

In addition, the amygdala and orbitofrontal cortex contain a record of the unpleasant experiences encountered throughout the person's lifetime. These experiences are encoded in the form of synaptic linkages between previously neutral stimuli associated with an unpleasant experience and the genetically determined collection of natural "punishers" that is already represented (Rolls 2005). For example, human infants quickly connect the sight of a syringe with pain and show signs of distress before immunizations. Many people with hypertension paradoxically increase their blood pressure just as it is about to be measured, because the measurement process has become associated with unpleasant outcomes in the past. This phenomenon, which involves arousal as a response to cognitive information, requires activation of the dorsal anterior cingulate gyrus (Critchley et al. 2003), which in turn triggers autonomic centers.

The anxious patient in front of the therapist is focused intensely on his or her set of symptoms and wonders how the therapist could possibly "understand" this distress, given the therapist's privileged position of power and success. Instinctively, and without any knowledge of neurobiology, the patient senses that it will be difficult for the therapist to internally model the subjective components of his or her singularly unpleasant mental state. The cognitive uncertainties of the initial meeting with the therapist can cause even more autonomic arousal through the combined action of the dorsolateral prefrontal cortex (DLPFC), which represents current cognitive contents, and the cingulate gyrus, which generates autonomic tone consistent with those contents (Critchley et al. 2003).

As the therapist works toward successful therapeutic engagement, critical steps must include relief of this initial cognitive tension through an exchange of cognitive and emotional signals, until the therapist is indeed capable of "understanding," or internally modeling, the patient's situation. If engagement is successfully negotiated, then the therapeutic process can proceed. Eventually, previously neutral stimuli related to the therapist may become linked to experiences of reward in the patient's brain. This process is also believed to involve synaptic modifications in the amygdala and orbitofrontal cortex, in a manner similar to what was described for unpleasant experiences (Rolls 2005).

As the patient begins to associate the therapist with symptom reduction and positive emotions, reward circuits and other areas in the patient's brain that represent gratifying social interactions are likely to be activated. For example, imaging studies have shown that internal representations of individuals perceived as "cooperative" in interactive situations elicit activation of the nucleus accumbens, which is at the center of reward circuitry (Viamontes and Beitman 2006b), as well as the orbitofrontal cortex, fusiform gyrus, superior temporal sulcus, and insula (Ferris et al. 2004). We can hypothesize that excessive activation of reward circuitry may underlie the strong emotional attachments that patients can develop toward therapists.

Within the trusting, confiding psychotherapeutic relationship, patients can frequently reflect upon their emotionally laden difficulties in ways that would have been impossible outside therapy. Secure relationships such as can be achieved in therapy are associated with enhanced resiliency, as suggested by studies of traumatized children (Main 1991). In response to major losses such as the death of a parent, divorce, or major parental illness, children who were securely attached to their mothers were more resilient and less affected by the stressors than were other children. To be resilient is to be able to recognize that the "map is not the territory" or, in other words, that neural representations of the outside world, which incorporate both external and internal contents, are not equivalent to reality. Experimental evidence suggests that secure attachment, as extrapolated from imaging studies of romantic love (Bartels and Zeki 2000) and mother–child affection (Bartels and Zeki 2004), is associated with reduction in amygdala firing (lessening anxiety), increases in nucleus accumbens activity (possibly related to enhanced reward representations), and lessening of orbitofrontal firing (possibly reducing inhibitions). Within the secure attachment achieved through basic psychotherapeutic engagement techniques, circuits associated with negative emotions, social judgment, and "mentalizing" (Viamontes and Beitman 2006a) can be activated safely through verbal means, and their consequences can be explored. This controlled activation of negative contents within the psychotherapeutic relationship helps liberate the patient from past constraints, permitting the exploration of new interpersonal concepts (Fonagy 2004). The common mechanism for such self-exploration is likely the activation of self-observation (Beitman and Soth 2006).

Self-Observation

Self-observation can produce knowledge about many internal states, such as intentions, expectations, feelings, thoughts, behaviors, and perceived effect on others. It can also enhance the capacity for introspection and anchor the person's understanding of his or her relationship with the environment (Stuss and Benson 1983). Self-observation increases the ability to "distinguish inner from outer reality, pretend from 'real' modes of functioning, and intrapersonal mental and emotional processes from interpersonal communications" (Greenspan 2004). Psychotherapy, specifically the psychotherapeutic relationship, offers the opportunity to create and function within a "reflective space" that enhances the power to explore current maps of reality and alter them. Self-observation is a distinct process that can be distinguished from consciousness, awareness, and self-awareness.

Consciousness, in the strictest neurological sense, refers simply to the waking state. This type of consciousness requires firing of the reticular activating system, as well as the integrity of basic homeostatic processes such as breathing, cardiac function, and autonomic tone. It represents the "general capacity that an individual possesses for particular kinds of mental representations and subjective experiences" that are "not directed at anything" (Wheeler et al. 1997, p. 335). One must be conscious in order to be aware.

Awareness—the "particular manifestation or expression" that "always has an object" (Wheeler et al. 1997, p. 337)—implies consciousness of content, such as a cloud, another person, or a painful experience. Self-awareness is a special type of awareness that is focused on the "object" of the self. The act of being self-aware encompasses the potential to observe the subjective neural representations of the self and to "model" internally an inferred representation of what others may think about the self (Beitman et al. 2005). Self-observation, in contrast, is an open-ended exploratory process that motivates the active scanning of one's inner world. In this context, observations can be made dispassionately, and without criticism or evaluation (Deikman 1982).

When observing oneself, one may focus attention on the totality of one's subjective reality, which includes representations of the self's experiences in the past, present, and future (Wheeler et al. 1997). The broad reflective potential of self-observation allows one to marshal the resources of self-awareness to alter prediction errors (Pally 2005). This capability provides a sense of agency, an "I" who is observing, planning, deciding, and evolving toward a future goal. Most psychotherapies help clients to activate their self-observational capacities, with the primary intention of altering faulty predictions and expectations (Beitman et al. 2005; Pally 2005).

The ability to observe the content of one's own mind depends on the healthy functioning of many different parts of the brain. To begin the process, one must be awake, with an intact brain stem and a functioning reticular activating system. Next, the objects of self-observation, which are neural representations in the various functional circuits that drive cognition, emotion, and behavior, must be accessed and integrated in working memory. The basic representation of the visceral self, along with a variety of internal states, can be obtained by accessing the insula; objects and space are represented in the temporal and parietal cortices; risk–reward considerations are continuously generated by the amygdala, orbitofrontal cortex, and nucleus accumbens; and episodic and semantic memories can be recalled by accessing the hippocampus and connected cortices. Cognitive considerations are generated in the lateral prefrontal cortices, and the strongest current focus of behavioral attention, whether internal or external, is represented by activity in the cingulate. Activity within regions along the border between the rostral anterior cingulate and the medial prefrontal cortex is associated with representations of mental states of the self (Frith and Frith 1999) and is consistently activated during self-reflective thought (Johnson et al. 2002). The top of this functioning pyramid of self-awareness appears to be the DLPFC, which potentiates executive function and working memory (Wheeler et al. 1997) and is capable of integrating the full range of sensory, affective, and memory data.

The ability to generate a coherent self with temporal continuity depends on the power of the DLPFC to project individuals both backward and forward in time (Wheeler et al. 1997). People with damage to the DLPFC may lose the temporal sense of themselves. They may not recall episodic representations of past experiences and may be unable to project themselves into the future. The DLPFC and the right parietal lobe help to define the person in space and time by placing the body in the three physical dimensions, as well as in the past, present, and future. Without this sense, the self erodes and merges with its environment. During meditation, the right parietal lobe may decrease its activity, which can induce dissolution of the sense of self in space and time (Newberg et al. 2002). Other studies have shown that disturbances of the temporoparietal region can generate "out of body" experiences, in which an individual has the sensation of floating above the ground and observing his or her body below (Blanke and Arzy 2005).

As part of its integrating function, the DLPFC receives inputs from a variety of internal monitors. The insula, for example (Phillips et al. 2003), monitors visceral sensations as well as emotional body states, whereas the anterior cingulate can focus attention for the process of self-monitoring (Gusnard et al. 2001). In a clinical context, the dysfunction of prefrontal circuits that characterizes schizophrenia is thought to play an important role in the clinical finding that many patients with schizophrenia lack awareness of their disorder (Flashman 2005).

The current interest in the study of mindful awareness is likely to be supplemented by an expansion of knowledge about the neural circuitry that underlies self-observation. As researchers continue to acquire and integrate this information, self-observation will come to be viewed as another brain-based skill that can be developed not only in clients, but also in psychotherapists. In psychotherapy, the primary intent of self-observation is to uncover dysfunctional patterns that, if changed, will lead to relief of symptoms and improved functioning.

Pattern Search

A major task of the central nervous system is to organize the linkage between internal representations of sensory information and adaptive responses (Mesulam 1998). The brain creates patterns from the huge array of sensory information that it processes, to make sense of the environment in ways that optimize individual- and species-survival functions, including homeostasis, reproduction, and energy acquisition and conservation (Viamontes et al. 2005). Smaller brains cope with this challenge by developing inflexible bonds between sensation and action that are resistant to change. Larger brains have more flexible stimulus–response connections and therefore can have a wider range of alternative responses to specific environmental cues (Tanaka 2003). Smaller brains represent the world at a much coarser level of resolution because they have fewer cortical columns to devote to each aspect of represented reality. The simplification of the brain that can result from chronic stress or illness (Teicher et al. 2002) is relevant to this discussion. Although such simplification conserves energy and facilitates rapid responses, it can theoretically decrease the "richness" of experiences by limiting the amount of complexity that is represented.

An important component of habitual behavior is the formation of internal patterns that can be used to organize external stimuli, determine their "meaning," and respond to them. Humans are remarkably adept at inductive reasoning, which is the ability to infer complete patterns from perception of just a small number of their elements. Even advanced computers have difficulty matching the inductive power of the brain. People can recognize a song from a few notes, a person from a few words, and a concept from a single phrase. Effective psychotherapists induce patterns from nonverbal cues, key reported events, transference behaviors, and countertransference reactions (Beitman and Yue 2004). Psychotherapists can then help patients become aware of their internal patterns and drive therapeutic change by crystallizing awareness of maladaptive stimulus–response connections and ways in which these might be altered.

Understanding the brain's mechanisms for pattern recognition represents a major challenge for computational and neural sciences. Among the many perplexing questions is whether computational neuroscientists should attempt to mimic the brain with respect to pattern recognition, or develop an entirely different set of algorithms. Important clues about the brain's ability to recognize patterns have been gleaned from studies of visual pattern recognition. The following description of this process is quite simplified—many of the described functions are not localized but rather widely distributed within the named area (Haxby et al. 2001)—but it provides important insights into pattern recognition.

Visual inputs are first transmitted to the occipital cortex and then routed to the lateral inferior occipital lobe, where a "prepattern" is developed—an intelligent organization of the inputs. The data are sent to the fusiform gyrus in the ventral temporal lobe, where they are divided into at least two categories—namely, faces or objects. From the fusiform gyrus, the data continue to be transmitted rostrally. At the temporal pole, the object's identity is further clarified and integrated with limbic information. Data about the object are transmitted simultaneously to the parietal cortex, where the object is placed in three-dimensional space. Processed information about the object is sent to the entorhinal cortex, where its past significance is determined, and also to the DLPFC, where its implications for the future are elaborated.

Our experiences are organized by the facilitated pathways for information processing that have been encoded in our brains throughout our lifetimes. These facilitated pathways organize our perceptions of reality and allow us to perform activities of daily living. These pathways or patterns in our brains create expectations: if this happens, then that will follow. A remarkable corollary of these experiential encodings is that they can induce the generation of expectations from neutral circumstances. We find what we seek because we expect it to be there. For example, the expectations of a person who believes that he or she will be rejected are inevitably fulfilled, in part because the expectation itself creates the circumstances for rejection.

Behavioral patterns are deeply ingrained and manifest themselves in many settings, from the therapist's office to the work environment, and certainly throughout the whole spectrum of personal relationships. Therapists also expect to find certain patterns: past–present connections, narcissistic injury, hidden anger, cognitive distortions, role–relationship conflicts, and many others. Some clinicians even have a "favorite" diagnosis, and a disproportionate number of their patients are identified as fitting its characteristic constellation of symptoms.

Patterns that organize perceptions and expectations in a maladaptive manner are at the core of many psychiatric disorders. In neurobiological terms, these faulty expectations are sometimes called pathological attractors, because input data are channeled toward them, and they invariably lead to maladaptive behavioral outputs. Angry, impulsive, passive, or anxious excesses are the products of inputs channeled through pathological attractors that connect to excessive outputs.

Consider the "black-and-white" thinking that is characteristic of many patients, especially those with borderline personality disorder. How might experience create black versus white attractors? One possible model involves the hippocampus, which may shrink in size with trauma (Teicher et al. 2002), although some controversy remains about this claim. The simplification of brain structures can have adaptive value in chronically stressful situations, as it conserves energy and shortens the stimulus-to-response interval. However, it also limits function.

If traumatic experiences do indeed cause hippocampal simplification, then when patients with borderline personality disorder suffer numerous traumatic events, the functions of their hippocampal circuitry are likely to be affected. Specifically, simplification of the CA3 (cornu ammonis region 3) may reduce dendritic and axonal arborization, fostering excessive compression and simplification of information. In addition, damage to the dentate gyrus limits new cell production, which in turn may hinder the process of encoding new, differentiated memory patterns (Kemperman 2002).

Brain Correlates of Classical Psychotherapeutic Concepts

Sigmund Freud (1923) defined *ego, superego,* and *id* to segregate three functional modalities whose interplay, in his estimation, were central drivers of human behavior. Even if one does not agree with Freud's theoretical constructs, it is not difficult to understand the neurobiology that motivated his basic conceptualizations. The constant tension between unconscious appetitive urges and higher control that characterizes Freud's visualization has a definable origin in neural circuitry.

The development of the human brain included the evolution of circuits that can evaluate multiple variables before deciding on a course of action, including circuits that can postpone the motivational drive of appetitive urges to satisfy higher demands. These circuits transcend the narrow focus of the reward system and promote the pursuit of reward in a manner that is consistent with contextual considerations, learned rules, and a vision of the future. Often, the motivational elements of appetitive networks and higher circuits lead in opposite directions, and this generates emotions and bodily sensations that provide a somatic representation of the conflict. The manner in which such conflicts are represented and resolved is an important determinant of psychopathology and a focus of the psychotherapeutic process.

The higher circuits that determine human behavior have important components in the prefrontal cortex. The term *prefrontal cortex* refers to the region of the brain directly in front of the premotor and motor strips. In humans, the prefrontal cortex represents 30% of the neocortex and facilitates transcendence of simple reward-driven behavior by permitting the consideration of an expanded set of variables before the initiation of actions. It coordinates adaptable, goal-directed behavior through the integration of internal and external circumstances, memory, applicable rules, and projected consequences.

Functional and anatomical considerations have demonstrated three distinct circuits in the prefrontal cortex that modulate complex behavior. These are the anterior cingulate, the orbitofrontal, and the dorsolateral circuits. The oculomotor circuit, which controls automatic eye movements, is a fourth prefrontal network, but it will not be discussed in this chapter. All the prefrontal circuits have nodes in the thalamus, cortex, basal ganglia, and globus pallidus and/or substantia nigra pars reticulata (Burruss et al. 2000; Mega and Cummings 2001). The circuits are somatotopically mapped and define numerous "channels" through each circuit component (Mega and Cummings 2001).

The common functional element of all three circuits is modulation of the thalamus. Thalamic circuitry is tonically inhibited by the globus pallidus (Mega and Cummings 2001). This inhibition can be removed for selected channels through the action of the basal ganglia, which can suppress default pallidal inhibition. Self-excitatory loops that sustain representations of interest in the brain can therefore be selectively activated. Additional "indirect" loops pass through the subthalamic nucleus and external globus pallidus and complement the circuitry described above (Mega and Cummings 2001). Descriptions of the three major behavioral circuits in the prefrontal cortex follow (Burruss et al. 2000; Mega and Cummings 2001).

1. The anterior cingulate circuit has nodes in

   - Dorsomedial nucleus of the thalamus
   - Brodmann area 24 of the anterior cingulate gyrus
   - Ventromedial caudate, ventral putamen, nucleus accumbens, and olfactory tubercle
   - Rostromedial and ventral globus pallidus

2. The orbitofrontal circuit has nodes in

   - Ventral anterior and dorsomedial nuclei of the thalamus
   - Brodmann area 11 and inferomedial Brodmann area 10
   - Ventromedial caudate
   - Dorsomedial globus pallidus and substantia nigra pars reticulata

3. The dorsolateral circuit has nodes in

   - Ventral anterior and dorsomedial nuclei of the thalamus
   - Brodmann area 9 and dorsolateral Brodmann area 10
   - Dorsolateral caudate
   - Dorsomedial globus pallidus and substantia nigra pars reticulata

The anterior cingulate circuit, which contains the cingulate gyrus, is involved primarily in the motivation of goal-directed actions. The cingulate gyrus is a heterogeneous area with specific processing modules for emotion, cognition, sensation, and movement (Bush et al. 2000). Important functions of the cingulate are thought to include the motivation of appropriate responses to internal and external stimuli, emotional–cognitive integration, "attention for action," motor preparation, and conflict monitoring (Bush et al. 2000).

The cingulate carries out these functions by triggering body states that focus attention on internal and external demands, and motivate appropriate action. It generates emotional motivation through its projections to autonomic, visceromotor, and endocrine systems (Critchley et al. 2003) and is an important component of reward circuitry. The cingulate receives cognitive data from the DLPFC (Barbas et al. 2003) and facilitates emotional–cognitive integration by generating emotional states appropriate to cognitive contents (Critchley et al. 2003). Conversely, it conveys emotional information to the DLPFC for cognitive processing. Damage to the cingulate gyrus can result in a state of apathy in which responses to internal and external stimuli are significantly diminished (Mega and Cummings 2001). At worst, severe cingulate damage results in "akinetic mutism," a state with little spontaneous movement or speech (Mega and Cummings 2001).

The cingulate can organize "attention for action" by modulating arousal, motivation, autonomic tone, and attentional focus to drive behavioral responses that address the most salient internal or external stimuli (Bush et al. 2000). Cingulate gyrus–nucleus accumbens circuitry figures prominently in addictive states. The cingulate gyrus is also thought to generate the autonomic tone necessary to support many types of movement, and it signals behavioral conflicts by increasing arousal and autonomic tone (Critchley et al. 2003).

The orbitofrontal circuit modulates the pursuit of reward by adding considerations of risk, context, and potential consequences to the behavioral equation. The orbitofrontal cortex is reciprocally connected to the amygdala, and both act in concert to generate emotional states relevant to the pursuit of reward and avoidance of risk. Both the orbitofrontal cortex and the amygdala receive a rich set of inputs from all five sensory cortices, as well as from the insula. This information is integrated into comprehensive views of both external and internal milieus. The inputs come primarily from downstream regions of the unimodal cortices, and therefore the information is probably at the whole object rather than the individual feature level (Barbas et al. 2003). In addition, sensory inputs are relatively blended and provide multidimensional views of the environment. The amygdala projects to the same sites in the orbitofrontal cortex that receive direct sensory inputs, and this arrangement may allow the orbitofrontal cortex to extract the emotional significance of sensory events (Barbas et al. 2003). Both the amygdala and the orbitofrontal cortex ignore neutral sensory inputs with no implications of risk or reward, and stop responding to any inputs that lose their motivational value (Barbas et al. 2003).

Barbas et al. (2003) have elucidated the layout of orbitofrontal–amygdalar circuitry through experimental work with nonhuman primates. The amygdala can exert both inhibitory and stimulatory influences on hypothalamic autonomic nuclei. The central nucleus of the amygdala normally inhibits the hypothalamic nuclei, whereas the basolateral nucleus stimulates it.

The orbitofrontal cortex can suppress autonomic centers through stimulation of the amygdala's central nucleus (Barbas et al. 2003). Activation of this nucleus causes autonomic inhibition. The opposite result, autonomic activation, can be achieved by the orbitofrontal cortex through stimulation of the intercalated cell masses of the amygdala, which diminishes the default inhibition of hypothalamic nuclei by the amygdala's central nucleus (Barbas et al. 2003).

Functionally, the orbitofrontal cortex induces anticipatory body states that promote reward seeking, as well as aversive body states that reduce the likelihood of risky actions (Mega and Cummings 2001). The orbitofrontal cortex probably evolved to prevent injury in the pursuit of reward, to facilitate behavioral restraint by animals at lower levels of the social hierarchy, to promote the preferential pursuit of low-risk rather than high-risk rewards that are consistent with internal needs, and to inhibit pursuit of contextually inappropriate rewards, such as seeking food when sated. Humans with orbitofrontal cortex damage usually demonstrate personality changes that include high impulsivity, social inappropriateness, explosive behavior, disregard for rules and consequences, and the inability to use aversive emotions to inhibit risky behavior (Mega and Cummings 2001).

The dorsolateral prefrontal circuit modulates executive functions. These include organization, problem solving, working memory and memory retrieval, self-direction, the ability to address novelty, and the use of language to guide behavior (Mega and Cummings 2001). The DLPFC, like the orbitofrontal cortex, receives sensory inputs, although these are primarily from visual, auditory, and somatosensory cortices (Barbas et al. 2003). The frontal eye fields (Brodmann area 8) receive low-level visual information with a degree of detail that rivals what is found in the visual unimodal cortex (Barbas et al. 2003). Sensory information is less integrated in the dorsolateral cortex than in the orbitofrontal cortex, possibly facilitating more detailed analysis of specific stimuli (Barbas et al. 2003).

Individuals with damage to the DLPFC have difficulty organizing behavior to meet internal or external demands, and tend to perseverate in their thoughts and speech. Their decision making is impaired, and they have a

strong tendency to be drawn toward objects and situations with high salience, even if the interaction is contextually inappropriate. These individuals often engage in *utilization behavior*, which is the indiscriminate
handling of any salient objects encountered. They have significant difficulty with problem solving and are unable to address novelty (Mega and
Cummings 2001).

The DLPFC is the entry point for verbal psychotherapeutic interventions, because it is essential for advanced reasoning and for modulating
behavior through the use of words. Mayberg et al. (1999) demonstrated
increases in limbic–paralimbic blood flow in the subgenual cingulate (Brodmann area 25) and anterior insula in individuals experiencing sadness. Sad
persons also demonstrated decreases in blood flow to the right DLPFC and
inferior parietal cortex (Mayberg et al. 1999). These imbalances can be corrected through psychotherapy (Mayberg et al. 1999).

The dorsolateral prefrontal circuit has many of the attributes of the ego.
It facilitates executive functions such as integration of perceptual information, problem solving, and decision making (Burruss et al. 2000; Mega and
Cummings 2001). Imaging studies have also shown that the DLPFC, possibly in conjunction with the cingulate gyrus, plays a key role in the suppression of unwanted memories (Anderson et al. 2004).

The manifestations of the id are very much a function of cingulate gyrus–
nucleus accumbens circuitry. This circuit amplifies signals that suggest the
attainability of reward, and generates body states that motivate pursuit of
potential pleasures. In the presence of remembered cues, this circuit can generate overwhelming motivational pressure to engage in reward-producing
behavior, as is the case in chemical dependence.

The functions of the superego are implemented through orbitofrontal–
amygdalar circuitry. This functional network evolved to temper the pursuit
of pleasure with considerations of context and risk. Orbitofrontal–amygdalar circuits are directly wired to autonomic centers and can produce body
states conducive to disengagement and withdrawal. The actions of this circuit set limits on risk taking and can convey the visceral feelings of potential
punishment or embarrassment.

Much of the apparent conflict among the prefrontal circuits in the determination of behavior is a result of parallel processing. Cognitive and
emotional centers process information simultaneously rather than sequentially. In addition, emotional processing often is completed before cognitive
evaluation. This can lead to the production of a body state that motivates
approach or withdrawal, followed by a cognitive assessment that dictates the
opposite. Harmonious integration of cognition and emotions often is not
possible even in common social and occupational situations, and the imbalance is even greater when psychopathological processes have altered the

relative contributions of emotional and cognitive circuits. High-functioning individuals can sense processing discrepancies and use them to advantage in defining behavior. The feeling that "something is not quite right" can be very valuable, for example, during problem solving or creative pursuits. Conversely, emotional-cognitive dissonance can lead to severely impaired occupational and social behavior, and is an important area of concern for the psychotherapist.

The prefrontal circuits described above, which support adaptive behavior by making it possible to consider many variables before responding to a stimulus, are important targets for the psychotherapist. The dorsolateral prefrontal circuit must be enlisted to use words as tools for shaping behavior. This circuit is also responsible for executive functions, including organization, problem solving, abstract thinking, creativity, strategic planning, and future orientation. Many common psychotherapeutic problems are rooted in suboptimal function within this circuit.

The generation of motivational and emotional states appropriate to context is an important function of the cingulate gyrus (Critchley et al. 2003). The amygdala and orbitofrontal cortex, by virtue of their connections to hypothalamic autonomic centers and other subcortical targets, also are able to generate emotional body states. One of the most common conditions for which people seek psychotherapy is emotional dysregulation. Imaging studies have shown that orbitofrontal and amygdalar circuits can be modulated through conscious cognitive processes, such as psychotherapeutic interactions (Ochsner et al. 2002).

The orbitofrontal circuit, in concert with the amygdala, is responsible for tempering the unbridled pursuit of reward or saliency. Deficits in this circuit can present as impulsivity, social inappropriateness, lack of empathy, lack of respect for social conventions, and little response to the threat of personal risk, embarrassment, or punishment. In cases of suspected orbitofrontal dysfunction, the psychotherapist must first determine whether there is any functionality present, and then decide whether to try to bolster representations of adverse consequences in connection with inappropriate behaviors. If this circuit appears to be completely nonfunctional, the prognosis for a psychotherapeutic "cure" is considered poor, as is the case in the treatment of antisocial personality disorder.

Neurobiological Empathy

Knowing the brain helps therapists to understand each patient's mind, which is, after all, a projection of the patient's brain processes into subjective and interpersonal space. A critical task for the therapist is to represent the minds of patients within his or her own. Through this process, the constellation of symptoms reported by the patient is categorized according to the structural elements stored in the therapist's neural circuits during psychotherapeutic training and practice. This representational effort is usually summarized in objective terms as a formulation, a diagnosis, or a case conceptualization. In subjective terms, the plight of the patient also arouses emotional activity within the therapist. In general, such activity is part of countertransference. More specifically, when the emotions and feelings generate a positive connection based on shared emotional experiences, the result is the subset of countertransference phenomena that we call empathy.

In the context of a neural infrastructure for understanding behavior, a new kind of empathy becomes possible, which we call neurobiological empathy. Interpreting the actions and problems of patients requires the development of explanatory constructs that define a framework of imputed causality within the patient's sphere of interactions. These constructs can be experiential, rational, or both. In other words, the psychotherapist "understands" the nature and impact of the client's problem by accessing memories of similar experiences and/or applying theoretical knowledge about how the client's condition distorts normal rules of causality. In addition, the therapist can use neurobiological understanding to validate the patient's subjective experience and begin a dialogue about treatment. This dialogue can begin with an explanation of what is known about the neural basis of the patient's condition. For example, a psychotherapist treating a patient with severe phobia might have difficulty empathizing in a conventional way if he or she has never experienced a similar problem. In such a case, the psychotherapist must apply relevant knowledge acquired from previous treatment of similar patients and from having studied the neurobiology as well as the course and prognosis of the disorder.

The concept of neurobiological empathy asserts that the addition of focused neurobiological knowledge to this process can amplify the psychotherapist's ability to understand the patient and to communicate this understanding. If we return to the phobia example, recent neuroimaging work (Straube et al. 2006) has demonstrated a phobia-specific distortion of the cause–effect matrix that defines responses to environmental objects. During conscious identification of the feared object, phobic individuals showed activation of left and right amygdala, the left insula, the left anterior cingulate gyrus, and the left dorsomedial prefrontal cortex. In addition, the right amygdala was strongly activated under conditions of attentional distraction, demonstrating amygdalar reactivity to the feared object even under conditions of subliminal perception. All of the regions that show activation have efferent projections that allow them to modulate autonomic arousal, and they represent critical nodes in the circuitry that turns previously neutral objects into perceived threats.

An understanding of the neural mechanisms that underlie phobia can be important in planning its treatment. An important point to consider is that both conscious and unconscious representations of the feared object will cause activation of fear circuitry in the brain. Knowledge of the patient's neural reactions to the feared object is also the basis of neurobiological empathy. The therapist can explain to the patient the nature of the brain processes behind the behavioral problems that are the focus of therapy. This knowledge gives tangible reality to the patient's experiences and conveys to the patient a sense of informed concern and understanding by the therapist. Under these circumstances, both therapist and patient can begin their work from a concrete position that has both focus and objectivity. As knowledge of the neural basis of psychiatric disorders accumulates, this information can become an invaluable resource for those therapists who are prepared to use it.

Mirror Neuron Systems

Mirror neurons are groups of frontal and parietal neurons in the brains of primates that fire both during the execution of purposeful movements and during observation of other individuals performing similar actions (Iacoboni and Dapretto 2006). Mirror neurons were originally discovered in the brains of macaque monkeys by Rizzolatti and coworkers (Rizzolatti et al. 1996). These neurons are part of the brain's mechanisms for attributing meaning to the actions of others. In general, "meaning" in the brain is defined operationally and subjectively. In other words, the meaning of objects and movements is defined in terms of their functional significance to the individual. To encode this in the brain, some of the circuits involved in potential use of the object or movement in question are activated. In the case of mirror neurons, the meaning of observed actions is encoded by activating some of the neurons that would normally fire in the observer's brain if he or she were preparing to perform the same action.

Mirror neurons in humans are located in two interconnected brain regions (Iacoboni and Dapretto 2006): 1) the pars opercularis of the inferior frontal gyrus (within Broca's area) in the frontal lobe and 2) the anterior area of the inferior parietal lobe. Frontoparietal circuits in general are thought to function in sensorimotor integration. In humans, these mirror neuron areas, together with the superior temporal sulcus, act as a key circuit that supports certain forms of motor imitation (see Iacoboni and Dapretto 2006). The superior temporal sulcus provides a detailed visual description of the action to be imitated, the inferior parietal lobe defines its motoric components, and the pars opercularis defines its perceived goal.

Mirror neurons also seem to be part of a system for understanding the intentions and emotional experiences of others. The system includes the following (Carr et al. 2003; Iacoboni and Dapretto 2006):

- Superior temporal cortex, which encodes visual description of observed action
- Posterior parietal mirror neurons, which encode the kinesthetics of the action's movement sequence
- Inferior frontal mirror neurons, which encode perceived goal of the action
- Dysgranular field of the insula, which connects mirror neurons to limbic circuitry, and which facilitates the generation of a subjective body state related to the perceived action
- Limbic circuitry, including the amygdala, which can respond emotionally to the perceived goals

The ability to be empathic may depend on the functioning of these and related systems of circuits, although the actual mechanisms by which mirror neuron systems support empathy remain speculative (Carr et al. 2003).

These early findings can be tentatively extended to create brain-based explanations of a number of psychotherapeutic concepts. For example, patients with autism and autism spectrum disorders show markedly decreased activity in mirror neuron systems when viewing the emotional expressions of others (Iacoboni and Dapretto 2006). The well-known theory of mind deficit in autistic disorders can therefore be connected to actual brain dysfunction. Effective treatment may focus on enhancing mirror neuron activation to the degree that this might be possible, therefore optimizing the internal processes that lead to self- and other awareness.

Mirror neuron systems have become the cornerstone of an emerging neurobiological explanation of empathy. The highly social human brain may rely on these systems to navigate the complex universe of social interactions. As autism spectrum disorders suggest, people vary in their ability to register the emotional-cognitive states of others, including their psychotherapists.

Mirror neuron systems suggest an explanation of how a therapist's empathic resonance can affect a patient. Successful psychotherapy probably involves repeated "mirrorings" between the brains involved. The patient may mirror the therapist's empathic resonance by modeling the therapist's "attitude" within his or her neural circuits. Therefore, for a period of time of psychotherapeutic attunement, the therapist can give the patient a new set of experiences of the self. For example, the subjective experience of unbearable emotion and its therapeutic transformation in the mirrored environment of therapist calm may provide the patient access to a new set of circuits for emotional tolerance and management (Siegel 2006). On the other hand, overly empathic therapists may burn the internal experiences of emotionally difficult patients into their own brains through intense, repetitive mirroring, and may themselves sustain secondary trauma.

Functional Imaging Studies of the Effects of Psychotherapy on the Brain

The brain encodes experiences by altering neuronal connections, and prepares to meet perceived environmental challenges by modulating a variety of circuits, some of which have been discussed above. Before it was possible to visualize the activity of the brain as it addresses behavioral challenges, the neural correlates of psychotherapeutic change were unknown. At present, however, the visualization of functional changes in brain circuitry brought about by psychotherapy has become a reality. Because the field is relatively new and studies are not fully comparable in terms of methodology, hard conclusions cannot yet be drawn. However, important data are beginning to accumulate from which a theoretical framework that defines the neurobiology of psychotherapy can be built.

Goldapple et al. (2004) examined the effects of cognitive-behavioral therapy (CBT) on the brains of patients with depression, and compared the result with paroxetine treatment. Brain analysis involved positron emission tomography scanning, performed before the first and after the last treatment sessions. Patients in the psychotherapy group received 15–20 CBT sessions over a period of 19–33 weeks, and patients in the medication group received paroxetine for a similar period of time. All patients had equivalent scores (an average of 20 at the outset) on the Hamilton Rating Scale for Depression, and response was defined as at least a 50% reduction in the score.

In this study, responders to CBT showed significant increases in hippocampal and dorsal cingulate (Brodmann area 24) metabolism, as well as decreases in frontal cortex metabolism in dorsal (Brodmann area 9, 46), ventral (Brodmann area 47, 11), and medial (Brodmann area 9, 10, 11) regions. In contrast, responders to paroxetine showed increases in prefrontal metabolism, along with decreases in hippocampal and subgenual cingulate metabolism.

A study by Anderson et al. (2004) may be relevant to understanding the results of Goldapple et al. (2004). In Anderson et al.'s work, healthy volunteers were shown lists of words and asked to remember or forget certain ones. Successful forgetting was associated with increased activity of the prefrontal cortex, including the anterior cingulate, and decreased hippocampal activation during the initial word presentation. Conversely, the combination of increased cingulate and hippocampal activity was found to be important for successfully storing target words in memory.

In this context, the results reported by Goldapple et al. (2004) for the paroxetine group may represent decreased recall of dysphoric memories, combined with increased executive function. In the case of patients treated with CBT, increases in cingulate and hippocampal activity might reflect the fact that CBT works by changing cognitive patterns, thus requiring cingulate and hippocampal effort, while at the same time other frontal regions that can recruit autonomic and emotional centers and which could have fueled the depressed state showed decreased activation.

Mayberg (2006), who was an investigator in the Goldapple et al. (2004) study, has reviewed imaging-based models of depression and its treatment, in light of her own work in the field. Mayberg conceptualizes the behavioral syndrome that we call depression as "a systems-level disorder affecting select cortical, subcortical, and limbic regions and their related neurotransmitter and molecular mediators" (Mayberg 2006, p. 259). She has analyzed brain responses to a variety of treatments for depression, including psychotherapy, medication, electroconvulsive therapy, and deep brain stimulation. According to Mayberg, "The best-replicated behavioral correlate of a resting state abnormality in depression is that of an inverse relationship between prefrontal activity and depression severity" (p. 262).

Roffman et al. (2005) conducted a comprehensive review of neuroimaging studies in psychotherapy. In one of the reviewed studies (Ochsner et al. 2002), subjects were asked to reappraise mood cognitively. This technique resulted in improved mood, and the improvements correlated with increased metabolism in dorsolateral and dorsomedial prefrontal cortices, as well as decreased activity in the orbitofrontal cortex and amygdala.

In general, imaging studies of depressed patients have tended to show decreased activity in the dorsal prefrontal cortex (including the DLPFC) and increased activity in ventral prefrontal regions (Roffman et al. 2005). Dorsal prefrontal areas tend to participate in cognitive circuits, whereas ventral prefrontal areas have significant links to emotional circuitry.

In addition to Goldapple et al.'s (2004) CBT results described above, studies comparing the treatment of depression with interpersonal psychotherapy and medication (paroxetine) have been reported. One such study (Brody et al. 2001) showed decreases in dorsal and ventral prefrontal activity in responders to interpersonal psychotherapy that were similar to those reported by Goldapple et al. (2004) with CBT. In contrast, however, Brody et al. (2001) also reported decreases in prefrontal metabolism in paroxetine responders.

Roffman et al. (2005) also reviewed imaging studies of the treatment of obsessive-compulsive disorder with behavior therapy. In general, patients with symptomatic obsessive-compulsive disorder respond to either psychotherapy or medication by showing a reduction in caudate nucleus metabolism (especially on the right). This finding has been confirmed by several studies and is consistent with the theoretical conceptualization of obsessive-compulsive disorder as a disorder that affects thalamocorticostriatal circuitry.

Studies of the treatment of phobia with CBT and medication were also reviewed by Roffman et al. (2005). In one study (Furmark et al. 2002), individuals with social phobia were asked to read a speech about a personal experience to a small audience. At baseline, such patients exhibited activation of limbic regions, including the amygdala, the hippocampus, and the adjacent temporal cortex. After 8 weeks of treatment with either CBT or citalopram, the baseline pattern of limbic activation was greatly attenuated. CBT, but not citalopram, also resulted in decreased activation of the periaqueductal gray, an area involved in fear and defensive responses. Citalopram, but not CBT, also resulted in reduced activity of thalamic and ventral prefrontal cortex metabolism.

Functional neuroimaging of the psychotherapeutic process is in its infancy. As a result, there are currently no comprehensive models of psychotherapy's effects on the brain. Nevertheless, information is accumulating rapidly on the circuit-based changes in neural information processing that underlie psychotherapy's beneficial effects, as reviewed above.

Psychotherapy is clearly a top-down process. In other words, it relies on higher levels of communication, including verbal and emotional expressions, to access and modify the patient's neural circuitry. As the patient's brain processes the targeted communications of the therapist, dysfunctional representations and their emotional connections are modified. In this manner, the therapist is able to reshape the patient's internal representations and their subjective meaning, leading to more adaptive behavior.

Conclusion

It has always been tacitly assumed that psychotherapy, whose ultimate aim is to modify behavior, exerts its therapeutic effects by modulating the brain. Unfortunately, through most of the history of psychotherapy, the nature of this modulation has been unknown. Recently, however, functional imaging and animal studies have begun to clarify some of the neural substrates that underlie the psychotherapeutic process. The following neural circuits appear to have special relevance to psychotherapists:

- Mirror neuron circuits, first defined by Rizzolatti et al. (2001), which are groups of frontal and parietal neurons in the brains of primates that fire both during the execution of purposeful movements and during observation of other individuals performing similar actions. These circuits are important in the attribution of meaning to the actions of others and in the development of empathy.
- Circuits that contain basic representations of internal states and the visceral self, including representations in the brain stem and insula.
- Risk–reward evaluation circuits with nodes in the amygdala, orbitofrontal cortex, cingulate gyrus, and nucleus accumbens.

- Circuits that can generate discrete body states through autonomic and hormonal activation.
- Memory circuits that involve the hippocampus (explicit memory), dorsolateral prefrontal cortex (working memory), amygdala and orbitofrontal cortex (secondary rewards and punishers), and basal ganglia (implicit memory).
- Executive and evaluative circuits centered on the DLPFC.

In addition to providing insights into some of the possible circuits that underlie the psychotherapeutic process, advances in neurobiology are also facilitating the conceptualization of classical psychotherapeutic constructs in terms of neural circuitry. For example, the concepts of ego, superego, and id as defined by Freud can be functionally mapped to three thalamocorticostriatal circuits: 1) the *ego* shares many functions with the cortical-subcortical circuit centered on the DLPFC, including problem solving, working memory, self-direction, the ability to address novelty, and the use of language to guide behavior; 2) the *superego* shares many functions with the cortical-subcortical circuit centered on the orbitofrontal cortex, including the ability to consider rules and potential consequences before acting, and to exert behavioral inhibition through the generation of aversive body states; and 3) the *id* shares many functions with the cortical-subcortical circuit centered on the cingulate gyrus and nucleus accumbens, including the generation of motivational drive for the pursuit of pleasure (this circuit features prominently in addictive states).

A concept called *neurobiological empathy* has been introduced in this chapter. Knowing the neurobiological basis of a patient's behavioral complaints and sharing this knowledge with the patient can establish a concrete starting point for psychotherapeutic intervention and validate the patient's subjective experience.

A scientific framework for psychotherapy is currently being developed, led by functional imaging studies of the successful treatment of a variety of psychiatric illnesses. Results to date have included the following: 1) in depression, psychotherapy can alter the metabolic activity of the prefrontal cortex, hippocampus, and cingulate gyrus (specific patterns of alteration have been variable across studies); 2) in obsessive-compulsive disorder, psychotherapy, like medication, has generally produced a reduction in caudate nucleus metabolism, especially on the right; and 3) in specific phobia, psychotherapy has produced attenuation of metabolic activity in the amygdala, hippocampus, and periaqueductal gray.

Special tools that can uncover the neurobiology of psychotherapy are currently being applied in a variety of experimental settings. As investigational conditions become standardized and technical approaches are refined, the scientific foundations of psychotherapy will be extended from its current behavioral roots to the level of neural function.

Key Points

- Psychiatric illness is associated with specific patterns of brain dysfunction, which are currently being defined with functional brain imaging.

- Successful psychotherapy brings about measurable changes in neurotransmission, which appear to be associated with its beneficial effects.

- As brain-based advances in the understanding and treatment of mental illness accumulate, it is important for psychotherapists to become conversant in basic neurobiology and to apply neurobiological knowledge to psychotherapeutic practice.

- Core psychotherapeutic concepts, such as engagement, self-awareness, pattern search, and behavioral change, can be tentatively associated with specific neural circuits that have been functionally defined.

- Psychotherapy is, by design, a top-down process. It relies on higher levels of communication, including verbal and emotional expressions, to access and modify a patient's neural circuitry. By producing beneficial changes in neurotransmission, psychotherapy can promote more adaptive patterns of behavior.

References

Ahn H, Wampold BE: Where oh where are the specific ingredients? A meta-analysis of component studies in counseling and psychotherapy. J Couns Psychol 48:251–257, 2001

Anderson MC, Ochsner KN, Kuhl B, et al: Neural systems underlying the suppression of unwanted memories. Science 303:232–235, 2004

Barbas H, Saha S, Rempel-Clower N, et al: Serial pathways from primate prefrontal cortex to autonomic areas may influence emotional expression. BMC Neurosci 4:25–37, 2003

Bartels A, Zeki S: The neural basis of romantic love. Neuroreport 11:3829–3834, 2000

Bartels A, Zeki S: The neural correlates of maternal and romantic love. Neuroimage 21:1155–1166, 2004

Beitman BD, Soth AM: Activation of self-observation: a core process among the psychotherapies. Journal of Psychotherapy Integration 16:383–397, 2006

Beitman BD, Yue D: Learning Psychotherapy: A Time-Efficient, Research-Based, Outcome-Measured Psychotherapy Training Program, 4th Edition. New York, WW Norton, 2004

Beitman BD, Nair J, Viamontes GI: What is self-awareness? in Self-Awareness Deficits in Psychiatric Patients. Edited by Beitman BD, Nair J. New York, WW Norton, 2005a, pp 3–23

Blanke O, Arzy S: The out-of-body experience: disturbed self-processing at the temporoparietal junction. Neuroscientist 11:16–24, 2005

Brody AL, Saxera S, Stoessel P, et al: Regional brain metabolic changes in patients with major depression treated with either paroxetine or interpersonal therapy: preliminary findings. Arch Gen Psychiatry 58:31–40, 2001

Burruss JW, Hurley RA, Taber KA, et al: Functional neuroanatomy of the frontal lobe circuits. Radiology 214:227–230, 2000

Bush G, Liu P, Posner MI: Cognitive and emotional influences in anterior cingulate cortex. Trends Cogn Sci 4:215–222, 2000

Carr L, Iacoboni M, Dubeau MC, et al: Neural mechanisms of empathy in humans: a relay from neural systems for imitation to limbic areas. Proc Natl Acad USA 100:5497–5502, 2003

Critchley HD, Mathias CJ, Josephs O, et al: Human cingulate cortex and autonomic control: converging neuroimaging and clinical evidence. Brain 126:1–14, 2003

Deikman AJ: The Observing Self. Boston, MA, Beacon, 1982

Etkin A, Pittenger C, Polan J, et al: Toward a neurobiology of psychotherapy: Basic science and clinical applications. J Neuropsychiatry Clin Neurosci 17:145–158, 2005

Ferris CF, Snowdon CT, King JA, et al: Activation of neural pathways associated with sexual arousal in non-human primates. J Magn Reson Imaging 19:168–175, 2004

Flashman LA: Disorders of insight, self-awareness, and attribution in schizophrenia, in Self-Awareness Deficits in Psychiatric Patients. Edited by Beitman BD, Nair J. New York, WW Norton, 2005, pp 129–158

Fonagy P: Psychotherapy: attachment and the brain. Paper presented at the annual meeting of the Society for Psychotherapy Research, Rome, Italy, June 2004

Freud S: The ego and the id (1923), in Standard Edition of the Complete Psychological Works of Sigmund Freud, Vol 19. Translated and edited by Strachey J. London, Hogarth Press, 1961

Frith CD, Frith U: Interacting minds: biological basis. Science 286:1692–1695, 1999

Furmark T, Tillfors M, Marteindottir I, et al: Common changes in cerebral blood flow in patients with social phobia treated with citalopram or cognitive-behavioral therapy. Arch Gen Psychiatry 59:425–433, 2002

Goldapple K, Segal Z, Garson Z, et al: Modulation of cortical-limbic pathways in major depression: treatment-specific effects of cognitive behavior therapy. Arch Gen Psychiatry 61:34–41, 2004

Greenspan, SI: The First Idea: How Symbols, Language, and Intelligence Evolved From Our Primate Ancestors to Modern Humans. New York, International Universities Press, 2004, pp 232–250

Gusnard DA, Akbudak E, Sulman GL, et al: Medial prefrontal cortex and self referential mental activity: relation to a default mode of brain function. Proc Natl Acad Sci USA 98:4259–4264, 2001

Haxby JV, Gobini MI, Furey ML, et al: Distributed and overlapping representation of faces and objects in the ventral temporal lobe. Science 293:2425–2430, 2001

Iacoboni M, Dapretto M: The mirror neuron system and the consequences of its dysfunction. Nat Rev Neurosci 7:942–951, 2006

Johnson SC, Baxter LC, Wilder LS, et al: Neural correlates of self-reflection. Brain 125:1808–1814, 2002

Kemperman G: Why new neurons? Possible functions for adult hippocampal neurogenesis. J Neurosci 22:635–638, 2002

Krupnick JL, Sotsky SM, Simmens S, et al: The role of the therapeutic alliance in psychotherapy and pharmacotherapy outcome: findings in the National Institute of Mental Health Treatment of Depression Collaborative Research Program. J Consult Clin Psychol 64:532–539, 1996

Lambert MJ, Bergin AE: The effectiveness of psychotherapy, in Handbook of Psychotherapy and Behavior Change, 4th Edition. Edited by Bergin AE, Garfield SL. New York, Wiley, 1994, pp 143–199

Lambert MJ, Shapiro DA, Bergin AE: Evaluation of therapeutic outcomes and processes, in Handbook of Psychotherapy and Behavior Change, 3rd Edition. Edited by Garfield SL, Bergin AE. New York, Wiley, 1986, pp 157–212

Main M: Metacognitive knowledge, metacognitive monitoring, and singular (coherent) vs multiple (incoherent) model of attachment: findings and directions for future research, in Attachment Across the Life Cycle. Edited by Harris P, Stevenson-Hinde J, Parkes C. New York, Routledge & Kegan Paul, 1991, pp 127–159

Mayberg HS: Defining neurocircuits in depression. Psychiatr Ann 36:259–268, 2006

Mayberg HS, Liotti M, Brannon SK, et al: Reciprocal limbic-cortical function and negative mood: converging PET findings in depression and normal sadness. Am J Psychiatry 156:675–683, 1999

Mega MS, Cummings JL: Frontal subcortical circuits: anatomy and function, in The Frontal Lobes and Neuropsychiatric Illness. Edited by Salloway SP, Mallory PF, Duffy JD. Washington, DC, American Psychiatric Press, 2001, pp 15–32

Mesulam M: From sensation to cognition. Brain 121:1013–1052, 1998

Newberg A, d'Aquili E, Rause V: Brain Machinery: Why God Won't Go Away. New York, Ballantine Books, 2002

Ochsner KN, Bunge SA, Gross JJ, et al: Rethinking feelings: an FMRI study of the cognitive regulation of emotion. J Cogn Neurosci 14:1215–1222, 2002

Pally R: Non-conscious prediction and a role for consciousness in correcting prediction errors. Cortex 41:643–662, 2005

Phillips ML, Drevets WS, Rauch SL, et al: Neurobiology of emotion perception I: the neural basis of normal emotion perception. Biol Psychiatry 54:504–514, 2003

Prochaska JO, Norcross JC: Systems of Psychotherapy: A Transtheoretical Analysis, 5th Edition. Pacific Grove, CA, Brooks/Cole, 2003

Rizzolatti G, Fadiga L, Fogassi L, et al: Premotor cortex and the recognition of motor actions. Cogn Brain Res 3:131–141, 1996

Rizzolatti G, Fogassi L, Gallese V: Neurophysiological mechanisms underlying the understanding and imitation of action. Nat Rev Neurosci 2:661–670, 2001

Roffman JL, Marci CD, Glick DM, et al: Neuroimaging and the functional anatomy of psychotherapy. Psychol Med 35:1–15, 2005

Rolls ET: The Brain and Emotion. Oxford, England, Oxford University Press, 1999

Rolls ET: Emotion Explained. Oxford, England, Oxford University Press, 2005

Siegel DJ: An interpersonal neurobiology approach to psychotherapy. Psychiatr Ann 36:248–256, 2006

Straube T, Mentzel HJ, Miltner WHR: Neural mechanisms of automatic and direct processing of phobogenic stimuli in specific phobia. Biol Psychiatry 59:162–170, 2006

Stuss DT, Benson DF: Emotional concomitants of psychotherapy, in Advances in Neuropsychology and Behavioral Neurology. Edited by Heilman KM, Staz P. New York, Guilford, 1983, pp 11–40

Tanaka K: Columns for complex visual object features in the inferotemporal cortex: clustering of cells with similar but slightly different stimulus selectivities. Cereb Cortex 13:90–99, 2003

Teicher MH, Andersen SL, Polcari A, et al: Developmental neurobiology of child-hood stress and trauma. Psychiatr Clin North Am 25:397–426, 2002

Viamontes GI, Beitman BD: Neural substrates of psychotherapeutic change, Part I: the default brain. Psychiatr Ann 36:225–237, 2006a

Viamontes GI, Beitman BD: Neural substrates of psychotherapeutic change, Part II: beyond default mode. Psychiatr Ann 36:239–246, 2006b

Viamontes GI, Beitman BD, Viamontes CT, et al: Neural circuits for self-awareness: evolutionary origins and implementation in the human brain, in Self-Awareness Deficits in Psychiatric Patients. Edited by Beitman BD, Nair J. New York, WW Norton, 2005, pp 24–111

Wampold BE: The Great Psychotherapy Debate: Models, Methods, and Findings. Mahwah, NJ, Erlbaum, 2001

Wheeler MA, Stuss DT, Tulving E: Toward a theory of episodic memory: the frontal lobes and autonoetic consciousness. Psychol Bull 121:331–354, 1997

Wolfe BE, Goldfried MR: Research on psychotherapy integration: recommendations and conclusions from an NIMH workshop. J Consult Clin Psychol 56:448–451, 1988

Suggested Readings

Beitman BD, Yue D: Learning Psychotherapy: A Time-Efficient, Research-Based, Outcome-Measured Psychotherapy Training Program, 4th Edition. New York, WW Norton, 2004

Mega MS, Cummings JL: Frontal subcortical circuits: anatomy and function, in The Frontal Lobes and Neuropsychiatric Illness. Edited by Salloway SP, Mallory PF, Duffy JD. Washington, DC, American Psychiatric Press, 2001, pp 15–32

Mesulam M: From sensation to cognition. Brain 121:1013–1052, 1998

Rizzolatti G, Fogassi L, Gallese V: Neurophysiological mechanisms underlying the understanding and imitation of action. Nat Rev Neurosci 2:661–670, 2001

Roffman JL, Marci CD, Glick DM, et al: Neuroimaging and the functional anatomy of psychotherapy. Psychol Med 35:1–15, 2005

Rolls ET: The Brain and Emotion. Oxford, England, Oxford University Press, 1999

Viamontes GI, Beitman BD: Neural substrates of psychotherapeutic change, Part I: the default brain. Psychiatr Ann 36:225–237, 2006

Viamontes GI, Beitman BD: Neural substrates of psychotherapeutic change, Part II: beyond default mode. Psychiatr Ann 36:239–246, 2006

Viamontes GI, Beitman BD, Viamontes CT, et al: Neural circuits for self-awareness: evolutionary origins and implementation in the human brain, in Self-Awareness Deficits in Psychiatric Patients. Edited by Beitman BD, Nair J. New York, WW Norton, 2005, pp 24–111

Chapter 30

Professional Boundaries in Psychotherapy

Glen O. Gabbard, M.D.

Psychotherapy, regardless of orientation, must take place in a context that is safe and conducive to therapeutic possibilities. Psychotherapy is a professional relationship that, above all, is focused on helping patients with problems that they identify. Psychotherapeutic treatments occur within an envelope that is often referred to as the *therapeutic frame*. However, the metaphor of a frame implies a rigidity that may not be in the best interest of the process. The concept of *professional boundaries*, with some degree of inherent flexibility, may be more suited to most discussions of sound psychotherapeutic practice than the concept of therapeutic frame. A simple definition of professional boundaries is that they are the parameters defining the limits of a fiduciary relationship in which one person (a patient) entrusts his or her welfare to another (a psychotherapist), who is paid for the provision of a service (Gabbard and Nadelson 1995). Boundaries suggest a professional distance and respect that is characteristic of ethical professional behavior, but they also allow for some degree of bending in the service of individualizing treatment.

The concept of professional boundaries is a relatively recent addition to the mental health literature. To a large extent, it grew out of concern about sexual misconduct, which led to malpractice suits, serious harm to patients, and severe damage to the reputation of the mental health professions (Gutheil and Gabbard 1993). Studies of cases of sexual misconduct, however, led to a growing awareness that instances in which psychotherapists engage in sexual relations with patients are typically preceded by a "slippery slope" involving a progressive series of nonsexual boundary violations (Gutheil and Gabbard 1993; Strasburger et al. 1992). As a result, increasing attention has been focused on such matters as the location of sessions; confidentiality; excessive self-disclosure; the professional role of the therapist; length and time of sessions; fees; the exchange of gifts and services; appropriate clothing and language; and nonsexual physical contact (Table 30–1).

Boundary Crossings Versus Boundary Violations

Nonsexual boundary violations are less absolute than sexual boundary violations. All practitioners can think of instances in which the transgression of a boundary led to productive therapeutic work and caused no harm. Therefore, the definitions involved in professional boundaries must take into account that both boundary crossings and boundary violations exist in the practice of psychotherapy.

Boundary crossings are generally benign phenomena that do not occur repetitively, are discussable between the therapist and the patient, and are not exploitative (Gabbard and Lester 2003; Gutheil and Gabbard 1993, 1998). Inherent in the notion of a boundary crossing is the idea that rigidity is generally antitherapeutic. A good psychotherapist adjusts the treatment to the patient rather than expecting the patient to adjust to the treatment. Beginning psychotherapists sometimes practice with such great concern about maintaining proper boundaries that they become remote and overly formal in their way of relating to the patient. Some patients will feel that they are talking to an automaton and will not return for the next visit. Rigidity about boundaries can lead to a failure to engage the patient.

In most therapeutic dyads, there is a period of adjustment in which a sensitive psychotherapist implicitly negotiates with the patient a comfortable level of closeness or distance so that an optimal context for the therapy is jointly constructed. Some patients are much more comfortable with a more talkative therapist, whereas others need a good listener. Some patients appreciate the use of humor, whereas others feel they are being laughed at when the therapist jokes. Good psychotherapists often comment that they are different with each patient during the course of a workday. They vary

---

TABLE 30–1.   Dimensions of professional boundaries

Professional role	Dual relationships
Location of sessions	Clothing
Time of sessions	Language
Length of sessions	Excessive self-disclosure
Fees	Absence of sexual contact
Gifts and services	Limited physical contact
Confidentiality	Business transactions

---

their therapeutic style depending on the particular patient's needs. Obviously, these variations are within the general parameters of ethical behavior and do not involve outrageous conduct.

Another aspect of boundary crossings is the recognition that extraordinary events occur that require humane responses. If the patient suffers a tragic loss and reaches out to the therapist for an embrace, most therapists will return the embrace, knowing that pushing the patient away might permanently destroy the therapeutic alliance. Moreover, no therapist is perfect, and at times even the best of therapists unconsciously enact something with the patient that may be outside of the usual technique. These enactments often reflect significant internal object relationships that have been mobilized within the therapeutic dyad.

> One psychotherapist, who had seen a depressed man in therapy for several weeks, noted that she was becoming increasingly bored with the sessions. The patient frequently fell silent, tended to make repeated self-recriminations, and referred to his situation as "hopeless." Even though he had improved with antidepressants, the patient seemed to be characterologically entrenched in his depression, and the therapist found him frustrating and irritating. She often dreaded the sessions and felt bored with the content. On one occasion, she announced that the session was over and said to the patient, "I'll see you next week." The patient hesitated and then left the room with a strange expression on his face. The therapist suddenly realized that she had ended the session 15 minutes early, thinking that 45 minutes had elapsed. She felt mortified, and she began reflecting on her own motives for such a countertransference enactment. She was able to acknowledge that she really did not want to hear him drone on and on, and she was acting out of her own needs rather than on the basis of what the patient needed. When the patient returned the following week, she apologized for the mistake and offered to make up for the time. The patient forgave her, but he then said it reminded him of how his wife frequently interrupted him during a conversation and said she had to do something else. When the therapist and the pa-

tient explored the two separate phenomena, the patient began to see a pattern of how his negativity might lead others to feel alienated or irritated with him.

Hence a boundary crossing based on unconscious factors in the therapist as well as certain characteristics of the patient led to a productive discussion in the therapy about an issue that had not been directly addressed.

Boundary violations, on the other hand, represent egregious phenomena that are usually repetitive, harmful to the patient, and exploitative of the patient's dependent position. Engaging in a sexual relationship with a patient would be the most extreme example, but taking financial advantage of the patient by soliciting money for an investment scheme may be just as exploitative. Another feature of boundary violations is that the therapist often refuses to discuss them with the patient. Therapists may claim that the unorthodox behavior is part of the "real relationship," and therefore no discussion is required.

The psychotherapeutic relationship is by definition a relationship with a power imbalance. The psychotherapist is being paid to deliver a service based on a special set of skills and a knowledge base acquired by specialized training. The patient entrusts the therapist to function with the patient's best interest in mind. Hence the patient may assume that whatever the therapist says or does is designed to help the patient. As a result, even an intelligent, nonpsychotic patient may agree to egregious boundary violations under the influence of that power differential and vulnerability. Moreover, transferences to the therapist may resemble past relationships with parents and other authority figures and can set up a situation where the patient feels that saying "no" is not an option. Some nefarious therapists have suggested that sexual relations might be helpful to the patient in the service of overcoming sexual inhibitions, and patients have complied under the assumption that they are receiving a therapeutic intervention.

At times, *boundary transgression* is used as an umbrella term that encompasses both boundary crossings and boundary violations. Another term in the literature is *boundary blurring,* which is used to describe instances in which the boundaries are confused but not necessarily enacted in the form of a boundary crossing or boundary violation.

Specific Dimensions of Professional Boundaries

Location

In any consideration of the professional boundaries that define psychotherapy, one dimension that must be taken into account is where the therapy takes place. Therapy usually takes place in an office, a clinic, or a hospital that is sufficiently private so that the patient feels comfortable disclosing embarrassing and shameful wishes, fears, and fantasies. However, the location of psychotherapy may vary within a setting. In a psychiatric hospital environment, for example, disturbed patients may feel confined and uncomfortable in a closed room and may find it much easier to talk while taking a walk on the hospital grounds. A medically ill patient in a general hospital may require therapy at the bedside.

The location of the psychotherapy also varies with the type of therapy that is indicated by the nature of the patient's pathology. A patient with an elevator phobia, for example, may require a behavioral approach that includes in vivo exposure. Hence the therapist may drive the patient to a skyscraper and spend time riding up and down the elevator during the therapy hour. This form of treatment is entirely within the community standards of behavioral approaches and has been shown to be efficacious.

In general, when one is contemplating a departure from community standards in terms of the setting, one must consider one's rationale for the departure. Therapists may usefully ask themselves, "Is this part of a thoughtfully considered treatment plan?" Therapists may also wish to engage a consultant before making such a departure to make sure that they are not acting on unconscious countertransference needs of their own.

Confidentiality

The fundamental principle that what is heard in psychotherapy is not repeated elsewhere makes the therapeutic process possible. Patients who come to psychotherapy, for whatever reasons, are often struggling with shame, guilt, remorse, self-loathing, fears of disapproval, and a host of other anxieties. The reassurance that what they say will be kept private between the two people in the consulting room allows them to open up in a manner that would not be possible otherwise. Hence, *confidentiality* is one of the most sacred professional boundaries.

The principle of confidentiality extends beyond simply not repeating what the patient says. Therapists are ethically bound not to act on information they receive in a therapeutic session. In other words, a therapist should not act on a stock market tip from a patient. If a therapist hears from a patient that a colleague of the therapist's is going through a divorce and her only source of information is that patient, the therapist must not acknowledge that she knows about the divorce in any other context. Numerous cases exist in which a third party realized that the only source of specific information could have been from the patient, and there were justifiable feelings of violation or breach of privacy. Confidentiality is protected by state statutes and ethics codes as well. A breach of confidentiality can make one vulnerable to litigation or to sanctions from professional boards or organizations.

Taking confidentiality seriously entails deception at times. Ironically, in the interest of maintaining privacy, therapists may have to deceive those they encounter outside the consulting room. If, for example, the therapist noted above knows about a colleague's divorce only through her patient, and she then encounters the colleague, she must pretend that she does not know, and if asked if she has heard the news, she must deny it. Otherwise, the patient's confidentiality has been violated. Over time, psychotherapists develop the capacity to compartmentalize certain information so as to keep it sequestered in a private sector of the psyche belonging to information heard in psychotherapy (Gabbard and Lester 2003).

Confidentiality is not an absolute boundary. In all states, one is required to break confidentiality to report child abuse. In some venues, a threat of imminent violence to an individual requires a "duty to warn" exception to confidentiality. Similarly, when a patient appears acutely suicidal and likely to act on the wish to die, many therapists choose to disclose suicidality to family members in the interest of saving the patient's life by enlisting a support system to monitor the patient's potentially lethal behavior. In a small number of states, therapists who hear of sexual misconduct by a fellow professional from a confidential source are required to report this matter to a licensing board. However, these regulations vary from state to state, and psychotherapists are well advised to consult their own state statutes when in doubt and to consult an attorney or knowledgeable colleague about the implications of a breach of confidentiality. Clinicians who decide to report without checking their regulatory statutes may think they are doing the right thing, only to end up with a lawsuit based on violation of confidentiality. A useful Web site to check civil and criminal codes is AdvocateWeb: Helping Overcome Professional Exploitation (http://www.advocateweb.org).

Gossiping psychotherapists are ubiquitous, and the delight in treating a well-known patient often leads certain psychotherapists to confide in colleagues about their secret pleasure of treating an illustrious person. However, the notion of confidentiality should be construed as meaning that one cannot even reveal whether a specific patient is in treatment or not. A formal consultation with a colleague is a different matter, of course, and requires the same level of confidentiality as treatment. The same is true of supervision. In most cases, the supervisee or consultee does not need to reveal the patient's name; in certain circumstances, however, doing so may be necessary for the supervisor or colleague to fully appreciate the difficulties the therapist is experiencing. There is nothing unethical about that type of revelation in the context of supervision or consultation.

However, when one presents a psychotherapy case for educational purposes or chooses to use clinical material in a publication, one must be careful to disguise identifying features of the patient. There are pros and cons of obtaining consent from the patient to present or publish, and those considerations have been thoroughly discussed elsewhere (Gabbard 2000b). Some will argue that patients cannot provide truly informed consent because of the power differential and the difficulty of refusing the therapist who requests that permission. Moreover, even if consent is offered, identifying features must still be disguised so that an audience or reader does not recognize the patient. Some professional organizations have specific criteria that must be followed in publications or presentations, and members of each professional discipline must consult those guidelines before making a decision on how to proceed. Similarly, professional journals may have specific guidelines that must be followed.

Excessive Self-Disclosure

The classical principle of psychoanalytic psychotherapy known as *anonymity* has undergone a significant rethinking in recent years. Therapists cannot be anonymous to the patient, no matter how hard they may try. The way they dress, the way they decorate their offices, their facial expressions in response to what the patient says, and the issues they choose to address when they speak all reveal a great deal about the therapists' subjectivity. Hence, the idea of the therapist as a "blank screen" is a myth that is no longer endorsed by mainstream therapists of any persuasion. The issue for the contemporary psychotherapist is not whether to self-disclose. The technical and boundary concern is how much, what, and when to self-disclose.

Feelings that the therapist may experience in the here and now with the patient may be revealed at times in a way that advances the therapy and provides useful feedback for the patient. For example, when a provocative patient is insulting or devalues the therapist over and over again, the patient may pick up on the fact that the therapist is becoming angry. If, in such situations, the patient asks the therapist, "Are you angry at me?" the therapist may be far better off to answer honestly than to conceal true feelings in an effort to avoid self-disclosure (Gabbard and Wilkinson 1994). A therapist in that situation might choose to say something like, "Yes, I think you're picking up on something. Let's look at the interaction and try to figure out what is going on between us that provoked feelings of irritation in me." In this way, the therapist transforms the countertransference anger into a topic that can be productively explored between the two parties in the therapeutic dyad. It would be far better to be honest in that situation than to be deliberately deceptive.

Therapists often communicate feelings nonverbally so that the patient may know what the therapist feels before the patient asks him or her.

Keisler (1988) developed interpersonal communication therapy, which involves what he termed *metacommunicative feedback*, which refers to therapist disclosure of inner covert reactions that are evoked by a patient's recurrent behaviors. He also developed a self-report inventory that measured distinctive internal reactions to guide therapists in providing feedback.

Not all feelings that the therapist has toward a patient are helpful to self-disclose. For example, even if a therapist feels genuine feelings of hate toward the patient, the act of saying, "I hate you," to the patient is unlikely to help the therapy or lead to further self-understanding on the part of the patient. Similarly, saying to a patient "I have sexual feelings for you" is also unlikely to be useful and might even be experienced as traumatizing or violating to some patients. In society when one person says to another, "I have sexual feelings for you," an action is usually implied to follow, namely sexual engagement. On the other hand, it is not true that physical involvement follows an expression of irritation. Therefore, one must be wary of the implications of any type of self-disclosure.

One way of implementing a boundary on self-disclosure is to deliberately avoid sharing with the patient any details about one's personal life or family. Superficial elements of one's personal life may be helpful at times. For example, a therapist working with an adolescent boy may find that forming a therapeutic alliance requires some chitchat about sports that are of mutual interest, so the therapist might tell a patient about a football game he went to the previous weekend, to strike up a relationship with the patient.

Self-disclosures about personal problems must be rigorously monitored, however, because they are frequently the first step on the slippery slope (Gabbard 1996; Gabbard and Lester 2003). Some disclosures may be initially received with open arms by the patient and therefore mislead the therapist into thinking that such information is productive and should be continued.

> Dr. A, a male therapist in his 40s, came to a session with Ms. B, a female patient in her 30s. He seemed excessively tired and inattentive. Ms. B eventually said to him, "Are you okay? You look distracted today." Dr. A responded, "No, I don't think I could conceal anything from you. You read me like a book. My wife left me, and I'm struggling to stay at work in the midst of a huge personal crisis in my life." Ms. B paused for a moment and then said, "I am so honored that you would tell me about what is happening in your life, so I can help you. You're always the one helping me, and it feels great for me to be able to offer you support for a change. I feel it's easier to open up to you when you open up to me." At the end of the session, Ms. B

gave Dr. A a hug and told him, "You'll get through this. Hang in there." After she left, Dr. A thought to himself, "That went much better than I thought it would. She was so understanding about it." Having entered into this self-deception about the value of burdening the patient with his personal problems, Dr. A continued to disclose the details of the divorce to Ms. B at each session of the therapy, until they were sitting on the couch together embracing, meeting outside for coffee, and ultimately entering into a sexual relationship. During the course of an evaluation ordered by a licensing board, Ms. B told the evaluator that she realized she was paying a fee to Dr. A to hear about his personal problems. She said it didn't seem right to her in retrospect, even though she wanted to help him.

This vignette illustrates how a single self-disclosure can escalate into major boundary violations because of the therapist's neediness and the capacity for self-deception about who is helping whom. As always, consultation with a colleague may be essential in a life crisis to prevent this type of transgression from occurring.

Professional Role

The concept of *professional role* is fundamental to boundaries. Because of the fiduciary relationship, the therapist functions as one who tries to help the patient address symptoms or problems that have been brought to treatment. That is the therapist's sole purpose. The therapist is not a mother, a father, a priest or rabbi, a lover, a friend, or a sibling. In the initial therapist–patient meeting, some discussion of professional role is usually necessary to clarify what therapy is and what therapy is not.

The therapist's professional role does not require that the therapist be excessively formal or inordinately depriving. Although it is entirely appropriate to begin a first meeting by referring to the patient as "Mr. Smith" or "Ms. Jones," if the patient prefers to be called by his or her first name, the therapist may accommodate the patient's wish to help the patient feel comfortable in the therapeutic setting. Similarly, the therapist should not hesitate to be warm and emotionally available to help the patient grow and to provide empathic resonance that may have been missing in the patient's development.

Length and Time of Sessions

Another limit imposed on the therapist–patient relationship involves the length and time of sessions. Winnicott (1954) once noted that both love and aggression are communicated in the treatment relationship. The therapist communicates the loving component by listening empathically and providing an opportunity for the patient to grow and change in the context of an accepting relationship. On the other hand, the therapist communicates the aggressive part of the equation by ending the hour on time and charging a fee for the services.

The time of the session is often 45–50 minutes but can be as brief as 15 minutes or as long as 90 minutes. In any case, the time parameters must be clear to the patient, and it is useful for the patient to understand from the beginning of the therapy that time constraints will always apply. Patients generally understand if the therapist explains that the session cannot be extended because there are other patients waiting to be seen. One cannot be totally rigid, however, and occasionally may need to go over a few minutes to accommodate an intense emotional reaction by a patient or other unusual circumstances.

Another important factor related to time is the hour of the day when the patient is seen. A number of cases of boundary violations have been preceded by scheduling a patient during the last hour of the day, when the office personnel in the clinic may have gone home and no other people are around. This setting may communicate to the patient that there is a potential for something other than a professional relationship (Gutheil and Gabbard 1993). Therefore, one should be mindful about scheduling patients at such times.

Fees

That therapists are paid for their services underscores the fact that the therapist is working. Therapy is hard work, and the therapist deserves to be paid. There are many settings in which the patient does not hand the therapist a check or is not even charged a fee. However, therapists are nevertheless paid a salary by the clinic or organization for which they work, and the patient is aware that the therapist makes a living through seeing patients.

The fact of being paid further differentiates the therapist from parent, lover, friend, and so on. When patients pay a fee, they are reminded that they have "rented" the therapist's time and should use it productively. One of the most common steps in the descent down the slippery slope is for the therapist to stop charging a fee or to allow the bill to accumulate. Another variation is to allow the patient a double session but expect payment for only one. In any case, therapists should carefully monitor their attitude about the patient's payment and the fee they are charging as a way of examining countertransference wishes to give the patient something for nothing. Billing problems often relate to feelings that the therapy is not worth anything or that the clinician is doing a poor job. Beginning therapists are typically conflicted about deserving a fee, and in training settings, supervisors should include collecting the fee as part of the training of future therapists.

Exchange of Gifts and Services

Grateful patients often wish to express their appreciation by bringing surprise gifts to their therapists. Some wealthy patients may wish to make a donation to the institution where a therapist works or to a project with which a therapist is involved. Accepting large gifts from patients opens a door to a variety of complications. Patients may consciously or unconsciously feel that they are entitled to special dispensation because they have given money or other material gifts to a therapist. Gifts may also mask aggression and negative feelings that the patient prefers to conceal. Sometimes the gift is an "unconscious bribe" to influence the therapist in one way or another (Gutheil and Gabbard 1993). Patients may think, "Maybe the therapist will not bring up shameful or unpleasant topics"; "Maybe the therapist won't expect me to change things that I really don't want to change"; "Maybe a check written out to the therapist's research project will stop the therapist from pushing me in directions I do not want to go."

Because of concerns about the potential of gifts to corrupt the therapeutic process, there has been a historical tendency to refuse all gifts. However, in recent years, the view on accepting small gifts has shifted to a much more reasonable perspective, with the recognition that some patients will be devastated when a small gift is refused. When a patient brings something handmade, a recommended book, or a small memento, many therapists simply thank the patient for the gift and talk about the particular meaning or symbolism of the gift. At the end of therapy, a patient may want to express appreciation with a small gift, and if the therapist refuses it, there may be no opportunity to discuss the impact of that refusal on the patient. Sometimes, the therapist may have doubts about whether it is right to accept the gift and may share the dilemma with the patient. In some instances, the therapist may explain that he or she would like to have the opportunity to think about it or talk about the gift with a consultant before making a decision.

Despite the complexity of the problem of gifts, there are several rules of thumb:

1. Do not accept donations to one's projects or the institution's projects during treatment.
2. Do not accept cash gifts.
3. Avoid accepting expensive gifts, and when the expense is in doubt, consider delaying the decision and possibly consulting with a colleague.
4. Always feel free to explore the meaning of any gift to see if the act of offering the present to the therapist can open up new areas for exploration in the therapy.

A corollary to gift giving is the offering of services. Patients who may not be able to afford a gift or feel that gifts are inappropriate will sometimes offer to provide services for the therapist. These may include such activities as painting a house, babysitting, enhancing features on the therapist's computer, or redecorating the therapist's office. These types of services are fraught with difficulties because the therapist is stuck if the service is done badly. What therapist would feel free to complain or critique the service, or refuse to pay? In general, services from patients blend into the area of business transactions and dual relationships, which are almost always problematic in psychotherapy.

Clothing and Language

Both clothing and language are aspects of the psychotherapist role that are often underemphasized as part of professional boundaries. Dressing in a professional manner conveys that the therapist does not consider the meeting as recreation. Patients sometimes quit after an initial meeting with a mental health professional because they feel that the clinician does not appear to be professional. Besides casual dress, seductive clothing can also create a problem in conveying professionalism to the patient. Some clinicians dress in a way that appears seductive to others without knowing it themselves. It is sometimes useful for therapists to speak to one another when they perceive a problem with the way a colleague dresses.

Informal or crude language can also work against professionalism. The use of slang to refer to genitals or sexuality may be problematic for some patients, and therapists must attempt to mentalize a patient's probable response before choosing to speak in such terms. Generally, one is on much firmer ground when using more technical terms for sex acts and anatomical parts.

Language can also be experienced as abusive to some patients, particularly those who have experienced verbal abuse in the past.

> A 19-year-old male who was insecure about sexuality talked with his older male therapist about how he was approaching a girl he desired. The young man told his therapist what he had said to the girl after a college class, and the therapist said, "Omigod! You sound like such a pussy when you talk that way." The young man felt humiliated and criticized and did not return to therapy. The therapist insisted he was trying to give the young man helpful feedback, but his choice of words and his tone sounded far too critical for the patient, who also referred to the therapist's language as "unprofessional."

This brief fragment of a therapy session illustrates more than how language can feel violating to a patient. The therapist's comment is also poor technique. Indeed, effective technique and the maintenance of professional boundaries work hand in hand and have many areas of overlap.

Physical Contact

In general, psychotherapy proceeds without physical contact. There is generally a handshake when a therapist and patient first meet. However, in most cases, the handshakes do not continue throughout the treatment. There are exceptions, of course, often based on cultural practices, so that some patients will initiate a handshake at the beginning and end of each session. Psychotherapists can return the handshake without concerns about boundaries in most cases. The only exception is if there is erotization in the transference, and the patient is using the handshake as a way of having sexualized physical contact with the therapist. Hence, these judgments must be made on a case-by-case basis.

As noted previously, one cannot make an absolutist statement that hugs are never acceptable in psychotherapy. In unusual situations, such as a significant loss, therapists may return a hug initiated by a patient. However, hugs on a regular basis are not part of psychotherapy and may cause the patient to misinterpret the therapist's intentions. Some therapists argue that a hug is sometimes needed by a patient, but people's capacity for self-deception is extraordinary. What a therapist may think is best for the patient may actually be a way of fulfilling the therapist's own needs.

It is important to remember that psychotherapists have chosen their profession for a myriad of unconscious reasons that may be incompletely understood (Gabbard 1996). A therapist may have a conscious intention of demonstrating caring to a patient. However, a hug, for example, that is intended by a male therapist to provide nurturance may be perceived by the female patient as a sexual overture, particularly if there is a history of sexual violation in that patient's past. The concept of a "nonsexual" hug is usually in the mind of the therapist but not necessarily in the mind of the patient.

This consideration of hugs leads to a basic tenet of psychotherapy that must be part of the training of every psychotherapist. The therapist's intent when engaging in a particular behavior may not be the same as the impact that behavior has on the patient. A corollary to this tenet is that therapists cannot always know the unconscious intent. The road to hell is paved with good intentions, and many serious boundary violations have begun with what the therapist thought was a benign hug or a pat on the shoulder.

The following are useful guidelines regarding physical contact:

1. Do not initiate hugs.
2. Respond to hugs initiated by a patient only under extraordinary circumstances.
3. If there is clearly an erotic transference that the patient is expressing, physical contact should be avoided.

4. Explore the meaning of any physical contact with the patient as part of the therapeutic process.

Posttermination Professional Boundaries

Although there is a broad consensus that sexual contact between the psychotherapist and a patient is always unethical, the idea of posttermination sexual relations has been somewhat more controversial. The American Psychiatric Association determined in 1993 that any sexual relationship between a psychiatrist and a former patient is unethical (American Psychiatric Association 2001). The American Psychological Association, on the other hand, allows for the possibility of a 2-year "cooling-off" period, after which it *might* be ethical for a therapist and patient to begin a romantic or sexual relationship. However, the burden rests on the psychologist to demonstrate that there is no exploitation of vulnerability or dependency after that 2-year period. In practice, however, the most common scenario one encounters is that psychotherapy is terminated for the specific purpose of embarking on a romantic relationship (Gabbard and Lester 2003). As discussed in the following sections, there are several sound arguments that are useful in supporting the idea of an absolute prohibition against sexual relationships between a therapist and a former patient (Gabbard 2002).

The Persistence of Transference

Transference involves the reexperiencing of the therapist as a powerful and authoritative figure from the past. Cognitive neuroscience suggests that representations of parents are laid down in neural networks that represent self and other from early in childhood, and then activated again and again by specific characteristics of current figures in one's life (Westen and Gabbard 2002). One implication of this understanding of transference is that transference is never completely resolved. Follow-up research has confirmed that transference persists long after the therapist–patient relationship is terminated. A series of studies (Buckley et al. 1981; Norman et al. 1976; Pfeffer 1963, 1993) have demonstrated that transference is instantly reestablished when patients are followed up after the ending of treatment, and there is still an active effort to process and work through persistent transference issues. In other words, the patient's dependency and vulnerability to exploitation does not disappear at termination of therapy. Even in psychotherapies that eschew transference work, the phenomenon of transference is activated.

The Power Differential

Some critics of an absolute prohibition against posttermination sexual relationships have argued that psychodynamic constructs such as transference are not included in the conceptual model of other psychotherapies, such as cognitive-behavioral therapy, and therefore the argument regarding transference is not relevant. The counterargument to this point is that a power differential and an emotional dependency are established in any therapeutic relationship because of its fiduciary nature. Patients place their mental health in the hands of a therapist and offer a fee for the therapist's expertise. That power differential, once established, will continue after the therapeutic relationship has ended (Gabbard 2002).

Destruction of the Therapeutic Relationship

Above all, psychotherapists wish to avoid harm to the patient. An ethics code is constructed to identify situations of potential harm and prevent them from entering into a therapeutic relationship. Hence, another argument in favor of an absolute prohibition is that the knowledge of that prohibition may prevent a corruption of the therapeutic process.

If posttermination sexual relationships were acceptable, one could imagine a scenario with a single therapist and a single patient that would involve a growing attraction to one another that confounded the therapeutic purpose (Gabbard 2002). The therapist might begin to think that the patient is someone ideally suited as a romantic partner and try to foster idealization. The therapist might, for example, avoid confrontation of any undesirable features to gain the patient's love and respect. The patient, on the other hand, if also attracted, might decide to conceal certain shameful episodes from the past so as not to disgust or turn off the therapist. The patient might even curry favor by expressing to the therapist great admiration of the therapist's skill. The result might be a mutual admiration society, in which important therapeutic issues are kept out of the dialogue.

If one or both members of the therapeutic dyad are aware that a romantic relationship is forever off limits, this knowledge frees the therapeutic dialogue of interference from that hoped-for future relationship. Indeed, the essence of the therapeutic relationship is that it will never be anything but psychotherapy, so that patients are free to say whatever they like without repercussions in another context in which they will see the therapist.

Possible Return of the Patient

As all experienced clinicians know, patients who terminate psychotherapy frequently return for further therapeutic work in the midst of a life crisis or a struggle with a new developmental phase that must be mastered. In one study of 71 successfully analyzed patients, for example, Hartlaub et al. (1986) found that two-thirds of the patients had recontacted their analysts within 3 years of termination. Hence, another argument for an absolute prohibition against romantic involvement following termination is that the therapist may be needed again in the professional role of psychotherapist rather than as a friend, business partner, or lover.

When the professional boundaries do not involve considerations of sexual contact, posttermination relationships are much less clearly defined. Psychotherapists may see former patients in various social situations and certainly should feel free to be warm and friendly with them. There may be areas of common interest that bring them together periodically as well. For example, patients and mental health professionals may serve on committees together or be involved in organizing a conference. Nevertheless, therapists are well advised to maintain some boundary involving personal problems such that they remain available as a potential therapist in the future.

Prevention of Boundary Violations

Education about professional boundaries is essential in the training of psychotherapists, but one must face the fact that serious boundary violations will never be eliminated entirely from the practice of psychotherapy. By its very nature, psychotherapy involves a radical form of privacy. Two people are meeting each other regularly behind closed doors, and one of them is confessing his or her darkest and most shameful secrets to the other. The atmosphere of emotional confession and acceptance fosters a rare kind of intimacy not often available outside of therapy. Some therapists will rationalize to themselves that a romantic relationship is possible and acceptable because there is no exploitation of the patient.

Nevertheless, education about professional boundaries may be useful in preventing some instances of boundary transgressions by providing therapists with a framework to think about the nature of a professional versus a personal relationship. Boundaries cannot be taught simply as a list of rules. They need to be taught as part of clinical wisdom, integrating boundary notions into discussions of technique and the choices a therapist must make.

Ongoing consultation throughout one's career is probably the best preventive measure that psychotherapists can build into their professional lives. There is something quasi-incestuous about sexual relations between therapist and patient. Like incest, the sexual behavior occurs in a dyad outside the view of any third party. By introducing a consultant into that dyad, the dynamics of the relationship change in such a way that the therapist has a colleague or partner to discuss the case with, and the radical privacy shifts. In training, therapists are accustomed to a triad rather than a dyad: patient–therapist–supervisor. This triad builds in a quality-control factor: the therapist knows that he or she is being "observed" by the supervisor and can talk to someone when anything unusual is happening in the therapy.

Isolation is a risk factor for professional boundary violations (Gabbard and Lester 2003), and the use of consultation, either individually or in a group format, also serves to relieve that isolation. The therapist must be sure to choose a consultant who is not simply a friend who will confirm the value of whatever the therapist is doing. Consultants must have two key qualities: the capacity to make the therapist feel comfortable and the capacity to confront the therapist when things are heading in problematic directions (Gabbard 2000a). One must always keep in mind that this preventive measure is not foolproof, because consultation can be misused. The therapist can conceal information from the consultant. The therapist can select a consultant who will confirm the course of the therapy. The therapist can even use consultation informally in a way that is not effective—the so-called curbside consultation.

In any case, prevention depends to a large extent on what the therapist does in private moments. A useful monitoring tool is for therapists to ask themselves, "Is what I'm doing something I can tell my consultant?" If the answer is no, the therapist knows that this behavior is the very thing that *should* be brought up to the consultant. In the final analysis, therapists must be their own watchdogs to avoid professional boundary violations.

Conclusion

In this overview of professional boundaries in psychotherapy, a set of helpful guidelines has been provided that should be used flexibly by a psychotherapist. Different forms of psychotherapy are going to require different emphases on the way that the boundaries are implemented. Within different techniques, one adjusts the boundaries to make the patient more accessible and more capable of collaborating with the therapist.

One of the most difficult aspects of psychotherapeutic practice is our incapacity to know the ultimate impact of departing from boundaries. We can rationalize rather dramatic exceptions to boundaries in certain situations, and while we may think we are being humane, the patient may feel he or she is no longer safe. Hence frank discussion of the boundaries between therapist and patient must be part of the therapeutic dialogue on a regular basis.

Key Points

- Professional boundaries are the parameters defining the limits of a fiduciary relationship in which one person (a patient) entrusts his or her welfare to another (a psychotherapist), who is paid for the provision of a service.

- Boundary crossings are generally benign phenomena that do not recur repetitively, are discussable between the therapist and the patient, are not exploitative, and may even help the therapeutic process.

- Boundary violations are egregious phenomena that are usually repetitive, harmful to the patient, and exploitative of the patient's vulnerable position. They are also generally not discussable with the therapist.

- Specific dimensions of professional boundaries include location, confidentiality, excessive self-disclosure, professional role, time of sessions, payment, gifts and services, clothing, language, and nonsexual physical contact.

- Posttermination sexual contact is generally considered unethical because of the persistence of transference, the power differential, the potential to destroy the therapeutic nature of the relationship, and the possible return of the patient.

- Education about professional boundaries is essential in the training of all psychotherapists, even though it will not entirely eliminate the problem.

- Ongoing consultation throughout one's career is probably the best preventive measure that psychotherapists can use to avoid serious boundary violations.

References

American Psychiatric Association: The Principles of Medical Ethics: With Annotations Especially Applicable to Psychiatry. Washington, DC, American Psychiatric Association, 2001

Buckley P, Karasu TB, Charles E: Psychotherapists view their personal therapy. Psychotherapy Theory, Research, Practice, Training 18:299–305, 1981

Gabbard GO: Lessons to be learned from the study of sexual boundary violations. Am J Psychother 50:311–322, 1996

Gabbard GO: Consultation from the consultant's perspective. Psychoanalytic Dialogues 10:209–218, 2000a

Gabbard GO: Disguise or consent: problems and recommendations concerning the publication and presentation of clinical material. Int J Psychoanal 81:1071–1086, 2000b

Gabbard GO: Post-termination sexual boundary violations. Psychiatr Clin North Am 25:593–603, 2002

Gabbard GO, Lester ET: Boundaries and Boundary Violations in Psychoanalysis. Washington, DC, American Psychiatric Publishing, 2003

Gabbard GO, Nadelson C: Professional boundaries in the physician-patient relationship. JAMA 273:1445–1449, 1995

Gabbard GO, Wilkinson SM: Management of Countertransference With Borderline Patients. Washington, DC, American Psychiatric Press, 1994

Gutheil TG, Gabbard GO: The concept of boundaries in clinical practice: theoretical and risk management dimensions. Am J Psychiatry 150:188–196, 1993

Gutheil TG, Gabbard GO: Misuses and misunderstandings of boundary theory in clinical and regulatory settings. Am J Psychiatry 155:409–414, 1998

Hartlaub GH, Martin GC, Rhine MW: Re-contact with the analyst following termination: a survey of 71 cases. J Am Psychoanal Assoc 34:885–910, 1986

Keisler DJ: Therapeutic Metacommunication: Therapist Impact Disclosure as Feedback in Psychotherapy. Palo Alto, CA, Consulting Psychologists Press, 1988

Norman HF, Blacker KH, Oremland JD, et al: The fate of the transference neurosis after termination of a satisfactory analysis. J Am Psychoanal Assoc 24:471–498, 1976

Pfeffer AZ: The meaning of the analyst after analysis: a contribution to the theory of therapeutic results. J Am Psychoanal Assoc 11:229–244, 1963

Pfeffer AZ: After the analysis: analyst as both old and new object. J Am Psychoanal Assoc 41:323–327, 1993

Strasburger LH, Jorgenson L, Sutherland P: The prevention of psychotherapist sexual misconduct: avoiding the slippery slope. Am J Psychother 46:544–555, 1992

Westen D, Gabbard GO: Developments in cognitive neuroscience, II: implications for theories of transference. J Am Psychoanal Assoc 50:88–131, 2002

Winnicott DW: Metapsychological and clinical aspects of regression within the psycho-analytic set-up (1954), in Collected Papers: Through Paediatrics to Psycho-analysis. New York, Basic Books, 1958, pp 278–294

Suggested Readings

Epstein R: Keeping Boundaries: Maintaining Safety and Integrity in the Psychotherapeutic Process. Washington, DC, American Psychiatric Press, 1994

Gabbard GO, Lester E: Boundaries and Boundary Violations in Psychoanalysis. Washington, DC, American Psychiatric Publishing, 2003

Index

Page numbers printed in **boldface** *type refer to tables or figures.*

829

Anxiety
Anna Freud's concept of, 13
anticipatory, 178, 179, 183
in borderline personality disorder, 766
cognitive vulnerability to anxiety proneness, 178
depressive, 17
as exclusion criteria for psychodynamic group therapy, 629
learned, neural circuitry of, 178
neural correlates of, 785–786
neurobiology of, 730–731
objective, 13
persecutory, 17, 18
supportive psychotherapy techniques for reduction of, 431–435
Anxiety disorders. *See also specific anxiety disorders*
cognitive theory of, 177–185
cognitive-behavioral therapy for, 174, 202, 219–223
combined with medication, 267
efficacy of, 244–250
dialectical behavior therapy for, 731
interpersonal psychotherapy for, 341, **342**, 352, 385
psychodynamic psychotherapy for
combined with medication, 140
efficacy of, **102–103**, 108
supportive psychotherapy for, 456–457
efficacy of, 449
Anxiety sensitivity, 178
Anxious-ambivalent attachment style, 295
Arbitrary interference, **173**, 212, **213**
Area of Change Questionnaire, 537
Arieti, Silvano, 303
Assimilative psychotherapy integration, 709–710
Attachment styles, 295

Attachment theory
of Bowlby, 81, 295, 400, 558–559, 560
emotionally focused couples therapy and, 555, 557
love as attachment bond, 558–562
mentalization and, 758
in borderline personality disorder, 762–763, 766
Autism
as defect of theory of mind processing, 760
mirror neuron systems in, 800
normal, in Mahler's developmental model, 13, 14
Automatic thoughts
identification of, **208**, 208–210
checklists, 210
imagery and role-play, 209–210
recognizing mood shifts, 209
repetitive patterns, 218
thought recording, 210, **211**
using guided discovery, 208–209
modification of, **208**, 210–216
applying reattribution techniques, 212
examining the evidence, 211–212
identifying cognitive errors, 212–213, **213**
using thought change records, 213–216, **214–215**
negative, 172–173
pain-related, 686–688, **690–691**, 697–698
Automatic Thoughts Questionnaire, 210
Autonomous functions, 399
Autonomous relationship drive, 16
Autonomy
depression and, 175
promotion of, in supportive psychotherapy, 442
Avoidant attachment style, 295